Cosmetics and Dermatological Problems and Solutions

Cosmetics and Dermatological Problems and Solutions

A Problem Based Approach

Third Edition

Zoe Diana Draelos, MD

Consulting Professor, Department of Dermatology,
Duke University School of Medicine, Durham, North Carolina, U.S.A.

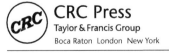

CRC Press
Taylor & Francis Group
Boca Raton London New York

CRC Press is an imprint of the
Taylor & Francis Group, an **informa** business

CRC Press
Taylor & Francis Group
6000 Broken Sound Parkway NW, Suite 300
Boca Raton, FL 33487-2742

First issued in paperback 2019

© 2011 by Taylor & Francis Group, LLC
CRC Press is an imprint of Taylor & Francis Group, an Informa business

No claim to original U.S. Government works

ISBN-13: 978-1-84184-740-5(hbk)
ISBN-13: 978-0-367-38245-2 (pbk)

Library of Congress Cataloging-in-Publication Data

Draelos, Zoe Diana.
  Cosmetics and dermatological problems and solutions : a problem based approach / Zoe Diana Draelos. -- 3rd ed.
    p. ; cm.
  Rev. ed. of: Cosmetics in dermatology / Zoe Diana Draelos. 2nd ed. 1995.
  Includes bibliographical references and index.
  ISBN 978-1-84184-740-5 (hb : alk. paper) 1. Cosmetics--Composition. 2. Dermatology. I. Draelos, Zoe Diana. Cosmetics in dermatology. II. Title.
  [DNLM: 1. Cosmetics. 2. Dermatologic Agents. 3. Hair--drug effects. 4. Nails--drug effects. 5. Skin--drug effects.
6. Skin Care--methods. QV 60]
  RL72.D73 2011
  616.5--dc23
                                                                                    2011021178

**Visit the Taylor & Francis Web site at
http://www.taylorandfrancis.com**

**and the CRC Press Web site at
http://www.crcpress.com**

I dedicate this book to everyone who has touched my life in the past 25 years of dermatology practice, especially my husband, Michael, who has been supportive of my writing efforts and infinitely inspirational to challenge me to think beyond with new ideas. I also dedicate this book to my boys, Mark and Matthew, who have opened my eyes to the electronic world and helped me immensely in the preparation of this text.

This third edition represents a life of learning as I have grown in the understanding of complex formulations in the cosmetic realm that impact the practice of dermatology.

Contents

Foreword

It is a great pleasure to write the foreward to the third edition of Dr. Zoe Draelos's textbook, *Cosmetics and Dermatological Problems and Solutions*. Zoe has a long interest in this area and has made major contributions to the field through the application of scientific principles to the evaluation of the efficacy of cosmetic products. Her training as an engineer, clinical researcher and clinical dermatologist are a unique combination in this field and the result is a new level of understanding of the wide variety of agents that are used as cosmetics.

This book is a testament to Dr. Draelos's commitment to educating dermatologists about the wide variety of products available to our patients and on the scientific basis for cosmetics. This is a benefit to all dermatologists as we attempt to answer the many questions our patients have regarding the vast array of products and confusing advertising that confront us all daily.

The third edition continues on the foundation of the first two editions. It is comprehensive, including the vast array of products that our patients may utilize. It is however more than a list, in that Zoe has included the proposed mechanisms of action of each product. Finally, this book is an independent effort including all products without regard to any specific member of the cosmetic industry. *Cosmetics and Dermatological Problems and Solutions* is an important contribution to our specialty and will be useful to the experienced dermatologist and residents alike.

Russell P. Hall
Department of Dermatology
Duke University School of Medicine
Durham, North Carolina, USA

Acknowledgment

Many people have contributed to my search for knowledge and preparation of this book. I am grateful to those who trained me to practice dermatology at the University of Arizona, namely Peter Lynch, MD, Norman Levine, MD, and Ron Hansen, MD. Peter Lynch, MD, was visionary in encouraging my knowledge development in the area of cosmetic dermatology during my residency and provided me with the opportunity to publish the first edition of this book in 1990. The second edition was published in 1995 and this is the third edition which is being published in 2011.

I am also grateful to my son, Matthew Draelos, who helped with the preparation of the references for this book and editing of the text and photographs. In short, this third edition acknowledges the cumulative efforts of many who have positively influenced my love of dermatology.

This book contains images of many products to illustrate the topics discussed. These are not product endorsements, but representations of widely available formulations in the present marketplace. An effort has been made to photograph products from many different manufacturers, unless there is only one company that dominates a certain market segment.

Introduction

As the understanding of skin, hair, and nail physiology has evolved, so too has the design of products to enhance the appearance of these external structures. This book is designed to aid the dermatologist in understanding and utilizing these products in daily practice. The book is organized first by structure in terms of the skin, hair, and nails. This layout was selected because dermatologists are the medical experts in charge of disease and appearance issues related to the skin, hair, and nails. After reading this book, the dermatologist should have a fundamental understanding of the formulation, application, side effects, and issues of special interest as related to nonprescription products to maintain and enhance appearance. All the products discussed are in the over-the-counter realm, not traditionally covered by dermatology textbooks. Yet, the maintenance of healthy skin, hair, and nails is accomplished solely by the use of over-the-counter products, which makes the reading of this book important. The dermatologists must learn to make recommendations and identify problems related to over-the-counter products.

Within the broad topics of skin, hair, and nails, there are several subdivisions. Skin is broken down into body areas of face and body. Great distinctions exist because the facial skin is adorned with colored cosmetics, whereas the body is only cleansed and moisturized; however, the control of armpit perspiration is also important. Differences between female and male skin needs, considering all variations of skin color, are explored and the products used for hygiene are also evaluated. The book goes a step further by discussing the use of cosmetics and skin care products in common, cosmetically relevant skin disease, such as acne, eczema, rosacea, and sensitive skin. Further, skin can be distinguished by age and the amount of oil production. All these variables influence cleanser and moisturizer selection while providing opportunities for manufacturers to customize formulations. These formulations are presented to better understand the subtle differences between the myriad of customized products that are available for purchase.

Within the face, there are unique hygiene and product application areas. The eyes are elaborately adorned with color cosmetics, but represent a sensitive skin area with a junction between cornified skin and mucosa. A similar junction exists around the mouth, but the vermillion is also adorned with lip cosmetics and subject to the trauma of speaking and chewing. The ears are discussed with attention to the health of the ear canal and earlobe. Finally, the face must be considered in terms of photoprotection needs to prevent both painful sunburn and photoaging. Sunscreens can be used as separate products or applied through moisturizers, facial foundations, or powders. Cosmetics can provide functionality beyond adornment through photoprotection.

Aesthetic issues of facial scarring, asymmetries, and the care of post-surgical facial skin are tackled, since there are needs for an understanding of camouflaging techniques. The use of artistic color to improve appearance through recontouring and the minimization of scarring with opaque cosmetics is part of the knowledge base of the dermatologist. Proper use of cosmetics can enhance patient satisfaction with healing following an invasive procedure or the final skin appearance after an incisional surgery.

Even though the hair and nails are nonliving structures, they are of tremendous cosmetic value. Hair grooming issues, such as shampooing and conditioning, for all types of hair architectures are important to hair appearance and also for the maintenance of scalp health following treatment of seborrheic dermatitis, psoriasis, postmenopausal dry scalp, and the alopecias. Improper hair styling procedures and products may cause hair breakage and loss, requiring special discussion, along with hair dyeing, permanent waving, and straightening. The chemistry behind hair cosmetic manipulations is complex and damaging to the unique keratin structure of the hair shaft. The desire for appearance alterations must be balanced with hair health, which sometimes requires compromise on the part of the patient. While abundant hair growth is desirable on the scalp, it is undesirable on the female face, armpits, and legs. This book also covers issues of hirsutism and hair removal options.

Nails are also addressed both from a functional and cosmetic standpoint. Brittle nails, nails in children, and toenails are discussed along with the use of nail cosmetics from polishes to prostheses. Nail health can be affected by improper grooming procedures and cosmetic elongation manipulations, but nail disease also be improved with the use of nail cosmetics.

In short, this book covers all aspects of cosmetic dermatology presented in a fashion that allows the dermatologist to use this material in everyday practice. This problem-oriented approach is not found in any other textbook on the subject and is a new addition to the third edition. When the first edition of this book was published some 20 years ago in 1990, a more encyclopedic approach was taken because it was the first book of its kind in dermatology to address the area of cosmetics. It was a paperback book with a few tables and line drawings. The second edition of the book was launched in 1995 into hardback with more tables, but only a black on white layout. The third edition of this book in 2011 is hardback and in full color with numerous textboxes, images, and tables and a digital layout. The advancements in publishing technology have supplemented the advancements in cosmetics, which are showcased in this third edition. The 20-year evolution of this book represents my growth as a person, as a dermatologist, and as a teacher. It is the culmination of my passion for learning and sharing. I hope you can sense my enthusiasm for the subject and the joys I experienced while developing the material. Writing, after all, is a unique undertaking. It is done in silence with focused thought and vigilant hands tapping on the keyboard using borrowed moments in the far reaches of the globe in all time zones. This book is the culmination of ideas that zip across the subconscious brain unexpectedly only to find their way into a framework of organization and logic. It is my hope that you will find illumination and enjoyment while we share together an increased understanding of the place that cosmetics has in dermatology!

Zoe Diana Draelos

I Facial cosmetic dermatology: Introduction

Facial skin receives the major attention in the realm of cosmetic dermatology as it is our outer expressive conduit to the world. It ages more rapidly than the rest of the skin due to its almost constant exposure to the sun. Decoration of the facial skin is a time-honored tradition among many of the world's peoples. Most modern cosmetics are used to highlight facial features and camouflage facial defects. The earliest cosmetic designed to cover facial blemishes was the beauty patch. These patches became popular in the 1600s as they were used to cover the permanent scars left behind on the faces of people who survived smallpox epidemics in Europe. These patches were black silk or velvet pieces shaped like stars, moons, and hearts that were carefully placed on the face. Patch boxes—shallow metal boxes with a mirror in the cover—were carried everywhere to keep replacements handy should a patch fall off in public. Modern facial cosmetics were developed from the decorative patches (1).

The concept of covering the face with a pigmented cream originated in the theater with a product known as "French White," which consisted of face powder incorporated into a liquid vehicle (2). This was considered a novel improvement over simply powdering the skin due to its superior adherence. Later, "grease paints" were developed as thick oily pigmented pastes, but they were not appropriate for wear outside the theater. The first major breakthrough in facial foundations for the average woman came when Max Factor developed cake make-up, which he patented in 1936 (3). This product camouflaged the underlying skin, providing a velvety texture with subtle color.

However, the face is not only adorned with cosmetics, but it is also cleansed and moisturized. Cosmetics are used not only for hygiene purposes but also to maintain and enhance skin beauty. Harley Procter developed the first widely marketed American facial cleansing soap in 1878 when he decided that his father's soap and candle factory should produce a delicately scented, creamy white soap to compete with imported European products. He accomplished this feat with the help of his cousin James Gamble, a chemist, who made a richly lathering product called "White Soap." By accident, they discovered that whipping air into the soap solution before molding resulted in a floating soap that could not be lost in the stream or bathtub (4). This resulted in a product known as "Ivory" soap, which is still manufactured today.

The excellent sebum removal afforded by the first soaps created the need for moisturizers to compensate for the flaking and dryness experienced. It is surprising that the very first American moisturizer is still in use and known as "Vaseline," as named by Robert A. Chesebrough who manufactured and patented the concoction in 1872. Chesebrough originally recommended petrolatum as a chemical to treat leather; however, its value was soon recognized as a remedy for chapped hands and as a hair pomade. Later, petrolatum was adapted by the pharmaceutical industry as a vehicle instead of lard.

It offered the benefit of preservative-free stability since lard frequently turned rancid.

Facial skin care has a rich history, but the modern formulations are clearly superior and better able to meet skin needs. This section of the text examines facial skin care from a disease-oriented approach. It examines the needs of the oily skin of acne, the dry skin of eczema, and the sensitive skin of rosacea. Cleansing, moisturizing, and the use of facial foundations are examined for these basic prototype groups. The discussion then turns to the large category of aging facial skin to additionally encompass the realm of cosmeceuticals. Finally, the section focuses on the special needs areas of the face, specifically the eyes and lips. It is hoped that at the end of this section, the dermatologist will be able to understand how these over the counter products fit into the medical armamentarium.

SKIN PHYSIOLOGY

A brief discussion of skin physiology is presented in order to understand the challenge in creating a healthy normal facial skin for patients of all skin colors, complexion types, and ages. This is particularly challenging when the constituents of "normal" skin have not been defined; rather there is a range of normal skins among all peoples of the world. Skin is the largest organ of the body possessing a regularly irregular surface composed of skin scales with intervening hairs, sweat ducts, and oil glands that reflect light to the eye, which is perceived as beauty. Unfortunately, with the passage of time the beauty of the skin fades, even though it may be considered "normal." Sun, smoking, stress, disease, scarring, and aging alter the structure of the skin and degrade its pristine appearance that is present at birth.

SKIN STRUCTURE

The skin is composed of two layers, the epidermis and the dermis, each with distinct functions (Fig. I.1). The outer epidermis forms a barrier to the world, keeping out water, sunlight, insects, bacteria, toxins, and allergens. It acts as a beautiful barrier between the body and the environment and is responsible for all the variations in skin appearance. Below the epidermis lies the dermis, accounting for more than 90% of skin mass and providing physical strength to the skin. The dermis is composed of the papillary dermis and the reticular dermis with the papillary dermis lying in direct contact with the epidermis. It is composed of collagen and elastin fibers containing blood vessels and lymphatic channels. In addition, there are connective tissue cells and glycosaminoglycans responsible for holding water in the dermis and maintaining skin hydration. Under the papillary dermis lies the reticular dermis, possessing fewer cells, relatively few blood vessels, dense collagen bundles, and coarse elastin fibers. The papillary dermis provides physical strength to the skin and is the location of the eccrine and apocrine sweat glands, sebaceous glands, and hair follicles.

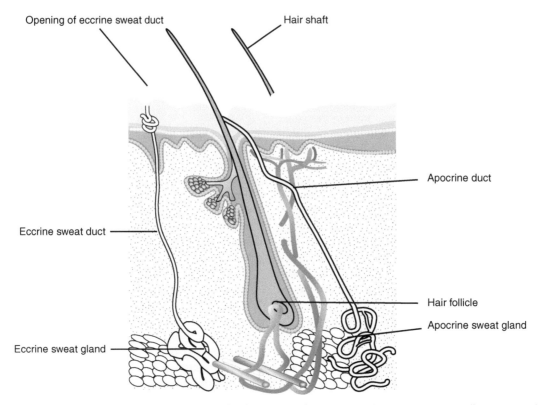

Figure I.1 The skin is composed of the epidermis and the dermis, with a thin nonliving layer known as the stratum corneum. All cosmetic products impact the stratum corneum, which is the basis for the visual beauty of the skin.

STRATUM CORNEUM

Perhaps the most important layer of the skin, from a cosmetic standpoint, is the stratum corneum, also known as the horny layer. This outermost layer of the epidermis is impacted by cleansing, moisturization, and other skin care treatments to the greatest degree. It is the layer assessed by the eye to arrive at the impression of a lovely skin, but is only 15 to 150 μm thick. The rest of the chapter will address this layer from a cosmetic viewpoint.

The stratum corneum is composed of helical polypeptides known as keratin protein arranged into corneocytes. The corneocytes have been termed the bricks in the "brick and mortar" construction of the skin barrier. The mortar is composed of the intercellular lipids that form a waterproof covering of the body to which cleansers, moisturizers, and cosmetics are applied. There are two types of lipids found in the skin: polar and nonpolar. The polar lipids possess an electrical charge and consist of phospholipids, glycolipids, and cholesterol. The uncharged nonpolar lipids are triglycerides, squalene, and waxes. The percentage breakdown of the intercellular lipids is given in Table I.1.

Moisturizers attempt to mimic the effect of the intercellular lipids, but they can only create a barrier that reduces the amount of water lost to the environment. Cleansers must allow these intercellular lipids to remain intact without

Table I.1 Intercellular Lipid Composition

Lipid	Quantity (%)
Triglycerides	12–25
Fatty acids	12–20
Waxes	6
Cholesterol, sphingolipids, ceramides	14–25

producing irritation or premature desquamation of the corneocytes. Finally, colored cosmetics and cosmeceuticals must enhance the appearance of the stratum corneum on the face to create the optical sensation of beauty. With this introduction, our attention now turns to the incorporation of these concepts into a patient treatment regimen.

REFERENCES

1. Panati C. Beauty patch and compact. In: Extraordinary Origins of Everyday Things. New York: Perennial Library, Harper & Row, 1987: 225–6.
2. Schlossman ML, Feldman AJ. Fluid foundations and blush make-up. In: deNavarre MG, ed. The Chemistry and Manufacture of Cosmetics, 2nd edn. Wheaton, IL: Allured Publishing Corporation, 1988: 741–65.
3. Wells FV, Lubowe II. Cosmetics and the Skin. New York: Reinhold Publishing Corporation, 1964: 141–9.
4. Panati C. Soap. In: Extraordinary Origins of Everyday Things. New York: Perennial Library, Harper & Row Publishers, 1987: 217–19.

1   Acne and cosmetics

Acne is the most common inflammatory condition treated by the dermatologist, using both prescription and over the counter (OTC) formulations. This chapter focuses on the OTC drugs and cosmetics that are used in conjunction with prescription medication and in the maintenance phase of therapy. Consumers spend about $100 million per year on OTC anti-acne products, which include cleansers, creams, and moisturizers (1).

OTC DRUG ACNE THERAPIES

Acne products listing an active ingredient are regulated by the US Food and Drug Administration as OTC drugs. Only certain ingredients can be used in acne products, which are listed in the final Acne Monograph. Some of the ingredients approved for this use in the monograph are salicylic acid, sulfur, sulfur combined with resorcinol, and benzoyl peroxide (2). These ingredients can only be used singly and not in combination. Their utility in the treatment of acne in combination with skin care products is discussed in this chapter.

Benzoyl Peroxide

The most effective and most commonly used active ingredient in OTC drug acne preparations is benzoyl peroxide. Eventually, even all prescription benzoyl peroxide products will be available as OTC drugs. About 23% of people aged 13 to 27 years have used an OTC benzoyl peroxide product (3). It is a member of the organic peroxide family consisting of two benzoyl groups joined by a peroxide group. Benzoyl peroxide is prepared by treating benzoyl chloride with sodium peroxide to yield benzoyl peroxide and sodium chloride. It is a radical initiator and is highly flammable, explosive, a possible tumor promoter, and a mutagen.

> Benzoyl peroxide is the most effective acne treatment ingredient in the OTC market.

Benzoyl peroxide has many properties pertinent to acne, including antibacterial, anti-inflammatory, and comedolytic effects (4). When benzoyl peroxide touches the skin, it breaks down into benzoic acid and oxygen, neither of which is problematic. It has antimicrobial properties against *Propionibacterium acnes* as demonstrated by a $2\log_{10}$ decrease in *P. acnes* concentration after two days of topical application of 5% benzoyl peroxide (5). This same antimicrobial effect was observed after applying 10% benzoyl peroxide cream for three days, which resulted in a mean $2\log_{10}$ decrease in the concentration of microbial organisms; however, after seven days, no further decline in *P. acnes* concentration was observed (6).

Benzoyl peroxide is an important antimicrobial agent that has a better potency against *P. acnes* than other topical antibiotics such as erythromycin or clindamycin. However, unlike topical antibiotics, benzoyl peroxide does not result in resistant organisms (7). Benzoyl peroxide also acts as an anti-inflammatory agent by reducing oxygen radicals. In addition, its ability to reduce the *P. acnes* population also reduces inflammation due to fewer bacterial induced monocytes producing tumor necrosis factor α, interleukin 1β, and interleukin 8 (8). This anti-inflammatory effect is perceived by the consumer as reduced redness and pain.

Finally, benzoyl peroxide is also a comedolytic, which is capable of producing a 10% reduction in comedones (9). Comedolytics allow the plug in the pore to loosen from the surrounding follicle restoring the normal flow of sebum to the skin surface. It was originally thought that higher concentration benzoyl peroxide preparations would provide superior comedolytic benefits; however, it now appears that even 2.5% benzoyl peroxide is effective. This is the strength most commonly found in products available in the consumer market. Higher concentration benzoyl peroxides may only increase skin irritation, resulting in peeling and redness (10). In addition, benzoyl peroxide causes allergic contact dermatitis in 1–2.5% of consumers, resulting in redness, swelling, oozing, and pain (11).

> 2.5% Benzoyl peroxide in small particulate size may be as effective as 5–10% benzoyl peroxide in acne treatment creams.

One of the major unresolved concerns regarding benzoyl peroxide is its safety. Benzoyl peroxide is a highly reactive molecule capable of causing explosions in concentrations of 20% or higher. The manufacture of benzoyl peroxide products requires a special facility, and stability problems are common in new formulations. Benzoyl peroxide is capable of producing DNA strand breaks, but rodent carcinogenicity studies have been negative (12). No correlation has been shown between benzoyl peroxide use and skin cancer in humans.

Current trends in benzoyl peroxide formulation have focused on the use of less irritating hydrogel formulations and smaller particle size benzoyl peroxide (13). Raw benzoyl peroxide is a particulate that must be solubulized into solution. It is only the benzoyl peroxide particles that touch the skin surface that are active in the killing of *P. acnes*. Although larger particles will yield higher concentrations in the formulation, most of the benzoyl peroxide particles will not touch the skin. A smaller particle size allows better skin coverage with less irritation, since the concentration is reduced. It is possible to create a 2.5% benzoyl peroxide formulation with an efficacy equal to that of a 10% benzoyl peroxide formulation based on skin contact with the active ingredient. A careful, creative formulation can minimize tolerability issues associated with OTC benzoyl peroxide formulations (Fig. 1.1).

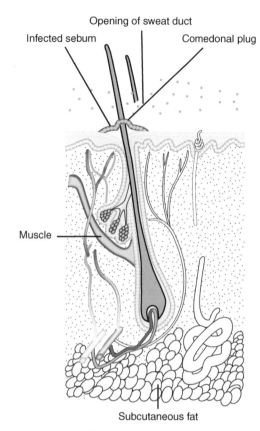

Opening of sweat duct
Infected sebum   Comedonal plug

Muscle

Subcutaneous fat

Figure 1.1 Benzoyl peroxide particles that contact the skin in and around the ostia provide a comedolytic and antibacterial effect by causing the skin to shed the comedonal "Plug," which seals the infected sebum and causes inflammation.

Salicylic Acid

Salicylic acid is another major comedolytic used as an active ingredient in OTC acne treatments in concentrations up to 2% (14). Salicylic acid is a colorless, crystalline, oil-soluble phenolic compound originally derived from the willow tree *Salix*. It is a β-hydroxy acid where the OH group is adjacent to the carboxyl group. The compound is synthesized by treating sodium phenolate, the sodium salt of phenol, with carbon dioxide at 100 atm pressure and 390 K temperature followed by acidification with sulfuric acid.

Salicylic acid is able to exfoliate in the oily milieu of the pore.

Salicylic acid, also known as 2-hydroxybenzoic acid, has a rich history in medicine. It is used as an anti-inflammatory inhibiting arachidonic acid, since it is chemically related to aspirin, a flavoring agent with the characteristic wintergreen taste, a liniment for sore muscles and an acne treatment. Salicylic acid can penetrate into the follicle and dislodge the comedonal plug from the follicular lining. It neither kills *P. acnes* nor does it prevent the development of antibiotic resistance. Thus, salicylic acid may be less effective than benzoyl peroxide in acne treatment, but it is also less irritating and less allergenic. Some proprietary salicylic acid preparations have shown parity to 5% benzoyl peroxide (15). Salicylic acid is sometimes used in hypoallergenic acne treatments and acne treatments for mature individuals.

Salicylic acid can be applied to the skin in a variety of different formulations (16). It can be applied as a solution in an alcohol-detergent vehicle or in the form of an impregnated pad (17,18). It can be formulated as a 2% salicylic acid scrub, with clinical data demonstrating a reduction in open comedones (19). Also, 10% and 20% salicylic acid peels are used to promote comedolysis.

Some individuals experience allergic reactions when salicylic acid is ingested; however, it is generally accepted as a safe ingredient. An overdose of salicylic acid can lead to salicylate intoxication, presenting as a state of metabolic acidosis with a compensatory respiratory alkalosis. This has not been reported with topical applications and salicylic acid acne preparations are considered safe and effective, even during pregnancy.

Sulfur

The oldest treatment for acne predating benzoyl peroxide and salicylic acid is sulfur. Sulfur is a known bacteriostatic and antifungal agent (20). It is a yellow, nonmetallic element that has been used for centuries to treat various dermatologic conditions. The mechanism of action for sulfur is not totally understood, but it is thought to interact with cysteine in the stratum corneum causing a reduction in sulfur to hydrogen sulfide. Hydrogen sulfide in turn degrades keratin, producing the keratolytic effect of sulfur (21). Sulfur has been labeled as a comedogen, but this is controversial (22). Sulfur is available in concentrations of 3–8% in OTC acne formulations. It has a characteristic foul odor and unusual yellow color. It stains clothing and is typically formulated as a thick paste.

Sulfur is thought to interact with cysteine in the stratum corneum causing a reduction in sulfur to hydrogen sulfide, which has a comedolytic effect beneficial in curing acne.

COSMETIC ACNE THERAPIES

In addition to the monographed acne treatment ingredients of benzoyl peroxide, salicylic acid, and sulfur, other substances have been used in the cosmetic treatment of acne, which are not monographed. These ingredients are found in cosmetic acne therapies and include hydroxy acids, retinol, triclosan, and tea tree oil.

Hydroxy Acids

Hydroxy acids, such as glycolic acid, are used in the cosmetic treatment of acne as desquamating agents. Glycolic acid is the smallest alpha hydroxy acid appearing as a colorless, odorless, hygroscopic crystalline solid. While glycolic acid can be obtained from the fermentation of sugar cane, it is more commonly synthesized by reacting chloroacetic acid with sodium hydroxide followed by re-acidification.

The efficacy of glycolic acid in treating acne is related to the free acid concentration (23). The free acid is able to dissolve the ionic bonds between the corneocytes forming the stratum corneum. This desquamation can remove the comedonal plugs; however, the water-soluble glycolic acid cannot enter the oily milieu of the pore. For this reason, salicylic acid is a much better comedolytic.

Glycolic acid is an exfoliant used in acne washes.

Glycolic acid can be delivered to the skin in the form of a cleanser, moisturizer, or peel. The rinse-off cleanser is less effective in acne therapy than the leave-on moisturizer. Higher concentrations such as 20–70% glycolic acid can be delivered to the skin in the form of a peel that is left on for 3–5 minutes and rinsed off later. The peels can also be used to improve the dark scarring associated with acne, known as post-inflammatory hyperpigmentation (24).

Triclosan

Topical antimicrobials may also be used in the treatment of acne. One common antimicrobial used in deodorant soaps and waterless hand sanitizers is triclosan. Triclosan is not on the US Acne Monograph, but is used for the treatment of acne in other countries, such as England. Triclosan decreases the *P. acnes* count on the skin surface, which accounts for the dermatologist recommendation that acne patients use deodorant soap as part of an acne treatment regimen. Other OTC delivery methods for triclosan, including hydrogel patch delivery, have been published (25).

Triclosan is an antibacterial used in many deodorant soaps popular with acne patients.

No bacterial resistance to triclosan has been identified to date, but the use of triclosan is increasing dramatically with the popularity of triclosan-containing antibacterial waterless hand sanitizers for consumer and hospital use. It is thought that triclosan interferes with lipid synthesis in the bacterial cell wall accounting for its wide ranging antibacterial effect.

OTC Retinoids

Vitamin A derivatives, known as retinoids, are used in the treatment of acne. Three prescription acne treatment retinoids exist: adapalene, tretinoin, and tazarotene. A variety of OTC retinoids exist that may be helpful in acne treatment. These retinoids include retinol and retinaldehyde. Retinol can be absorbed by keratinocytes and reversibly oxidized into retinaldehyde. Retinaldehyde is irreversibly converted into all-trans retinoic acid, also known as tretinoin. Tretinoin is transported into the keratinocyte nucleus modulating follicular keratinization. Large, multicenter, double blind, placebo-controlled studies on the use OTC retinoids in acne treatment are yet to be conducted. However, retinol has been shown to be 20 times less potent than topical tretinoin but exhibits greater penetration than tretinoin (26).

Retinol and retinaldehyde are used in some cosmetic acne treatment creams, but they do not have a similar effect on microcomedones like tretinoin.

Tea Tree Oil

Tea tree oil is the most common herbal essential oil used for acne treatment. Tea tree oil, obtained from the Australian tree *Melaleuca alternifolia*, contains several antimicrobial substances such as terpinen-4-ol, alpha-terpineol, and alpha-pinene (27).

The oil has a pale golden color with a fresh camphoraceous odor. It is used for medicinal purposes as an antiseptic, antifungal, and antibacterial (28).

The antibacterial activity of 10% tea tree oil has been shown against *Staphylococcus aureus*, including methicillin-resistant *Staphylococcus aureus*, without resistance (29). Lower concentrations, however, have demonstrated bacterial resistance. Tea tree oil has been found to be as effective in the treatment of acne as 5% benzoyl peroxide based on a reduction in comedones and inflammatory acne lesions; however, the onset of action is slower for tea tree oil (30). The tea oil group did experience fewer side effects than the benzoyl peroxide group. Another randomized, 60-subject placebo-controlled study in subjects with mild to moderate acne found 5% topical tea tree oil produced a statistically significant reduction in total lesion count and acne severity index as compared to placebo (31). Tea tree oil may also reduce the amount of inflammation present around acne lesions thereby reducing the redness (32).

Tea tree oil is used as an antibacterial in some natural botanical cosmetic acne treatment products.

Tea tree oil is toxic when swallowed. It also has produced toxicity when applied topically in high concentrations to cats and other animals (33). Its use in low concentration topically for the treatment of acne has not produced toxicity problems. However, tea tree oil is a known cause of allergic contact dermatitis. An Italian study of 725 subjects patch tested with undiluted, 1%, and 0.1% tea tree oil found that 6% of the subjects experienced a positive reaction to undiluted tea tree oil, one subject experienced an allergic reaction to 1% tea tree oil, and none of them had any reaction to the 0.1% dilution (34). Thus, the incidence of allergic reactions to tea tree oil is concentration dependent.

Miscellaneous Acne Ingredients

An ingredient of some interest in acne treatment is zinc. It has been applied topically, since zinc salts are bacteriostatic to *P. acnes*, and orally ingested as a homeopathic acne therapy (35). A study by Dreno et al., demonstrated that zinc salts in the culture media of *P. acnes* prevented the development of organisms resistant to erythromycin. Since many *P. acnes* organisms are resistant to topical erythromycin, which has been largely replaced by topical clindamycin, this may be an important mechanism for preventing bacterial resistance (36). Zinc taken orally with nicotinamide orally for acne reduces inflammation. It is theorized that they reduce inflammation by inhibiting leukocyte chemotaxis, lysosomal enzyme release, and mast cell degranulation (37).

The value of topical nicotinamide in acne has been reported along with its use orally (38,39). A commercially available OTC vitamin preparation, based on nicotinamide, has been shown to produce acne improvement in eight weeks (40). Topically, nicotinamide 4% was shown to be comparable to clindamycin gel 1% in the treatment of moderate acne (41).

SKIN CARE IN ACNE PATIENTS

Beyond the acne treatments discussed earlier, skin care products and cosmetics can aid in acne therapy or contribute to disease worsening. These ancillary skin care products include cleansers, astringents, exfoliants, facial scrubs, epidermabrasion, textured cloths, mechanized skin care devices, and face masks.

Cleansers

A variety of cleansers are useful in removing sebum and normalizing the acne biofilm. Soaps are some of the major cleansers used in acne treatment. These include true soaps that are composed of long chain fatty acid alkali salts, with a pH of 9–10. Many of the milder acne soaps are composed of synthetic detergents, known as syndets. These cleansers contain less than 10% soap with a more neutral pH adjusted to 5.5–7.0 (42). Some of the most popular soaps for acne patients are combars composed of alkaline soaps to which surface active agents with a pH of 9–10 have been added. These combars also contain triclosan, a potent antibacterial helpful in acne, discussed earlier.

Beyond traditional soaps that are used in acne treatment, specialized formulations known as facial scrubs are commonly used. Facial scrubs are mechanical exfoliants, as opposed to the glycolic acid chemical exfoliants previously discussed, employing small granules in a cleansing base to enhance corneocyte desquamation. The scrubbing granules may be polyethylene beads, aluminum oxide, ground fruit pits, or sodium tetraborate

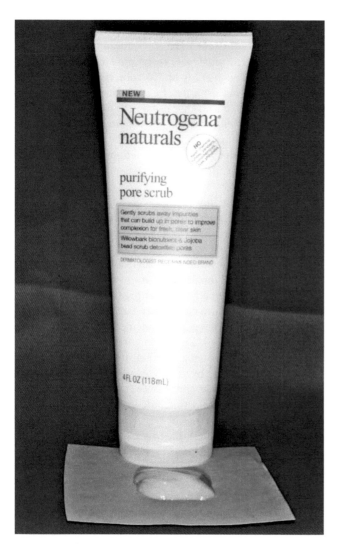

Figure 1.2 Scrubs are used in OTC acne cleansers for increased exfoliation in and around the pore.

decahydrate granules aiding in the removal desquamating stratum corneum from the face (Fig. 1.2) (43). Sibley et al. considered abrasive scrubbing creams effective in controlling excess sebum and removing desquamating tissue (44). However, they can cause epithelial damage if used too vigorously. This view is held by Mills and Kligman, who noted that the products produced peeling and erythema with no reduction in comedones. Aluminum oxide and ground fruit pits provide the most abrasive scrub due to their rough edged particles, followed by polyethylene beads, which are smoother and produce less stratum corneum removal. Sodium tetraborate decahydrate granules become softer and dissolve during rubbing, providing the least abrasive scrub.

> Acne scrub creams may contain polyethylene beads, aluminum oxide, ground fruit pits, or sodium tetraborate decahydrate granules.

A currently popular trend in facial exfoliant scrubs is the production of warmth. These products are labeled as "self-heating" scrubs. Heat is produced as part of an exothermic reaction resulting in the heat byproduct. The heat does not increase the exfoliant efficacy, but is added for consumer comfort and marketing purposes. Sometimes these heated exfoliant scrubs are preceded by a self-administered hydroxy acid peel, thus combining both chemical and physical exfoliation in one kit.

Astringents and Exfoliants

Astringents and exfoliants are used in cosmetic acne treatment regimens marketed by many companies. Astringents are liquids applied to the face following cleansing and are used widely in cosmetic acne treatments. They comprise a broad category of formulations known by many terms: toners, clarifying lotions, controlling lotions, protections lotions, skin fresheners, toning lotions, T-zone tonics, etc. Originally, astringents were developed to remove alkaline soap scum from the face following cleansing with lye-based soaps and high-mineral-content well water. The development of synthetic detergents and public softened water systems greatly decreased the amount of post-washing residue. A new use for astringents was found when cleansing cream became a preferred method of removing facial cosmetics and environmental dirt. The astringent then became an effective product for removing the oily residue left behind following cleansing cream use.

Astringent formulations are presently available for all skin types (oily, normal, dry, sensitive, photoaged, etc.); with a variety of uses, their primary benefit is in oily skin afflicted with acne (45). Oily skin astringents contain a high concentration of alcohols, water, and fragrance functioning to remove any sebum left behind after cleansing, to produce a clean feel, and possibly apply some treatment product to the face. For example, 2% salicylic acid or witch hazel may be added for a keratolytic and drying effect on the facial skin of acne patients. Clays, starches, or synthetic polymers may be added to absorb sebum and minimize the appearance of facial oil.

> Cosmetic acne treatment astringents may contain 2% salicylic acid as the active ingredient.

Exfoliants are similar to astringents, but these are solutions, lotions, or creams applied to the face after cleansing and after the application of an exfoliant designed to hasten stratum corneum exfoliation and assist in comedolysis in the acne patient. Their exfoliant effect is based on the use of alpha, poly, or beta hydroxy acids, thus inducing chemical exfoliation. The goal is to loosen the retained comedonal plug chemically from the lining of the pore. Many cosmetic acne treatment exfoliants use this theory to support claims and purport efficacy. Glycolic acid exfoliants based on alpha hydroxy acids may be useful in patients with acne and photoaged skin to improve appearance; however, the salicylic beta hydroxy acid exfoliants are more effective. This is due to their inherent oil solubility that allows them to exfoliate in the oily milieu of the pore. Polyhydroxy acid exfoliants based on gluconolactone are also marketed with the main claim of reduced irritation. Their large molecular weight impedes skin penetration and reduces irritation.

Epidermabrasion and Textured Cloths

Epidermabrasion and textured clothes are used to induce mechanical exfoliation of comedonal plugs as opposed to the exfoliants that induce chemical exfoliation. Durr and Orentreich termed mechanical exfoliation as epidermabrasion, who examined the use of a nonwoven polyester fiber web sponge for the removal of keratin excrescences and trapped hairs in pilosebaceous ducts (46–47). Other epidermabrasion implements include rubber puffs, sea sponges, and loofahs, and the most recent addition of textured fiber face cloths. The fiber face cloths have come to be a major segment of the current epidermabrasion marketplace and are discussed in detail.

Fiber cloths are extremely versatile dermatologic devices. They can be premoistened and impregnated with surfactants to cleanse the face; can be perfumed containing volatile solvents to freshen the face; they can be packaged dry with lipids and detergents to clean the face, and they can be covered with a plastic film pouch that has microscopic holes to time release an active acne ingredient onto the skin surface. Also, they can be textured with patterns to physically exfoliate the skin. Even though the use of facial fiber cloth as a cosmetic acne treatment is new, the cloth has been around for 30 years (Fig. 1.3).

Fiber cloths are useful in cleansing the face of acne patients to clean in and around the pores.

Modern fiber cloth technology focused on creating a soft wipe with excellent strength to prevent tearing. The fibers used are a combination of polyester, rayon, cotton, and cellulose fibers held together via heat through a technique known as thermobonding. Additional strength is imparted to the wipe by hydroentangling the fibers. This is achieved by entwining the individual rayon, polyester, and wood pulp fibers with high pressure jets of water. Thermobonding and hydroentangling have eliminated the use of adhesive binders thereby creating a soft, strong cloth suitable for facial use.

Face cloths are available both dry and moist. The dry packaged cloths are impregnated with a cleanser that foams modestly when the cloth is water moistened. The type of cleanser in the cloth can effect an aggressive sebum removal for oily skin and contain salicylic acid. Humectants and emollients can also be added to the cloth to decrease barrier damage or to smooth the xerotic skin scale common in acne patients who are on prescription therapy.

In addition to the composition of the ingredients preapplied to the dry cloth, the weave of the cloth will also determine its acne effect. Two types of fiber weaves are used in facial acne cloths: open weave and closed weave. Open weave cloths are so named because of the 2–3 mm windows in the cloth between the adjacent fiber bundles. These cloths are used in persons with dry and/or sensitive skin and acne to increase the softness of the cloth and decrease the surface area contact between the cloth and the skin yielding a milder exfoliant effect. Closed weave cloths, on the hand, are designed with a much tighter weave and are double sided. One side of the closed weave cloth is textured and impregnated with a synthetic detergent cleanser designed to optimize the removal of sebum, cosmetics, and environmental dirt while providing an exfoliant effect. The opposite side of the cloth is smooth and designed for rinsing the face and possibly applying skin conditioning or acne agents.

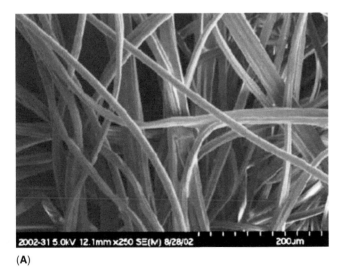

(A)

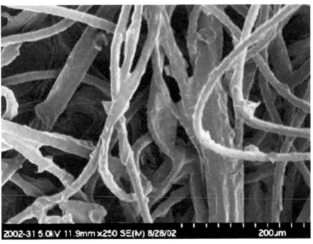

(B)

Figure 1.3 (**A**) A scanning electron microscopy image of a fiber cloth prior to cleansing showing the entangled fibers compressed to form a continuous fabric. (**B**) A used cleansing cloth showing the skin scale and debris attached to the fibers prior to rinsing.

The texture of the cloth provides gentle mechanical exfoliation that may be valuable in the patient who cannot tolerate chemical exfoliation with hydroxy acids. The mechanical exfoliation can be achieved on the skin surface and around the follicular ostia due to the ability of the textured cloth to traverse the irregular topography of the skin more effectively than the hands or a wash cloth. The degree of exfoliation achieved is dependent on the cloth weave, the pressure with which the cloth is stroked over the skin surface, and the length of time the cloth is applied. The cloth can aid in the removal of comedonal plugs.

Mechanized Skin Care Devices

Mechanization of the epidermabrasion process is known as microdermabrasion. This is a procedure performed by estheticians and paramedical personnel, where small particulates, such as aluminum, silica, baking soda, etc., are sprayed against the skin surface and simultaneously removed with a vacuum. Microdermabrasion simply is another technique to induce stratum corneum exfoliation.

> Mechanized cleansing devices can rotate, vibrate, or sonicate to aid in removal of skin scale and sebum.

A variety of devices are available to exfoliate the facial skin. These include rotary brushes that drag synthetic bristles across the skin surface to physically remove the stratum corneum. These devices are sold with a special cleanser to remove sebum and clean the bristles simultaneously. A variant of this technology used scrubbing pads of varied roughness to produce exfoliation. The scrubbing pads were held on the device head with adhesive and could be replaced when worn. These devices vibrated instead of rotating to remove skin scale.

A third type of facial cleansing device produces a sonicating motion, similar to that of sonicating electric toothbrushes. The hand-held device runs on a rechargeable battery that is attached to a miniaturized motor creating an oscillatory motion of the brush head. This oscillatory sonic motion allows the brush bristles to traverse the dermatoglyphics, facial pores, and facial scars more adeptly than other mechanized cleansing methods. These devices may be useful in acne patients with facial scarring.

Face Masks

Face masks are also used in the cosmetic treatment of acne. Typically, a face mask is applied on a weekly basis to provide a more aggressive type of acne treatment, but the medical benefits may be minimal. The masks that are used in acne treatment are earth based. Earth-based masks, also known as paste masks or mud packs, are formulated from absorbent clays such as bentonite, kaolin, or china clay. The clays produce an astringent effect on the skin making this mask most appropriate for oily-complected patients. The astringent effect of the mask can be enhanced through the addition of other substances such as magnesium, zinc oxide, salicylic acid, etc. The masks can be applied as a cloth that is laid over the entire face or as a paste that is scooped from a jar. The mask is left on the face for 15–30 minutes and then rinsed away with water.

COMEDOGENICITY AND SKIN CARE FORMULATIONS

The issue of comedogenicity in relation to cosmetics arose in 1972 when Kligman and Mills described a low-grade acne characterized by closed comedones on the cheeks of women aged 20–25 years (48). They labeled this phenomenon "acne cosmetica." Many of these women had not experienced adolescent acne. The authors proposed that substances present in cosmetic products induced the formation of closed comedones and, in some cases, a papulopustular eruption. This led to the concept that skin care products and cosmetics could cause acne.

Further research on cosmetic-induced acne led to the development of the rabbit ear comedogenicity model, which is still sometimes used by cosmetic companies to test products. The cosmetic is applied to the ears of New Zealand white albino rabbits. One ear serves as a control while the other ear receives one-half mL of the test substance five days per week for two consecutive weeks. Visual observations of enlarged pores and hyperkeratosis are made daily. At the completion of the study, the skin is biopsied to look for hyperkeratosis of the sebaceous follicles (49).

While this model was the standard test for comedogenicity for many years, it is currently out of favor as animal testing has been abandoned by many cosmetic companies and there are inherent problems with the model (50). First, some studies do not perform a biopsy and rely on the visual inspection of the rabbit ear, which is less sensitive than the microscopic examination. Microcomedones, now known to be important acne precursor lesions, can only be identified through microscopic examination. Second, some studies have confused follicular dilation with comedone formation. Follicular dilation is a side effect of cutaneous irritation and is not necessarily the same as comedone formation. Third, the use of immature or aged rabbits may not yield accurate data since sebum production is reduced in rabbits not in their prime. Fourth, the rabbit ear may not accurately simulate the human face: many substances that produce comedones in the rabbit ear model produce pustules and inflammatory papules, not comedones, on the human face.

> The follicular biopsy has become the standard technique for assessing comedogenicity in skin care formulations.

Due to the aforementioned limitations with the rabbit ear model, many cosmetic companies are now using the upper back of male and female volunteers for comedogenicity assessment (51). The volunteers are first checked for the ability to produce comedones by taking a follicular biopsy. This is done by placing a drop of cyanoacrylate glue on a microscope slide and letting it dry on the back of the subject. The microscope slide is then pulled from the skin removing comedonal plugs that appear as waxy mountains when the slide is viewed with a dissecting 5× microscope. Occlusive patch tests are used to apply the material to the upper back for 30 days with repeated daily changing. Follicular biopsies are repeated at the end of the test period and the slides are examined for an increase in the presence of comedonal plugs (52). A negative no-treatment patch is applied and a positive treatment patch containing coal tar is also used. This test for

Table 1.1 A Standard List of Possible Comedogenic Substances

Butyl stearate
Cocoa butter
Corn oil
D&C red dyes
Decyl oleate
Isopropyl isostearate
Isopropyl myristate
Isostearyl neopentanoate
Isopropyl palmitate
Isocetyl stearate
Lanolin, acetylated
Laureth-4
Linseed oil
Mineral oil
Myristyl ether propionate
Myristyl lactate
Myristyl myristate
Methyl oleate
Oleic acid
Oleyl alcohol
Olive oil
Octyl palmitate
Octyl stearate
Peanut oil
Petrolatum
Propylene glycol stearate
Safflower oil
Sesame oil
Sodium lauryl sulfate
Stearic acid

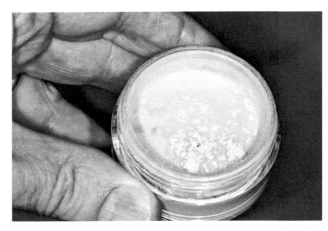

Figure 1.4 It is impossible to determine whether a cosmetic is comedogenic or acnegenic based on the appearance or from the ingredient disclosure. Clinical testing is required.

comedogenicity is also performed in addition to pre- and post-marketing surveillance.

The established lists of comedogenic substances, such as those shown in Table 1.1, are used by watch dog websites and some companies to show marketing advantages. These lists were generated many years ago by studying the material in concentration of 100% in the rabbit ear assay, which may not be relevant to actual cosmetic formulations. Giving patients this list of comedogenic substances to avoid is not very useful, since it is practically impossible to find formulations that possess none of these ingredients. The list contains some of the most effective emollients (octyl stearate, isocetyl stearate), detergents (sodium lauryl sulfate), occlusive moisturizers (mineral oil, petrolatum, sesame oil, cocoa butter), and emulsifiers found in the cosmetic industry (53). A product line that avoided all of these substances would not perform well on the skin and would possess a low cosmetic acceptability. Comedogenicity can only be evaluated in light of the patient's susceptibility to the formation of comedonal plugs. Some individuals have never developed a comedone in their life and use cocoa butter daily as a facial moisturizer. For some reason, it is not yet understood why certain patients develop fewer comedones than others (54,55).

Lists of comedogenic substances are not particularly helpful in selecting skin care product formulations for acne patients.

ACNEGENICITY AND SKIN CARE FORMULATIONS

Acnegenicity is a completely separate issue from comedogenicity. Substances that are comedogenic cause comedones, or blackheads, whereas substances that are acnegenic cause papules and pustules. Comedogenicity is due to follicular plugging whereas acnegenicity is due to follicular irritation (56). Thus, substances that are comedogenic are not necessarily acnegenic and vice versa (Fig. 1.4).

At first glance, acnegenicity also may seem rather simple. A list of substances that irritates the follicular ostia could be generated and then used to pick skin care products and cosmetics for patient use. Unfortunately, lists of acnegenic substances are useless since the interaction of ingredients, as well as their concentration, is important. But of more importance, is the individual patient susceptibility to acne formation. Cosmetics that are acnegenic in one patient are not necessarily acnegenic in another patient.

It is interesting to note that, in a general dermatologist's practice, the phenomenon of acnegenicity due to cosmetics is a more common occurrence than that of comedogenicity due to cosmetics. This makes acnegenicity a more important issue than comedogenicity. However, the incidence of comedone and acne formation due to cosmetics is rare, considering the number of persons who use such products on a daily basis.

SUMMARY

This chapter has discussed the various ingredients and ancillary skin care products for acne treatment in the current marketplace. Astringents represent a broad category and may impart both cleansing and moisturizing effects to the skin, depending on the formulation and skin type. Exfoliants, which became popular when glycolic acid was introduced to the cosmetic acne treatment marketplace, can contain both chemical and physical exfoliating ingredients to enhance the desquamation of the stratum corneum. Physical exfoliating agents are commonly packaged as particulate facial scrubs, woven sponges, or textured cloths. Textured cloths are the most recent introduction and can function like disposable washcloths or may leave behind ingredients on the skin surface. Mechanized skin care devices attempt to deliver at home microdermabrasion with rotary, vibrating, or sonicating motors. Finally, face masks deliver skin care benefits. These are popular acne ingredients and devices that should be understood by a dermatologist.

REFERENCES

1. Management of acne. Agency for healthcare research and quality. 2001 March 2001 Contract No.: 01-E018.
2. 21 CFR Part 333.350(b)(2), 21 CFR (1991).
3. Kraus AL, Munro IC, Orr JC, et al. Benzoyl peroxide: an integrated human safety assessment for carcinogenicity. Regul Toxicol Pharmacol 1995; 21: 87–107.
4. Tanghetti E. The evolution of benzoyl peroxide therapy. Cutis 2008; 82: 5–11.
5. Bojar RA, Cunliffe WJ, Holland KT. Short-term treatment of acne vulgaris with benzoyl peroxide: effects on the surface and follicular cutaneous microflora. Br J Dermatol 1995; 132: 204–8.
6. Pagnoni A, Kligman AM, Kollias N, Goldberg S, Stoudemayer T. Digital fluorescence photography can assess the suppressive effect of benzoyl peroxide on Propionibacterium acnes. J Am Acad Dermatol 1999; 41 (5 Pt 1): 710–16.
7. Leyden JJ. Current issues in antimicrobial therapy for the treatment of acne. J Eur Acad Dermatol Venereol 2001; 15(Suppl 3): 51–5.
8. Kim J, Ochoa M, Krutzik S, et al. Activation of toll-like receptor 2 in acne triggers inflammatory cytokine responses. J Immunol 2002; 169: 1535–41.
9. Bojar RA, Cunliffe WJ, Holland KT. Short-term treatment of acne vulgaris with benzoyl peroxide: effects on the surface and follicular cutaneous microflora. Br J Dermatol 1995; 132: 204–8.
10. Mills OH Jr, Kligman AM, Pochi P, Comite H. Comparing 2.5%, 5%, and 10% benzoyl peroxide on inflammatory acne vulgaris. Int J Dermatol 1986; 25: 664–7.
11. Morelli R, Lanzarini M, Vincenzi C. Contact dermatitis due to benzoyl peroxide. Contact Dermatitis 1989; 20: 238–9.
12. Kraus AL, Munro IC, Orr JC, et al. Benzoyl peroxide: an integrated human safety assessment for carcinogenicity. Regul Toxicol Pharmacol 1995; 21: 87–107.
13. Tanghetti E, Popp KF. A current review of topical benzoyl peroxide: new perspectives on formulation and utilization. Dermatol Clin 2009; 27: 17–24.
14. Eady EA, Burke BM, Pulling K, Cunliffe WJ. The benefit of 2% salicylic acid lotion in acne. J Dermatol Ther1996; 7: 93–6.
15. Bissonnette R, Bolduc C, Seite S, et al. Randomized study comparing the efficacy and tolerance of a lipophilic hydroxy acid derivative of salicylic acid and 5% benzoyl peroxide in the treatment of facial acne vulgaris. J Cosmet Dermatol 2009; 8: 19–23.
16. Chen T, Appa Y. Over-the-Counter Acne Medications. In: Draelos ZD, Thaman LA, eds. Cosmetic Formulations of Skin Care Products. New York: Taylor & Francis, 2006: 251–71.
17. Shalita AR. Treatment of mild and moderate acne vulgaris with salicylic acid in an alcohol-detergent vehicle. Cutis 1981; 28: 556–8.
18. Zander E, Weisman S. Treatment of acne with salicylic acid pads. Clin Ther 1992; 14: 247–53.
19. Pagnoni A, Chen T, Duong H, Wu IT, Appa Y. Clinical evaluation of a salicylic acid containing scrub, toner, mask and regimen in reducing blackheads. 61st meeting, American Academy of Dermatology. 2004 February 2004; Poster 61.
20. Gupta AK, Nicol K, Gupta AK, Nicol K. The use of sulfur in dermatology. J Drugs Dermatol 2004; 3: 427–31.
21. Lin AN, Reimer RJ, Carter DM. Sulfur revisited. J Am Acad Dermatol 1988; 18: 553–8.
22. Mills OH Jr, Kligman AM. Is sulphur helpful or harmful in acne vulgaris? Br J Dermatol 1972; 86: 620–7.
23. Berardesca E, Distante F, Vignoli GP, Oresajo C, Green B. Alpha hydroxy-acids modulate stratum corneum barrier function. Br J Dermatol 1997; 137: 934–8.
24. Garg VK, Sinha S, Sarkar R. Glycolic acid peels versus salicylic acid peels in active acne vulgaris and post-acne scarring and hyperpigmentation: a comparative study. Dermatol Surg 2009; 35: 59–65.
25. Lee TW, Kim JC, Hwang SJ. Hydrogel patches containing triclosan for acne treatment. Eur J Pharm Biopharm 2003; 56: 407–12.
26. Duell EA. Unoccluded retinol penetrates human skin in vivo more effectively than unoccluded retinyl palmitate or retinoic acid. J Invest Dermatol 1997; 109.
27. Raman A. Antimicrobial effects of tea-tree oil and its major components on Staphylococcus aureus, Staph. epidermidis and Propionibacterium acnes. Lett Appl Microbiol 1995; 21: 242–5.
28. Hammer KA, Carson CF, Riley TV. Susceptibility of transient and commensal skin flora to the essential oil of Melaleuca alternifolia. Am J Infect Control 1996; 24: 186–9.
29. Shemesh A, Mayo WL. Australian tea tree oil: a natural antiseptic and fungicidal agent. Aust J Pharm 1991; 72: 802–3.
30. Bassett IB, Pannowitz DL, Barnetson RS. A comparative study of tea-tree oil versus benzoyl peroxide in the treatment of acne. Med J Aust 1990; 153: 455–8.
31. Enshaieh S, Jooya A, Siadat AH, Iraji F. Indian J Dermatol Venereol Leprol 2007; 73: 22–5.
32. Koh KJ, Pearce AL, Marshman G, Finlay-Jones JJ, Hart PH. Tea tree oil reduces histamine-induced skin inflammation. Br J Dermatol 2002; 147: 1212–17.
33. Bischoff K, Guale F. Australian tea tree oil poisoning in three purebred cats. J Vet Diag Invest 1998; 10: 208.
34. Lisi P, Melingi L, Pigatto P, et al. Prevalenza della sensibilizzazione all'olio exxenziale di Melaleuca. Ann Ital Dermatol Allergol 2000; 54: 141–4.
35. Elston D. Topical antibiotics in dermatology: emerging patterns of resistance. Dermatol Clin 2009; 27: 25–31.
36. Dreno B, Trossaert M, Boiteau HL, Litoux P. Zinc salts effects on granulocyte zinc concentration and chemotaxis in acne patients. Acta Derm Venereol 1992; 72: 250–2.
37. Fivenson DP. The mechanisms of action of nicotinamide and zinc in inflammatory skin disease. Cutis 2006; 77(1 Suppl): 5–10.
38. Ottte N, Borelli C, Korting HC. Nicotinamide biologic actions of an emerging cosmetic ingredient. Int J Cosmet Sci 2005; 27: 255–61.
39. Niren NM. Pharmacologic doses of nicotinamide in the treatment of inflammatory skin conditions: a review. Cutis 2006; 77(1 Suppl): 11–16.
40. Niren NM, Torok HM. The Nicomide Improvement in Clinical Outcomes Study (NICOS): results of an 8-week trial. Cutis 2006; 77 (1 Suppl): 17–28.
41. Shalita AR, Smith JG, Parish LC, Sofman MS, Chalker DK. Topical nicotinamide compared with clindamycin gel in the treatment of inflammatory acne vulgaris. Int J Dermatol 1999; 34: 434–7.
42. Wortzman MS, Scott RA, Wong PS, et al. Soap and detergent bar rinsability. J Soc Cosmet Chem 1986; 37: 89–97.
43. Mills OH, Kligman AM. Evaluation of abrasives in acne therapy. Cutis 1979; 23: 704–75.
44. Sibley MJ, Browne RK, Kitzmiller KW. Abradant cleansing aids for acne vulgaris. Cutis 1974; 14: 269–74.
45. Wilkinson JB, Moore RJ. Astringents and skin toners. In: Harry's Cosmeticology, 7th edn. New York: Chemical Publishing, 1982: 74–81.
46. Durr NP, Orentreich N. Epidermabrasion for acne. Cutis 1976; 17: 604–8.
47. Mackenzie A. Use of But-Puf and mild cleansing bar in acne. Cutis 1977; 20: 170–1.
48. Kligman AM, Mills OH. Acne cosmetica. Arch Dermatol 1972; 106: 843.
49. Kaufman PJ, Rappaport MJ. Skin care products. In: Whittam JH, ed. Cosmetic Safety a Primer for Cosmetic Scientists. New York: Marcel Dekker, Inc, 1987: 179–204.
50. Frank SB. Is the rabbit ear model, in its present state, prophetic of acnegenicity? J Am Acad Dermatol 1982; 6: 373.
51. Mills OH, Kligman AM. A human model for assessing comedeogenic substances. Arch Dermatol 1982; 118: 903–5.
52. Kaufman PJ, Rappaport MJ. Skin care products. In: Whittam JH, ed. Cosmetic Safety a Primer for Cosmetic Scientists. New York: Marcel Dekker, Inc, 1987: 179–204.
53. Fulton JE, Pay SR, Fulton JE. Comedogenicity of current therapeutic products, cosmetics, and ingredients in the rabbit ear. J Am Acad Dermatol 1984; 10: 96–105.
54. Fulton JE, Bradley S, Aqundez A, Black T. Non-comedogenic cosmetics. Cutis 1976; 17: 344.
55. Report of the 1988 American Academy of Dermatology Invitational Symposium on Comedogenicity. J Am Acad Dermatol 1989; 20: 272–7.
56. Mills OH, Berger RS. Defining the susceptibility of acne-prone and sensitive skin populations to extrinsic factors. Dermatol Clin 1991; 9: 93–8.

SUGGESTED READING

Barker MO. Masks and astringents/toners (Chapter 13). In: Baran R, Maibach H, eds. Textbook of Cosmetic Dermatology, 2nd edn. Martin Dunitz Ltd, 1998: 155–65.

Cunliffe WJ, Holland DB, Clack SM, Stables GI. Comedogenesis: some new aetiological, clinical and therapeutic strategies. Br J Dermatol 2000; 142: 1084–91.

Cunliffe WJ, Holland DB, Jeremy A. Comedone formation: etiology, clinical presentation, and treatment. Clin Dermatol 2004; 22: 367–74.

Draelos ZD. A Re-evaluation of the Comedogenicity Concept. J Am Acad Dermatol 2006; 54: 507–12.

Draelos ZD. Cosmetics in acne and rosacea. Semin Cutan Med Surg 2001; 20: 209–14.

Draelos ZD. Treating the patient with multiple cosmetic product allergies. A problem-oriented approach to sensitive skin. Postgrad Med 2000; 107: 70–2, 75–7.

Draelos ZD, DiNardo JC. A re-evaluation of the comedogenicity concept. J Am Acad Dermatol 2006; 54: 507–12.

Katsambas AD, Stefanaki C, Cunliffe WJ. Guidelines for treating acne. Clin Dermatol 2004; 22: 439–44.

Kiken DA, Cohen DE. Contact dermatitis to botanical extracts. Am J Contact Dermat 2002; 13: 148–52.

Klock J, Ikeno H, Ohmori K, et al. Sodium ascorbyl phosphate shows in vitro and in vivo efficacy in the prevention and treatment of acne vulgaris. Int J Cosmet Sci 2005; 27: 171–6.

Leyden JJ. Antibiotic resistance in the topical treatment of acne vulgaris. Cutis 2004; 73 (6 Suppl): 6–10.

Mirshahpanah P, Maibach HI. Models in acnegenesis. Cutan Ocul Toxicol 2007; 26: 195–202.

Nguyen SH, Dang TP, Maibach HI. Comedogenicity in rabbit: some cosmetic ingredients/vehicles. Cutan Ocul Toxicol 2007; 26: 287–92.

Zatulove A, Konnerth NA. Comedogenicity testing of cosmetics. Cutis 1987; 39: 521.

2 Rosacea and cosmetics

The use of cosmetics in a rosacea patient is very important to minimize inflammation as well as to camouflage facial redness. Rosacea patients form a subset of sensitive skin, making the selection of skin care products and cosmetics problematic. Ingredients that typically cause no difficulty in an average patient can cause severe stinging and burning in a rosacea patient. Sometimes the adverse reaction can be invisible; more typically, it is characterized by the rapid onset of facial flushing. For this reason, developing a methodology for product recommendations in a rosacea patient becomes important. This chapter will discuss a rationale for the selection of cleansers, moisturizers, cosmeceuticals, and facial cosmetics for rosacea patients.

Many skin care and cosmetic products are labeled as appropriate for sensitive skin, including the rosacea patient, but this term does not have any scientific definition. Most manufacturers who make this claim will test sensitive skin care products on a population consisting of at least 30% rosacea sufferers. Of the entire population, approximately 40% consider themselves to possess the characteristics of sensitive skin (1). Sensitive skin can be defined in both subjective and objective terms. Subjective perceptions of sensitive skin are derived from patient observations regarding stinging, burning, pruritus, and tightness following various environmental stimuli. These symptoms may be noticed immediately following product application or delayed by minutes, hours, or days (2). Furthermore, the symptoms may only result following a cumulative product application or in combination with concomitant products. Objective perceptions of sensitive skin include the onset of facial flushing and/or inflammatory papules following application. An adverse reaction to a cosmetic or skin care product may elicit subjective and/or objective signs in a rosacea patient.

TESTING OF FACIAL PRODUCTS IN ROSACEA PATIENTS

Skin care and cosmetic products designed for rosacea patients must be specially tested as appropriate for sensitive skin. One method of testing is simply to employ an in-use model by enrolling 40–60 subjects with mild to moderate rosacea and asking them to use the newly developed product for four weeks while recording their perceptions in a diary. A dermatologist investigator can also assess the state of the subject's rosacea at two-week intervals for improvement or worsening related to the study product. This is the most basic type of test that should be performed.

> The facial sting test is useful for the testing of skin care and cosmetic products to find out whether they are appropriate for rosacea sufferers.

A more sophisticated testing method should be performed to evaluate subsets of rosacea patients who may have a more sensitive skin and a higher incidence of cosmetic problems. This method of evaluating product appropriateness for rosacea is to use a modification of the lactic acid facial stinging test (3). This test provokes a flare of rosacea by exposing the skin to an irritating chemical, accompanied by heat. The test is performed by placing the rosacea patient in a warm facial sauna for 15 minutes or until profuse sweating and redness appears, followed by an application of a 5% aqueous solution of lactic acid at room temperature to one randomized nasolabial fold using brisk rubbing strokes of a cotton-tipped applicator. The product in question is applied to the other nasolabial fold and the subject is asked to rate the stinging of both application areas. The subject is blinded as to the identity of the applied products, so as not to bias the stinging response. The patient rates the stinging at 2.5 and 5 minutes after application on an ordinal 4-point scale (0 = no stinging, 1 = slight stinging, 2 = moderate stinging, 3 = severe stinging) (4,5). Even though this test is quite artificial, it appears to correlate well with skin care and cosmetic products that might cause difficulty in rosacea patients, but this remains controversial (6). This type of challenge testing can be adapted for use in the dermatology office.

The most important part of the product testing for rosacea patients is the need to expose the facial skin to the cosmetic during a rosacea flare when active inflammation is present. Vasodilation and inflammatory mediator release must be present to get an accurate assessment. Products that sting on the face of a rosacea patient may provoke a flare, which is undesirable, and they should not be marketed as appropriate for sensitive skin. In general, rosacea patients can use skin care and cosmetic products from reputable manufacturers that are labeled as appropriate for sensitive skin.

FACIAL CLEANSERS

Proper skin care can enhance rosacea treatment or, in some cases, totally negate a positive effect. No skin care act is more important than cleansing. Since *Demodex* and *Propionibacterium acnes* may be contributory in some forms of rosacea, skin cleansing is the first step to restoring and maintaining a healthy biofilm. Thorough cleansing is also necessary to control the growth of *Pityrosporum* species in patients with the overlap syndrome of rosacea and seborrheic dermatitis. In short, the goals of cleansing in a rosacea patient are to remove excess sebum, environmental debris, desquamating corneocytes, unwanted organisms, and old skin care and cosmetic products while leaving the skin barrier untouched. This can be a challenge since cleansers cannot distinguish between sebum and intercellular lipids, meaning that products that clean too well may be problematic (Fig. 2.1). This discussion focuses on the use of the cleansers in rosacea patients with a

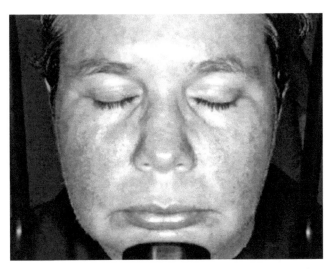

Figure 2.1 The typical inflamed appearance of a rosacea patient with an excessive-cleansing-induced irritation from surfactant barrier damage.

variety of skin needs to include oily, normal, and dry skin. Cosmetic removal, cleansing devices, and problematic products are also discussed.

> Facial cleansing assumes great importance in rosacea to maintain a healthy biofilm without damaging the skin barrier.

Oily Skin

Many rosacea patients with a highly sebaceous skin produce abundant sebum. Even though the skin is oily, overcleansing will result in shiny, flaky skin. This is due to the barrier disruption created by the removal of the intercellular lipids that causes premature corneocyte desquamation followed by the subsequent reacummulation of sebum. The face becomes overdry immediately after cleansing, but turns oily again two to four hours after cleansing. This is a challenging situation, since cleansing does not reduce sebum production; it only removes the sebum present at the time of cleansing. This observation accounts for the ill-founded belief of some rosacea patients that skin cleansing produces redness and increased sebum.

The most basic cleanser for oily skin is soap, created as a reaction between a fat and an alkali resulting in a fatty acid salt with detergent properties (7). Soap is composed of long-chain fatty acid alkali salts with a pH between 9 and 10 (8). The high pH thoroughly removes sebum, but can also damage the intercellular lipids. For persons with extremely oily skin, this type of cleanser may be appropriate (Ivory, Procter & Gamble). Aggressive scrubbing with a washcloth or other implements should be avoided when trying to remove copious sebum, since the manipulation of the skin may provoke a rosacea flare. A better solution is to wash the face twice, each time removing more sebum. Gentle massaging of the cleanser into the skin with the hands followed by lukewarm water rinsing is the best. It is important to avoid exposing the face to water temperature extremes, which could provoke flushing.

Normal Skin

There is no definition of normal skin; however, for this discussion the term will refer to patients without oily or dry skin.

Soap may remove too much sebum in this population, making syndet cleansers the preferred choice. Syndets, also known as synthetic detergents, contain less than 10% soap with an adjusted pH of 5.5–7. The neutral pH, closer to the natural pH of the skin, produces less irritation. In general, all beauty bars, mild cleansing bars, and sensitive skin bars are of the syndet variety (Oil of Olay, Procter & Gamble; Dove, Unilever; Cetaphil Bar, Galderma). The most commonly used detergent is sodium cocoyl isethionate. These cleansers also possess excellent rinsability, meaning that a soap scum film is not left behind on the skin when used with water of varying hardness. This is an important property in the sensitive-skin rosacea patients where the soap film might produce irritation.

For rosacea patients who are concerned about body odor and desire a "squeaky-clean" skin feel, another type of cleanser, known as a combar, is available. Combars are produced by combining an alkaline soap with a syndet to produce less aggressive sebum removal than a soap, but more aggressive sebum removal than a syndet. Most of the combars also add an antibacterial, such as triclosan, to provide odor control properties. These cleansers are commonly labeled as deodorant soaps (Dial, Dial Corporation; Irish Spring, Colgate Palmolive) (9). For rosacea patients with abundant sebum production and difficult–to-control pustules, this type of cleanser may be beneficial. Triclosan is not approved as an acne ingredient in the U.S.A., but is used in Europe for this purpose. For patients with normal sebum production, the deodorant cleanser can be used once daily or once every other day to provide antibacterial effects without overly aggressive sebum production.

Dry and/or Sensitive Skin

Many rosacea patients possess a sensitive skin that must be gently cleaned due to limited sebum production. These patients are usually mature postmenopausal women. Lipid-free cleansers represent a cleansing alternative for this population. Lipid-free cleansers are liquids that clean without fats, a point which distinguishes them from soaps (Cetaphil Cleanser, Galderma; CeraVe, Coria; Aquanil, Person & Covey). The cleanser is applied to dry or moistened skin, rubbed to produce a slight lather, and rinsed or wiped away. These products may contain water, glycerin, cetyl alcohol, stearyl alcohol, sodium laurel sulfate, and occasionally propylene glycol. They leave behind a thin moisturizing film, but do not possess strong antibacterial properties. For this reason, lipid-free cleansers are excellent for the dry face, but are not recommended for cleansing the groin or armpits. They also are not good at removing excessive environmental dirt or sebum.

Cosmetic Removal

Lipid-free cleansers may also be used to remove cosmetics in the rosacea patient (Cetaphil, Galderma; CeraVe Cleanser, Valeant). They can be applied dry and rubbed over the eyelids, cheeks, and lips to remove both water-removable and water-resistant cosmetics and rinsed off with lukewarm water. If necessary, another cleanser can be used for additional cleaning. Many of the commercially marketed cosmetic removers contain solvents that are volatile and damaging to the intercellular lipids, thus provoking rosacea.

Lipid-free or low-foaming cleansers are excellent for makeup removal in rosacea patients.

Another product for cosmetic removal is the cleansing cream. A cleansing cream is composed of water, mineral oil, petrolatum, and waxes (Albolene) (10). The most common variant of the cleansing cream, known as cold cream, is created by adding borax to mineral oil and beeswax (Pond's Cold Cream) (11). These products are popular among mature women as they do cosmetic removal and mild cleansing in one step.

Cleansing Devices

Cleansing devices combine a cleanser with an implement for washing the skin. The most common cleansing device is a disposable cleansing cloth impregnated with a cleanser. The cloth can be of polyester, rayon, cotton, and cellulose fibers, which are heated to produce a thermobond. Additional strength is imparted to the cloth by hydroentangling the fibers with high pressure jets of water, which eliminates the need for adhesive binders. This creates a soft durable cloth. The cloth can be packaged dry or wet typically with a syndet cleanser. Dry cloths are wetted before use.

Open weave cleansing cloths can be used to gently but thoroughly cleanse the face of rosacea patients.

The amount of sebum removal achieved by the cloth can be varied based on the amount of cleanser as well as the type of the weave of the cloth. There are two types of fiber weaves used in facial cloths: open weave and closed weave. Open weave cloths possess 2–3 mm windows between adjacent fiber bundles. These cloths are used on dry and/or sensitive skin as it increases the softness of the cloth and decreases the cleansing surface area. Closed weave cloths, on the hand, are designed with a much tighter weave and provide a more thorough cleansing, but also induce exfoliation. The exfoliation is intended to remove desquamating corneocytes. While this may be beneficial in some rosacea patients, it may be problematic in others. The degree of exfoliation achieved is dependent on the cloth weave, the pressure with which the cloth is stroked over the skin surface, and the length of time the cloth is applied. Individuals with sensitive skin may wish to consider using an open weave cloth gently over the face once weekly for mild exfoliation.

Moisturizing cleansing cloths are also available and may be the preferable choice in rosacea patients. The cloth contains two sides, which may be differently designed to deliver different benefits. The moisturizing cloths contain a cleanser on the textured side and a moisturizer on the smooth side. The cloth is dipped in water to wet it; the textured side of it is used first to clean and gently exfoliate the skin; then the cloth is rinsed. The cloth is then turned over and the face is rinsed and moisturized simultaneously. This cloth technology can also be used for cosmetic removal in some patients.

A variant of the cleansing cloth is the cleansing pouch. Fusing two cleansing cloths around skin cleansing and conditioning ingredients creates the cleansing pouch. A plastic membrane is placed between two fiber cloths containing holes of various diameters to control the release of ingredients onto the skin surface. Many times the cleansing pouches contain a variety of botanicals, which may be problematic in rosacea patients.

Problematic Cleansers and Cleansing Implements

Other cleansers and cleansing implements may also be problematic in rosacea patients. Products that induce aggressive exfoliation, such as abrasive scrubs, may provoke flushing. Abrasive scrubs incorporate polyethylene beads, aluminum oxide, ground fruit pits, or sodium tetraborate decahydrate granules to induce various degrees of exfoliation (12). The most aggressive exfoliation is produced by irregularly shaped aluminum oxide particles and ground fruit pits, which should be avoided by rosacea patients. Milder exfoliation is produced by polyethylene beads, which possess a smooth rounded surface. The least aggressive exfoliation is produced by sodium tetraborate decahydrate granules, which soften and dissolve during use.

Aggressive facial cleansers and scrubbing implements should be avoided in a rosacea patient.

Another form of aggressive exfoliation is produced by sponges composed of nonwoven polyester fibers (Buf Puf) (13). These sponges are too aggressive for most of the rosacea patients. Rosacea patients have sensitive skin that must be handled gently like a fine silk scarf. Pulling, tugging, rubbing vigorously, and strong cleansers will ruin a silk scarf immediately and are not recommended for the rosacea patient with sensitive skin. Some rosacea sufferers scrub their face mercilessly hoping to cleanse away the inflammatory lesions and redness, when in actuality they are only worsening the barrier damage. However, barrier damage repair can be facilitated with moisturizers, the next topic for discussion.

FACIAL MOISTURIZERS

Moisturizers are important to provide an environment suitable for barrier repair in the rosacea patient. Facial moisturizers are the most important cosmetic in the prevention of a facial rosacea flare (Fig. 2.2). These moisturizers attempt to mimic the effect of sebum and the intercellular lipids composed of sphingolipids, free sterols, and free fatty acids. They intend to provide an environment allowing the stratum corneum barrier to heal by replacing the corneocytes and the intercellular lipids. Yet, the moisturizing substances must not occlude the sweat ducts, or miliaria will result in; must not produce irritation at the follicular ostia, or else an acneiform eruption will break out; and must not initiate comedone formation. Furthermore, the facial moisturizer must not produce noxious sensory stimuli, which may also provoke a rosacea flare.

Moisturizers are used to heal the barrier-damaged skin by minimizing transepidermal water loss (TEWL) and creating an environment optimal for rosacea control. Three categories of substances that can be combined to enhance the water content of the skin are occlusives, humectants, and hydrocolloids. Occlusives are oily substances that retard TEWL by placing an oil slick over the skin surface, while humectants are substances

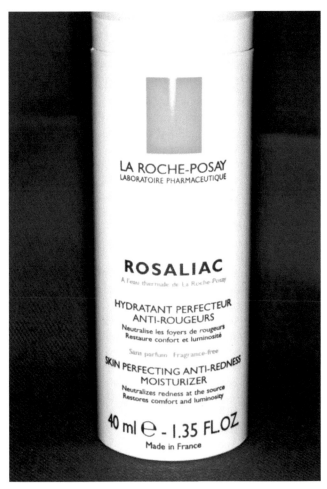

Figure 2.2 An example of a variety of anti-inflammatory facial moisturizers, typically labeled as redness-reducing moisturizers, that are available for rosacea patients.

that attract water to the skin, not from the environment, unless the ambient humidity is 70%, but rather from the inner layers of the skin. Humectants draw water from the viable dermis into the viable epidermis and then from the nonviable epidermis into the stratum corneum. Lastly, hydrocolloids are physically large substances, which cover the skin thus retarding TEWL.

> Moisturizers to prevent facial rosacea flares combine with occlusive agents and humectant agents to prevent water loss and to attract water and facilitate barrier repair, respectively.

The best moisturizers to prevent facial rosacea flares combine occlusive and humectant ingredients. For example, a well-formulated moisturizer might contain petrolatum, mineral oil, and dimethicone as occlusive agents. Petrolatum is the synthetic substance mostly like intercellular lipids, but too high a concentration will yield a sticky greasy ointment. The aesthetics of petrolatum can be improved by adding dimethicone, which is also able to prevent water loss, but reduces the petrolatum concentration and yields a thinner more acceptable formulation. Mineral oil is not quite as greasy as petrolatum, but still an excellent barrier repair agent; it further improves the ability of the moisturizer to spread, yielding enhanced aesthetics. The addition of glycerin to the formulation attracts

water from the dermis speeding up hydration. It is through the careful combination of these ingredients that facial moisturizers can be constructed to prevent a rosacea flare.

FACIAL COSMECEUTICALS

Cosmeceuticals are over-the-counter moisturizers with a variety of active ingredients designed to enhance the appearance of the skin. Most of the cosmeceuticals designed for rosacea patients contain anti-inflammatory agents that are intended to reduce redness. The anti-inflammatory agents are botanical extracts that may complement prescription therapy in the maintenance phase of rosacea treatment. Commonly used botanical anti-inflammatory agents in the current marketplace include ginkgo biloba, green tea, aloe vera, allantoin, and licochalcone. Their rationale for use in redness-reducing cosmeceuticals is discussed.

> Cosmeceuticals for rosacea patients generally contain anti-inflammatory agents to reduce facial redness.

Ginkgo Biloba

Ginkgo biloba leaves contain unique polyphenols such as terpenoids (ginkgolides, bilobalides), flavonoids, and flavonoid glycosides with anti-inflammatory effects. These anti-inflammatory effects have been linked to antiradical and antilipoperoxidant effects in experimental fibroblast models. Ginkgo leaves are also purported to alter skin microcirculation by reducing blood flow at the capillary level and inducing a vasomotor change in the arterioles of the subpapillary skin plexus. Taken together, these changes may lead to decreased skin redness.

Green Tea

Green tea, also known as *Camellia sinensis*, is another anti-inflammatory botanical agent containing polyphenols, such as epicatechin, epicatechin-3-gallate, epigallocatechin, and epigallocatechin-3-gallate. The term "green tea" refers to the manufacture of the botanical extract from fresh leaves of the tea plant by steaming and drying at elevated temperatures avoiding oxidation and polymerization of the polyphenolic components. A study by Katiyar et al. demonstrated the anti-inflammatory effects of topical green tea application on C3H mice (14). A second study by the same authors found that topically applied green tea extract containing epigallocatechin-3-gallate reduced the UVB-induced inflammation as measured by double skin-fold swelling (15). Green tea extracts are the most commonly used botanical anti-inflammatory cosmeceutical at the time of this writing.

Aloe Vera

The second most commonly used anti-inflammatory botanical herb is aloe vera. The mucilage is released from the plant leaves as a colorless gel and contains 99.5% water and a complex mixture of mucopolysaccharides, amino acids, hydroxy quinone glycosides, and minerals. Compounds isolated from aloe vera juice include aloin, aloe emodin, aletinic acid, choline, and choline salicylate. The reported cutaneous effects of aloe vera relevant to rosacea include reduced inflammation, decreased skin bacterial colonization, and enhanced wound healing. The anti-inflammatory effects of aloe vera may result from its ability to inhibit cyclooxygenase as part of the arachidonic acid pathway through the choline salicylate component of the juice. However, the final concentration of aloe vera in any moisturizer must be at least 10% to achieve a cosmeceutical effect relevant for rosacea patients.

Allantoin

Allantoin is oldest anti-inflammatory ingredient added to many moisturizers labeled as appropriate for sensitive skin. It is found naturally in the comfrey root, but usually synthesized by the alkaline oxidation of uric acid in a cold environment. It is a white crystalline powder readily soluble in hot water, making it easy to formulate in cream and lotion moisturizers designed for sensitive skin. It is called a skin protectant and may be helpful in redness reduction.

Licochalcone A

Licochacone A is isolated by heating from the root of the Glycyrrhiza inflata licorice plant. It possesses anti-inflammatory properties as evidenced by its in vitro ability to inhibit the keratinocyte release of PGE_2 in response to UVB-induced erythema and the lipopolysaccharide-induced release of PGE_2 by adult dermal fibroblasts (16). Licochalcone A is the active agent in one of the largest product lines currently sold internationally for redness reduction (Eucerin, Beiersdorf).

FACIAL CAMOUFLAGE COSMETICS

Many times a complete redness reduction with pharmaceuticals and skin care products is impossible due to the presence of telangiectasias, which cannot be addressed with either treatment modality. This leaves colored cosmetics as a viable alternative for all female rosacea patients, and possibly some males. The cosmetics can camouflage the underlying redness by either blending colors or concealing the underlying skin to achieve a more desirable appearance.

> Green moisturizers are useful in rosacea patients, in minimizing facial redness under a facial foundation.

The art of blending colors to minimize facial redness utilizes a color complementary to red, which is green. Moisturizers with a slight green tint are applied after the prescription medication and well blended. Since the mixture of red and green produce brown, the sheer green tint will tone down bright red cheeks. Sometimes, over the green tint a tan facial foundation is applied that matches the desired skin color. The green tint allows a sheer facial foundation to better camouflage the red tones. If the red remains apparent, a more translucent or even opaque facial foundation can be used.

TROUBLESHOOTING FACIAL COSMETICS AND SKIN CARE IN ROSACEA PATIENTS

Occasionally, a rosacea patient will present who cannot use any topical medications and skin care or cosmetic products without an adverse effect. The dermatologist may at first think that the patient is histrionic, since these patients present with a basket full of problematic products and will have usually seen multiple dermatologists. In this case, it may be worthwhile to embark on a logical elimination scheme to determine

which products can and cannot be tolerated. This discussion introduces an algorithm for dealing with these difficult patients, based more on the art of medicine than the science that first discontinues all unnecessary products and then reintroduces them systematically. The algorithm is outlined below:

1. Discontinue all topical cosmetics, over-the-counter treatment products, cleansers, moisturizers, and fragrances. Use only a lipid-free cleanser and a bland moisturizing cream for two weeks.
2. Discontinue all topical prescription medications for two weeks. Especially, avoid medications containing retinoids, benzoyl peroxide, glycolic acid, and propylene glycol. Oral medications for rosacea may be continued.
3. Eliminate all sources of skin friction by selecting loose, soft clothing.
4. Discontinue any physical activities that involve skin friction, such as weight lifting, running, horseback riding, etc.
5. Evaluate the patient at two weeks to determine whether any improvement has occurred or whether any concommitant dermatoses are present. If an underlying dermatosis, such as seborrheic dermatitis, psoriasis, eczema, atopic dermatitis, or perioral dermatitis appear, treat as appropriate until two weeks after all visible signs of the newly diagnosed skin disease have disappeared.
6. Patch test the patient to elicit any allergens with the standard dermatologic patch test substances. Determine which of these allergens are clinically relevant and make avoidance recommendations.
7. Evaluate the patient's mental status especially, noting signs of depression, menopause, or psychiatric disease.
8. Allow the female patient to add one facial cosmetic in the following order: lipstick, face powder, blush.
9. Test all remaining cosmetics used by the patient by applying nightly to a 2-cm area lateral to the eye for at least five consecutive nights. Cosmetics should be tested in the following order: mascara, eye liner, eyebrow pencil, eye shadow, facial foundation, blush, facial powder, and any other colored facial cosmetics.
10. Lastly, test all topical rosacea medications by applying nightly to a 2-cm area lateral to the eye for five consecutive nights.
11. Analyze all data and present the patient with a list of medications, skin care products, and cosmetics that are appropriate for use.

This is indeed a time-consuming undertaking, but it is a thorough approach to determining the topical products that are appropriate for the challenging patient.

SUMMARY

Rosacea patients are a challenge to the dermatologist who aims to give practical advice on the selection of skin care and cosmetic products. This chapter has discussed the variety of cleansers, moisturizers, and cosmeceuticals in the current marketplace that may or may not be appropriate for rosacea patients. Key to success lies in customizing a skin treatment regimen for each patient. Identifying the skin needs and prescribing products that match those needs will not only treat rosacea but satisfy the patient. An approach for identifying products suitable for the problematic patient has also been presented. The ideas discussed in this chapter should provide ideas for supplementing traditional rosacea therapy with skin care and cosmetic products.

REFERENCES

1. Jackson EM. The science of cosmetics. Am J Contact Dermat 1993; 4: 108–10.
2. Draelos ZD. Sensitive skin: perceptions, evaluation, and treatment. Contact Derm 1997; 8: 67.
3. Facial Sting Task Group, ASTM Committee E-18.03.01.
4. Grove G, Soschin D, Kligman AM. Guidelines for performing facial stinging tests. In: Proc 12th Congress Internat Fed Soc of Cosmet Chem. Paris: September 13–17, 1982.
5. Laden K. Studies on irritancy and stinging potential. J Soc Cosmet Chem 1973; 24: 385–93.
6. Basketter DA, Griffiths HA. A study of the relationship between susceptibility to skin stinging and skin irritation. Contact Derma 1993; 29: 185–8.
7. Willcox MJ, Crichton WP. The soap market. Cosmet Toilet 1989; 104: 61–3.
8. Wortzman MS. Evaluation of mild skin cleansers. Dermatol Clin 1991; 9: 35–44.
9. Wortzman MS, Scott RA, Wong PS, et al. Soap and detergent bar rinsability. J Soc Cosmet Chem 1986; 37: 89–97.
10. deNavarre MG. Cleansing creams. In: deNaarre MG, ed. The Chemistry and Manufacture of Cosmetics. Vol. 3, 2nd edn. Wheaton, Illinois: Allured Publishing Corporation, 1975: 251–64.
11. Jass HE. Cold creams. In: deNaarre MG, ed. The Chemistry and Manufacture of Cosmetics. Vol. 3, 2nd edn. Wheaton, Illinois: Allured Publishing Corporation, 1975:237–49.
12. Mills OH, Kligman AM. Evaluation of abrasives in acne therapy. Cutis 1979; 23: 704–5.
13. Durr NP, Orentreich N. Epidermabrasion for acne. Cutis 1976; 17: 604–8.
14. Katiyar SK, Elmets CA. Green tea and skin. Arch Dermatol 2000; 136: 989.
15. Katiyar SK, Elmets CA, Agarwal R, et al. Protection against ultraviolet-B radiation-induced local and systemic suppression of contact hypersensitivity and edema responses in C3H/HeN mice by green tea polyphenols. Photochem Photobiol 1995; 62: 861.
16. Kolbe L, Immeyer J, Batzer J, et al. Anti-inflammatory efficacy of Licochalcone A: correlation of clinical potency and in vitro effects. Arch Derm Res 2006; 298: 23–30.

3　Facial moisturizers and eczema

Facial moisturizers are some of the most important over-the-counter skin care products. Dramatic changes are induced in the skin through the addition or removal of water. A well-hydrated facial skin is soft, smooth, and beautiful while a poorly hydrated facial skin is rough, harsh, and unattractive (Fig. 3.1). The main effect produced by most cosmeceuticalsthat are designed to minimize the appearance of wrinkles is excellent skin hydration. Conditions ranging from facial wrinkles of dehydration to facial eczema are treated by moisturization.

Various terms are used by the cosmetics industry to describe the effects of creams and lotions: lubricants, moisturizers, repair or replenishing products, emollients, etc. These terms do not have a scientific meaning since the mechanisms for rehydrating dry skin or rejuvenating damaged skin remain to be elucidated. In basic terms, lubricants refer to those products that increase skin slip in dry skin that is rough and flaky; moisturizers impart moisture to the skin by increasing the skin flexibility; and repair or replenishing products are intended to reverse the appearance of aging skin. All three classes of products are based on emollients. An understanding of the function of facial moisturizers and their formulation is essential to the dermatologist who must maintain the health of facial skin once the dermatitis has resolved (1).

PHYSIOLOGY OF XEROSIS
Xerosis is a result of decreased water content of the stratum corneum which leads to abnormal desquamation of corneocytes (Fig. 3.2). For the skin to appear and feel normal, the water content of this layer must be above 10% (2). Water is lost through evaporation to the environment under low humidity conditions and must be replenished by water from the lower epidermal and dermal layers (3). The stratum corneum must have the ability to maintain this moisture or the skin will feel rough, scaly, and dry. However, this is indeed a simplistic view as there are minimal differences between the amount of water present in the stratum corneum of dry and normal skin (4). Xerotic skin is due to more than simply low water content (5). Electron micrographic studies of dry skin demonstrate a stratum corneum that is thicker, fissured, and disorganized (Fig. 3.3).

> Water is lost through evaporation to the environment under low humidity conditions and must be replenished by water from the lower epidermal and dermal layers.

There are three intercellular lipids implicated in epidermal barrier function: sphingolipids, free sterols, and free fatty acids (6). In addition, it is thought that the lamellar bodies (Odland bodies, membrane-coating granules, and cementsomes), containing sphingolipids, free sterols, and phospholipids, play a key role in barrier function and are essential to trap water and prevent excessive water loss (7,8). The lipids are necessary for barrier function since solvent extraction of these chemicals leads to xerosis, directly proportional to the amount of lipid

removed (9). The major lipid by weight found in the stratum corneum is ceramide, which becomes sphingolipid if glycosylated via the primary alcohol of sphingosine (10). Ceramides have most of the long-chain fatty acids and linoleic acid in the skin. Perturbations within the barrier result in rapid lamellar body secretion and a cascade of cytokine changes associated with adhesion molecule expression and growth factor production (11). If skin with barrier perturbations is occluded with a vapor-impermeable wrap, the expected burst in lipid synthesis is blocked. However, occlusion with a vapor-permeable wrap does not prevent barrier recovery (12). Therefore, transepidermal water loss (TEWL) is necessary to initiate synthesis of lipids to allow barrier repair (13,14).

> The three intercellular lipids implicated in epidermal barrier function are sphingolipids, free sterols, and free fatty acids.

Remoisturization of the skin must then occur in four steps: initiation of barrier repair, alteration of surface cutaneous moisture partition coefficient, onset of dermal-epidermal moisture diffusion, and synthesis of intercellular lipids (15). It is generally thought in the cosmetics industry that a stratum corneum containing 20–35% water will exhibit the softness and pliability of normal stratum corneum (16).

Other disease states, such as facial atopic dermatitis, also demonstrate abnormal barrier function due to ceramide distribution (17,18). Interestingly enough, xerosis tends to increase with age due to a lower, inherent water content of the stratum corneum (19). But this does not totally account for the scaliness and roughness of the aged skin, probably an abnormal desquamatory process is also present (20).

There are other lipids present in the stratum corneum, besides those previously discussed, that are worth mentioning: cholesterol sulfate, free sterols, free fatty acids, triglycerides, sterol wax/esters, squalene, and n-alkanes (21). Cholesterol sulfate only comprises 2–3% of the total epidermal lipids, but is important in corneocyte desquamation (22). It appears that corneocyte desquamation is mediated through the desulfation of cholesterol sulfate (23). Fatty acids are also important since it has been demonstrated that barrier function can be restored by topical or systemic administration of linoleic acid-rich oils in essential fatty-acid-deficient rats (24).

> The primary two methods for remoisturization of the skin are occlusives and humectants.

MECHANISMS OF MOISTURIZATION
There are four mechanisms by which the stratum corneum can be rehydrated: occlusives, humectants, hydrophilic matrices, and sunscreens (25).

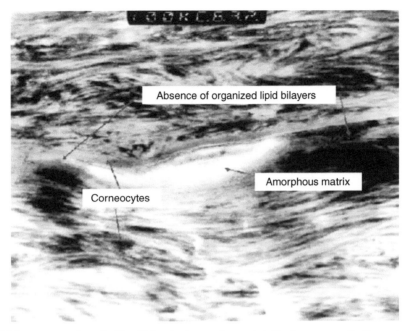

Figure 3.1 A SEM appearance of xerotic skin with barrier damage demonstrated by the presence of a disorganized lipid bilayer.

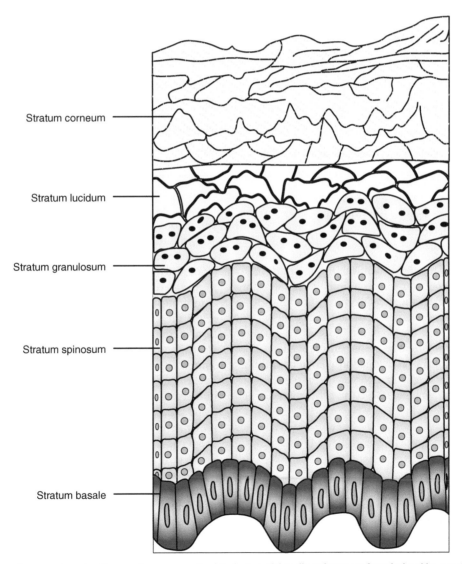

Figure 3.2 The process of corneocyte maturation requires a progressive dehydration of the cells as they move from the basal layer to the stratum corneum.

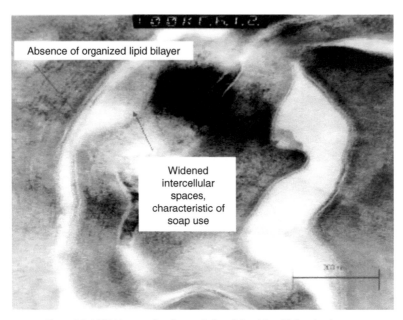

Figure 3.3 A SEM image of surfactant-induced dry skin with barrier damage.

Occlusives

There are 20 different generic classes of chemicals that can function as occlusives to retard TEWL . Each chemical imparts a different feel and thickness to the moisturizer. Listed below are some of the more widely used substances (26):

1. Hydrocarbon oils and waxes: petrolatum, mineral oil, paraffin, and squalene
2. Silicone oils
3. Vegetable and animal fats
4. Fatty acids: lanolin acid and stearic acid
5. Fatty alcohol: lanolin alcohol and cetyl alcohol
6. Polyhydric alcohols: propylene glycol
7. Wax esters: lanolin, beeswax, and stearyl stearate
8. Vegetable waxes: carnauba and candelilla
9. Phospholipids: lecithin
10. Sterols: cholesterol

The most occlusive of the above chemicals is petrolatum (27). It appears, however, that a total occlusion of the stratum corneum is undesirable. While the TEWL can be completely halted, once the occlusive is removed, water loss resumes at its preapplication level. Thus, the occlusive moisturizer has not allowed the stratum corneum to repair its barrier function (28). But, petrolatum does not appear to function as an impermeable barrier; rather it permeates throughout the interstices of the stratum corneum allowing the barrier function to be reestablished (29).

Petrolatum remains the most effective occlusive moisturizing agent.

While petrolatum is a very effective facial moisturizer, it is not commonly used, except in formulations for very dry skin. It is very greasy and does not allow makeup to perform well. It also does not allow sweat to evaporate from the skin surface creating the feeling of warmth. Finally, it stains clothing. Petrolatum is used in small amounts in facial moisturizers, but is usually mixed with dimethicone and cetyl alcohol to make a more cosmetically acceptable formulation. This need for cosmetic elegance has led to all the countless facial moisturizers on the market today.

Humectants

Another concept in rehydrating the facial stratum corneum is the use of humectants. Humectants have been used in cosmetics for many years to increase the shelf life by preventing product evaporation and subsequent thickening due to variations in temperature and humidity. For example, humectants are a necessary part of all oil-in-water creams to maintain their required water content. Substances that function as humectants are glycerin, honey, sodium lactate, urea, propylene glycol, sorbitol, pyrrolidone carboxylic acid, gelatin, hyaluronic acid, vitamins, and some proteins (26,30).

Cosmetic chemists have theorized that humectants could be used to draw water from the environment, under conditions where the ambient humidity exceeds 70%, and more commonly from the deeper epidermal and dermal tissues to rehydrate the stratum corneum. Water that is applied to the skin in the absence of a humectant is rapidly lost to the atmosphere (31). Humectants may also allow the skin to feel smoother by filling holes in the stratum corneum through swelling (32). However, under low humidity conditions, humectants such as glycerin will actually draw moisture from the skin and increase TEWL (33). Therefore, a good moisturizer should combine both occlusive and humectant properties.

Glycerin is mixed with occlusive petrolatum and dimethicone in many facial moisturizers to aid in drawing water to the skin surface that is held in place by the artificial barrier. Too much glycerin can make the facial moisturizer sticky by holding sweat to the skin surface. Other humectants, such as vitamins and proteins, are added to complement the effect of glycerin. While the patient may believe that the proteins or peptides are affecting skin collagen, they are in actuality preventing facial skin water loss by humectancy. This is the art of facial moisturizer formulation.

Hydrophilic Matrices

Hydrophilic matrices are large molecular weight substances that physically retard water loss from the face. Some of the more recent advances in facial moisturization have been in this category. Topical hyaluronic acid is a high-molecular-weight substance that is one of the newer hydrophilic matrices found in facial moisturizers. It sits on the skin surface not only blocking water loss physically but also functioning as a humectant to hold water. Many proteins also function as humectants and hydrophilic matrices simultaneously. One manufacturer produces a facial moisturizer based on colloidal oatmeal, familiar to dermatologists from the oatmeal bath, which also physically prevents water loss. Hydrophilic matrices are the least commonly used moisturizing mechanism in facial moisturizers.

> Hydrophilic moisturizers are large molecular weight substances that impede water loss.

Sunscreens

The most potent antiaging ingredient in any facial moisturizer is sunscreen. As a matter of fact, most of the claims that deal with aging are supported by the sunscreen primarily and the moisturizer secondarily. It is widely felt that protection against UVB and UVA radiation is beneficial in the prevention of skin aging, but this theory has never been tested, only observed. Sunscreens are listed as moisturizers because they prevent cellular damage and thus prevent dehydration. Sunscreens are considered moisturizing ingredients, but do not alter facial skin water loss in the profound manner of occlusive and humectant ingredients.

MECHANISMS OF EMOLLIENCE

Emollience is another important characteristic of moisturizers independent of their ability to increase skin hydration. Emollients function by filling the spaces between the desquamating corneocytes with oil droplets (34), but their effect is only temporary. They make the skin feel smooth and soft, which is the primary facial moisturizer attribute addressed by most patients (Fig. 3.4). Some moisturizing ingredients are emollients, but not all emollients are moisturizing ingredients.

> Emollients function by filling the spaces between the desquamating corneocytes making the skin feel smooth and soft.

Emollients can be divided into several categories: protective emollients, fattening emollients, dry emollients, and astringent emollients (35). Protective emollients are substances such as diisopropyl dilinoleate and isopropyl isostearate that remain on the skin longer than average time and allow the skin to feel smooth immediately upon application. Fattening emollients, such as castor oil, propylene glycol, jojoba oil, isostearyl isostearate, and octyl stearate, also leave

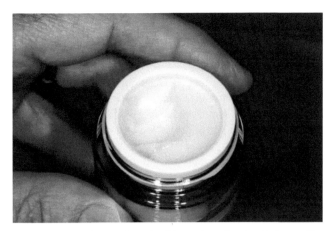

Figure 3.4 Most patients evaluate the efficacy of a moisturizer for its emollient properties, not for its barrier repair properties.

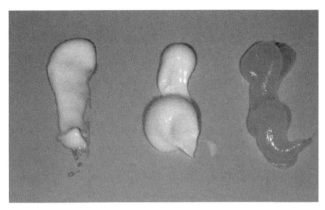

Figure 3.5 The ability of a moisturizer to create an environment for facial barrier repair cannot be assessed by visually inspecting the viscosity properties of the product.

a long lasting film on the skin, but may feel greasy. Dry emollients such as isopropyl palmitate, decyl oleate, and isostearyl alcohol do not offer much skin protection but produce a dry feel. Lastly, astringent emollients, such as dimethicones and cyclomethicones, isopropyl myristate and octyl octanoate, have minimal greasy residue and can reduce the oily feel of other emollients.

> Dimethicone can function as an emollient and as an occlusive moisturizer.

FACIAL MOISTURIZER FORMULATION

Most moisturizers consist of water, lipids, emulsifiers, preservatives, fragrance, color, and specialty additives. Interestingly enough, water accounts for 60–80% of any moisturizer; however, externally applied water does not remoisturize the face. In fact, the rate of water passage through the skin increases with increased hydration (36). The water functions as a diluent and evaporates leaving the active agents behind. Emulsifiers are generally soaps in concentrations of 0.5% or less and function to keep the water and lipids in one continuous phase. Parabens are the most commonly used preservatives in moisturizers, usually combined with one of the formaldehyde donor preservatives (15). The variety of specialty additives incorporated into moisturizers is endless, limited only by the imagination of the cosmetic chemist (Fig. 3.5).

Facial moisturizers consist of water, lipids, emulsifiers, preservatives, fragrance, color, and specialty additives.

A marketable moisturizer facial formulation must fulfill three criteria: it must increase the water content of the skin (moisturization), it must make the skin feel smooth and soft (emollience), and it must protect injured or exposed skin from harmful or annoying stimuli (skin protection).

Facial moisturizers and related products are the fastest growing cosmetic market (Fig. 3.6). There are two basic formulations: oil-in-water emulsions in which water is the dominant phase and water-in-oil emulsions in which oil is the dominant phase. Oil-in-water formulations are used for the thinner daytime facial moisturizers and water-in-oil formulations are used for night creams or facial replenishing creams. Oil-in-water emulsions can be identified by their cool feel and nonglossy appearance while water-in-oil emulsions can be identified by their warm feel and glossy appearance (37). Daytime moisturizers are generally composed of mineral oil, propylene glycol, and water in sufficient quantity to form a lotion (Fig. 3.7). Night creams are composed of mineral oil, lanolin alcohol, petrolatum, and water to form a cream (Fig. 3.8). Specialized eye creams are night creams with some of the more irritating ingredients removed to prevent eye stinging. The differences between products thus lie in the addition of fragrances, exotic oils, vitamins, protein or amino acid products, and other minor moisturizing aids.

The plethora of facial moisturizers has made categorization of the various products difficult; however, a brief look at the claims and composition of some key products is valuable. The cosmetic companies market facial moisturizers based on skin types. Naturally, products designed for oily complexions are oil-free or contain small amounts of light oils. Products for normal skin contain moderate amounts of light oils, and products for dry skin contain increased amounts of heavier oils. The lighter oil used is generally mineral oil and the heavier oil is petrolatum. Thus, moisturizing products can be developed for all skin types based on varying water-to-oil ratios.

Oily complexion moisturizers are oil-free and composed of water and silicone derivatives, such as cyclomethicone or dimethicone.

Oily complexion products that are oil-free are composed of water and silicone derivatives, such as cyclomethicone or dimethicone. This combination has been shown to be noncomedogenic in the rabbit ear assay. These products are nongreasy since the bulk of the product evaporates from the face. Many oily complexion moisturizers also claim to provide oil control, which is accomplished through the use of oil-absorbing substances such as talc, clay, starch, or synthetic polymers.

Products designed for normal or combination skin contain predominantly water, mineral oil, and propylene glycol with very small amounts of petrolatum. These products leave a greater oily residue on the face than oil-free formulations. Moisturizers in this line are also called antiwrinkle lotions, protective creams, or sport creams if they contain sunscreening agents.

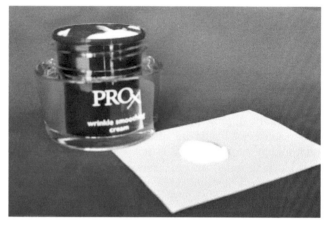

Figure 3.6 Facial moisturizers improve appearance by hydrating fine lines of dehydration, especially around the eyes.

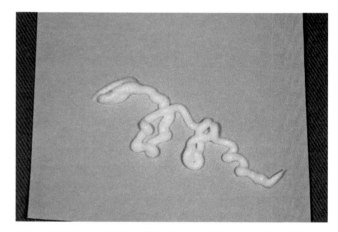

Figure 3.7 A demonstration of the viscosity of a day cream formulation.

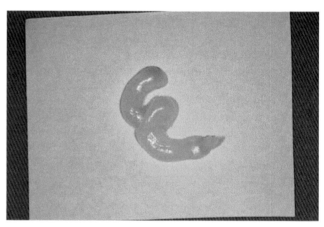

Figure 3.8 A demonstration of the viscosity of a night cream formulation.

Normal skin facial moisturizers are composed predominantly of water, mineral oil, and propylene glycol with very small amounts of petrolatum.

Dry skin moisturizers contain water, mineral oil, propylene glycol, and larger amounts of petrolatum or lanolin in addition to low concentrations of numerous additives claiming to rebuild, renew, or replenish. The patients should realize that there is no perfect skin moisturizer. Creams and lotions that

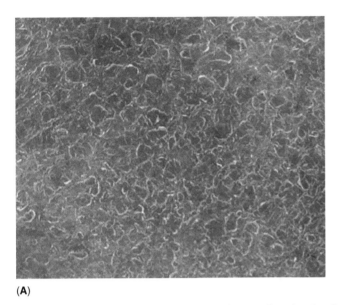 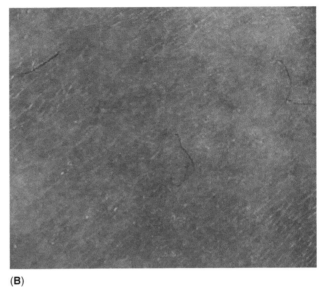

(A)   (B)

Figure 3.9 (**A**) The appearance of dry skin prior to application of a moisturizer. (**B**) The same dry skin in (**A**) immediately following moisturizer application which has smoothed the skin scale temporarily and improved the appearance.

claim to restore or rebuild tissue in the dermis do not penetrate deeply to have any effect. The extremely high cost of some moisturizers is not justified by the value of the ingredients. Patients are buying a certain feel, fragrance, or image. If the patient achieves more self-confidence or an increased sense of well being after using a certain facial cream, the money has been well spent. The role of the physician should be to identify which cosmetic claims are unfounded so that the patient has a medical perspective on the product he or she chooses to purchase.

Dry skin facial moisturizers contain water, mineral oil, propylene glycol, and larger amounts of petrolatum.

It is important that the patient select the appropriate facial moisturizer for his or her skin type. Most cosmetic companies clearly label which moisturizers are for oily, normal, and dry skin. Even though patients with oily skin may be hesitant to use a moisturizer, a product that contains oil-absorbing talc or kaolin can decrease the facial shine. Patients with the oily skin often use a soap containing benzoyl peroxide to remove unwanted oil and aid in acne treatment. These soaps can leave the face scaly with the subsequent washing immediately interfering with the foundation application. An oil-free moisturizer can help flatten the scale enabling smooth foundation application rather than preferentially adhering to skin scale. Patients selecting an oil-free foundation must use an oil-free moisturizer to ensure maximum foundation wear and minimal color drift.

Patients with dry skin will benefit from the selection of an appropriate moisturizer. Fine wrinkling due to cutaneous dehydration and roughness due to skin scale can be improved (Fig. 3.9).

FACIAL MOISTURIZER EFFICACY EVALUATION
The efficacy of facial moisturizers can be difficult to assess; however, several excellent noninvasive methods have been developed: regression analysis, profilometry, squametry, in vivo image analysis, corneometry, and evaporimetry (38).

These methods are used to evaluate the benefits of a given moisturizer formulation without injury to the skin.

Regression analysis is a method of evaluating moisturizer efficacy under clinical conditions. Here patients are selected and treated by an objective observer with moisturizers at a predetermined test site for two weeks. The test site is evaluated on days 7 and 14. If an improvement is noted, the moisturizer application is discontinued and the test site is evaluated daily for two weeks, or until the baseline skin dryness has reappeared (39). This method is particularly valuable since the efficacy of all facial moisturizers is excellent immediately following application, but the true effectiveness can only be assessed with the passage of time (40).

Regression analysis evaluates the longevity of the effect of a moisturizer on the skin.

Profilometry involves the analysis of silicone rubber (Silflo) replicas of the skin surface. These silicone replicas are then cast into plastic positives, which are then measured with a computerized stylus instrument that provides a contour tracing of the surface. Thus, a two- or three-dimensional topogram is created. Unfortunately, this method can be inaccurate since the silicone application to the skin surface tends to flatten and disturb the desquamating skin scale (41). The use of actual silicone replicas is now sometimes replaced with the video imaging of the skin surface, but the replicas remain the more accurate standard.

Video imaging and silicone replicas examine the skin surface topography.

Squametry involves the analysis of skin squames harvested by pressing a sticky tape against the skin. The outermost, loosely adherent skin scale is then removed. The tape provides a specimen that retains the topographical relationships of the skin surface and the pattern of desquamation. Image processing is then used to evaluate the scaliness of the skin (42).

This technique is very useful when evaluating the effect of facial moisturizers on patients with desquamatory defects. Squametry can also be used to harvest corneocytes in a painless manner for extraction of ceramides and lipids to determine the effect of facial moisturizers on intercellular lipid composition. Further, the squames can be dissolved with a solvent to examine the penetration of externally applied moisturizers into the skin. Multiple squames removed successively provide a penetration map for the moisturizer.

> Squametry can be used to track the penetration of a moisturizing ingredient into the stratum corneum.

In vivo image analysis uses a video microscope to magnify the skin surface and examine the condition of the facial corneocytes in real time (43). Care is necessary to standardize lighting and camera angles to insure accurate data for analysis. In vivo imaging can also measure pigmentation and erythema to examine the effect of skin lightening preparations or the erythema of rosacea.

Finally, two techniques are available to measure the amount of water present in the skin or that coming out of the skin. The amount of water in the skin can be assessed by evaluating the conductance of the skin with a technique known as corneometry. Corneometry puts a low voltage current into the skin with an electrode consisting of pins. One set of pins delivers the current while the second set of pins senses the current. The more water there is in the skin, the more hydration that is present. Thus, increased corneometry readings indicate an increased skin hydration (44,45). Evaporimetry measures the amount of water coming out of the skin known as TEWL (46). This is accomplished by using two humidity meters spaced at known distance from the skin and evaluating the passage of water vapor per time past the probe. More occlusive substances would be expected to lower water loss while humectants, such as glycerin, actually increase water loss (47,48). Lower evaporimetry measurements mean that the skin barrier is better, while higher evaporimetry measurements mean that the skin barrier is damaged.) A quality moisturizer would be expected to lower TEWL and decrease the evaporimetry reading.

> Corneometry evaluates the amount of water in the skin while evaporimetry evaluates the amount of water leaving the skin.

Even though these sophisticated noninvasive methods of cutaneous evaluation sound appealing, there is no substitute for the opinion of a trained unbiased observer when evaluating moisturizer effectiveness. Mechanistic evaluation can be easily biased to produce data that serves the best interest of the manufacturer. Computers cannot yet accurately synthesize all the tactile and visual information that can be obtained with human evaluation. The noninvasive techniques simply present another tool for assessing facial moisturizer function (49).

FACIAL MOISTURIZER: ADVERSE REACTIONS

Many patients with dry skin will claim that they are "allergic" to most moisturizers as a result of skin stinging experienced following application. This may represent an irritant contact dermatitis rather than a true allergic contact dermatitis (50). These patients should avoid moisturizers containing propylene glycol, which may cause burning upon application to damaged skin. Other substances found in facial moisturizers that cause stinging include benzoic acid, cinnamic acid compounds, lactic acid, urea, emulsifiers, formaldehyde, and sorbic acid.

Moisturizing ointments, creams, lotions, and gels should be patch tested "as is." If an irritant reaction is experienced with closed patch testing, the product should be retested with open patch testing and provocative use testing (51).

SUMMARY

Facial moisturizers are one of the most important categories of skin care products. They can reduce wrinkles and minimize dry skin. Their composition is simple, but their effects are profound. Using occlusive and humectant ingredients, they can improve the look and feel of the skin within minutes. Moisturizers also form the basis for all prescription topical formulations and can supplement or hinder the functioning of drugs.

REFERENCES

1. Goldner R. Moisturizers: a dermatologist's perspective. J Toxicol Cut Ocular Toxicol 1992; 11: 193–7.
2. Boisits EK. The evaluation of moisturizing products. Cosmet Toilet 1986; 101: 31–9.
3. Wu MS, Yee DJ, Sullivan ME. Effect of a skin moisturizer on the water distribution in human stratum corneum. J Invest Dermatol 1983; 81: 446–8.
4. Wildnauer RH, Bothwell JW, Douglass AB. Stratum corneum biomechanical properties. J Invest Dermatol 1971; 56: 72–8.
5. Pierard GE. What does "dry skin" mean? Int J Dermatol 1987; 26: 167–8.
6. Elias PM. Lipids and the epidermal permeability barrier. Arch Dermatol Res 1981; 270: 95–117.
7. Holleran WM, Man MQ, Wen NG, et al. Sphingolipids are required for mammalian epidermal barrier function. J Clin Invest 1991; 88: 1338–45.
8. Downing DT. Lipids: their role in epidermal structure and function. Cosmet Toilet 1991; 106: 63–9.
9. Grubauer G, Elias PM, Feingold KR. Transepidermal water loss: the signal for recovery of barrier structure and function. J Lipid Res 1989; 30: 323–33.
10. Petersen RD. Ceramides key components for skin protection. Cosmet Toilet 1992; 107: 45–9.
11. Nickoloff BJ, Naidu Y. Perturbation of epidermal barrier function correlates with initiation of cytokine cascade in human skin. J Am Acad Dermatol 1994; 30: 535–46.
12. Elias PM. Epidermal lipids, barrier function, and desquamation. J Invest Dermatol 1983; 80: 44s–9s.
13. Jass HE, Elias PM. The living stratum corneum: implications for cosmetic formulation. Cosmet Toilet 1991; 106: 47–53.
14. Holleran W, Feingold K, Man MQ, et al. Regulation of epidermal sphingolipid synthesis by permeability barrier function. J Lipid Res 1991; 32: 1151–8.
15. Jackson EM. Moisturizers: What's in them? How do they work? Am J Contact Dermatitis 1992; 3: 162–8.
16. Reiger MM. Skin, water and moisturization. Cosmet Toilet 1989; 104: 41–51.
17. Motta S, Monti M, Sesana S, et al. Abnormality of water barrier function in psoriasis. Arch Dermatol 1994; 130: 452–6.
18. Imokawa G, Abe A, Jin K, et al. Decreased level of ceramides in stratum corneum of atopic dermatitis: an etiologic factor in atopic dry skin? J Invest Dermatol 1991; 96: 523–6.
19. Potts RO, Buras EM, Chrisman DA. Changes with age in the moisture content of human skin. J Invest Dermatol 1984; 82: 97–100
20. Wepierre J, Marty JP. Percutaneous absorption and lipids in elderly skin. J Appl Cosmetol 1988; 6: 79–92.

21. Brod J. Characterization and physiological role of epidermal lipids. Int J Dermatol 1991; 30: 84–90.

22. Lampe MA, Williams ML, Elias PM. Human epidermal lipids: characterization and modulation during differentiation. J Lipid Res 1983; 24: 131–40.

23. Long SA, Wertz PW, Strauss JS, et al. Human stratum corneum polar lipids and desquamation. Arch Dermatol Res 1985; 277: 284–7.

24. Elias PM, Brown BE, Ziboh VA. The permeability barrier in essential fatty acid deficiency: Evidence for a direct role for linoleic acid in barrier function. J Invest Dermatol 1980; 75: 230–3.

25. Baker CG. Moisturization: new methods to support time proven ingredients. Cosmet Toilet 1987; 102: 99–102.

26. De Groot AC, Weyland JW, Nater JP. Unwanted Effects of Cosmetics and Drugs Used in Dermatology, 3rd edn. Amsterdam: Elsevier, 1994: 498–500.

27. Friberg SE, Ma Z. Stratum corneum lipids, petrolatum and white oils. Cosmet Toilet 1993; 107: 55–9.

28. Grubauer G, Feingold KR, Elias PM. Relationship of epidermal lipogenesis to cutaneous barrier function. J Lipid Res 1987; 28: 746–52.

29. Ghadially R, Halkier-Sorensen L, Elias PM. Effects of petrolatum on stratum corneum structure and function. J Am Acad Dermatol 1992; 26: 387–96.

30. Spencer TS. Dry skin and skin moisturizers. Clin Dermatol 1988; 6: 24–8.

31. Rieger MM, Deem DE. Skin moisturizers II The effects of cosmetic ingredients on human stratum corneum. J Soc Cosmet Chem 1974; 25: 253–62.

32. Robbins CR, Fernee KM. Some observations on the swelling of human epidermal membrane. JSCC 1983; 37: 21–34.

33. Idson B. Dry skin: moisturizing and emolliency. Cosmet Toilet 1992; 107 69–78.

34. Wehr RF, Krochmal L. Considerations in selecting a moisturizer. Cutis 1987; 39: 512–15.

35. Brand HM, Brand-Garnys EE. Practical application of quantitative emolliency. Cosmet Toilet 1992; 107: 93–9.

36. Warner RR, Myers MC, Taylor DA. Electron probe analysis of human skin: Determination of the water concentration profile. J Invest Dermatol 1988; 90: 218–24.

37. Idson B. Moisturizers, emollients, and bath oils. In: Frost P, Horwitz SN, eds. Principles of Cosmetics for the Dermatologist. St. Louis: CV Mosby Company, 1982: 37–44.

38. Grove GL. Noninvasive methods for assessing moisturizers. In: Waggoner WC, ed. Clinical Safety and Efficacy Testing of Cosmetics. New York: Marcel Dekker, Inc, 1990: 121–48.

39. Kligman AM. Regression method for assessing the efficacy of moisturizers. Cosmet Toilet 1978; 93: 27–35.

40. Lazar AP, Lazar P. Dry skin, water, and lubrication. Dermatol Clin 1991; 9: 45–51.

41. Grove GL, Grove MJ. Objective methods for assessing skin surface topography noninvasively. In: Leveque JL, ed. Cutaneous Investigation in Health and Disease. New York: Marcel Dekker, 1988: 1–32.

42. Grove GL. Dermatological applications of the Magiscan image analysing computer. In: Marks R, Payne PA, eds. Bioengineering and the Skin. Lancaster, England: MTP Press, 1981: 173–82.

43. Prall JK, Theiler RF, Bowser PA, Walsh M. The effect of cosmetic products in alleviating a range of skin dryness conditions as determined by clinical and instrumental techniques. Int J Cosmet Sci 1986; 8: 159–74.

44. Tagami H. Electrical measurement of the water content of the skin surface. Cosmet Toilet 1982; 97: 39–47.

45. Grove GL. The effect of moisturizers on skin surface hydration as measured in vivo by electrical conductivity. Curr Ther Res 1991; 50: 712–19.

46. Idson B. In vivo measurement of transdermal water loss. J Soc Cosmet Chem 1976; 29: 573–80.

47. Rietschel RL. A method to evaluate skin moisturizers in vivo. J Invest Dermatol 1978; 70: 152–5.

48. Rietschel RL. A skin moisturization assay. J Soc Cosmet Chem 1979; 30: 360–73.

49. Grove GL. Design of studies to measure skin care product performance. Bioeng Skin 1987; 3: 359–73.

50. Lazar PM. The toxicology of moisturizers. J Toxicol Cut Ocular Toxicol 1992; 11: 185–91.

51. Maibach HI, Engasser PG. Dermatitis due to cosmetics. In: Fisher AA, ed. Contact Dermatitis. 3rd edn. Phildelphia: Lea & Febiger, 1986: 371.

SUGGESTED READING

Altemus M, Rao B, Dhabhar F, Ding W, Granstein R. Stress-induced Changes in Skin Barrier Function in Healthy Women. J Invest Dermatol 2001; 117: 309–17.

Ananthapadmanabhan KP, Subramanyan K, Rattinger GB. Moisturizing cleansers (Chapter 20). In: Leyden JJ, Rawlings AV, eds. Skin Moisturization. Vol. 25. Marcel Dekker, Inc., 2002: 405–32.

Arct J, Gronwald M, Kasiura K. Possibilities for the Prediction of an Active Substance Penetration through Epidermis. IFSCC Magazine 2001; 4: 179–83.

Atrux-Tallau N, Romagny C, Padois K, et al. Effects of Glycerol on Human Skin Damaged by Acute Sodium Lauryl Sulphate Treatment. Arch Dermatol Res 2009; [Epub ahead of print].

Barton S. Formulation of Skin Moisturizers (Chapter 25). In: Leyden JJ, Rawlings AV, eds. Skin Moisturization. Vol. 25. Marcel Dekker, Inc., 2002: 547–75.

Bikowski J. The use of therapeutic moisturizers in various dermatologic disorders. Cutis 2001; 68 (5 Suppl): 3–11.

Bissonnette R, Maari C, Provost N, et al. A Double-Blind Study of Tolerance and Efficacy of a New Urea-Containing Moisturizer in Patients with Atopic Dermatitis. J Cosmet Dermatol 2010; 9: 16–21.

Buraczewska I, Berne B, Lindberg M, Torma H, Loden M. Changes in skin barrier function following long-term treatment with moisturizers, a randomized controlled trial. Br J Dermatol 2007; 156: 492–8.

Chamlin SL, Kao J, Frieden IJ, et al. Ceramide-dominant Barrier Repair Lipids Alleviate Childhood Atopic Dermatitis: Change in Barrier Function Provide a Sensitive Indicator of Disease Activity. J Am Acad Dermatol 2002; 47: 198–208.

Coderch L, Lopez O, de la Maza A, Parra JL. Ceramides and Skin Function. Am J Clin Dermatol 2003; 4: 107–29.

Crowther JM, Sieg A, Clenkiron P, et al. Measuring the effects of topical moisturizers on changes in stratum corneaim thickness, water gradients and hydration in vivo. Br J Dermatol 2008; 159: 567–77.

Denda M, Kumazawa N. Negative electric potential induces alteration of ion gradient and lamellar body secretion in the epidermis, and accelerates skin barrier recovery after barrier disruption. J Invest Dermatol 2002; 118: 65–72.

Draelos ZD. Concepts in skin care maintenance. Cutis 2005; 76 (6 Suppl): 19–25.

Draelos ZD. The ability of onion extract gel to improve the cosmetic appearance of postsurgical scars. J Cosmet Dermatol 2008; 7: 101–4.

Draelos ZD. Therapeutic moisturizers. Dermatol Clin 2000; 18: 597–607.

Draelos ZD, Ertel K, Berge C. Niacinamide-containing facial moisturizer improves skin barrier and benefits subjects with rosacea. Cutis 2005; 76: 135–41.

Endo K, Suzuki N, Yoshida O, et al. Two factors governing transepidermal water loss: barrier and driving force components. IFSCC Magazine 2003; 6: 9–13.

Fluhr JW, Bornkessel A, Berardesca E. Glycerol—Just a Moisturizer? (Chapter 20). In: Loden M, Maibach HI, eds. Biological and Biophysical Effects. Dry Skin and Moisturizers, 2nd edn. Taylor & Francis Group, LLC, 2006: 227–43.

Fluhr J, Holleran WM, Berardesca E. Clinical effects of emollients on skin (Chapter 12). In: Leyden JJ, Rawlings AV, eds. Skin Moisturization. Vol. 25. Marcel Dekker, Inc., 2002: 223–43.

Ghali FE. Improved clinical outcomes with moisturization in dermatologic disease. Cutis 2005; 76 (6 Suppl): 13–18.

Giusti F, Martella A, Bertoni L, Seidernari S. Skin Barrier, Hydration, and pH of the Skin of Infants Under 2 years of Age. Pediatr Dermatol 2001; 18: 93–6.

Hannuksela A, Kinnunen T. Moisturizers prevent irritant dermatitis. Acta Derm Venereol 1992; 72: 42–4.

Hannuksela M. Moisturizers in the prevention of contact dermatitis. Curr Probl Dermatol 1996; 25: 214–20.

Harding CR. The stratum corneum: structure and function in health and disease. Derm Ther 2004; 17: 6–15.

Harding CR, Rawlings AV. Effects of natural moisturizing factor and lactic acid isomers on skin function (Chapter 18). In: Loden M, Maibach HI, eds. Dry Skin and Moisturizers. 2nd edn. Taylor & Francis Group, LLC, 2006: 187–209.

Hawkins SS, Subramanyan K, Liu D, Bryk M. Cleansing. Moisturizing, and sun-protection regimens for normal skin, self-perceived sensitive skin, and dermatologist-assessed sensitive skin. Derm Ther 2004; 17: 63–8.

Held E, Lund H, Agner T. Effect of different moisturizers of SLS-irritated human skin. Contact Dermatitis 2001; 44: 229–34.

Held E, Sveinsdottir S, Agner T. Effect of long-term use of moisturizer on skin hydration, barrier function and susceptibility to irritants. Acta Derm Venereol 1999; 79: 49–51.

Held E, Agner T. Effect of moisturizers on skin susceptibility to irritants. Acta Derm Venereol 2010; 81: 104–7.

Herman S. Lipid Assets. GCI. 2001 Dec: 12–14.

Herman S. The new polymer frontier. GCI. January 2002.

Jemec GB, Wulf HC. Correlation between the greasiness and the plasticizing effect of moisturizers. Acta Derm Venereol 1999; 79: 115–17.

Johnson AW. Overview: fundamental skin care—protecting the barrier. Derm Ther 2004; 17: 1–5.

Kao JS, Garg A, mao-Qiang M, et al. Testosterone perturbs epidermal permeability barrier homeostasis. J Invest Dermatol 2001; 116: 443–50.

Kraft JN, Lynde CW. Moisturizers: what they are and a practical approach to product selection. Skin Ther Lett 2005; 10: 1–8.

Lachapelle JM. Efficacy of protective creams and/or gels. Curr Probl Dermatol 1996; 25: 182–92.

Lebwohl M, Herrmann LG. Impaired skin barrier function in dermatologic disease and repair with moisturization. Cutis 2005; 76 (6 Suppl): 7–12.

Le Fur I, Reinberg A, Lopez S, et al. Analysis of Circadian and Ultradian Rhythms of Skin Surface Properties of Face and Forearm of Healthy Women. J Invest Dermatol 2001; 117: 718–24.

Leyden JJ, Rawlings AV. Humectants (Chapter 13). In: Leyden JJ, Rawlings AV, eds. Skin Moisturization. Vol. 25. Marcel Dekker, Inc., 2002: 245–66.

Lipozencic J, Pastar Z, Marinovic-Kulisic S. Moisturizers. Acta Dermatovenerol Croat 2006; 14: 104–8.

Loden M. Barrier recovery and influence of irritant stimuli in skin treated with a moisturizing cream. Contact Dermatitis 1997; 36: 256–60.

Loden M. Do moisturizers work? J Cosmet Dermatol 2003; 2: 141–9.

Loden M. Hydrating Substances (Chapter 20). In: Paye M, Barel AO, Maibach HI, eds. Handbook of Cosmetic Science and Technology. 2nd edn. Informa Healthcare USA, Inc., 2007: 265–80.

Loden M. Role of topical emollients and moisturizers in the treatment of dry skin barrier disorders. Am J Clin Dermatol 2003; 4: 771–88.

Loden M. Skin Barrier Function: Effects of Moisturzers. C & T.

Loden M. The clinical benefit of moisturizers. J Eur Acad Dermatol Venereol 2005; 19: 672–88; quiz 686–7.

Loden M. Urea-containing moisturizers influence barrier properties of normal skin. Arch Dermatol Res 1996; 288: 103–7.

Loden M, Andersson AC, Lindberg M. Improvement in skin barrier function in patients with atopic dermatitis after treatment with a moisturizing cream (Canoderm). Br J Dermatol 1999; 140: 264–7.

Lynde CW, Moisturizers: What They are and How They Work. Skin Terapy Lett 2001; 6: 3–5.

Madison KC. Barrier Function of the Skin: "La Raison d'Etre" of the Epidermis. J Invest Dermatol 2003; 121: 231–41.

Maes DH, Marenus KD. Main finished products: moisturizing and cleansing creams (Chapter 10). In: Baran R, Maibach HI, eds. Textbook of Cosmetic Dermatology. 2nd edn. Martin Dunitz Ltd, 1998: 113–24.

Mandawgade SD, Patravale VB. Formulation and evaluation of exotic fat based cosmeceuticals for skin repair. Indian J Pharm Sci 2008; 70: 539–42.

Norlen L. Skin barrier formation: the membrane folding model. J Invest Dermatol 2001; 117: 823–36.

Prasch TH, Schlotmann K, Schmidt-fonk K, Forster Th. The influence of cosmetic products on the stratum corneum by infrared and spectroscopy. IFSCC Magazine 2001; 4: 201–3.

Rawlings AV, Canestrari DA, Dobkowski B. Moisturizer technology versus clinical performance. Dermatol Ther 2004; 17 (Suppl 1): 49–56.

Rawlings AV, Harding CR. Moisturization and skin barrier function. Dermatol Ther 2004; 17: 43–8.

Rieger M. Moisturizers and humectants. In: Rieger MM, ed. Harry's Cosmeticology. 8th edn. Chemical Publishing Co., Inc., 2000.

Simion FA, Abrutyn ES, Draelos ZD. Ability of moisturizers to reduce dry skin and irritation and to prevent their return. J Cosmet Sci 2005; 56: 427–44.

Simion FA, Starch MS, Witt PS, Woodford JK, Edgett KJ. Hand and body lotions (Chapter 24). In: Baran R, Maibach HI, eds. Textbook of Cosmetic Dermatology. 2nd edn. Martin Dunitz Ltd, 1998: 285–308.

4 Sensitive skin and contact dermatitis

Treating sensitive skin can indeed present a challenge to the dermatologist, since formulations that are typically not problematic for the general population cause intense stinging, burning, and redness in individuals with sensitive skin. Patients with sensitive skin can present with either skin that appears normal to the eye or overt skin disease. Those with overt skin disease are sometimes easier to evaluate, since visual inspection can provide an idea of how to approach the problem. Invisible sensitive skin is a tremendous challenge as there is nothing to evaluate, except for the patient's history. This is most disconcerting to the dermatologist who only relies on history when all else has failed and the diagnosis is still not forthcoming. This is the perplexing part of treating sensitive skin and this chapter will discuss methods of treating both invisible and visible sensitive facial skin (1). It will then segue into contact dermatitis and its relationship with cosmetics and skin care products.

> Visible sensitive skin is characterized by eczema, atopic dermatitis, and rosacea.

VISIBLE SENSITIVE FACIAL SKIN

Visible sensitive facial skin is the easiest condition to diagnose, since the outward manifestations of erythema, desquamation, lichenification, and inflammation identify the presence of a severe barrier defect (Fig. 4.1). Any patient with a barrier defect will possess the signs and symptoms of sensitive skin until complete healing occurs. The three most common causes of barrier defect-induced facial sensitive skin are eczema, atopic dermatitis, and rosacea. These three diseases nicely illustrate the three components of sensitive skin, which include barrier disruption, immune hyper-reactivity, and heightened neurosensory response.

> The three components of visible sensitive skin are barrier disruption, immune hyper-reactivity, and heightened neurosensory response.

Eczema

Eczema is characterized by barrier disruption, which is the most common cause of facial sensitive skin. The barrier can be disrupted chemically through the use of cleansers and cosmetics that remove intercellular lipids, or physically through the use of abrasive substances that induce stratum corneum exfoliation. In some cases, the barrier may be defective either due to insufficient sebum production, inadequate intercellular lipids, abnormal keratinocyte organization, etc. The end result is the induction of the inflammatory cascade accompanied by erythema, desquamation, itching, stinging, burning, and possibly pain. The immediate goal of treatment is to stop the inflammation through the use of topical, oral, or injectable corticosteroids, depending on the severity of the eczema.

Newer topical options for the treatment of eczema-induced sensitive facial skin include the calcineurin inhibitors, pimecrolimus, and tacrolimus.

However, the resolution of the inflammation is not sufficient for the treatment of eczema. Proper skin care must also be instituted to minimize the return of the conditions that led to the onset of eczema. This includes the selection of skin care maintenance products, such as cleansers and moisturizers. Thus, the care of sensitive skin involves not only the treatment of the acute skin disease but also the prevention of recurrence through proper skin care maintenance.

Atopic Dermatitis

Sensitive facial skin due to eczema is predicated only on physical barrier disruption, while the sensitive facial skin associated with atopic dermatitis is predicated both on a barrier defect and an immune hyper-reactivity, as manifested by the association of asthma and hay fever. Patients with atopic dermatitis not only have sensitive skin on the exterior of the body but also sensitive mucosa lining the eyes, nose, and lungs. Thus, the treatment of sensitive facial skin in the atopic population involves topical and systemic considerations. There is also a prominent link between the worsening of hay fever and the onset of skin symptoms, requiring broader treatment considerations.

All of the treatments previously described for eczema also apply to atopic dermatitis, but additional therapy is required to minimize the immune hyper-reactivity. While this may take the form of oral or injectable corticosteroids, antihistamines (hydroxyzine, cetirizine hydrochloride, diphenhydramine, and fexofenadine hydrochloride, etc.) are typically added to decrease cutaneous and ocular itching. Antihistamines also improve the symptoms of hay fever and may prevent a flare should the patient be exposed to pollens or other inhaled allergens. The avoidance of sensitive skin in the atopic patient is largely predicated on avoidance of inciting substances. This means creating an allergy-free environment by removing old carpet, nonwashable drapes, items likely to collect dust, feather pillows and bedding, stuffed animal toys, heavy pollinating trees and plants, live pets, etc. The prevention of the release of histamine is the key to controlling the sensitive facial skin of atopic dermatitis.

Rosacea

Rosacea is an example of the third component of sensitive facial skin, which is a heightened neurosensory response. This means that patients with rosacea experience stinging and burning more frequently than the general population do to minor irritants. Whether this sensitive facial skin is due to nerve alterations from chronic photodamage, vasomotor instability, altered systemic effects to ingested histamine, or central facial lymphedema is unclear.

The treatments for rosacea-induced sensitive facial skin are much different than those for eczema or atopic dermatitis (2).

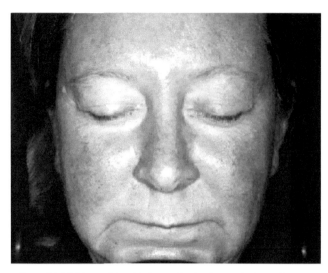

Figure 4.1 Visible sensitive skin is easy for the dermatologist to diagnose.

Anti-inflammatories in the form of oral and topical antibiotics form the therapeutic armamentarium. Antibiotics of the tetracycline family are used most commonly orally, while azelaic acid, metronidazole, sulfur, and sodium sulfacetamide are the most popular topical agents. However, the effect of the anti-inflammatory antibiotic can be enhanced through the use of complementary skin care products that enhance barrier function.

> Invisible sensitive skin is characterized by itching, stinging, burning, and possibly pain.

INVISIBLE SENSITIVE SKIN

Eczema, atopic dermatitis, and rosacea are in some ways the easiest forms of sensitive skin to treat. The skin disease is easily seen and the treatment success can be monitored visibly. If the skin looks more normal, generally the symptoms of itching, stinging, burning, and pain will also be improved. Unfortunately, there are some patients who present with sensitive facial skin and no clinical findings. These patients typically present with a bag full of skin care products they claim cannot be used because they cause facial acne, rashes, and/or discomfort. This situation presents a challenge for the physician, since it is unclear how to proceed.

Several treatment ideas are worth considering. The patient may have subclinical barrier disruption. For this reason, treatment with an appropriate-strength, topical corticosteroid for two weeks may be advisable. If symptoms improve, then the answer is clear. The patient may have subclinical eczematous disease. If the symptoms do not improve, it is then worthwhile to examine the next most common cause of invisible sensitive skin, which is contact dermatitis.

SENSITIVE FACIAL SKIN PRODUCT GUIDELINES

In many cases, it is impossible to determine the exact cause of the sensitive skin. No obvious skin disease is present, yet the patient experiences intense stinging and burning sensation whenever skin care products or cosmetics are applied to the skin. Frequently, patch testing reveals no obvious source of irritant or allergic contact dermatitis. This then leaves the physician to use empiric methods to make product recommendations to

Table 4.1 Considerations for the Minimization of Contact Dermatitis from Skin Care Products and Cosmetics

1. Eliminate common allergens and irritants, or reduce their concentration.
2. Select products from a reputable manufacturer that uses high-quality, pure ingredients free of contaminants.
3. Products should be well preserved to prevent the formation of auto-oxidation byproducts.
4. Paraben preservatives have proven to be the least problematic.
5. Avoid solvents, volatile vehicles, vasodilatory substances, and sensory stimulators in all products.
6. Minimize the use of surfactants and select minimally irritating emulsifier systems.

the patient. Products must be carefully selected based on the use of ingredients that are least likely to damage the skin barrier, elicit a noxious sensory response, or alter the skin structure (Table 4.1). Products with botanical anti-inflammatories may be helpful, but most patients want specific suggestions on how to select skin care products and cosmetics. This section discusses the approach I use in my practice for product selection for the sensitive skin patient who has not responded to any of the previously outlined treatment modalities.

> Products for sensitive skin must be carefully selected based on the use of ingredients that are least likely to damage the skin barrier, elicit a noxious sensory response, or alter the skin structure.

Even patients with sensitive skin require basic hygiene. The face and body must be cleansed. There is no doubt that the synthetic detergent cleansers, also known as syndets, provide the best skin cleansing while minimizing barrier damage. Bars based on sodium cocoyl isethionate appear to perform the best (Fig. 4.2). There are some patients, however, who only require the use of a facial syndet cleanser occasionally since the sebum production and physical activity are minimal. For these patients, a lipid-free cleanser is preferable because it can be used without water and wiped away. These products may contain water, glycerin, cetyl alcohol, stearyl alcohol, sodium laurel sulfate, and occasionally propylene glycol. They leave behind a thin moisturizing film and can be used effectively in persons with excessively dry, sensitive, or dermatitic skin. They do not have strong antibacterial properties, however, and may not remove odor from the armpit or groin. Lipid-free cleansers are best used where minimal cleansing is desired.

After completing cleansing, the sensitive skin patient requires moisturization. The moisturizer should create an optimal environment for barrier repair, while not inducing any type of skin reaction. For example, the product should not contain any mild irritants that may present as an acneiform eruption in a sensitive skin patient due to the presence of follicular irritant contact dermatitis. The best moisturizers are simple oil-in-water emulsions. The most common oil used is white petrolatum, but dimethicone and cyclomethicone are also acceptable oils in the sensitive skin population for decreasing the greasiness of a simple petrolatum and water formulation. As mentioned previously, the fewer ingredients the better.

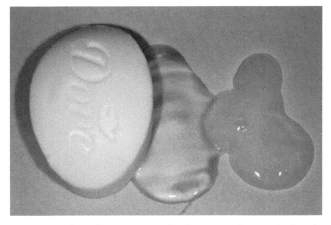

Figure 4.2 Synthetic detergents or syndet cleansers produce gentle cleansing for patients with sensitive skin. From left to right, they are available as bars, opaque liquids, or foaming clear washes.

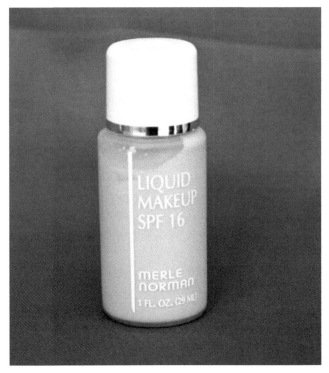

Figure 4.3 Facial foundations can be tested for sensitive skin suitability by applying a small amount to the lateral eye for five consecutive nights.

Sensitive skin products should contain as few ingredients as possible.

Sensitive skin women also require recommendations on proper cosmetic selection. This can be a challenge for the physician, since cosmetic formulations change rapidly as dictated by the needs of fashion. The best method for evaluating problematic facial cosmetics is the provocative use test, performed by applying a 2-cm area of product lateral to the eye for 5 consecutive nights (Fig. 4.3). This allows the isolation of the cosmetic products one at a time on the most sensitive part of the face, which has the highest yield of uncovering the problem. Powder cosmetics overall appear to have the fewest ingredients and present the least problems (Fig. 4.4).

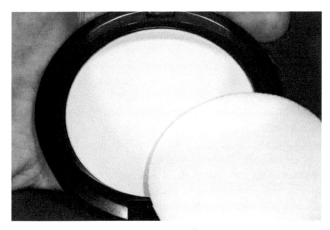

Figure 4.4 Powder cosmetics are preferred in sensitive skin.

CONTACT DERMATITIS

The use of cosmetics and skin care products can occasionally result in contact dermatitis. This is certainly a minor issue, but no discussion of cosmetic dermatology could be complete without addressing this important aspect of patient care. With the tremendous variety of products available for purchase, it is easy for the consumer to simply discard or return any product that has produced an untoward reaction. Occasionally, however, a patient finds that he or she experiences numerous reactions or severe reactions requiring the expertise of a dermatologist skilled in the diagnosis and treatment of contact dermatitis. Contact dermatitis can be classified as irritant contact dermatitis, allergic contact dermatitis, contact urticaria, phototoxic contact dermatitis, and photoallergic contact dermatitis. Each of these subjects is discussed in the framework of skin care products and cosmetics.

Irritant Contact Dermatitis

Irritant contact dermatitis, the most commonly encountered adverse reaction to cosmetics and skin care products, is manifested as erythematous, burning, pruritic skin that may develop microvesiculation and later desquamation. The dermatitis is characterized by stratum corneum damage without immunologic phenomena. The irritancy may be due to the presence of chemical factors with excessively high or low pH, or by volatile vehicles that dissolve protective sebum (3). Physical factors including the rubbing necessary to apply cosmetics or abrasive particles within cosmetics may cause irritancy. Most importantly, a damaged stratum corneum may not be able to provide a protective barrier, so that any cosmetic applied to the damaged skin will cause irritation. This is the case in patients with atopic dermatitis, xerotic eczema, or neurodermatitis. These patients frequently will describe numerous products that produce "allergic" symptoms. In actuality, there is no immunologic basis for the dermatitis, but an irritancy heightened by a damaged stratum corneum. Any cosmetic applied to dermatitic skin may produce irritation; therefore, patients should not wear cosmetics or use personal care items until the dermatitis has resolved.

Any cosmetic applied to dermatitic skin may produce irritation.

Allergic Contact Dermatitis

It is difficult to differentiate allergic contact dermatitis from irritant contact dermatitis clinically, but the distinction is essential for good patient care. Both conditions may present as erythematous plaques; however, acute allergic contact dermatitis may exhibit more vesiculation. In some cases, late-stage allergic and irritant contact dermatitis cannot be differentiated clinically or histologically. Allergic contact dermatitis is an immunologic phenomenon requiring antigen-presenting and antigen-processing cells irrespective of the condition of the protective stratum corneum. Therefore, an intact stratum corneum cannot prevent the development of allergic contact dermatitis in sensitized individuals. The only course is avoidance of the allergen (4). The most common cosmetic-induced causes of allergic contact dermatitis as determined by the North American Contact Dermatitis Group are listed by product category (Table 4.2) and ingredient (Table 4.3) (5). Other studies have also been published by the European dermatologic community (6,7).

An intact stratum corneum cannot prevent the development of allergic contact dermatitis in sensitized individuals.

Contact Urticaria

Contact urticaria may be an immunologic or nonimmunologic reaction to cosmetics and skin care products. It is characterized by the development of a wheal-and-flare response to a topically applied chemical. The spectrum of clinical presentation ranges form itching and burning to generalized urticaria to anaphylaxis. Nonimmunologic contact urticaria is induced when histamine is released by a direct contactant and thus passive transfer is not possible. It is more commonly encountered than immunologic contact urticaria where immunologic mechanisms are involved in histamine release, thus the phenomenon can only be elicited in sensitized individuals and passive transfer is possible. However, there are some chemicals that produce contact urticaria due to uncertain mechanisms. Table 4.4 lists the nonimmunologic and immunologic causes

Table 4.2 Causes of Allergic Contact Dermatitis as per North American Contact Dermatitis Group

Skin care products	28%
Hair care products	24%
Facial cosmetics	11%
Nail cosmetics	8%
Fragrance products	7%

Source: Data from Ref. 5.

Table 4.3 Ingredients Causing Allergic Contact Dermatitis in Order of Decreasing Incidence

Fragrances
Preservatives
p-Phenylenediamine (hair dye component)
Lanolin
Glyceryl thioglycolate (permanent wave solution component)
Propylene glycol
Toluenesulfonamide/formaldehyde resin (nail polish component)
Sunscreens

Source: Data from Ref. 5.

of contact urticaria to substances encountered in cosmetics (8). Testing for contact urticaria should be carried out under carefully controlled conditions with nearby resuscitation facilities since anaphylaxis due to topically applied chemicals has occurred in sensitized individuals.

Contact urticaria is characterized by the development of a wheal-and-flare response to a topically applied chemical.

Phototoxic and Photoallergic Dermatitis

Phototoxic and photoallergic dermatitis are limited to areas exposed to light. Phototoxic reactions are based on nonimmunologic mechanisms and usually appear as sunburns that may be followed by hyperpigmentation and desquamation. The molecules that produce phototoxicity are generally of low molecular weight and possess highly resonant structures that readily absorb mainly UVA radiation (9). Photoallergic dermatitis, on the other hand, is less common and immunologically mediated; generally requires repeat exposure and can be passively transferred. It is characterized by erythema, edema, and vesiculation. Photoallergens are generally low-molecular-weight, lipid-soluble substances that possess highly resonant structures absorbing energy over a wide range of wavelengths, but again predominantly UVA. The light energy photochemically converts the photosensitizer into its active form (10). Less ultraviolet radiation energy is required to elicit a photoallergic reaction compared with a phototoxic reaction (11). Differentiating between the two may be difficult, however, especially if a severe phototoxic reaction results in vesiculation. Substances found in cosmetics that may cause photoallergic

Table 4.4 Substances Used in Cosmetics that Cause Contact Urticaria

Nonimmunologic
    Acetic acid
    Alcohols
    Balsam of Peru
    Benzoic acid
    Cinnamic acid
    Cinnamic aldehyde
    Formaldehyde
    Sodium benzoate
    Sorbic acid
Immunologic
    Acrylic monomer
    Alcohols
    Ammonia
    Benzoic acid
    Benzophenone
    Diethyltoluamide
    Formaldehyde
    Henna
    Menthol
    Parabens
    Polyethylene glycol
    Polysorbate 60
    Salicylic acid
    Sodium sulfide
Uncertain
    Ammonium persulfate
    Para-phenylenediamine

reactions include fragrances such as methylcoumarin and musk ambrette and antibacterial agents and the para-aminobenzoic acid esters such as sunscreening agents (12).

> Photoallergens are low-molecular-weight, lipid-soluble substances that possess highly resonant structures which absorb energy over a wide range of wavelengths.

PATCH TESTING

Patch testing is performed to determine the source of allergic contact dermatitis (13). Generally, the appropriate substances for patch testing are selected from the dermatologic patch test tray (Table 4.5) and applied to filter paper discs affixed to a strip of polyethylene-coated aluminum foil (Al-test) or placed in 8-mm aluminum chambers affixed to a nonwoven textile tape (14). The prepackaged TRUE test can also be used. The healthy skin of the upper back is selected and marked for placement of the tape strips, which are worn for 48 hours. During this time, the patient should not get the patches wet or engage in activities that induce heavy sweating. The tests are initially evaluated at 20 minutes after removal and again at two to seven days (15). Table 4.6 shows the method of evaluation used by the North American Contact Dermatitis Group.

Table 4.5 Substances on a Standard Patch Test Tray

1. Benzocaine 5% petrolatum
2. Imidazolidinyl urea 2% aqueous
3. Thiram mix 1% petrolatum
4. Lanolin alcohol 30% petrolatum
5. Neomycin sulfate 20% petrolatum
6. p-Phenylenediamine 1% petrolatum
7. Mercaptobenzothiazole 1% petrolatum
8. P-tert-butylphenol formaldehyde resin 1% in petrolatum
9. Formaldehyde 1% aqueous
10. Carba mix 3% petrolatum
11. Rosin (colophony) 20% petrolatum
12. Black rubber mix 0.6% petrolatum
13. Ethylenediamine dihydrochloride 1% petrolatum
14. Quaternium-15 2% petrolatum
15. Mercapto mix 1% petrolatum
16. Epoxy resin 1% petrolatum
17. Balsam of Peru 25% petrolatum
18. Potassium dichromate 0.25% petrolatum
19. Nickel sulfate 2.5% petrolatum
20. Cinnamic aldehyde 1% petrolatum

Table 4.6 Evaluation of Patch Test Reactions

+?	=	Doubtful reaction; possibly caused by a weak irritant effect: the reaction shows only a weak erythema without infiltration
+	=	Weak reaction; erythema with infiltration and possibly papules
++	=	Strong reaction; erythema, infiltration, papules, vesicles
+++	=	Extreme reaction; erythema, infiltration, papules, confluent vesicles or bullae
−	=	Negative reaction
IR	=	Irritant reaction
NT	=	Not patch tested

There are two other methods of patch testing that are useful in patients with suspected cosmetics or skin care product sensitivities: open patch tests and provocative use tests. Open patch testing is useful when the test chemical is suspected of being a cutaneous irritant. The chemical is applied to the skin on the outer aspect of the arms above the elbow unoccluded twice daily for two or more days without washing the test site. The site is evaluated in the same manner as illustrated in Table 4.6. False-negative results may occur with this method, however. Provocative use testing is valuable in confirming positive reactions to cosmetic products containing ingredients that were previously found to be sources of allergic contact dermatitis with standard patch testing. The product is applied twice daily to the skin 3 cm in diameter above or below the antecubital fossae for one week. A modification of this test for eye cosmetics is application to the skin lateral to the eye twice daily for one week. Reactions are also evaluated as illustrated in Table 4.6.

> Two additional methods of patch testing useful in patients with suspected cosmetics or skin care product sensitivities are the open patch test and provocative use test.

ADDITIONAL SENSITIVITY TESTING

Testing beyond patch testing may be required to ensure the complete safety of cosmetic and skin care products. Ingredients used in cosmetics are evaluated by the Cosmetic Ingredient Review committee who makes recommendations for use and concentration of the chemical in question.

Draize Test

The Draize test is an evaluation of dermal irritation using an animal model (16) Semiocclusive patch tests of the evaluation substance are placed at 100% concentration on both intact and abraded albino rabbit skin. Readings are performed at 24 and 72 hours after leaving the skin uncovered for 30 to 60 minutes to allow local effects to subside. The sites are evaluated for erythema and edema to determine the degree of irritancy (17). This test is required by law for cosmetics and skin care products under the Federal Hazardous Substances Act (18) to predict the toxicity of chemicals to humans in a manner that overestimates the risk (19,20).

Repeat Insult Patch Test

Repeat insult patch testing evaluates skin sensitization by repeating chemical exposure at the same site on the body. Ten patches are applied to the same site at 48-hour intervals for a three- to four-week period. The skin is allowed to rest for two weeks and then a repeat challenge of the same chemical to the skin is applied for 48 hours and read. This method is commonly used by reputable cosmetic companies in evaluating ingredients and final products for minor sources of sensitization prior to manufacturing them on a large scale.

Cumulative Irritancy Test

The cumulative irritancy test is designed to assess the irritancy of an ingredient, such as those found in a cosmetic or skin care item, or a final product. The test involves daily application of the same substance to the test site under occlusion for 21 days (21).

The repeat application is designed to maximize the irritant reactions.

Eye Irritancy Test

The eye irritancy test is important for cosmetic products since cosmetics may accidentally enter into eyes. This test assesses the irritant effects of substances on the conjunctivum, cornea, and iris of Albino rabbits. This is similar to patch testing; however, 0.10 mL of the test substance is instilled into the eye. In one group of rabbits, the treated eyes are left unwashed; in the second group the treated eyes are washed with 20 mL of lukewarm water after 2 seconds and in the third group the eyes are washed with 20 mL of lukewarm water after 4 seconds. Evaluation of the eyes are performed at 24 hours, 48 hours, 72 hours, 4 days, and 7 days after treatment, or for as long as the injury persists (22). Human subjects are also used to assess the irritant capacity of products introduced into or around the eye. Cosmetics and skin care products should be tested in this manner to ensure human safety.

Photopatch Testing

Photopatch testing is performed when photosensitivity evaluation is required. Two patch test pads are placed with the suspected chemical: one on a site to be irradiated and the other on a protected site. The pads are placed on the skin for 48 hours (23). One site is subjected to ultraviolet radiation of the wavelength desired and read in 24 to 48 hours. This process may be repeated if desired. A phototoxic reaction consists of erythema and usually arises within six hours. A photoallergic reaction is characterized by erythema, papules, and vesicles. If only the irradiated site is positive, a diagnosis of photoallergy can be made. If both the irradiated and the protected sites are positive, a diagnosis of allergic contact dermatitis can be made. If the irradiated site is more positive than the protected site, then a diagnosis of allergic contact dermatitis and photoallergy can be made. Substances that cause photoallergic dermatitis found in cosmetics are tested as follows: methylcoumarin 5% in petrolatum, musk ambrette 5% in petrolatum, and para-aminobenzoic acid esters 10% in petrolatum.

Cutaneous Stinging

There is a group of patients who note stinging or burning within several minutes after applying a cosmetic that intensifies over 5 to 10 minutes and then resolves after 15 minutes. These patients are known as "stingers" and will not tolerate certain cosmetic products even though patch testing for allergic contact dermatitis is negative and no evidence of irritant contact dermatitis is present. Patients who are stingers can be identified by inducing sweating (110°F and 80% relative humidity or exposure to a desktop facial sauna machine) and applying a 5–10% aqueous solution of lactic acid to the nasolabial fold. Those who develop stinging for at least 5 to 10 minutes are identified as "stingers." These individuals can then be used as test panel subjects to evaluate the stinging capacity of cosmetic ingredients or finished products by applying the test substance on one nasolabial fold and a bland control on the other nasolabial fold. Substances that can induce stinging are listed in Table 4.7 (24).

Table 4.7 Substances that Induce Stinging

Slight stingers
  Benzene
  Phenol
  Salicylic acid
  Resorcinol
  Phosphoric acid
Moderate stingers
  Sodium carbonate
  Trisodium phosphate
  Propylene glycol
  Propylene carbonate
  Propylene glycol diacetate
  Dimethylacetamide
  Dimethylformamide
  Dimethyl sulfoxide
  Diethyltoluamide
  Dimethyl phthalate
  2-ethyl-1,3-hexanediol
  Benzoyl peroxide
Severe stingers
  Crude coal tar
  Phosphoric acid
  Hydrochloric acid
  Sodium hydroxide
  2-ethoxyethyl p-methoxy-cinnamate

Source: Table adapted from Ref. 24.

SUMMARY

The diagnosis and treatment of a sensitive skin is a medical challenge. Any treatment must address the barrier disruption, immune hyper-reactivity, and heightened sensory responsiveness that characterize the sensitive skin. If the sensitive skin is due to a visible dermatosis, the treatment can be streamlined, but if it is an invisible sensitive skin, a long treatment algorithm must be followed to further elucidate valuable diagnostic information. Patch testing may be necessary if irritant or allergic contact dermatitis is suspected. Finally, basic skin care and cosmetic recommendations can be made to the sensitive skin patient to minimize the chances of encountering a problem.

REFERENCES

1. Draelos ZD. Sensitive skin: perceptions, evaluation, and treatment. Contact Dermatitis 1997; 8: 67.
2. Draelos ZD. Noxious sensory perceptions in patients with mild to moderate rosacea treated with azelaic acid 15% gel. Cutis 2004; 74: 257.
3. Jackson EM. Irritation and sensitization. In: Waggoner WC, ed. Clinical Safety and Efficacy Testing of Cosmetics. New York: Marcel Dekker, Inc, 1990: 23–42.
4. Baer RL. The mechanism of allergic contact hypersensitivity. In: Fisher AA, ed. Contact Dermatitis, 3rd edn. Philadelphia: Lea & Febiger, 1986: 1–8.
5. Adams RM, Maibach HI. A five-year study of cosmetic reactions. J Am Acad Dermatol 1985; 13: 1062–9.
6. De Groot AC, Beverdam EGA, Ayong CT, Coenraads PJ, Nater PJ. The role of contact allergy in the spectrum of adverse effects caused by cosmetics and toiletries. Contact Dermatitis 1988; 19: 195–201.
7. De Groot AC. Contact allergy to cosmetics: causative ingredients. Contact Dermatitis 1987; 17: 26–34.
8. Fisher AA. Contact Dermatitis, 3rd edn. Philadelphia: Lea & Febiger, 1986: 686–709.
9. Billhimer WL. Phototoxicity and photoallergy. In: Waggoner WC, ed. Clinical Safety and Efficacy Testing of Cosmetics. New York: Marcel Dekker, Inc, 1990: 43–74.

10. Stephens RJ, Bergstresser PR. Fundamental concepts in photoimm-
    unology and photoallergy. In: Jackson EM, ed. Photobiology of the Skin
    and Eye. New York, Marcel Dekker, 1986: 41–66.
11. Epstein JH. Phototoxicity and photoallergy in man. J Am Acad Dermatol
    1983; 8: 141–7.
12. DeLeo VA, Harber LC. Contact photodermatitis. In: Fisher AA, ed.
    Contact Dermatitis, 3rd edn. Philadelphia: Lea & Febiger, 1986: 454–69.
13. Nethercott JR. Sensitivity and specificity of patch tests. Am J Contact
    Dermatitis 1994; 5: 136–42.
14. Goldner R. Clinical tests. In: Jackson EM, Goldner R, eds. Irritant Contact
    Dermatitis. New York: Marcel Dekker, Inc, 1990: 201–18.
15. Fowler JF. Reading patch tests: some pitfalls of patch testing. Am J Contact
    Dermatitis 1994; 5: 170–2.
16. Draize JH, Woodard G, Calvary HO. Methods for the study of irritation
    and toxicity of substances applied topically to the skin and mucous
    membranes. J Pharmacol Exp Ther 1944; 82: 377–419.
17. Bronaugh RL, Maibach HI. Primary irritant, allergic contact, phototoxic,
    and photoallergic reactions to cosmetics and tests to identify problem
    products. In: Frost P, Horwitz SN, eds. Principles of cosmetics for the
    dermatologist. St. Louis: CV Mosby Company, 1982: 223–43.
18. Method of testing primary irritant substances, United States Code of
    Federal Regulations, 16 CFR, 1500.41, 1979, Consumer Product Safety
    Commission, Washington, DC.
19. Philips L, Steingerg M, Maibach HI, Akers WA. A comparison of rabbit
    and human skin response to certain irritants. Toxicol Appl Pharmacol
    1972; 21: 369.
20. Gabrial KL. In vivo preclinical tests. In: Jackson EM, Goldner R, eds.
    Irritant Contact Dermatitis. New York: Marcel Dekker, Inc, 1990: 191–9.
21. Kligman AM, Wooding WM. A method for the measurement and
    evaluation of irritants in human skin. J Invest Dermatol 1967; 49: 78–
    94.
22. Wortzman MS. Eye products. In: Whittam JH, ed. Cosmetic Safety A primer
    for Cosmetic Scientists. New York: Marcel Dekker, Inc, 1987: 205–20.
23. DeLeo VA. Photocontact dermatitis in photosensitivity. In: DeLeo VA, ed.
    New York: Igaku-Shoin, 1992: 84–99.
24. Frosch PJ, Kligman AM. A method for appraising the stinging capacity of
    topically applied substances. J Soc Cosmet Chem 1977; 28: 197–209.

SUGGESTED READING
Adams RM, Maibach HI. A five-year study of cosmetic reactions. J Am
    Dermatol 1985; 13: 1062–9.
Basketter DA, Briatico-Vangosa G, Kaestner W, Lally C, Bontinck WJ. Nickel,
    cobalt and chromium in consumer products: a role in allergic contact der-
    matitis? Contact Dermatitis 1993; 28: 15–25.
Campbell L, Zirwas MJ. Triclosan. Dermatitis 2006; 4: 204–7.
Davari P, Maibach HI. Contact Urticaria to Cosmetic and Industrial Dyes. Clin
    Exp Dermatol 2010; [Epub ahead of print].
de Groot AC. Contact allergy to cosmetics: causative ingredients. Contact
    Dermatitis 1987; 17: 26–34.
de Groot AC, Bruynzeel DP, Bos JD, et al. The allergens in cosmetics. Arch
    Cermatol 1988; 124: 1525–9.

de Groot AC, Frosch PJ. Adverse reactions to fragrances. A clinical review.
    Contact Dermatitis 1997; 36: 57–86.
de Groot AC, Liem DH, Weyland JW, Kathon CG. Cosmetic allergy and patch
    test sensitization. Contact Dermatitis 1985; 12: 76–80.
Diepgen TL, Weisshaar E. Contact dermatitis: epidemiology and frequent sensitizers
    to cosmetics. J Eur Acad Dermatol Venereol 2007; 21 (Suppl 2): 9–13.
Distante F, Rigano L, D'Agostina R, Bonfigli A. Intra-and Inter-Individual
    Differences in Sensitive Skin. Cosmet Toilet 2002; 117: 39–43.
Draelos ZD. Cosmetic Selection in the Sensitive-Skin Patient. Dermatol Ther
    2001; 14: 175–7.
Elias PM, Feingold KR. Does the tail wag the dog? Role of the barrier in the
    pathogenesis of inflammatory dermatoses and therapeutic implications.
    Arch Dermatol 2001; 137: 1079–81.
Hachem JP, De Paepe. K, Vanpee E, et al. The effect of two moisturizers on skin
    barrier damage in allergic contact dermatitis. Eur J Dermatol 2002; 12:
    136–8.
Johansen JD. Fragrance contact allergy: a clinical review. Am J Clin Dermatol
    2003; 4: 789–98.
Larsen W, Nakayama H, Lindberg M, et al. Fragrance contact dermatitis:
    a worldwide multicenter investigation(Part 1). Am J Contact Dermatitis
    1996; 7: 77–83.
Mehta SS, Reddy BS. Cosmetic dermatitis-current perspectives. Int J Dermatol
    2003; 42: 533–42.
Nardelli A, Carbonez A, Ottoy W, Drieghe J, Goossens A. Frequency of and
    trends in fragrance allergy over a 15-year period. Contact Dermatitis
    2008; 58: 134–41.
Nigram PK. Adverse Reactions to Cosmetics and Methods of Testing. Indian
    J Dermatol Venereol Leprol 2009; 75: 10–18.
Orton DI, Wilkinson JD. Cosmetic allergy: incidence, diagnosis, and manage-
    ment. Am J Clin Dermatol 2004; 5: 327–37.
Ortiz KJ, Yiannias JA. Contact dermatitis to cosmetics, fragrances, and
    botanicals. Dermatol Ther 2004; 17: 264–71.
Pascoe D, Moreau L, Sasseville D. Emergent and Unusual Allergens in
    Cosmetics. Dermatitis 2010; 21: 127–37.
Ramirez Santos A, Fernandez-Redondo V, Perez Perez L, Concheiro Cao J,
    Toribio J. Contact allergy from vitamins in cosmetic products. Dermatitis
    2008; 19: 154–6.
Rastogi SC, Johansen JD. Significant exposures to isoeugenol derivatives in
    perfumes. Contact Dermatitis 2008; 58: 278–81.
Rastogi SC, Johansen JD, Bossi R. Selected important fragrance sensitizers in
    perfumes-current exposures. Contact Dermatitis 2007; 56: 201–4.
Scheinman PL. Is it really fragrance-free? Am J Contact Dermatitis 1997; 8:
    239–42.
Tomar J, Jain VK, Aggarwal K, Dayal S, Gupta S. Contact allergies to cosmetics:
    testing with 52 cosmetic ingredients and personal products. J Dermatol
    2005; 32: 951–5.
Warshaw EM, Belsito DV, DeLeo VA, et al. North American Contact Dermatitis
    Group patch-test results, 2003–2004 study period. Dermatitis 2008; 19:
    129–36.
Yokota T, Matsumoto M, Sakamaki T, et al. Classification of Sensitive Skin and
    Development of a Treatment System Appropriate for Each Group. IFSCC
    Magazine 2003; 6: 303–7.

5 Aging skin and cosmeceuticals

The cosmeceutical category is an undefined, unclassified, and unregulated area of dermatology that is yet in its infancy (1). Traditional cosmeceuticals involve the topical application of biologically active ingredients, which affect the skin barrier and overall skin health. The ability of these ingredients to enhance skin functioning depends on how they are formulated into creams, lotions, etc., to maintain the integrity of the active agent, deliver it in a biologically active form to the skin, reach the target site in sufficient quantity to exert an effect, and properly release from the carrier vehicle. In the United States, cosmeceuticals are sold as cosmetics making marketing, packaging, and aesthetic appeal important considerations. Ideally, the cosmeceutical should be clinically tested for efficacy to ensure a proven skin benefit, but also to substantiate marketing claims. The recognition that there are governmental limitations on efficacy claims restricts cosmeceutical development, since products can only be assessed in terms of their ability to improve skin appearance, but not function. Improving function would remove the cosmeceutical from cosmetic category and place it in the drug category. Herein rests the challenge of defining the cosmeceutical category, the topic of this chapter.

When the cosmeceutical category was first introduced to the dermatologist, cosmeceuticals were prescription items that addressed appearance issues (2). The first cosmeceutical that met these criteria was topical tretinoin. Tretinoin has been a significant force in dermatology, but is not as popular as some of the cosmetic formulations containing less biologically effective retinol. Why? Unfortunately, tretinoin produces no short-term benefits. As a matter of fact, tretinoin produces short-term setbacks in skin appearance due to the peeling and redness that occur during the first two weeks of use, requiring the encouragement of a dermatologist for compliance. The long-term benefits of tretinoin take at least six months to realize. While the functional benefits of tretinoin are great, there are no aesthetic benefits. This has led to the proliferation of over-the-counter (OTC) retinol, retinyl propionate, and retinaldehyde moisturizers that cannot deliver the ultimate collagen regeneration benefits of prescription tretinoin, but do not cause irritation and peeling. Thus, a modern cosmeceutical must combine the aesthetics of a cosmetic with the efficacy of a drug.

The next cosmeceutical introduced to the dermatologist was topical minoxidil. This product demonstrated a functional benefit in terms of hair growth, but at least six months of use was necessary to perceive any increase in hair fullness. In order to achieve topical minoxidil penetration, a high concentration of propylene glycol was required, which produced scalp itching and dryness. The established safety profile of this prescription drug allowed reclassification into the OTC drug market, but the lack of immediate aesthetic benefits prevented this formulation from reaching its full potential for use among patients with male or female pattern alopecia. Thus, a modern

cosmeceutical must produce an immediate benefit like a cosmetic, but also a long-term benefit like a drug.

The world of the prescription cosmeceutical has virtually come to a standstill following the approval of tretinoin and minoxidil. Yet, the concept of cosmeceuticals is alive and well. Patients are well educated via the mass media, periodicals, and the Internet demanding sophistication in products they purchase. These demands have led to the new concept of cosmeceuticals, which can be most accurately described as multifunctional cosmetics, products that are purchased without a prescription that do more than scent or color the skin. These modern cosmeceuticals are expected to have superior feel and smell while providing a visibly perceivable improvement in skin appearance. Our review of cosmeceuticals and skin care products begins with a discussion of aging skin.

AGING SKIN
Aging of the skin can be classified into two components: intrinsic and extrinsic aging. As the names imply, intrinsic aging is due to genetically controlled senescence and extrinsic aging is due to environmental factors superimposed on intrinsic aging. Environmental factors known to accelerate extrinsic aging are sun exposure and cigarette smoking. Cutaneous aging due to sun exposure is known as photoaging (3).

Youthful skin is characterized by its unblemished, evenly pigmented, smooth, and pink appearance. This is in contrast to intrinsically aged skin, which is thin, inelastic, and finely wrinkled with deepening of facial expression lines (4). These changes are evident histologically as a thinned epidermis and dermis with the flattening of the rete pegs at the dermoepidermal junction (5). Extrinsically aged, sun-exposed skin appears clinically as blemished, thickened, yellowed, lax, rough, and leathery (6). These changes may begin as early as the second decade (7) and can be used to divide photoaged skin into four groups known as the Glogau Classification (Table 5.1). It may also contain precancerous and cancerous growths, as well as telangiectasias and lentigines (8). Some of the propensity toward cancerous growths may be due to a decrease in Langerhans cells and their function (9). Photoaged skin is characterized histologically by epidermal dysplasia with varying degrees of cytologic atypia, loss of keratinocyte polarity, an inflammatory infiltrate, decreased collagen, increased ground substance, and elastosis. Elastosis is the degradation of elastic material, which, in early photoaging, is increased in amount and seen microscopically as thickened, twisted, degraded elastic fibers (10). These fibers degenerate into an amorphous mass as photoaging progresses (11). Thus, intrinsic aging of the skin results in atrophy while extrinsic photoaging results in hypertrophy. This distinction is not always clinically apparent, but in ideal cases intrinsically aged skin has fine wrinkling while photoaged skin demonstrates coarse wrinkling and furrowing (12) (Fig. 5.1). Many substances have been put forth to treat aging skin, perhaps the first being hormone creams, which is discussed next.

AGING AND HORMONES

Since the beginning of time, man has searched for topicals and ingestibles that promise to deliver the magic of youth. Prior to the 1930s, many products were sold door to door promising to be a youth elixir, but some contained toxic ingredients such as arsenic and mercury. One of the most popular antiaging preparations at the time the Cosmetics and Toiletries Act was penned in the 1930s was the facial moisturizers containing estrogen (Fig. 5.2). The introduction of legislation defining cosmetics as products that do not alter the structure or function of the skin reclassified hormone creams as drugs and they were removed from the consumer market. However, the past 70 years have brought an increased understanding of skin physiology and the recognition that even water can alter the structure and function of the skin. This has created a renewed interest in cosmeceuticals, especially in the realm of hormone therapy.

There is no doubt that hormone therapy is effective for improving the appearance of aging skin, as supported by the article published in this issue by Wolff, Narayan, and Taylor. Not only do estrogens improve skin rigidity and decrease wrinkling, but they also increase skin thickness as measured by ultrasound (13), increase skin sebum production as measured by a sebumeter (14), increase skin elasticity as measured by skin deformability using a suction device (15), increase skin hydration as measured by corneometry (16), and increase skin collagen content as measured by skin biopsy (17). Many methods that assess the skin function point to oral and/or transdermal estrogen as a valuable replacement hormone.

A variety of studies have also examined estrogen delivery topically. Estrogen is readily soluble in a creamy vehicle and easily penetrates the stratum corneum due to its small molecular size. It is the ideal cosmeceutical for topical application. Topical estrogen has been shown to increase the production of type III collagen and the overall collagen fiber count after six months of application (18). It also increased the acid mucopolysaccharide and hyaluronic acid levels in the skin, which are important for maintaining skin hydration and barrier function (19). The combination of increased dermal volume, due to more collagen fibers, and increased dermal hydration, due to more hyaluronic acid, may explain the decreased wrinkling apparent in women using estrogens. It is important to note that there is currently no other substance available to the cosmetic formulator that delivers such documentable reproducible results in women.

Table 5.1 Glogau Classification of Photoaging Groups

Group 1 Mild
  No keratosis
  Little wrinkling
  No scarring
  Little or no makeup
  Usually age 28–35 yrs
Group 2 Moderate
  Early actinic keratoses
  Slight yellow skin discoloration
  Early wrinkling (parallel smile lines)
  Mild scarring
  Little makeup
  Usually age 35–50 yrs
Group 3 Advanced
  Actinic keratoses
  Obvious yellow skin discoloration with telangiectasia
  Wrinkling present at rest
  Moderate acne scarring
  Always wears makeup
  Usually age 50–65 yrs
Group 4 Severe
  Actinic keratoses and skin cancers have occurred
  Wrinkling of actinic gravitational and dynamic origin
  Severe acne scarring
  Wears makeup, but does not cover well
  Usually age 60–75 yrs

Phytoestrogens, such as genistein, daidzein, and glycitein, are found in fermented soy and can be consumed in the form of roasted soy nuts or tofu.

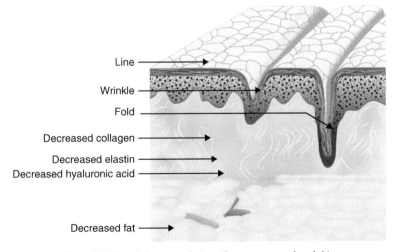

Line
Wrinkle
Fold
Decreased collagen
Decreased elastin
Decreased hyaluronic acid

Decreased fat

Figure 5.1 Many defects contribute to the appearance of aged skin.

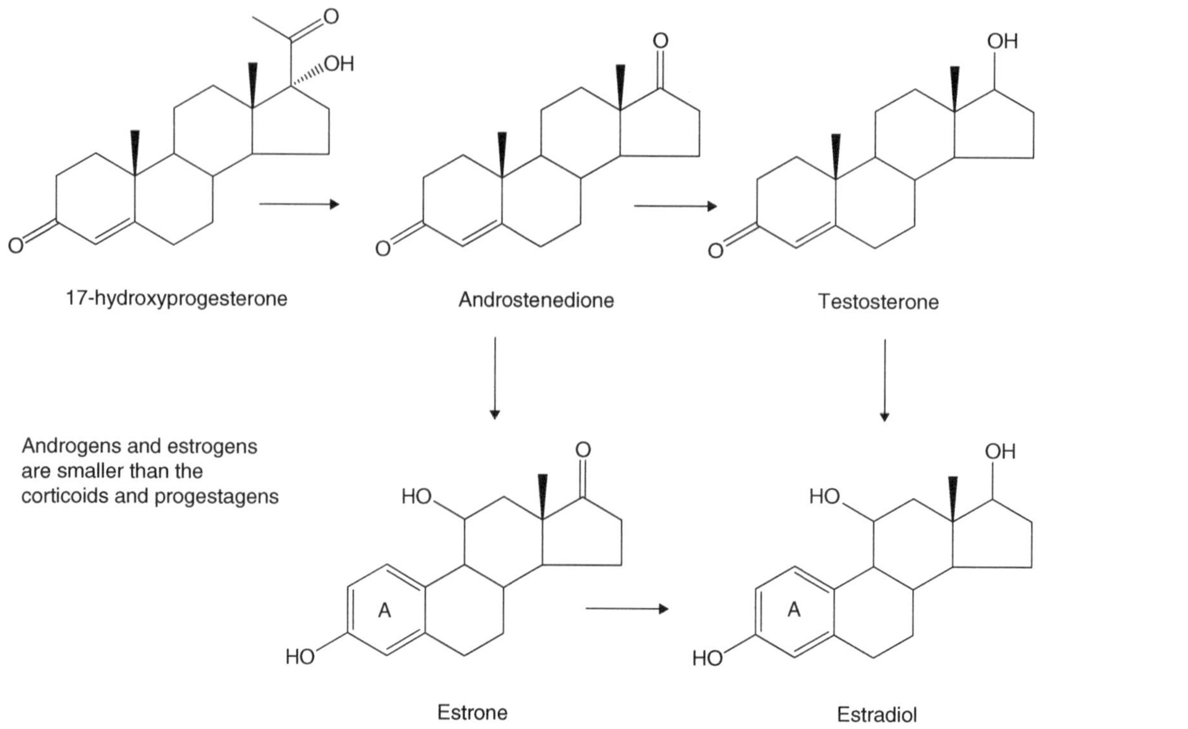

Figure 5.2 Estrogen creams were the first cosmeceutical facial moisturizer for aging skin.

The legal restriction on OTC estrogen has led to an interest in phytoestrogens, especially those derived from soy. Phytoestrogens, such as genistein, daidzein, and glycitein, are found in fermented soy and can be consumed in the form of roasted soy nuts or tofu. Soy protein supplements have been investigated for their benefit in a variety of postmenopausal symptoms, but the data is somewhat inconsistent. One controlled study by Kotsopoulos et al., found that a soy protein supplement had no statistically significant effect over placebo on dry skin (20). Yet, genistein is one of the most popular botanical additives to skin care products promising to decrease the appearance of fine lines on the face. It can be difficult, however, to determine whether the decreased wrinkling advertised by the manufacturer is due to the vehicle moisturizer decreasing the lines of dehydration and altering light reflection from the skin surface or true changes in skin collagen production and decreased wrinkling due to increased dermal thickness. In the current regulatory climate, no cosmetic manufacturer wants to determine the answer to this question. Moisturizing the skin and changing the optical characteristics is the realm of cosmetics, but enhancing collagen production is the realm of a drug. Any soy product that documented an increased collagen production would certainly be removed from the market by the Food and Drug Administration (FDA). It is for this reason that research is lacking in the topical application of phytoestrogens.

The question then remains as to why topical estrogen creams and estrogen replacement therapy are so controversial when the skin benefits have been well documented. There have been some concerns that estrogens predispose women to malignant melanoma in the literature, although the reports are contradictory. A study by Smith et al., demonstrated no link between melanoma and oral contraceptives or replacement estrogens (21). Topical estrogens are even more controversial, since they are theoretically linked to breast cancer and cancer of other female organs. No company wants to market a topical product with such tremendous opportunity for lawsuits, since cause and effect are hard to demonstrate or negate. Topical estrogens are also associated with facial telangiectasias, which is undesirable.

One area of estrogen benefit for skin appearance is rarely discussed in the literature. This is the decrease in facial bone mass. Many articles allude to the benefit of oral estrogens in bone mineral density, but few have studied the mineralization of the facial bones (22). Much of the wrinkling experienced with advancing age is not due to skin effects, but due to loss of the underlying subcutaneous tissue and bony architecture. Loss of facial bone structure also contributes to wrinkling, which may be improved through oral estrogen supplementation.

DEVELOPMENT OF COSMECEUTICALS

Since the removal of the first cosmeceutical, topical estrogen, from the market, many other cosmeceutical formulations have been introduced. There is nothing special about cosmeceuticals, which are classified by industry as functional cosmetics. This means that the ingredients that are included in formulations must come from a list of raw materials that are generally recognized as safe, or the cosmeceutical would be classified as a drug. The easiest source of new cosmeceutical ingredients is the plant kingdom. Plants are rich in endogenous antioxidants, because they must survive in an environment rich in UV radiation insults. Plant extracts are also felt to be safe and meet the FDA criteria for substances that can be put in OTC formulations. It is generally felt that substances that are safe for oral consumption can be assumed safe when applied topically. This has led to a renewed interest in herbal preparations, which form the basis for functionality in many cosmeceuticals (Fig. 5.3).

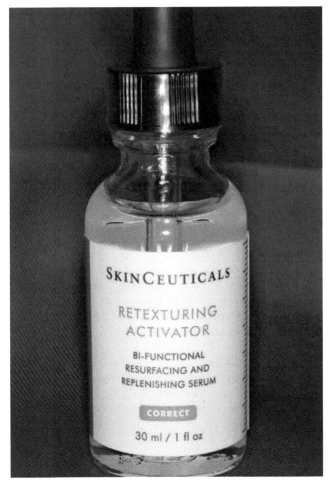

Figure 5.3 Botanicals form the basis for many cosmeceutical formulations.

Cosmeceuticals are moisturizers that contain active agents commonly derived from plant materials, such as flowers, seeds, roots, leaves, twigs, and berries.

The search for novel herbals has led to the gathering of flowers, seeds, roots, leaves, twigs, and berries from plants all over the world. This can be a complex process, since the constituents of a plant extract are influenced by the season in which the plant material is picked, the growing conditions, and the processing of the botanical ingredient. The popular sources for botanical cosmeceutical ingredients are summarized in Table 5.2. Once a possible functional cosmeceutical active agent has been identified and synthesized, it is typically applied to a fibroblast gene chip to determine whether it affects any key cellular event. After the demonstration of a presumed physiologic effect, the active agent is tested in vitro to determine its effect on cultured fibroblasts. If positive data are obtained, the active agent is studied in a mouse model for confirmation. It is then placed in a vehicle suitable for human application, and clinical studies are undertaken. Successful human clinical studies pave the way for successful introduction into the marketplace via ingredient licensing arrangements. These steps for cosmeceutical development are summarized in Table 5.3.

An important consideration in cosmeceutical development is safety. Cosmeceuticals are considered cosmetics by the US

Table 5.2 Botanical Sources of Cosmeceutical Functional Ingredients

1. Plant source leaves, roots, fruits, berries, stems, twigs, barks, flowers
2. Growing conditions: soil composition, amount of available water, climate variations, plant stress
3. Harvesting conditions: time from harvest to transport, care of plant materials during shipping, storage conditions prior to manufacture
4. Preparation methods: crushing, grinding, boiling, distilling, pressing, drying
5. Final extract status: liquid, powder, paste, syrup, crystal
6. Concentration sufficient amount of active agent to produce the biologic effect

Table 5.3 Steps in Cosmeceutical Development

1. New botanical material received in the laboratory.
2. Various fractions of the botanical extracted.
3. Fractions analyzed for relationship to known chemical compounds.
4. Purified fraction exposed to gene array chip.
5. Analysis completed for upregulation or downregulation of key events in cellular oxidation, inflammation, or irritation.
6. New isolate studied in an in vitro model of cell culture for confirmation of gene array results.
7. Positive in vitro findings lead to isolate analysis in mouse model focusing on markers of possible cutaneous benefit.
8. Positive mouse findings lead to formulation in a vehicle suitable for human use.
9. Human model testing conducted to determine whether the active agent has any cutaneous value.
10. Formulation fine-tuned and patented.
11. New ingredient licensed to cosmetic manufacturer.
12. New technology enters the marketplace.

government and as such are unregulated. However, the cosmetic industry does an excellent job of self-policing the safety of products introduced into the marketplace. No reputable cosmetic manufacturer wants to introduce problematic formulations that would tarnish the hard earned reputation of the company. Most of the quality cosmeceuticals are formulated from ingredients that already have a proven safety record in the marketplace. This may be due to their extraction from foods, such as topical lycopene from tomatoes or topical avocadin from avocados. Alternatively, extensive animal testing may be undertaken by the raw material supplier to determine that the new ingredient is appropriate for human use. In the case of botanicals, most are assumed safe based on their ubiquitous nature.

Cosmeceuticals are unregulated and presently considered cosmetics in the U.S.A.

COSMECEUTICAL OVERVIEW

A tremendous variety of ingredients can be incorporated into cosmeceuticals, far beyond the reach of this text. For an in-depth discussion, the reader is referred to a book I edited on Cosmeceuticals published by Elsevier in second edition in

2009. In this chapter, I would like to highlight a few cosmeceutical ingredients that are of particular interest. They belong to three families of substances including carotenoids, flavonoids, and polyphenols. These are the major categories of antioxidants, which have excellent evidence to support their oral ingestion, but less impressive evidence to support their topical application.

The three major families of antioxidants found in cosmeceuticals are carotenoids, flavonoids, and polyphenols.

Carotenoids

Carotenoids are derivatives of vitamin A and have found widespread use in cosmeceuticals due to the established topical antiaging benefits associated with the prescription retinoid tretinoin. The carotenoids are a large family of orange-, red-, and yellow-appearing substances that perform vital antioxidant roles when ingested and are less well established as topical antioxidants.

Astaxanthin

Astaxanthin is a pink carotenoid found in high concentration in salmon, accounting for the characteristic pink color of the fish. This is the rationale for antiaging diets recommending the ingestion of a serving of salmon five times weekly (23). For topical application purposes, astaxanthin is obtained from the marine microalgae *Haematococcus pluvialis*. The efficacy of astaxanthin is attributed to its cell membrane that is composed of two external lipid layers, which has been touted to possess stronger antioxidant abilities than vitamin E (24). It is both water and oil soluble only being produced by algae when exposed to intense UV radiation.

Few topical studies exist to confirm the topical effect of astaxanthin (25), but it has been studied extensively as an oral supplement (26). It is used as a homeopathic treatment for macular degeneration because, unlike canthaxanthin, another carotenoid, it does not crystallize in the eye. It crosses the blood–brain barrier and has been studied in brain dysfunction, to include spinal cord injuries and Parkinson's disease (27). Even though other carotenoids, such as beta-carotene, have been proven ineffective in reducing the oxidative stress associated with cardiovascular disease, astaxanthin is currently undergoing further investigation (28).

Astaxanthin in concentrations of 0.03–0.07% produces a pink color cream. This limits the concentration that can be used, but no topical adverse reactions have been associated with this carotenoid. The topical antioxidant benefits of astaxanthin have not been established.

Lutein

Another carotenoid found in topical cosmeceuticals is lutein. It is naturally found in green leafy vegetables, such as spinach and kale. Lutein is an antioxidant in the plant kingdom, also being used for blue light absorption. In the animal kingdom, lutein is found in egg yolks, animal fats, and the corpus luteum. It is a lipophilic molecule, not soluble in water, characterized by a long polyene side chain composed of conjugated double bonds. These double bonds are degraded by light and heat, a universal characteristic of carotenoids to a greater or lesser degree (29).

Lutein is used as a natural colorant due to its orange-red color resulting from the absorption of blue light. Its largest use is as a food supplement for chickens, which results in more vivid yellow yolks. In humans, lutein is concentrated in the macula and has been linked to the prevention of macular degeneration (30). It has been available as a nutritional supplement since 1996 and can be administered as a sublingual spray for elderly patients with macular degeneration.

The question remains as to whether lutein applied topically is of value. Again no data are available to support this, but an excess lutein intake can result in carotenodermia and an excess topical application results in bronzing of the skin.

Lycopene

Another potent carotenoid is lycopene, found in most fruits and vegetables with a red color including, tomatoes, watermelon, pink grapefruit, papaya, gac, red bell pepper, and pink guava. The highest lycopene containing food is ketchup, but lycopene is not an essential human nutrient. The Mayo Clinic website rates the evidence for the use of lycopene as an antioxidant as a C, since is it not clear if lycopene has these effects on the human body.

Lycopene is a highly unsaturated hydrocarbon containing 11 conjugated and 2 unconjugated double bonds, which makes it a longer molecule than any other carotenoid. This makes its absorption into the skin doubtful. It undergoes cis-isomerization when exposed to sunlight making it an unlikely topical ingredient.

Flavonoids

Flavonoids are aromatic compounds, frequently with a yellow color, which occur in higher plants. Five thousand flavonoids have been identified with a similar chemical structure possessing 15 carbon atoms and a variety of biologic activities (31) (Fig. 5.4). Flavonoids can be divided into flavones, flavonols, isoflavones, and flavanones, each with a slightly different chemical structure (Fig. 5.5). Common flavonoids include curcumin, silymarin, and pycnogenol.

Curcumin

Curcumin is a popular natural yellow food coloring used in everything from prepackaged snack foods to meats. It is sometimes used in skin care products as a natural yellow coloring in products that claim to be free of artificial ingredients. Curcumin comes from the rhizome of the turmeric plant and is consumed orally as an Asian spice, frequently found in rice dishes to color the otherwise white rice yellow. However, this yellow color is undesirable in cosmetic preparations, since yellowing of products is typically associated with oxidative spoilage. Tetrahydrocurcumin, a hydrogenated form of curcumin, is off-white in color and can be added to skin care product. It not only functions as a skin antioxidant but also prevents the lipids in the moisturizer from becoming rancid. The antioxidant effect of tetrahydrocurcumin is said to be greater than that of vitamin E by cosmetic chemists. It is said to provide antioxidant skin benefits by quenching oxygen radicals and inhibiting nuclear factor-KB (32,33). The effects of curcumin as a topical antioxidant in the skin have not been studied so well.

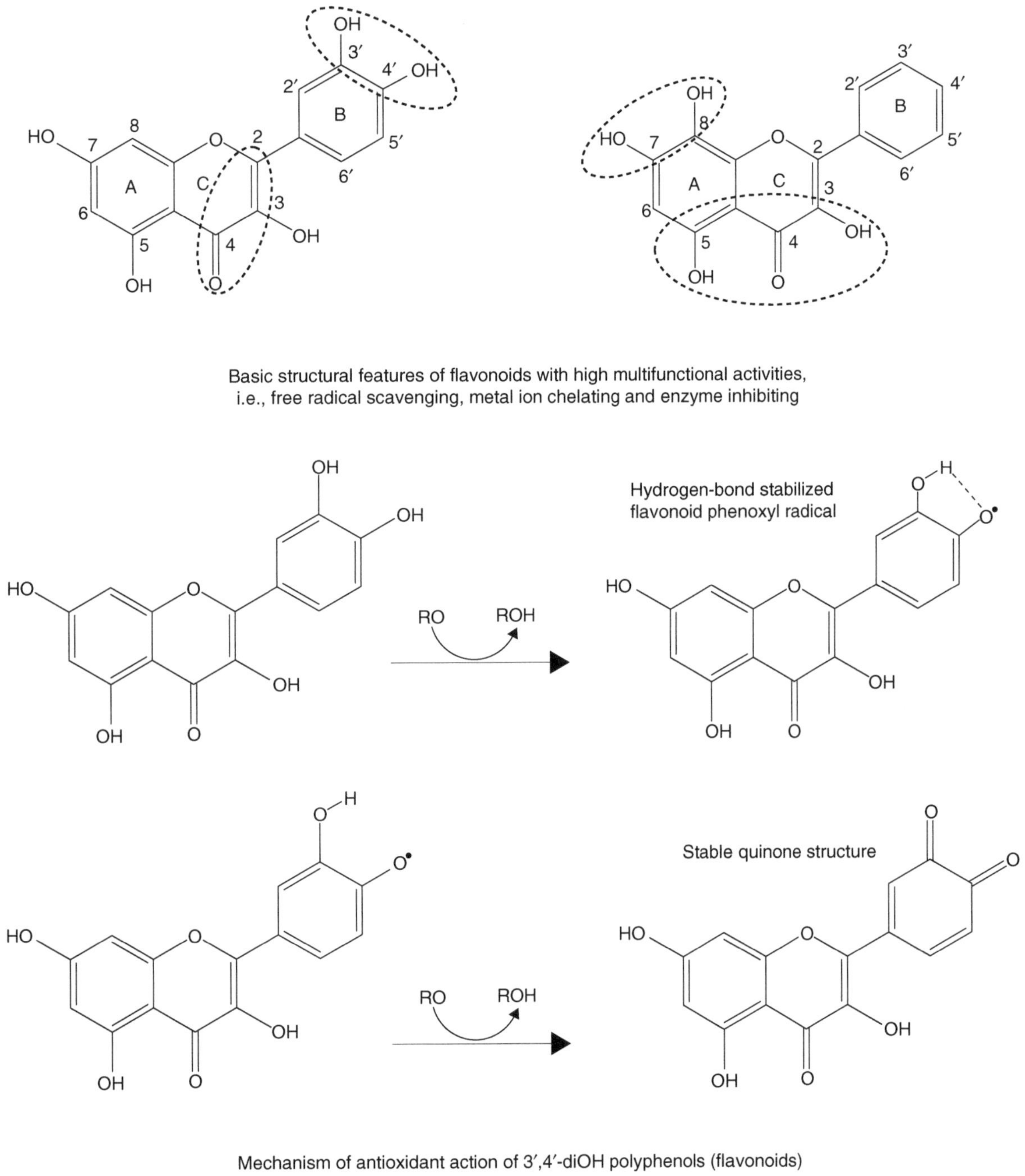

Basic structural features of flavonoids with high multifunctional activities, i.e., free radical scavenging, metal ion chelating and enzyme inhibiting

Mechanism of antioxidant action of 3',4'-diOH polyphenols (flavonoids)

Figure 5.4 The chemical structure of flavonoids illustrating their ability to function as antioxidants.

Silymarin

Silymarin is an extract of the milk thistle plant (*Silybum marianum*), which belongs to the aster family of plants including daisies, thistles, and artichokes. The plant is named milk thistle because the oldest recorded use of the extract was to enhance human lactation, and the plant produces a white milky sap. The extract consists of three flavonoids derived from the fruit, seeds, and leaves of the plant. These flavonoids are silybin, silydianin, and silychristin. Homeopathically, silymarin is used to treat liver disease, but it is a strong antioxidant preventing lipid peroxidation by scavenging free radical species. Its antioxidant effects have been demonstrated topically in hairline mice by the 92% reduction of skin tumors following UVB

exposure (34,35). The mechanism for this decrease in tumor production is unknown, but topical silymarin has been shown to decrease the formation of pyrimidine dimers in a mouse model (36). It has also been found to improve the healing of burns in albino rats (37).

Silymarin is found in a number of high-end moisturizer for benign photoaging to prevent cutaneous oxidative damage and to reduce facial redness. A double-blind placebo-controlled study in 46 subjects with stage I to III rosacea found improvement in skin redness, papules, itching, hydration, and skin color (38). This was felt to be due to its direct activity on modulating cytokines and angiokines. Other well-controlled human trials are lacking.

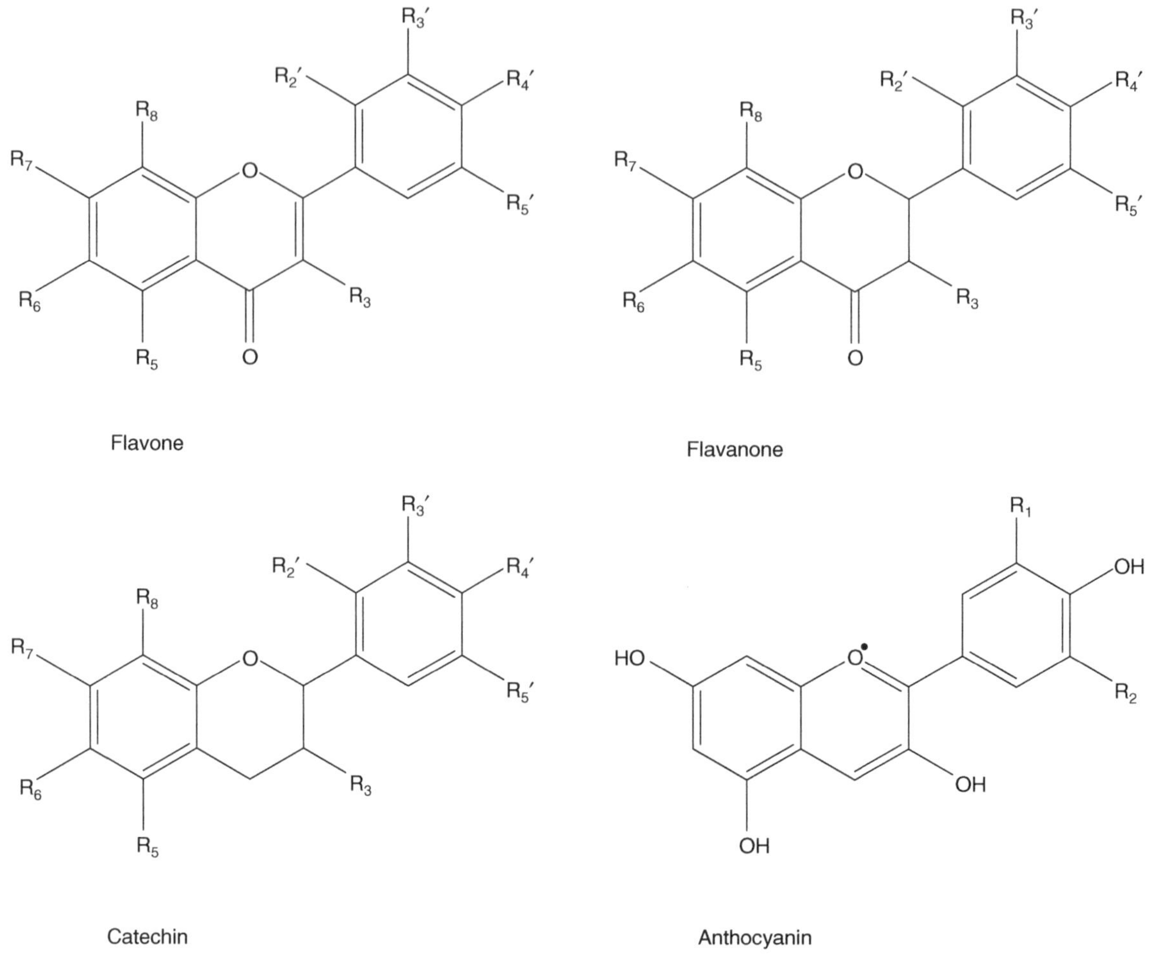

Flavone

Flavanone

Catechin

Anthocyanin

Figure 5.5 The chemical structures of common flavonoids.

Pycnogenol

Pycnogenol is an extract of French marine pine bark (*Pinus pinaster*), which grows only on the southwest coast of France in Les Landes de Gascogne. The extract is a water-soluble liquid containing several phenolic constituents, including taxifolin, catechin, and procyanidins. It also contains several phenolic acids, including p-hydroxybenzoic, protocatechuic, gallic, vanillic, p-couric, caffeic, and ferulic (39). It is a trademarked ingredient that is sold for oral consumption as a preventative for cardiovascular disease (40), a treatment for diabetic microangiopathy (41), and a pain reliever for muscle cramps (42). It is a potent-free radical scavenger that can reduce the vitamin C radical, returning the vitamin C to its active form (43). The active vitamin C in turn regenerates vitamin E to its active form maintaining the natural oxygen scavenging mechanisms of the skin intact.

Pycnogenol is the ideal antiaging additive since it demonstrates no chronic toxicity, mutagenicity, teratogenicity, or allergenicity (44). It is consumed orally to enhance the production of nitric oxide, which inhibits platelet aggregation in coronary artery disease, thus it is also deemed safe for topical use. Its use for skin indications is less well documented, however. In B16 melanoma cells, it was shown to inhibit tyrosinase activity and melanin biosynthesis (45). Many discussions of antioxidant flavonoids include a mention of pycnogenol, but only few quality data are presented (46).

Polyphenols

Polyphenols are a subset of flavonoids used in many cosmeceuticals. Two main sources of polyphenols are tea and fruits. Pomegranate is used as an example of a commonly used polyphenol cosmeceutical.

Pomegranate

Similar to lycopene, another oral supplement appearing in health drinks and vitamin is pomegranate extract. Pomegranate, botanically known as *Punica granatum*, is a deciduous tree bearing a red fruit native to Afghanistan, Pakistan, Iran, and northern India (47). It was brought to California by the Spanish settlers in 1769 and is commercially cultivated for its juice. The pomegranate became famous in Greek mythology when Persephone was kidnapped by Hades and taken to the Underworld to be his wife. Persephone had consumed four pomegranate seeds while in the Underworld and thus had to spend four months every year in Hades, during which time nothing would grow. This gave rise to the season of winter.

Pomegranate juice, commonly consumed in the Middle East, provides about 16% of the adult requirement of vitamin C per 100 mg serving. It also contains pantothenic acid, also known as vitamin B5, potassium, and antioxidant polyphenols. These substances have been demonstrated to protect against UVA- and UVB-induced cell damage in SKU-1064 human skin fibroblasts (48). Pomegranate juice has also been

Vitamin A metabolites	Vitamin A	Vitamin A esters
Retinoic acid R = COOH	Retinol R = CH$_2$OH	Retinyl acetate R = CH$_2$OOCCH$_3$
Retinaldehyde R = CHO		Retinyl propionate R = CH$_2$OOCC$_2$H$_5$
Tazarotene		Retinyl palmitate R = CH$_2$OOCC$_{15}$H$_{31}$

Figure 5.6 The family of over-the-counter and prescription retinoids.

purported to reduce oxidative stress and affect LDL and platelet aggregation in humans and apolipoprotein E-deficient mice (49,50). It has also been studied for improving the levels of hyperlipidemia in diabetic patients (51).

> Unfortunately, there is little evidence to support the use of most cosmeceutical active ingredients. The vehicle moisturizer remains the active agent in most cases.

Retinoids

Retinoids represent one of the most important categories of cosmeceuticals both in the prescription and the OTC realm (Fig. 5.6). Prescription retinoids, such as tretinoin, can reverse photo-induced skin changes (52–54). Tretinoin has been shown to transform an atrophic epidermis into a hyperplastic, thicker epidermis resulting in the improvement of skin wrinkling (55). Tretinoin also induces papillary dermal collagen synthesis, new blood vessel formation, increased glycosaminoglycan deposition, and exfoliation of retained stratum corneum (56,57). These histologic changes translate clinically into skin with less yellow and more pink hues accompanied by increased tactile smoothness (58). Changes may be perceived in four months in some patients who use topical tretinoin daily, but more improvement is seen with a longer therapy. Naturally, more improvement is visible in patients with severe photoaging, but results are also seen in non-sun-exposed elderly skin (59). It is interesting to note improved psychosocial status in patients who undergo topical tretinoin therapy (60).

> Retinoids represent one of the most important categories of cosmeceuticals both in the prescription and the OTC realm.

Tretinoin must be applied daily to the face to achieve reversal of photoaging. Patients who initiate treatment may experience varying degrees of erythema and dermatitis for the first two to six weeks of therapy. It is thought that the skin eventually "hardens" to the irritating effect of the tretinoin, with the disappearance of burning, pruritus, and desquamation (61). This hardening effect is lost when application is discontinued.

Topical tretinoin is the most commonly used cutaneous prescription cosmeceutical. However, successful use may require alterations in skin care products and cosmetics. During the phase of retinoid dermatitis, a mild cleansing bar may need to be substituted for a deodorant soap to prevent further xerosis and irritation. The use of all drying agents, such as astringents and toners, exfoliants, abrasive scrubbers, and cleansing masks, should be discontinued. Oil-free or water-based facial foundations will tend to adhere preferentially to facial scale, necessitating the use of an appropriate moisturizer to smooth the desquamating stratum corneum prior to application of foundation. Where possible, foundations with a higher oil content designed for dry skin can be selected. These alterations in skin care may facilitate the use of tretinoin.

In addition to prescription retinoids, OTC retinoids are found in some cosmeceuticals in the form of retinol, retinyl palmitate, retinyl propionate, and retinaldehyde. It is theoretically possible to interconvert the retinoids from one form to another. For example, retinyl palmitate and retinyl propionate, chemically known as retinyl esters, can become biologically active following a cutaneous enzymatic cleavage of the ester bond and subsequent conversion to retinol. Retinol is the naturally occurring vitamin A form found in red, yellow, and orange fruits and vegetables. Although the pigment is responsible for the vision, it is highly unstable (Fig. 5.7). Retinol can be oxidized to retinaldehyde and then oxidized to retinoic acid, also known as prescription tretinoin. It is this cutaneous conversion of retinol to retinoic acid that is responsible for the biologic activity of some of the new stabilized OTC vitamin A preparations designed to improve the appearance of benign photodamaged skin (62). Unfortunately, only small amounts of retinyl palmitate and retinol can be converted by the skin, accounting for the increased efficacy seen with prescription preparations containing retinoic acid.

> OTC retinoids include retinol, retinyl palmitate, retinyl propionate, and retinaldehyde.

The main problem with prescription retinoids is their irritancy. Unfortunately, as the biological efficacy of the retinoid increases, so does the irritancy. This is also the case with the OTC retinoids. Retinol is a greater irritant than the retinyl esters and is also more unstable. It is for this reason that cosmeceutical formulations not manufactured under strict oxygen-free conditions prefer to add retinyl palmitate to moisturizing creams. However, the retinyl palmitate may act as an antioxidant for the lipids present in the moisturizer.

The topical benefit of retinol has been documented by well-controlled studies (63). It is commonly felt among

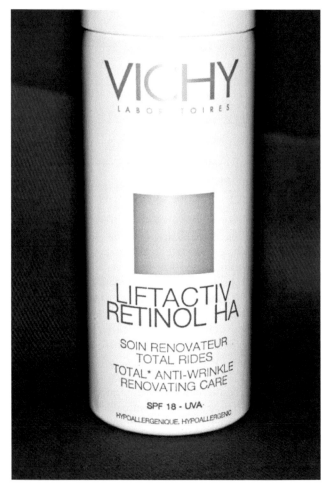

Figure 5.7 Retinol is the most popular OTC retinoid used in cosmeceutical formulations.

Table 5.4 Glycolic Acid: Different Concentrations with Different pH Levels

Concentration (%)	pH
5	1.7
10	1.6
20	1.5
30	1.4
40	1.3
50	1.2
60	1.0
70	0.6

The alpha hydroxy acids include glycolic, lactic, citric, malic, mandelic, and tartaric acids.

dermatologists that retinol is of benefit (64), but it is difficult in moisturizer studies that do not include vehicle control to separate the retinol benefit from the moisturizer benefit. Nevertheless, of all the carotenoids available for formulation, retinol has the greatest evidence to support topical application efficacy.

Hydroxy Acids

No discussion of cosmeceuticals would be complete without the mention of the hydroxy acids. The hydroxy acids were some of the first substances to initiate interest in cosmeceuticals. Interestingly, hydroxy acids represent the oldest facial cosmeceuticals. It is said that Cleopatra used the debris at the bottom of the wine barrels to massage her face. Chemically, this was the tartaric acid, thus Cleopatra was the first woman recorded to routinely apply facial alpha hydroxy acids. Alpha hydroxy acids represent a group of chemicals consisting of organic carboxylic acids in which a hydroxy group is at the alpha position. Members of this group include glycolic, lactic, citric, malic, mandelic, and tartaric acid. Glycolic acid is derived from sugar cane, lactic acid is derived from fermented milk, citric acid is found in citrus fruits, malic acid is found in unripe apples, mandelic acid is an extract of bitter almonds, and tartaric acid is found in fermented grapes (65). The acids are now produced synthetically for cosmetic use.

Glycolic acid is the most popular of the alpha hydroxy acids for antiaging purposes available in OTC and physician-dispensed products. Its pH varies with concentration, as demonstrated in Table 5.4. This acidic pH is sometimes buffered for facial application with phosphoric acid and monosodium phosphate or neutralized with sodium hydroxide (66). A desirable pH for facial application lies between 2.8 and 4.8. Glycolic acid is finding its way into formulations for facial moisturizers, cleansers, and toners. Additionally, it is used alone, or in combination with other chemicals, at various concentrations for facial peels (67–69). The epidermal effects of glycolic acid are manifested by decreased keratinocyte cohesion, which may be due to alterations in ionic bonding (70), while the dermal effects lead to increased mucopolysaccharide and collagen synthesis (71). Visibly this translates into less cutaneous wrinkling and dyspigmentation (72). Furthermore, glycolic acid may act as an antioxidant, as demonstrated by its ability to alleviate the erythema observed after ultraviolet radiation exposure to the skin (73).

Alpha hydroxy acids and tretinoin can be combined as therapy for photoaged skin since the combination is well tolerated and the effects may be additive (74). They act very different chemically since the hydrophilic alpha hydroxy acids diffuse freely throughout the watery intercellular phase while the hydrophobic retinoids require proteins in the plasma and skin to act as carriers (75). Current trends use an 8% glycolic acid moisturizer in the morning, accompanied by a bedtime use of the highest strength of tretinoin tolerated. This treatment can be supplemented with biweekly to monthly glycolic acid face peels in concentrations of 20%, 35%, 50%, and 70%. Better-controlled clinical studies with histologic evaluation are required before the optimum therapy for photoaged skin emerges (Fig. 5.8).

SKIN CARE IN MATURE PATIENTS

This chapter closes with an examination of skin care products in mature patients. These products include color cosmetics, face masks, and exfoliants. Color cosmetics are necessary to camouflage photoaging while face masks can be used to improve skin texture. Exfoliants can smooth the skin surface by minimizing the effect of the desquamatory failure found in mature skin.

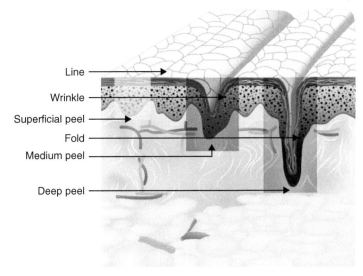

Line
Wrinkle
Superficial peel
Fold
Medium peel
Deep peel

Figure 5.8 Alpha hydroxy acid peels produce superficial skin peeling to temporarily improve skin texture and induce exfoliation.

Color cosmetics, face masks, and exfoliants can be used to improve the appearance of mature skin.

Color Cosmetics

Cutaneous sun exposure accelerates and exaggerates the clinical changes associated with advanced age (76). Thus, individuals turn to cosmetics, which can aid in the camouflage of telangiectasias and lentigines, but cannot conceal the deep wrinkling found in photoaging. Facial foundations become difficult to apply evenly and tend to migrate into cutaneous furrows. The yellow skin hue imparted by elastosis can be improved by the use of a purple undercover cosmetic, but again uniform application is difficult. The patient may attempt to solve these problems by using a high-coverage cream foundation. Unfortunately, thicker facial foundations, which can cover skin color abnormalities, only accentuate the deep wrinkling and furrows. One possible cosmetic solution is to use a white eyeliner pencil to line the depths of each furrow and a subsequent application of a moderate-coverage facial foundation appropriate for the patient's skin type. The white pigment placed at the depth of each furrow will make the recessed skin less shadowed, depending on the concept of facial contouring. Lining each furrow is time-consuming but can improve, although not eliminate, the photoaged skin appearance.

Face Masks

Face masks consist of substances applied to the face for an extended period for therapeutic and/or esthetic purposes. Masks are available for domestic and professional uses. They may be packaged in a jar or bottle for immediate application to the face or as dry ingredients in a pouch for mixing with water. Typically, a mask is applied on a weekly basis to provide a time for relaxation, an esthetically pleasing sensation, and skin benefits. There are four basic mask formulations: wax based, vinyl or rubber based, hydrocolloid, and earth based.

Wax Masks

Wax masks are popular among women who visit professional spas for their warm, esthetically pleasing feel. They are composed of beeswax or, more commonly, paraffin wax to which petroleum jelly and cetyl or stearyl alcohols have been added to provide a soft, pliable material for facial application with a soft brush. The wax is heated in a pot placed in a water bath to control the temperature and prevent burning. Sometimes the wax is dipped from the pot and painted over the face and other times it may be brushed over thin cotton gauze draped over the face. Gauze is commonly used to enable the facial technician to remove the wax in one piece (77). Gauze also prevents the wax from sticking to the vellus hairs on the face, which may be painfully epilated as the wax is peeled off the face.

Wax-based face masks temporarily impede cutaneous transepidermal water loss. This effect is limited only to the time the mask is in direct contact with the face, unless a suitable occlusive moisturizer is applied immediately following mask removal. For this reason, they are popular in persons with dry skin.

Vinyl- and Rubber-Based Masks

Vinyl and rubber-based masks are popular masks for home use, since they are easily squeezed from a pouch onto the face and removed in one piece. Rubber-based masks are usually based on latex while vinyl-based masks are based on film-forming substances, such as polyvinyl alcohol or vinyl acetate. Because of the concern over latex allergy, there are no true rubber-based masks for home use.

Vinyl masks are squeezed premixed from a tube or pouch and applied with fingertips or a wooden applicator to the face. Upon evaporation of the vehicle, a thin flexible vinyl film remains behind on the face. The mask is generally left in contact with the skin for 10 to 30 minutes and then peeled off in one sheet by loosening the edges from the face.

Vinyl and rubber masks are appropriate for all skin types. The evaporation of the vehicle from the wet mask creates a cooling sensation and the shrinking of the mask with drying may give the impression that the skin is actually tightening. These masks can temporarily impede transepidermal water loss while they are in contact with the skin.

Hydrocolloid Masks

Hydrocolloid masks are used both in professional salons and at home. Hydrocolloids are substances, such as oatmeal, that are of large molecular weight and thus interfere with transepidermal water loss. These masks are formulated from gums and humectants and enjoy tremendous popularity since many specialty ingredients are easily incorporated into their formulation. They are marketed in the form of dry ingredients in a sealed pouch that must be mixed with warm water prior to application. The resulting paste is then smeared over the face with the hands or a wooden blade and allowed to dry (78).

Hydrocolloid masks leave the skin feeling smooth, and create the sensation of skin tightening as the water evaporates and the mask dries. Temporary moisturization can occur while the mask is on the skin. Specialty additives such as honey, egg whites, chamomile flowers, aloe vera, almond oil, zinc oxide, sulfur, avocado, witch hazel, etc. may be used to customize the mask. Many spas have their own special concoction. By varying the ingredients, masks can be created for all skin types. In addition, herbal medicine can be practiced by combining various healing plants into a poultice for facial application.

Earth-Based Masks
Earth-based masks, also known as paste masks or mud packs, are formulated of absorbent clays such as bentonite, kaolin, or china clay. The clays produce an astringent effect on the skin making this mask most appropriate for oily-complected patients. The astringent effect of the mask can be enhanced through the addition of other substances such as magnesium, zinc oxide, salicylic acid, etc.

Exfoliants

Exfoliants containing hydroxy acids produce both epidermal and dermal changes. The epidermal changes are immediate and occur at the junction of the stratum corneum and stratum granulosum. They constitute a reduction in the thickness of the hyperkeratotic stratum corneum due to decreased corneocyte adhesion (79). The dermal effects, which are delayed, consist of increased glycosaminoglycan synthesis (80). These effects are most pronounced with the alpha hydroxy acids (glycolic acid, lactic acid, and malic acid), which rapidly penetrate the epidermis to enter the dermis. Individuals with sensitive skin may not be able to tolerate the low pH of 3 required to cause this epidermal renewal (81). This has led to development of polyhydroxy acids (gluconolactone, lactobionic acid, and ferulic acid), which are larger-molecular-weight hydroxy acids that do not penetrate as rapidly to the dermis. This produces less irritation; therefore, polyhydroxy acid is suitable for persons with sensitive skin, eczema, and atopic dermatitis.

Another mechanism for reducing the irritation of chemical exfoliants is through neutralization or buffering. Irritation can also be minimized by raising the exfoliant pH through sodium hydroxide neutralization; however, this also reduces the exfoliation produced. The use of buffering agents, such as phosphoric acid or monosodium phosphate, is preferable since the buffer maintains the product at a desired pH (82). Ideally, the pH of an exfoliant solution should not be lower than 3. Exfoliation is induced more with a lower pH, since the hydroxy acid concentration is increased, but a greater irritation in the form of stinging and burning is also expected.

Beta hydroxy acids, such as salicylic acid, may also be used, but do not produce dermal penetration. Salicylic acid is technically not a beta hydroxy acid; it is rather a phenolic compound, but the marketing nomenclature has popularized this terminology. Salicylic acid is an oil-soluble acid, as compared with the alpha hydroxy acids that are mainly water soluble, and remains on the skin surface. Since exfoliation occurs on the skin surface, this is a desirable characteristic that minimizes irritation.

Exfoliants provide the quickest way to improve the appearance of aging skin. They can improve skin smoothness, skin color, and skin light reflection. This can result in the aggressive use of these products, but the benefits decline if used continuously.

SUMMARY

Cosmeceuticals form an important part of the OTC skin treatment market in aging skin. It is felt that cosmeceutical development has been stymied largely due to the failure of the FDA to develop a new classification system. It is thought that a new "quasi-drug" category, similar to the Japanese designation, would allow the introduction of more robust active ingredients into cosmeceuticals. These more robust ingredients would provide enhanced consumer-perceived skin benefits, supporting stronger claims.

In summary, I believe that cosmeceuticals will become an ever-increasing part of the fund of knowledge of dermatology. We are now only at the beginning of the cosmeceutical story. Cosmeceuticals were derived from the cosmetic industry's desire to go beyond simply adorning the skin. They wanted to improve the appearance of the skin by tackling important functional issues to meet the demands of consumers. Now, the cosmeceutical category needs to learn from the drug category. The principles of the scientific method must be applied to the clinical study of cosmeceuticals. No longer can in vitro data be used to extrapolate visible clinical results, nor can 15-subject studies be used to determine the value of a specific ingredient. Trends without statistical significance are of no use anymore, to confirm the skin effect of a given formulation. Dermatology will move the cosmeceutical category forward and the cosmeceutical category will move dermatology forward.

REFERENCES

1. Vermeer BJ, Gilchrest BA. Cosmeceuticals. A proposal for rational definition, evaluation and regulation. Arch Dermatol 1996; 132: 337.
2. Kligman AM. Cosmeceuticals as a third category. Cosmet Toilet 1998; 113: 33.
3. Gilchrest BA. Cellular and molecular changes in aging skin. J Geriatr Dermatol 1994; 2: 3–6.
4. Hurley HJ. Skin in senescence: a summation. J Geriatr Dermatol 1993; 1: 55–61.
5. West MD. The cellular and molecular biology of skin aging. Arch Dermatol 1994; 130: 87–95.
6. Griffiths CEM, Wag TS, Hamilton TA, Voorhees JJ, Ellis CN. A photonumeric scale for the assessment of cutaneous photodamage. Arch Dermatol 1992; 128: 347–51.
7. Kligman AM. Early destructive effects of sunligt on human skin. J Am Med Assoc 1969; 210: 2377–80.
8. Majmudar G, Nelson BR, Mazany KD, Billard M, Johnson TM. Cutaneous aging and collagen. J Geriatr Dermatol 1994; 2: 36–44.
9. Suader DN. The immunology of aging skin. J Geriatr Dermatol 1994; 2: 15–18.
10. Kligman LH, Kligman AM. Ultraviolet radiation-induced skin aging. In: Lowe NJ, Shaath NA, eds. Sunscreens Development, Evaluation and Regulatory Aspects. New York: Marcel Dekker, Inc., 1990: 55–60.
11. Braverman IM, Fonferko E. Studies in cutaneous aging. I. The elastic fiber network. J Invest Dermatol 1982; 78: 434–44.

12. Uitto JJ. Intrinsic aging changes in the dermis. J Geriatr Dermatol 1994; 2: 7–14.

13. Chotnopparatpattara P, Panyakhamlerd K, Taechakraichana N, et al. An effect of hormone replacement therapy on skin thickness in early post-menopausal women. J Med Assoc Thai 2001; 84: 1275–80.

14. Callens A, Vaillant L, Lecomte P, et al. Does hormonal skin aging exist? A study of the influence of different hormone therapy regimens on the skin of postmenopausal women using non-invasive measurement techniques. Dermatology 1996; 193: 289–94.

15. Sumino H, Ichikawa S, Abe M, et al. Effects of aging, menopause, and hormone replacement therapy on forearm skin elasticity in women. J Am Geriatr Soc 2004; 52: 945–9.

16. Pierard-Franchimont C, Letawe C, Goffin V, Pierard GE. Skin water holding capacity and transdermal therapy for menopause: a pilot study. Maturitas 1995; 22: 151–4.

17. Sauerbronn AV, Fonseca AM, Bagnoli VR, Saldiva PH, Pinotti JA. The effects of systemic hormonal replacement therapy on the skin of post-menopausal women. Int J Gynaecol Obstet 2000; 68: 35–41.

18. Schmidt JB, Binder M, Demschik G, Bieglmayer C, Reiner A. Treatment of aging skin with topical estrogens. Int J Dermatol 1996; 35: 669–74.

19. Shah MG, Maibach HI. Estrogen and skin. An overview. Am J Clin Dermatol 2001; 2: 143–50.

20. Kotsopoulos D, Dalais FS, Liang YL, McGrath BP, Teede HJ. The effects of soy protein containing phytoestrogens on menopausal symptoms in post-menopausal women. Climacteric 2000; 3: 161–7.

21. Smith MA, Fine JA, Barnhill RL, Berwick M. Hormonal and reproductive influences and risk of melanoma in women. Int J Epidemiol 1998; 27: 751–7.

22. Sumino H, Ichikawa S, Abe M, et al. Effects of aging and postmenopausal hypoestrogenism on skin elasticity and bone mineral density in Japanese women. Endocr J 2004; 51: 159–64.

23. Hussein G, Sankawa U, Goto H, Matsumoto K, Watanabe H. Astaxanthin, a carotenoid with potential in human health and nutrition. J Nat Prod 2006; 69: 443–9.

24. Karppi J, Rissanen TH, Nyyssonen K, et al. Effects of astaxanthin supplementation of lipid peroxidation. Int J Vitam Nutr Res 2007; 77: 3–11.

25. Seki T. Effects of astaxanthin on human skin. Fragrance J 2001; 12: 98–103.

26. Higuera-Ciapara I, Felix-Valenzuela L, Goycoolea FM. Astaxanthin: a review of its chemistry and applications. Crit Rev Food Sci Nutr 2006; 46: 185–96.

27. Tso MO, Lam TT. Method of retarding and ameliorating central nervous system and eye damage. US Patent #5527533. Board of trustees of the University of Illinois, USA, 1996.

28. Pashkow FJ, Watumull DG, Campbell Cl. Astaxanthin: a novel potential treatment for oxidative stress and inflammation in cardiovascular disease. Am J Cardiol 2008; 101: 58D–68D.

29. Alves-Rodrigues A, Shao A. The science behind lutein. Toxical Lett 2004; 150: 57–83.

30. Barclay L. Lutein Improves Visual Function in Age-Related Macular Degeneration. Medscape Medical News. [Available from: http://www.medscape.com]

31. Arct J, Pytokowska K. Flavonoids as components of biologically active cosmeceuticals. Clin Dermatol 2008; 26: 347–57.

32. Hatcher H, Planalp R, Cho J, Torti FM, Torti SV. Curcumin: from ancient medicine to current clinical trials. Cell Mol Life Sci. 2008; 65: 1631–52.

33. Jagetia GC, Aggarwal BB. "Spicing up" of the immune system by curcumin. J Clin Immunol 2007; 27: 19–35.

34. Katiyar SK, Korman NJ, Mukhtar H, Agarwal R. Protective effects of silymarin against photocarcinogenesis in a mouse skin model. J Natl Cancer Inst 1997; 89: 556–66.

35. Katiyar SK. Silymarin and skin cancer prevention: anti-inflammatory, antioxidant and immunomodulatory effects (Review). Int J Oncol 2005; 26: 169–76.

36. Chatterjee L, Agarwal R, Mukhtar H. Ultraviolet B radiation-induced DNA lesions in mouse epidermis: an assessment sing a novel 32P-postlabeling technique. Biochem Biophys Res Commun 1996; 229: 590–5.

37. Toklu HZ, Tunali-Akbay T, Erkanli G, et al. Silymarin, the antioxidant component of Silybum marianum, protects against burn-induced oxidative skin injury. Burn 2007; 33: 908–16.

38. Berardesca E, Cameli N, Cavallotti C, et al. Combined effects of silymarin and methyisulfonylmethane in the managementof rosacea: clinical and instrumental evaluation. J Cosmet Dermatol. 2008; 7: 8–14.

39. [Available from: http://www.drugs.com/npp/pyconogenol.html], accessed December 7, 2008.

40. Devaraj S, Vega-Lopez S, Kaul N, et al. Supplementation with a pine bark extract rich in polyphenols increases plasma antioxidant capacity and alters the plasma lipoprotein profile. Lipids 2002; 37: 931–4.

41. Cesarone MR, Belcaro G, Rohdewald P, et al. Improvement of diabetic microangiopathy with pycnogenol: a prospective, controlled study. Angiology 2006; 57: 431–6.

42. Vinciguerra G, Belcaro G, Cesarone MR, et al. Cramps and muscular pain: prevention with pycnogenol in normal subjects, venous patients, athletes, claudicants and in diabetic microaniopathy. Angiology 2006; 57: 331–9.

43. Cossins E, Lee R, Packer L. ESR studies of vitamin C regeneration, order of reactivity of natural source phytochemical preparations. Biochem Mol Biol Int 1998; 45: 583–98.

44. Schonlau F. The cosmetic pycnogenol. J Appl Cosmetol 2002; 20: 241–6.

45. Kim YJ, Kang KS, Yokozawa T. The anti-melanogenic effect of pycnogenol by its anti-oxidative actions. Food Chem Toxicol 2008; 46: 2466–71.

46. Rona C, Vailati F, Berardesca E. The cosmetic treatment of wrinkles. J Cosmet Dermatol 2004; 3: 26–34.

47. Jurenka JS. Therapeutic applications of pomegranate (Punica granatum L.): a review. Altern Med Rev 2008; 13: 128–44.

48. Pacheco-Palencia LA, Noratto G, Hingorani L, Talcott ST, Mertens-Talcott SU. Protective effects of standardized pomegranate (Punica granatum L.) polyphenolic extract in ultraviolet-irradiated human skin fibroblasts. J Agric Food Chem 2008; 56: 8434–41.

49. Aviram M, Rosenblat M, Gaitini D, et al. Pomegranate juice consumption for 3years by patients with carotid artery stenosis reduces common carotid intima-media thickness, blood pressure and LDL oxidation. Clin Nutr 2004; 23: 423–33.

50. Aviram M, Dornfeld L, Rosenblat M, et al. Pomegranate juice consumption reduces oxidative stress, atherogenic modifications to LDL, and platelet aggregation: studies in humans and in atherosclerotic apolipoprotein e-deficient mice. Am J Clin Nutr 2000; 71: 1062–76.

51. Esmaillzadeh A, Tahbaz F, Gaieni I, et al. Concentrated pomegranate juice improves profiles in diabetic patients with hyperlipidemia. J Med Food 2004; 7: 305–8.

52. Kligman AM, Grove GL, Hirose R, Leyden JJ. Topical tretinoin for photoaged skin. J Am Acad Dermatol 1986; 15: 836–59.

53. Weiss JS, Ellis CN, Headington JT, et al. Topical tretinoin improves photoaged skin. JAMA 1988; 259: 527.

54. Weiss JS, Ellis CN, Headington JT, Voorhees JJ. Topical tretinoin in the treatment of aging skin. J Am Acad Dermatol 1988; 19: 169–75.

55. Hermittte R. Aged skin, retinoids, and alpha hydroxy acids. Cosmet Toilet 1992; 107: 63–7.

56. Goldfarb MT, Ellis CN, Weiss JS, Voorhees JJ. Topical tretinoin therapy: its use in photoaged skin. J Am Acad Dermatol 1989; 21: 645–50.

57. Bhawan J, Gonzalez-Serva A, Nehal K, et al. Effects of tretinoin on photodamaged skin. Arch Dermatol 1991; 127: 666–72.

58. Olsen EA, Katz HI, Levine N, et al. Tretinoin emollient cream: a new therapy for photodamaged skin. J Am Acad Dermatol 1992; 26: 215–24.

59. Kligman AM, Dogadkina D, Lavker RM. Effects of topical tretinoin on non-sun-exposed protected skin of the elderly. J Am Acad Dermatol 1993; 29: 25–33

60. Gupta MA, Goldfarb MT, Schork NJ, et al. Treatment of mildly to moderately photoaged skin with topical tretinoin has a favorable psychosocial effect: a prospective study. J Am Acad Dermatol 1991; 24: 780–1.

61. Weinstein GD, Nigra TP, Pochi PE, Savin RC. Topical tretinoin for treatment of photodamaged skin. Arch Dermatol 1991; 127: 659–65.

62. Duell EA, Derguini F, Kang S, Elder JT, Voorhees JJ. Extraction of human epidermis treated with retinol yields retro-retinoids in addition to free retinol and retinyl esters. J Invest Dermatol 1996; 107: 178–82.

63. Kafi R, Swak HS, Schumacher WE, et al. Improvement of naturally aged skin with vitamin A (retinol). Arch Dermatol 2007; 143: 606–12.

64. Hruza GJ. Retinol benefits naturally aged skin. J Watch Dermatol 2007.

65. Rosan AM. The chemistry of alpha-hydroxy acids. Cosmet Dermatol Suppl 1994: 4–11.

66. Yu RJ, Van Scott EJ. Alpha-hydroxy acids: science and therapeutic use. Cosmet Dermatol Suppl 1994: 12–20.

67. Moy LS, Murad H, Moy RL. Glycolic acid peels for the treatment of wrinkles and photoaging. J Dermatol Surg Oncol 1993; 19: 243–6.

68. Moy LS, Murad H, Moy RL. Glycolic acid therapy: evaluation of efficacy and techniques in treatment of photodamage lesions. Am J Cosmet Surg 1993; 10: 9–13.

69. Elson ML. The art of chemical peeling. Cosmet Dermatol Suppl 1994: 24–8.

70. Van Scott JE, Yu RJ. Hyperkeratinization, corneocyte cohesion and alpha hydroxy acids. J Am Acad Dermatol 1984; 11: 867–79.
71. Van Scott JE, Yu RJ. Alpha hydroxyacids: therapeutic potentials. Can J Dermatol 1989; 1: 108–12.
72. Van Scott EJ, Yu RJ. Alpha hydroxy acids: procedures for use in clinical practice. Cutis 1989; 43: 222–8.
73. Perricone NV. An alpha hydroxy acid acts as an antioxidant. J Geriatr Dermatol 1993; 1: 101–4.
74. Kligman AM. Compatibility of a glycolic acid cream with topical tretinoin for the treatment of the photo damaged face of older women. J Geriatr Dermatol 1993; 1: 179–81.
75. Hermittte R. Aged skin, retinoids, and alpha hydroxy acids. Cosmet Toilet 1992; 107: 63–7.
76. Gilchrest BA. Overview of skin aging. J Cutan Aging Cosmet Dermatol 1988; 1: 1–3.
77. Gerson J. Milady's Standard Textbook for Professional Estheticians. Buffalo, NY: Milady, 1992: 240–2.
78. Draelos ZD. Cosmetics in Dermatology, 2nd edn. Edinburgh: Churchill Livingstone (WB Saunders), 1995: 213.
79. Dietre CM, Griffin TD, Murphy CF, et al. Effects of alpha-hydroxy acids on photoaged skin. J Am Acad Dermatol 1996; 34: 187–95.
80. Van Scott JE, Yu RJ. Hyperkeratinization, corneocyte cohesion and alpha hydroxy acids. J Am Acad Dermatol 1984; 11: 867–79.
81. Smith WP. Hydroxy acids and skin aging. Cosmet Toilet 1994; 109: 41–8.
82. Yu RJ, Van Scott EJ. Alpha hydroxy acids: science and therapeutic use. Cosmet Dermat Suppl 1994: 12–20.

SUGGESTED READING

Babamiri K, Nassab R. Cosmeceuticals: the evidence behind the retinoids. Aesthet Surg J 2010; 30: 74–7.
Beer K, Kellner E, Beer J. Cosmeceuticals for rejuvenation. Facial Plast Surg 2009; 25: 285–9.
Briden ME. Alpha-hydroxyacid chemical peeling agents: case studies and rationale for safe and effective use. Cutis 2004; 73: 18–24.
Bruce S. Cosmeceuticals for the attenuation of extrinsic and intrinsic dermal aging. J Drugs Dermatol 2008; 7 (2 Suppl): s17–22.
Choi CM, Berson DS. Cosmeceuticals. Semin Cutan Med Surg 2006; 25: 163–8.
Contet-Audonneau J-L, Danoux L, Gauche D, Pauly G. Stress, apoptosis and ageing in human skin. IFSCC Magazine 2001; 4: 115–24.
Draelos ZD. Clinical situations conducive to proactive skin health and anti-aging improvement. J Invest Dermatol Symp Proc 2008; 13: 25–7.
Draelos ZD. Concepts in a multiprong approach to photoaging. Skin Ther Lett 2006; 11: 1–3.
Draelos ZD. The cosmeceutical realm. Clin Dermatol 2008; 26: 627–32.
Draelos ZD. Concepts in skin care maintenance. Cutis 2005; 76 (6 Suppl): 19–25.
Fisher G, Kang S, Varani J, et al. Mechanisms of photoaging and chronological skin aging. Arch Dermatol 2002; 138: 1462–70.
Gao XH, Zhang L, Wei H, Chen HD. Efficacy and safety of innovative cosmeceuticals. Clin Dermatol 2008; 26: 367–74.
Giacomoni PU. Advancement in skin aging: the future cosmeceuticals. Clin Dermatol 2008; 26: 364–6.
Gilchrest B. Skin aging 2003: recent advances and current concepts. Cutis 2003; 72: 5–10.
Glaser DA. Anti-aging products and cosmeceuticals. Facial Plast Surg Clin North Am 2004; 12: 363–72, vii.
Green BA, Edison BL, Lee Y. Treatment of Photoaged Hands. C & T.
Grimes P, Green BA, Wildnauer RH, Edison BL. The use of polyhydroxy acids(PHAs) in photoaged skin. Cutis 2004; 73: 3–13.
Katsambas AD, Katoulis AC. Topical retinoids in the treatment of aging of the skin. Adv Exp Med Biol 1999; 455: 477–82.
Kawi N. Phytoestrogens: applications of soy isoflavones in skin care. Cosmet Toilet Magazine 2003; 118: 73–80.
Kennedy C, Bastiaens M, Bajdik C, et al. Effect of smoking and sun on the aging skin. J Invest Dermatol 2003; 120: 548–54.
Kligman A. The treatment of photoaged human skin by topical tretinoin. Drugs 1989; 38: 1–8.
Kligman AM. Topical treatments for photoaged skin. Separating the reality from the hype. Postgrad Med 1997; 102: 115–8, 123–6.
Kligman A, Grove G, Hirose R, Leyden J. Topical tretinoin for photoaged skin. J Am Acad Dermatol 1986; 15 (4 pt 2): 836–59.
Kockaert M, Neumann M. Systemic and topical drugs for aging skin. J Drugs Dermatol 2003; 2: 435–41.
Kullavanijaya P, Lim H. Photoprotection. J Am Acad Dermatol 2005; 52: 937–58.
Larrabee WF Jr, Caro I. The aging face. Why changes occur, how to correct them. Postgrad Med 1984; 76: 37–9, 42–6.
Mukherjee S, Date A, Patravale V, et al. Retinoids in the treatment of skin aging: an overview of clinical efficacy and safety. Clin Interv Aging 2006; 1: 327–48.
Petkovich PM. Retinoic acid metabolism. J Am Acad Dermatol 2001; 45: S136–42.
Pinnell S. Cutaneous photodamage, oxidative stress, and topical antioxidant protection. J Am Acad Dermatol 2003; 48: 1–20.
Rivers JK. The role of cosmeceuticals in antiaging therapy. Skin Ther Lett 2008; 13: 5–9.
Robinson LR, Fitzgerald NC, Doughty DG, et al. Topical palmitoyl pentapeptide provides improvement in photoaged human facial skin. Int J Cosmet Sci 2005; 27: 155–60.
Sadick NS. Cosmeceuticals. Their role in dermatology practice. J Drugs Dermatol 2003; 2: 529–37.
Scully K. Topical agents for the aging face. J Cutan Med Surg 1999; 3 (Suppl 4): 51–6.
Serri R, Iorizzo M. Cosmeceuticals: focus on topical retinoids in photoaging. Clin Dermatol 2008; 26: 633–5.
Singh M, Griffiths CE. The use of retinoids in the treatment of photoaging. Dermatol Ther 2006; 19: 297–305.
Sorg O, Antille C, Kaya G, Saurat JH. Retinoids in cosmeceuticals. Dermatol Ther 2006; 19: 289–96.
Stratigos AJ, Katsambas AD. The role of topical retinoids in the treatment of photoaging. Drugs 2005; 65: 1061–72.
Thornton MJ. The biological actions of estrogens on skin. Exp Dermatol 2002; 11: 487–502.

6   Facial scarring and camouflaging

Special color cosmetics are available for individuals with acquired or congenital contour and color defects of the face. These cosmetics are known as camouflage cosmetics since they attempt to recreate a more attractive appearance. They do not, however, duplicate the appearance of a freshly washed, unadorned face. It is obvious to all that the individual is wearing a cosmetic. Therefore, camouflage cosmetics are designed to minimize facial defects while accentuating the attractive features of the face (1).

Paramedical camouflage artists, estheticians, dermatologists, plastic surgeons, and cosmetic consultants use camouflaging cosmetics. Their successful use requires a well-formulated, quality product applied with the skill of a stage makeup technician and the artistic abilities of a painter.

CAMOUFLAGING OF FACIAL DEFECTS

Key to understanding the importance and use of camouflage cosmetics is a basic discussion of the types of facial defects that can occur. There are defects of contour, pigmentation, or a combination of both.

> Camouflaging is required for facial defects of contour, pigmentation, or a combination of both.

Defects of contour are defined as areas where the scar tissue is hypertrophied or atrophied. In addition, the scar tissue may also demonstrate a texture difference due to absence of follicular ostia and hair. Pigmentation defects are abnormalities solely in the color of the skin and not in the texture. Some pigmentation abnormalities arise from tumors of the skin while others are due to systemic abnormalities or extrinsic effects, such as sun exposure (Table 6.1) (2,3).

These defects can be camouflaged using principles that are adapted from stage makeup texts. Camouflaging is the art of illusion and demands that the cosmetics be applied both with skill and artistic ability. Fortunately, the cosmetics can be easily applied and removed providing opportunity for experimentation and easy alteration of a bad result.

Facial Scar Recontouring

The basic concept of facial scar recontouring is predicated on the fact that dark colors make surfaces recede while light colors make surfaces appear to project (4). Thus, lighter colors will minimize depressed areas of scarring while darker colors will minimize protuberant areas of the scar.

> Facial scar contouring is predicated on the fact that dark colors make surfaces recede while light colors make surfaces appear to project.

Figure 6.1 demonstrates how this technique works on a patient who has sustained a depressed scar following a surgery for the removal of a skin cancer on the nose. The scar itself is

lightened to compensate for decreased light reflection while the sides and tip of the nose are darkened to draw attention away from the surgical defect.

Camouflaging of Pigmentation Defects

Pigmentation defects can be camouflaged by either applying an opaque cosmetic that allows none of the abnormal underlying skin tones to be appreciated or by applying foundations of complementary colors (Fig. 6.2). For example, red pigmentation defects can be camouflaged by applying a green foundation, which is the complementary color to red. The blending of the red skin with the green foundation yields a brown tone, which can be readily covered by a more conventional facial foundation. Furthermore, yellow skin tones can be blended with a complementary colored purple foundation to also yield brown tones. Skin areas that are lighter or darker than desired complexion can be camouflaged by applying facial foundations with the appropriate amount of brown pigment to hide the defect (5) (Fig. 6.3).

> Pigmentation defects can be camouflaged either by applying an opaque cosmetic that allows none of the abnormal underlying skin tones to be appreciated or by applying foundations of complementary colors.

CAMOUFLAGE COSMETICS

There are many companies in the U.S.A. and Europe, who manufacture cosmetics specifically designed for camouflaging purposes. A good camouflage artist will generally purchase a color palette from at least two different companies to provide the necessary mixture of cosmetic shades required to match a given patient's skin tone (6).

Different formulations of camouflaging cosmetics are designed to meet the needs of each defect to be concealed. The basic products required for camouflaging are makeup bases, lining colors, and rouges. Makeup bases or facial foundations are designed to create the desired skin color. They are available as hard grease paints, soft grease paints, pancakes, and liquids. Hard grease paints come in stick form and consist of pigments in an anhydrous, waxy base. Application requires great skill and is more time consuming than other makeup bases. This product is extremely long-wearing, but mainly reserved for theatrical uses.

Soft grease paints come in a jar or are squeezed from a tube and have a creamy texture due to the incorporation of low viscosity oils in addition to waxes in the anhydrous preparation (Fig. 6.4). They usually contain a high proportion of titanium dioxide to provide superior coverage (7). These products tend to have a high shine and do not survive body heat, thus some type of setting preparation is required to prolong wear.

Pancake products are packaged in a flat, round container. The product is removed from the compact by stroking with a wet sponge (Fig. 6.5). It is composed of talc, kaolin, zinc oxide, precipitated chalk, titanium dioxide, and iron oxide (8). This product dries quickly and possesses a matte, or dull, finish. Unfortunately, it is easily removed with body warmth and perspiration, but is easy to retouch, if necessary (Fig. 6.6).

Liquid foundations for camouflaging are similar to those marketed for general use; however, increased amounts of titanium dioxide provide a superior coverage. Also, these products usually contain higher concentration oils to allow a complete color development and improved wearability. Special liquid cosmetics are available for application under a traditional facial foundation. These products, as discussed previously, are formulated with green and purple pigments to camouflage red and yellow color defects, respectively.

> Liquid foundations for camouflaging are similar to those marketed for general use; however increased amounts of titanium dioxide provide superior coverage.

Special colors are required in localized facial areas to provide shading and highlighting for contour defects. Products used for this purpose are known as lining colors, also called moist rouges, and dry rouges, otherwise called powdered rouges. Lining colors are available in all shades of gray, maroon, red, brown, green, blue, white, and black. They are packaged both in hard sticks and soft tins. These products can be mixed to obtain the desired final specialty color for use. Dry rouges are compressed powder compacts and are available in shades of red. They do not wear as long as their oil-containing counterparts, but are easily used for quick touch-ups and final shading purposes.

APPLICATION OF CAMOUFLAGE COSMETICS
The most popular camouflage facial foundations are the creamy products, which are scooped from a jar or tin with a spatula and applied to the hand for warming. These products are the easiest to use since they exhibit a long playtime, good blending characteristics, minimal application skill, excellent coverage, and adequate wearability for most individuals (9).

Initially, a makeup base must be selected that is closest to the patient's natural skin color. Blending usually is necessary, but no more than three colors should be combined as this produces a final muddy color quality. If the patient has an underlying pigmentation problem, this counts as one color. In this case, the pink color of the wound due to an increased vascular supply to promote healing, counts as one color. Other color abnormalities may be due to increased melanin, producing a brown color, or increased hemosiderin, producing a rust color, or degenerated facial elastin, producing a yellow color, etc.

Depending on the situation, it may be desirable to camouflage the red hues by initially applying a green undercover cosmetic and then a traditional facial foundation, thus

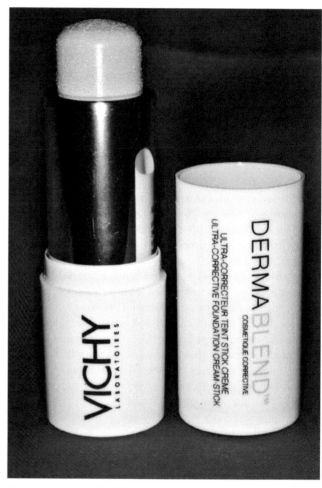

Figure 6.2 An opaque facial foundation that camouflages underlying pigmentation abnormalities can be easily applied from a roll-up tube.

Table 6.1 Facial Pigmentation Defects

Facial color	Disease process	Foundation color
Red	Psoriasis, lupus, rosacea	Green undercover foundation
Yellow	Solar elastosis, chemotherapy, dialysis	Purple undercover foundation
Brown hyperpigmentation	Chloasma, lentigines, nevi	White undercover foundation
Hypopigmentation and depigmentation	Post-inflammatory, congenital, vitiligo	Brown undercover foundation

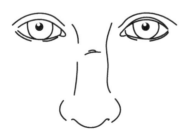 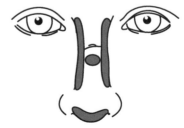

Figure 6.1 Cosmetic camouflaging of a depressed scar on the nose.

avoiding the surgical products. If, however, the color contrast is too prominent, a high coverage surgical foundation that covers all underlying skin tones may be a better camouflaging makeup selection.

Once the closest foundation color has been selected, it may necessary to blend in yellow, if the individual has a sallow complexion, or red, if the patient has a ruddy complexion, etc. All facial tones should be represented in the final foundation blend if a good color match is to be obtained. Blending is

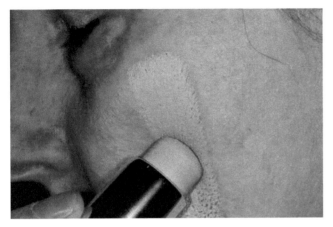

Figure 6.3 The brown facial foundation can be stroked directly over the facial pigmentation defect.

usually done by applying a small amount of the makeup to the back of the hand. This provides a good surface for blending, which can be easily held up to the face to evaluate the color match, and also warms the product which allows an easier mixing and application.

The final foundation color mix is then dabbed, not rubbed, over the scarred area and then applied from the central face outward into the hairline for approximately 0.25 inch and blended over the ears and beneath the chin. It is necessary to feather the cosmetic where the application ends to achieve a more natural appearance. The importance of dabbing cannot be overemphasized since scars do not contain appendageal structures, such as follicular ostia, that are necessary for good cosmetic adherence. Rubbing will remove the makeup as it is applied. The cosmetic should be actually pressed into the skin and allowed to dry for five minutes.

Following this brief drying period, the cosmetic must be set with an unpigmented, finely ground, talc-based powder to prevent smudging, improve wearability, provide waterproof characteristic, and impart a matte finish. Camouflaging make-ups are designed to be worn with this powder and do not function properly without it. The powder should be pressed, not dusted, on top of the foundation.

Lastly, shading and highlighting principles are employed to minimize the scar contour abnormalities. Unfortunately,

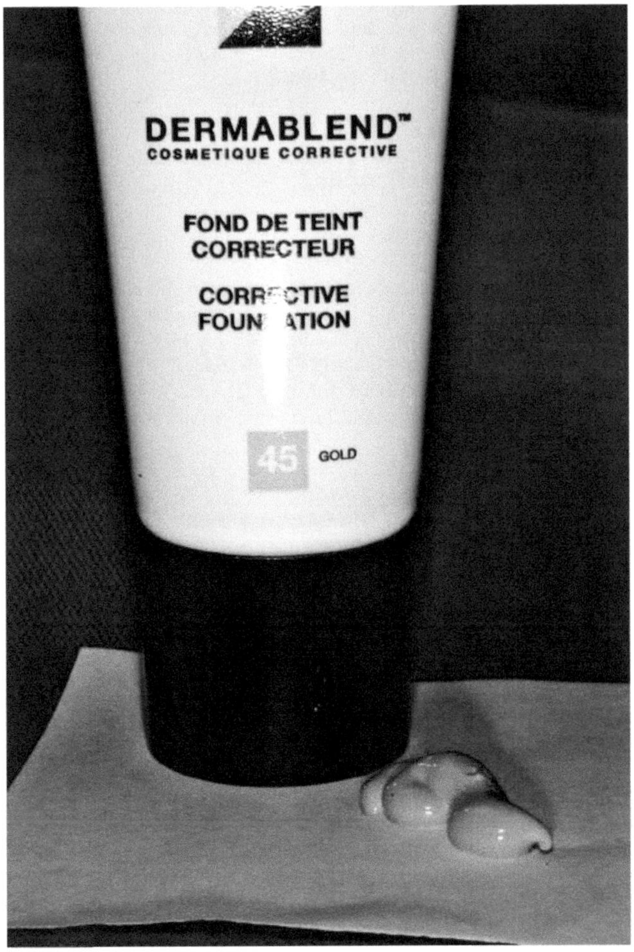

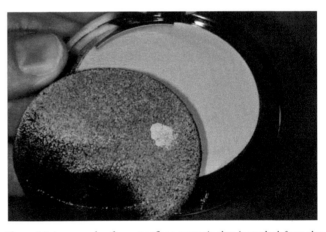

Figure 6.5 An example of a camouflage cosmetic that is stroked from the compact with a wet sponge.

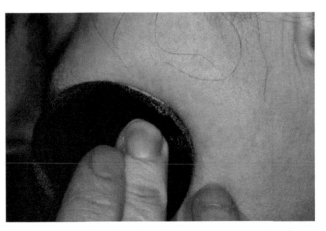

Figure 6.6 The cream foundation is stroked from a sponge onto the entire face or just the areas where camouflage is required.

Figure 6.4 Camouflage cosmetics can be squeezed from a tube for application to the face.

the camouflage foundation may actually accentuate the surface irregularities of the scar and normal skin structures, such as pores and wrinkles. Depressed scars usually appear darker than the surrounding skin even though the same color foundation has been applied, due to the presence of shadows. Figure 6.1 demonstrates areas to be highlighted in an atrophic scar. Thus, a lighter powdered rouge is applied over the scar. If the scar is elevated, a darker powdered rouge needs to be applied. Lastly, a reddish powdered rouge is dusted over the central face (central forehead, nose, and chin) and upper cheeks to mimic natural color variations of the face. Unfortunately, the high-coverage surgical makeup also covers these facial landmarks resulting in a flat, mask-like face. Other colored facial cosmetics (eye shadow, eyeliner, mascara, etc.) are usually necessary to give an attractive final appearance (10).

In general, the removal of camouflaging cosmetics requires more than soap and water washing because of the waterproof nature of the product. Most companies provide an oily cleanser for cosmetic removal and then recommend soap and water cleansing of the skin. The cosmetic should only be worn when needed and definitely thoroughly removed at bedtime (11).

Camouflage cosmetics are generally used by patients without difficulty. Usually, a specially trained paramedical camouflage artist or esthetician will train the patient in proper blending and application of the makeup. Two to three hourly session are enough to solve most of the problems encountered with the cosmetic, but sometimes special difficulties arise. Most camouflage foundations contain a high concentration of oils which may rarely cause comedone formation in predisposed individuals. Evaluating ingredient lists for the absence or presence of comedogenic oils is not of much practical value; rather the foundation should be tested by the patient. This is accomplished by applying a little amount of the cosmetic to the upper lateral cheek for two to four weeks, followed by a dermatologic evaluation.

Acne can also arise in certain susceptible individuals who use camouflaging foundations. Camouflaging cosmetics are much more likely to be acnegenic than comedogenic, since they are worn for a prolonged period of time and must be occlusive to provide adequate coverage and waterproof properties. The occlusion may also lead to miliaria formation. However, allergic contact dermatitis to camouflage makeups is rare since the formulation is generally fragrance-free with a low preservative concentration. It is possible, however, for both allergic and irritant contact dermatitis to occur from the use of camouflage cosmetics. These products can be open or closed patch tested "as is."

BODY CAMOUFLAGING

Camouflaging cosmetics appropriate for covering macular pigmentation defects on the legs, arms, and body are also available. The easiest products to apply are thinner creams squeezed from a tube that spread better over larger areas, but provide less coverage than the thicker facial products. Unfortunately, application is difficult and unsatisfactory in body areas densely covered with hair. Application with a sponge is recommended followed by loose powder to improve wearability and impart a better waterproof finish. A special removal product is required.

Camouflaging cosmetics appropriate for covering macular pigmentation defects on the legs, arms, and body are also available.

These products use either zinc oxide or titanium dioxide for coverage, iron pigments for color, methyl cellulose or other waxes for viscosity, and glycerin or other nonevaporating substances for increased adherence of the product to the skin. They are a rare cause of irritant or allergic contact dermatitis and can be open or closed patch tested "as is."

SUMMARY

Camouflaging techniques are important to the dermatologist who may need to counsel patients on temporary use or permanent use. For temporary redness or discoloration of the skin that may occur after a surgery or laser resurfacing, a camouflage cosmetic will be used for a limited period until the skin heals. Other patients may experience permanent contour or pigmentation problems that require continued use of camouflaging techniques. This chapter has highlighted the theory, application, and removal of cosmetics for camouflaging purposes.

REFERENCES

1. Stewart TW, Savage D. Cosmetic camouflage in dermatology. Br J Dermatol 1972; 86: 530–2.
2. Draelos ZK. Cosmetic camouflaging techniques. Cutis 1993; 52: 362–4.
3. Benmaman O, Sanchez JL. Treatment and camouflaging of pigmentary disorders. Clin Dermatol 1988; 6: 50–61.
4. Helland JR, Schneider MF. Special features. New York: M Evans and Company, 1985: 41–6.
5. Draelos ZD. Use of cover cosmetics for pigmentation abnormalities. Cosmet Dermatol 1989; 2: 14–16.
6. Rayner V. Clinical cosmetology: a medical approach to esthetics procedures. Albany, New York: Milady Publishing Company, 1993: 116–22.
7. Schlossman ML, Feldman AJ. Fluid foundation and blush makeup. In: deNavarre MG, ed. The Chemistry and Manufacture of Cosmetics. Wheaton, Illinois: Allured Publishing Company, 1988: 748–51.
8. Wilkinson JB, Moore RJ. Harry's cosmeticology, 7th edn. New York: Chemical Publishing, 1982: 304–7.
9. Reisch M. Masking agents as adjunct therapy in cutaneous disorders. Clin Med 1961; 8.
10. Draelos ZD. Cosmetics have a positive effect on the postsurgical patient. Cosmet Dermatol 1991; 4: 11–14.
11. Thomas RJ, Bluestein JL. Cosmetics and hairstyling as adjuvants to scar camouflage. In: Thomas RJ, Richard G, eds. Facial scars, St. Louis: CV Mosby, 1989: 349–51.

SUGGESTED READING

Akerson J, Imokawa G. Miscellaneous skin care products; skin bleaches and others (Chapter 19). In: Reiger MM, ed. Harry's Cosmeticology, 8th edn. Chemical Publishing Co., Inc., 2000: 393–413.
Antoniou C, Stefanaki C. Cosmetic camouflage. J Cosmet Dermatol 2006; 5: 297–301.
Aydogdu E, Misirlioglu A, Eker G, Akoz T. Postoperative camouflage therapy in facial aesthetic surgery. Aesthetic Plast Surg 2005; 29: 190–4.
Balkrishnan R, McMichael AJ, Hu JY, et al. Corrective cosmetics are effective for women with facial pigmentary disorders. Cutis 2005; 75: 181–7.
Benmaman O, Samchez JL. Treatment and camouflaging of pigmentary disorders. Clin Dermatol 1988; 6: 50–61.
Boehncke WH, Ochsendorf F, Paeslack I, Kaufmann R, Zollner TM. Decorative cosmetics improve the quality of life in patients with disfiguring skin diseases. Eur J Dermatol 2002; 12: 577–80.

Draelos ZD. Camouflaging techniques and dermatologic surgery. Dermatol Surg 1996; 22: 1023–7.

Draelos ZD. Degradation and migration of facial foundations. J Am Acad Dermatol 2001; 45: 542–3.

Draelos ZD. Colored facial cosmetics. Dermatol Clin 2000; 18: 621–31.

Draelos ZK. Cosmetic camouflaging techniques. Cutis 1993; 52: 362–4.

Draelos ZK. Cosmetics in the postsurgical patient. Dermatol Clin 1995; 13: 461–5.

Draelos ZD, Ertel K, Schnicker M, Bacon R, Vickery S. Facial foundation with niacinamide and N-acetylglucosamine improves skin condition in women with sensitive skin. J Am Acad Dermatol 2009; 60 (Suppl 1): AB82.

Fesq H, Brockow K, Strom K, et al. Dihydroxyacetone in a new formulation – a powerful therapeutic option in vitiligo. Dermatology 2001; 203: 241–3.

Grimes PE. Skin and hair cosmetic issues in women of color. Dermatol Clin 2002; 18: 659–65.

Hakozaki T, Minwalla L, Zhuang J, et al. The effect of niacinamide on reducing cutaneous pigmentation and suppression of melanosome transfer. Br J Dermatol 2002; 147: 20–31.

Hamed S, Sriwiriyanont P, deLong MA, et al. Comparative efficacy and safety of deoxyarbutin, a new tyrosinase-inhibiting agent. J Cosmet Sci 2006; 57: 291–308.

Hell B, Frangillo-Engler F, Heissler E, et al. Camouflage in head and neck region-a non-invasive option for skin lesions. Int J Oral Maxillofac Surg 1999; 28: 90–4.

Holme SA, Beattie PE, Fleming CJ. Cosmetic camouflage advice improves quality of life. Br J Dermatol 2002; 147: 946–9.

Hsu S. Camouflaging vitiligo with dihydroxyacetone. Dermatol Online J 2008; 14: 23.

Ichihashi M, Funasaka Y, Oka M, Keishi A, Ando H. UV-melanogenesis and cosmetic whitening. IFSCC Magazine 2003; 6: 279–86.

Iredale J, Linder J. Mineral makeup and its role with acne and rosacea. J Cosmet Dermatol 2009; 22: 407–12.

Johnson BA. Requirements in cosmetics for black skin. Dermatol Clin 1988; 6: 489–92.

Korichi R, Pelle-de-Queral D, Gazano G, Aubert A. Why women use makeup: implication of psychological traits in makeup functions. J Cosmet Sci 2008; 59: 127–37.

Loden M, Buraczewska I, Halvarsson K. Facial anit-wrinkle cream: influence of product presentation on effectiveness: a randomized and controlled study. Skin Res Technol 2007; 13: 189–94.

Paine C, Sharlow E, Liebel F, et al. As alternative approach to depigmentation by soybean extracts via inhibitions of the PAR-2 pathway. J Invest Dermatol 2001; 116: 587–95.

Rayner VL. Camouflage cosmetics (Chapter 35). In: Baran R, Maibach H, eds. Textbook of Cosmetic Dermatology, 2nd edn. Martin Dunitz Ltd., 1998: 417–32.

Rayner VL. Camouflage therapy. Dermatol Clin 1995; 13: 467–72.

Sarwer DB, Crecand CE. Body image and cosmetic medical treatments. Body Image 2004; 1: 99–111.

Seiberg M, Paine C, Sharlow E, et al. Inhibition of melanosome transfer results in skin lightening. J Invest Dermatol 2000; 15: 162–7.

Stewart TW, Savage D. Cosmetic camouflage in dermatology. Br J Dermatol 1972; 86: 530–2.

Tanioka M, Miyachi Y. Camouflaging vitiligo of the fingers. Arch Dermatol 2008; 144: Correspondence.

Taylor SC. Cosmetic problems in skin of color. Skin Pharmacol Appl Skin Physiol 1999; 12: 139–43.

Tedeschi A, Dall'Oglio F, Micali G, Schwartz RA, Janniger CK. Corrective camouflage in pediatric dermatology. Cutis 2007; 79: 110–12.

Zhai H, Maibach HI. Skin-whitening products (Chapter 37). In: Paye M, Barel A, Maibach H, eds. Handbook of Cosmetic Science and Technology, 2nd edn. Informa Healthcare USA, Inc., 2007: 457–63.

Zhu W-Y, Zhang R-Z. Skin lightening techniques (Chapter 13). In: Draelos ZD, Thaman LA, eds. Cosmetic formulation of skin care products. Vol. 30. Taylor & Francis Group, LLC, 2006: 205–17.

7 Ethnic skin and pigmentation

Beneath the stratum corneum and epidermis, skin is the same, although skin complexions and tones vary. The dermis appears a creamy white in persons of all cultural backgrounds, thus ethnic skin concerns focus primarily on the interaction between melanin production, melanin transfer, and factors affecting melanogenesis (Fig. 7.1). Light reflection from the skin surface and within the skin accounts for the blending of brown melanin, red hemoglobin, and yellow collagen. Subtle differences in melanin allow skin to appear almost black when the concentration is high and a reddish-white when the concentration is low. Melanin is produced in two forms: pheomelanin, a polymer of benzothiazine which is red, and eumelanin, a polymer of dihydroxyindole and dihydroxyindole carboxylic acid, and their reduced forms, which is a dark brown (Fig. 7.2). Eumelanin is the ancestral brown-black melanin formed as an oblong or spherical granule about $0.9\,\mu m$ long and $0.3\,\mu m$ wide. Pheomelanin is the red-yellow pigment formed as a spherical granule about $0.7\,\mu m$ in diameter. It is a less common form of melanin found in higher concentration in the female lips, areola, and genitalia. It is the various combinations of these two pigments that produce the diversity of skin colors observed in modern society. This chapter examines the ethnic skin and pigmentation issues.

> Subtle differences in melanin concentration allow the skin to appear almost black when the melanin concentration is high and a reddish-white when the melanin concentration is low.

MELANIN AND SKIN COLOR

Melanin production is the primary differentiating factor in multicultural skin. Skin color is determined by several genes, including the recently discovered SLC24A5, which accounts for the average difference of 30 melanin units between European and African skin. Another important gene is the MC1R, also known as melanocortin-1-receptor, which is a hormone produced by the pituitary gland that stimulates melanin production. The MC1R gene consists of 954 nucleotides. Among Africans there are no differences in the amino acid sequences of the receptor proteins, but 18 differences were noted among light-skinned populations in Ireland, England, and Sweden. While it has been thought that light skin was a genetic mutation to allow adequate vitamin D production by the body, this theory has been questioned.

> Skin color is determined by several genes, including the recently discovered SLC24A5, which accounts for the average difference of 30 melanin units between European and African skin.

Melanin is produced in response to sun exposure, transforming harmful UV radiation into heat. This explains the uncomfortable skin warmth when dark skin is exposed to the sun, which is not the case with poorly melanized skin, accounting for the preponderance of light-complected persons engaging in tanning practices. Tanning is a boon for skin injury and not a health benefit.

The number of melanocytes, typically $1000-2000/mm^2$ of skin, does not differ between skin colors, but their ability to produce and transfer melanin is different. Melanocytes are located at the lower level of the epidermis transferring melanin to skin cells in packages known as melanosomes. Melanosomes in recipient cells accumulate atop the cellular nucleus, where they protect nuclear DNA from ionizing radiation damage and the resultant cellular mutations. These cellular mutations contribute to photoaging when mild, precancerous changes when moderate, and photocarcinogenesis when severe. Irregular melanin transfer results in a mottled pigmentation characteristic of photoaged skin.

> The number of melanocytes, typically $1000-2000/mm^2$ of skin, does not differ between skin colors, but the ability to produce and transfer melanin is different.

Melanogenesis can be affected by many factors that differ cross culturally. Irregular melanin production is of prime cosmetic importance. Increased melanin production can occur in response to a variety of different stimuli, including UV radiation, injury, and hormone production. Melanogenesis can be epidermal or dermal. Epidermal melanogenesis is due to the release and subsequent oxidation of arachidonic acid to prostaglandins, leukotrienes, and other inflammatory mediators, which initiate pigment production. If the inflammation disrupts the basal cell layer, the melanin is released and trapped by macrophages in the dermis. Dermal pigment, also known as pigmentary incontinence, is not amenable to cosmetic intervention while epidermal pigment can be effectively modulated. The difference can be detected visually, since epidermal pigment can vary from light brown to dark black while dermal pigment has a grayish appearance.

Besides skin color appearance, there are other differences of cosmetic importance between Caucasian skin and African-American skin. These include the presence of more mixed apocrine and eccrine sweat glands (1), increased blood and lymphatic vessels (2), a predisposition to hyperpigmentation (3), a denser and more compact stratum corneum (4), an increased transepidermal water loss following irritation (5) and possibly an increased skin sensitivity to irritants in African-American skin (6,7).

SKIN LIGHTENING

Skin lightening is an important cosmetic need that has been poorly addressed to date. Many prescription and nonprescription skin lightening agents have been developed, but none

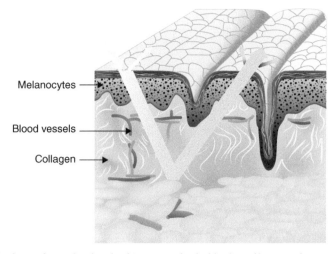

Figure 7.1 Light reflection from the skin surface and within the skin account for the blending of brown melanin, red hemoglobin, and yellow collagen.

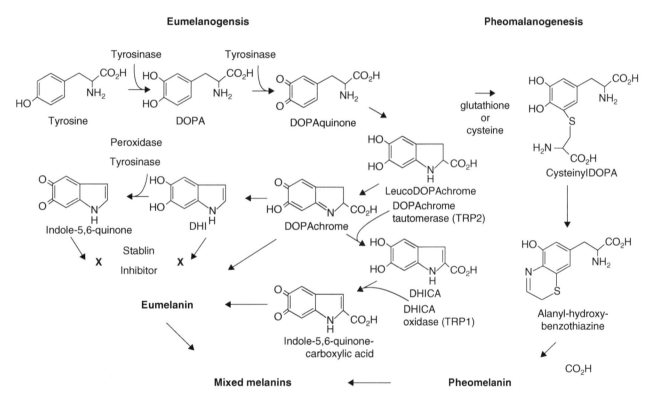

Figure 7.2 The biosynthetic pathway for melanin demonstrating the differences between eumelanin and pheomelanin. DOPA, L-3,4-dihydroxyphenylalanine.

work efficiently to completely lighten the skin. A brief review of these substances used in over-the-counter (OTC) skin lightening preparations is discussed.

The gold standard for pigment lightening in the U.S.A. remains hydroquinone.

Hydroquinone

The gold standard for hyperpigmentation therapy in the U.S.A. remains hydroquinone. This substance is actually quite controversial having been removed from the OTC markets in Europe and Asia. Concern arose because oral hydroquinone has been reported to cause cancer in mice that are fed large amounts of the substance. While oral consumption probably is not related to topical application, hydroquinone remains controversial because it actually is toxic to melanocytes. Hydroquinone, a phenolic compound chemically known as 1,4 dihydroxybenzene, functions by inhibiting the enzymatic oxidation of tyrosine and phenol oxidases (Fig. 7.3). It covalently binds to histidine or interacts with copper at the active site of tyrosinase. It also inhibits RNA and DNA synthesis and may alter melanosome formation, thus selectively damaging melanocytes. These activities suppress the melanocyte metabolic processes inducing a gradual decrease in melanin pigment production (8).

Hydroquinone is available both as an OTC and prescription drug in the US markets. The maximum concentration in OTC

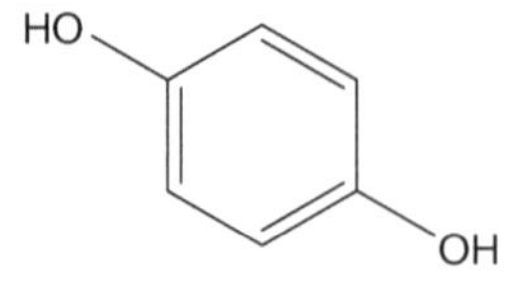

Figure 7.3 The chemical structure of hydroquinone.

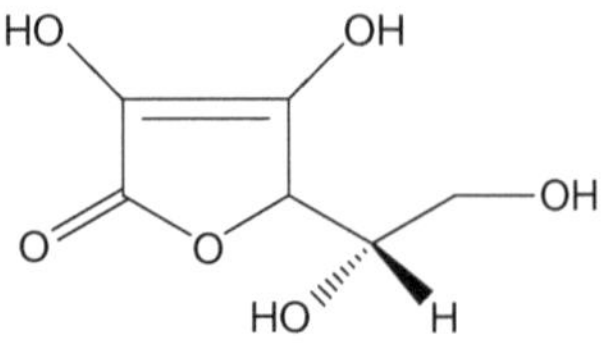

Figure 7.4 The chemical structure of highly photosensitive vitamin C.

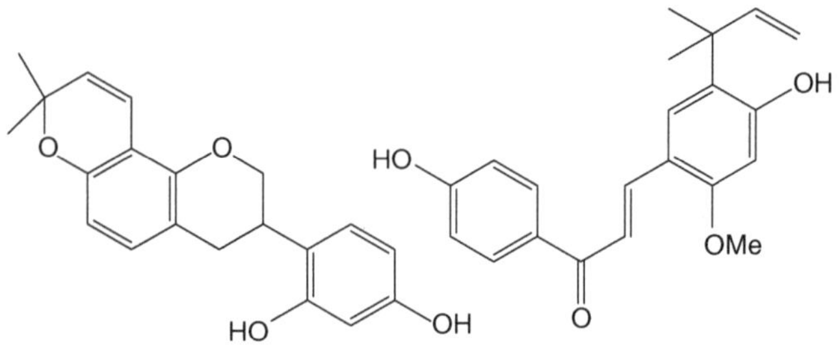

Figure 7.5 A licorice extract used in skin care products.

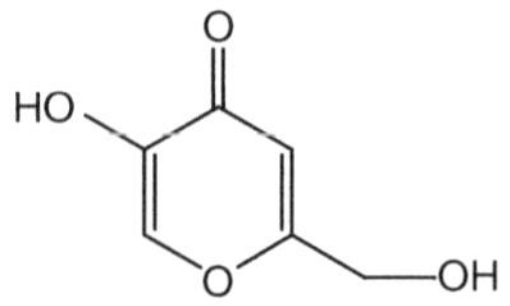

Figure 7.6 Kojic acid is a highly effective skin lightening agent widely used in the cosmetic industry.

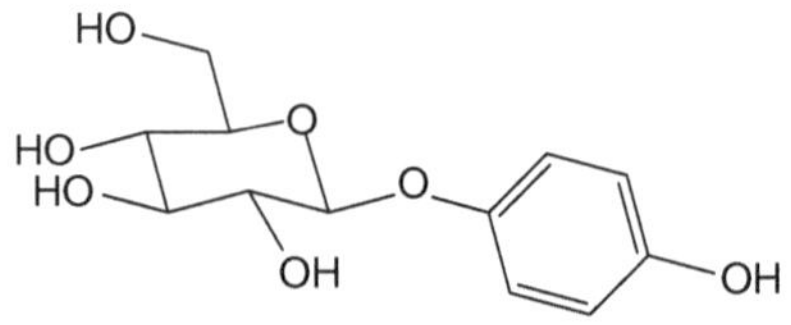

Figure 7.7 Arbutin is a botanical, skin lightening agent that is not toxic to melanocytes.

formulations is 2% while most prescription formulations have 4%. In all formulations, hydroquinone is unstable turning brown upon contact with air. Once the hydroquinone has oxidized, it is no longer active and should be discarded.

Ascorbic Acid

Ascorbic acid, also known as vitamin C, is used in the treatment of hyperpigmentation (Fig. 7.4). It interrupts the production of melanogenesis by interacting with copper ions to reduce dopaquinone and blocking dihydrochinindol-2-carboxyl acid oxidation (9). Ascorbic acid, an antioxidant, is rapidly oxidized when exposed in air and is of limited stability. High concentrations of ascorbic acid must be used with caution as the low pH can be irritating to the skin.

Licorice Extract

Licorice extracts are being used as topical anti-inflammatory preparations to decrease skin redness and hyperpigmentation (Fig. 7.5). The active agents are known as liquiritin and isoliquertin, which are glycosides containing flavonoids (10). Liquiritin induces skin lightening by dispersing melanin. It is typically applied to the skin in a dose of 1 g/day for four weeks to see the clinical result. Irritation is not a side effect.

Alpha Lipoic Acid

Alpha lipoic acid is found in a variety of antiaging cosmeceuticals to function as an antioxidant, but it may also have very limited pigment lightening properties. It is a disulfide derivative of octanoic acid that is able to inhibit tyrosinase. However, it is a large molecule and therefore, cutaneous penetration to the level of the melanocyte is challenging for the acid.

Kojic Acid

Kojic acid, chemically known as 5-hydroxymethyl-4H-pyrane-4-one) is one of the most popular cosmeceutical skin lightening agents found in the cosmetic-counter skin lightening cream distributed worldwide (Fig. 7.6). It is a hydrophilic fungal derivative obtained from *Aspergillus* and *Penicillium* species. It is the most popular agent employed in the Orient for the treatment of melasma (11). Some studies indicate that kojic acid is equivalent to hydroquinone in pigment lightening ability (12). The activity of kojic acid is attributed to its ability to prevent tyrosinase activity by binding to copper.

Kojic acid is a popular cosmetic skin-lightening ingredient.

Aleosin

Aleosin is a low-molecular-weight glycoprotein obtained from the aloe vera plant. It is a natural hydroxymethylchromone functioning to inhibit tyrosinase by competitive inhibition at the DOPA (L-3,4-dihydroxyphenylalanine) oxidation site (13,14). In contrast to hydroquinone, it shows no cell cytotoxicity; however, it has a limited ability to penetrate the skin due to its hydrophilic nature. It is sometimes mixed with arbutin, our next topic of discussion, to enhance its skin lightening abilities.

Arbutin

Arbutin is obtained from the leaves of the *Vaccinicum vitisidaea* and other related plants (Fig. 7.7). It is a naturally occurring gluconopyranoside that causes decreased tyrosinase activity without affecting the messenger RNA expression (15). It also inhibits melanosome maturation. Arbutin is not toxic to melanocytes and is used in a variety of pigment lightening preparations in Japan at a concentration of 3%. Higher concentrations are more efficacious than lower concentrations, but a paradoxical pigment darkening may occur.

ETHNIC COSMETICS FOR SKIN OF COLOR

The formulations and types of facial cosmetics available to patients with darker skin tones are the same as those formulated for lighter skin tones. Some cosmetic companies that traditionally cater to light-skinned customers have now enlarged their color selection to include darker skin tones. But, many new cosmetic companies are producing product lines specifically created for women of color (16).

The unique aspect of color cosmetic formulation for darker skin tones is the blending of pigments with the underlying skin color. Fair-skinned individuals, with little underlying skin pigment, can select a color cosmetic and expect it to look similar in the packaging and on the skin. However, women of color can expect the cosmetic to look entirely different in the package than on the skin. For example, a light pink blush that provides cheek highlights in a Caucasian patient is imperceptible on a Fitzpatrick type V skin. Therefore, cosmetics for skin of color generally contain vivid pigments to provide the desired result.

> It is estimated that 35 shades of facial foundation are necessary to match skin of color while only 7 shades of facial foundation are necessary to match Caucasian skin.

Facial foundations for women of color are found both at the cosmetic counter and in mass merchandisers. It is estimated that there are over 35 different colors of dark skin requiring tremendous color selection for complexion matching (17). This is compared to the 7 basic colors of Caucasian skin. African-American women traditionally wear facial foundations to blend uneven facial tones, whereas fair-skinned individuals wear facial foundations to add color to the skin. A greater emphasis is placed on skin of color foundations for dry skin, as pigmented skin is more subject to the ashy appearance of dry skin scale due to its higher rate of transepidermal water loss (5,18). Many women of color consider their skin to be extremely "sensitive," even though studies do not demonstrate a genetic predisposition to contact dermatitis. This may be due to the long lasting postinflammatory hyperpigmentation seen with skin care product irritation in women of color (19,20).

> The description of skin of color requires consideration of value, intensity, and undertone.

The description of deeply pigmented skin requires a more complex discussion of color in terms of value, intensity, and undertone (21). The value of a color is a measure of its light reflectivity. Dark skin with blue/black or mahogany hues may appear deeper in color due to the low value of these colors. Intensity refers to the brightness or dullness of a color. True colors, without the addition of white, brown or black pigments, tend to have higher intensity than mixed colors. For example, primary red has a greater intensity than brick red produced by the mixing of primary red with brown. This is an important concept in selecting facial foundations for dark skin, since too many pigments can leave the skin muddy appearing due to reduced color intensity. Lastly, undertones are extremely important. The undertones account for the tremendous variation seen in skin of color. Red, yellow, and orange undertones are said to give the skin a warm appearance while blue, purple, and green undertones are said to give the skin a cool appearance. Based on an analysis of undertones skin of color can be further classified as jet black, blue/black, purple/black, brown/red, bronze, honey, etc.

Color cosmetics applied to the face in women of color must contain deeper pigments. Popular eye shadow colors include deep blue, lilac, wine, gold, or emerald. Facial highlighter and blush colors for facial contouring in skin of color are deep plum, bronze, deep orange, coral, wine, or burgundy. The color selected depends upon the skin color shade, for example:

wine or plum blush for jet-black skin, coral, or deep orange for brown skin and pink or peach for light brown skin. The eye and face contouring methods, however, are the same for light- and dark-skinned patients.

SUMMARY
This chapter has examined the unique needs of skin of color, including OTC, pigment lightening preparations. It has assessed the use of color cosmetics for facial adornment. Even though the genetic differences among various skin colors are minimal, cosmetic formulations must be tailored to suit all skin colors.

REFERENCES
1. Anderson KE, Maibach HI. African-American and white skin differences. J Am Acad Dermatol 1979; 1: 276–86.
2. Montagna W, Carlisle K. The architecture of black and white facial skin. J Am Acad Dermatol 1991; 24: 929–37.
3. McLaurin DI. Unusual patterns of common dermatoses in blacks. Cutis 1983; 32: 352–60.
4. Weigand DA, Haygood C, Baylor JR. Cell layers and density of negro and caucasian stratum corneum. J Invest Dermatol 1974; 62: 563–8.
5. Wilson D, Berardesca E, Maibach HI. In vitro transepidermal water loss: differences between black and white human skin. Br J Dermatol 1988; 119: 647–52.
6. Stephens TJ, Oresajo C. Ethnic sensitive skin. Cosmet Toilet 1994; 109: 75–80.
7. Berardesca E, Maibach HI. Sensitive and ethnic skin. A need for special skin care agents? Dermatol Clin 1991; 9: 89–92.
8. Halder RM, Richards GM. Management of dischromias in ethnic skin. Dermatol Ther 2004; 17: 151–7.
9. Espinal-Perez LE, Moncada B, Castanedo-Cazares JP. A double blind randomized trial of 5% ascorbic acid vs 4% hydroquinone in melasma. Int J Dermatol 2004; 43: 604–7.
10. Amer M, Metwalli M. Topical liquiritin improves melasma. Int J Dermatol 2000; 39: 299–301.
11. Lim JT. Treatment of melasma using kojic acid in a gel containing hydroquinone and glycolic acid. Dermatol Surg 1999; 25: 282–4.
12. Garcia A, Fulton JE. Jr. The combination of glycolic acid and hydroquinone or kojic acid for the treatment of melasma and related conditions. Dermatol Surg 1996; 22: 443–7.
13. Choi S, Lee SK, Kim JE, et al. Aloesin inhibits hyperpigmentation induced by UV radiation. Clin Exp Dermatol 2002; 27: 513–15.
14. Jones K, Hughes J, Hong M, et al. Modulation of melanogenesis by aloesin: a competitive inhibitor of tyrosinase. Pigment Cell Res 2002; 15: 335–40.
15. Hori I, Nihei K, Kubo I. Structural criteria for depigmenting mechanism of arbutin. Phytother Res 2004; 18: 475–69.
16. Chester J, Dixon M. Ethnic market feels growth. Manufacturing Chemist 1988; 59: 32.
17. McLaurin CI. Cosmetic for blacks a medical perspective. Cosmet Toilet 1983; 98: 47–53.
18. Hood HL, Wickett RR. Racial differences in epidermal structure and function. Cosmet Toilet 1992; 107: 47–8.
19. Maibach HI. Racial and skin color differences in skin sensitivity. Cosmet Toilet 1990; 105: 35–6.
20. Berardesca E, Maibach HI. Racial differences in sodium lauryl sulphate induced cutaneous irritation: black and white. Contact Dermatitis 1988; 18: 65.
21. Patton JE. Color to Color. New York: Fireside, 1991: 31–3.

SUGGESTED READING
Abdel-Malek Z, Suzuki I, Tada A, Im S, Akcali C. The melanocortin-1 receptor and human pigmentation. Ann NY Acad Sci 1999; 885: 117–33.
Badreshia-Bansal S, Draelos ZD. Insight into skin lightening cosmeceuticals for women of color. J Drugs Dermatol 2007; 6: 32–9.
Baumann L, Rodriguez D, Taylor SC, Wu J. Natural considerations for skin of color. Cutis 2006; 76 (6 Suppl): 2–19.
DeLeo VA, Taylor SC, Belsito DV, et al. The effect of race and ethnicity on patch test results. J Am Acad Dermatol 2002; 46 (2 Suppl): S107–S112.

Halder RM, Nootheti PK. Ethnic skin disorders overview. J Am Acad Dermatol 2003; 48 (6 Suppl): S143–8.

Halder RM, Richards GM. Management of dyschromias in ethnic skin. Dermatol Ther 2004; 17: 151–7.

Hillebrand GG, Schnell B, Miyamoto K, et al. The age-dependent changes in skin condition in Japanese females living in Northern versus Southern Japan. IFSCC Magazine 2001; 4: 89–96.

Holloway VL. Ethnic cosmetic products. Dermatol Clin 2003; 21: 743–9.

Johnson BA. Requirements in cosmetics for black skin. Dermatol Clin 1988; 6: 489–92.

Levin CY, Maibach H. Exogenous ochronosis. An update on clinical features, causative agents and treatment options. Am J Clin Dermatol 2001; 2: 213–17.

Martín RF, Sánchez JL, González A, Lugo-Somolinos A, Ruiz H. Exogenous ochronosis. P R Health Sci J 1992; 11: 23–6.

Mahe A, Ly F, Aymard G, Dangou JM. Skin disorders associated with the cosmetic use of bleaching products in women from Dakar, Senegal. Br J Dermatol 2003; 148: 493–500.

Olumide YM, Akinkugbe AO, Altraide D, et al. Complications of chronic use of skin lightening cosmetics. Int J Dermatol 2008; 47: 344–53.

Ortonne JP, Bissett DL. Latest insights into skin hyperpigmentation. J Invest Dermatol Symp Proc 2008; 13: 10–14.

Petit A, Cohen-Ludmann C, Clevenbergh P, Bergmann JF, Dubertret L. Skin lightening and its complications among African people living in Paris. J Am Acad Dermatol 2006; 55: 873–8.

Pichon LC, Corral I, Landrine H, Mayer JA, Norman GJ. Sun-protection behaviors among African Americans. Am J Prev Med 2010; 38: 288–95.

Rawlings AV. Ethnic skin types: are there differences in skin structure and function? IFSCC Magazine 2006; 9: 3–11.

Stephens TJ, Oresajo C. Ethnic sensitive skin. Cosmet Toilet 1994; 109: 75–80.

Sugden D, Davidson K, Hough KA, Teh MT. Melatonin, melatonin receptors and melanophores: a moving story. Pigment Cell Res 2004; 17: 454–60.

Taylor SC. Enhancing the care and treatment of skin of color, part 1: the broad scope of pigmentary disorders. Cutis 2005; 76: 249–55.

Taylor SC. Enhancing the care and treatment of skin of color, part 2: understanding skin physiology. Cutis 2005; 76: 302–6.

Taylor SC. Cosmetic problems in skin of color. Skin Pharmacol Appl Skin Physiol 1999; 12: 139–43.

Yamaguchi Y, Hearing VJ. Physiological factors that regulate skin pigmentation. Biofactors 2009; 35: 193–9.

8 Male skin care

The male skin care market is rapidly expanding in the United States because of new product development and aggressive marketing tactics. Manufacturers see male skin care as a large area for economic growth as the female skin care market has shown sales for a number of years. Much of the interest in male skin care has focused on the concept of the "metrosexual" man. The metrosexual man is concerned with fashion, hair care, nail appearance, skin treatments, and cosmetic products. This image is in contrast to the "urban" man who is a low-maintenance person and uses toothpaste, bar soap, mass-market shampoo, and shaving cream as the sum total of his products. The advertising push to popularize the image of a metrosexual man is seen as a way to boost the sale of hair, skin, and nail care products and services by creating an image for which men of all ages can aspire.

Men use many of the same skin care products as women. Do these formulations need to be different or can the same moisturizer with a more masculine fragrance be used on the male face? Is male skin that different from the female skin? This chapter examines the unique issues differentiating male and female skin care.

> Male facial skin is thicker than female facial skin due to the presence of terminal hair follicles.

MALE VS. FEMALE SKIN

The differences between the skin of men and women are obvious to the human eye. Male skin is thicker than female skin, in part due to the presence of terminal hair follicles over much of the body. This difference is most pronounced on the face where women have only vellus hairs, which are fine and colorless, while men have fully developed terminal hairs, which are coarse and pigmented, taking up space within the skin. The presence of male facial hair is partially responsible for the more favorable appearance of mature men over mature women. As UV radiation activates collagenase to destroy dermal collagen, the male beard allows the skin to resist wrinkling. Thus, photoaged males do not exhibit the pronounced redundant facial skin seen in photoaged females.

What does the thicker male skin mean for the skin care market? It means that photoaging does not appear as early in men as it does in women. While women are eager at a young age to engage in the purchase of wrinkle creams, men are more resistant. The rugged coarse look is valued as a sign of masculinity and maturity. The thicker male skin is also less able to respond to beneficial effects of moisturization, especially on the hair-bearing upper cheeks. Wrinkle creams simply do not appeal to men immediately, due to their perceived lack of need and poor immediate efficacy.

The male beard also gives the skin a coarse texture hiding surface cosmetic irregularities, such as scarring, pigmentation changes, and broken capillaries. If the beard containing skin of the male face is stretched, many of these problems become apparent. Thus, women are much more anxious to "fix" problems than men who do not see skin changes as easily or as early in life.

Some of the resistance of male skin to aging is due to its inherent ability to diffuse UV radiation, especially in the UVA range. UVA radiation is the wavelength responsible for photoaging, which penetrates more deeply in women causing a greater damage in female skin. This allows women to age more rapidly than men, a phenomenon magnified by the media preference for younger leading women paired with older leading men.

> Male skin is more resistant to adverse reactions.

MALE SKIN AND ADVERSE REACTIONS

The difference in skin thickness also affects the decreased frequency of adverse product reactions experienced by men. Women experience adverse reactions more commonly than men. The thinner skin may allow irritants and allergens to penetrate deeper in female skin, but the increased incidence may also be due to greater product usage. Women overall use more skin care products and cosmetics than men. This increased usage magnifies the chances of contacting an irritant or an allergen. Women are also more likely to undergo procedures that destroy the skin barrier, such as facial peels, microdermabrasion, spa treatments, etc. This may account for the sensitive skin appeal of products marketed to women, which does not necessarily resonate with the male skin care market. In general, male skin is less subject to irritation and adverse reactions than female skin.

HORMONAL CONSIDERATIONS IN MALE SKIN CARE

The discussion to this point has focused on the most obvious visual difference, which is skin thickness and the presence of the male beard, but other equally important considerations also merit mention that affect product formulation. Perhaps one of the most important unique features of male skin is the dominance of testosterone. Testosterone secretion rises at puberty in males, with constant levels throughout life. Testosterone causes the production of facial and body sebum, which sets the stage for the growth of *Propionibacterium acnes* and the onset of acne. Acne is generally more severe in men than women.

Since testosterone secretion is present throughout life in men, it means that sebum production also remains high. This provides skin moisturization making the needs for facial and body creams for men somewhat different. While men do indeed develop dry skin about age 60 years and beyond, dry skin is a much greater concern for females. The male need for emollience is perhaps greater in middle age than for moisturization, unless skin disease is present.

Men prefer deodorant cleansers with antibacterials, since bacteria rapidly degrade the abundant apocrine sweat produced.

Testosterone not only triggers the onset of abundant sebum production but also increases the secretion of apocrine sweat in the eyelids, breasts, scalp, buttocks, and armpits. Both sebum and apocrine sweat create different skin cleansing needs. Odor must be controlled, but the formulator must also consider the interaction of the sebum and sweat with skin care products. It is for this reason that fragrance must be carefully considered in male skin care. Men typically prefer deodorant soaps and antibacterial products, since bacteria degrade the apocrine sweat rapidly creating a characteristic musty smell. This apocrine sweat, mixed with sebum rich in testosterone, creates a locker room smell that can ruin the most carefully balanced fragrance. This means that male products need more careful fragrance development for body odor than female products.

MALE SKIN AND HAIR REMOVAL

While male body hair provides excellent sunscreen, better than anything packaged in a bottle, it also requires grooming. Shaving is the most common method used for body hair management, but some men have embraced laser hair removal. One of the problems with laser hair removal is that it changes the apparent skin color and texture. Loss of the hair in the follicular ostia eliminates brown tones, the most common color of male facial hair, leaving the skin appearing lighter. Loss of the hair also eliminates the coarse texture of the male facial skin and predisposes to wrinkling, as discussed earlier. It is unlikely that shaving will be abandoned by the entire male community for these reasons. A more detailed discussion of shaving is found in the chapter on hair removal techniques.

Shaving is the most effective physical method of exfoliation.

Shaving also produces some unexpected skin benefits. It is probably the most effective physical method of exfoliation, better than topical hydroxy acids, hand-held microdermabrasion devices, or mechanical brushes. It efficiently removes desquamating corneocytes along with beard debris. Shaving also is an effective method of removing open comedones from the skin, providing acne treatment. However, improper shaving techniques result in razor burn and pseudofolliculitis barbae. Razor burns result from the removal of the skin around where the hair exits, an opening known as the follicular ostia. Newer razors with spring-mounted blades and shaving gels that reduce friction can minimize the occurrence of razor burn. Pseudofolliculitis barbae is seen in individuals with kinky facial hair where the sharp edge of the cut hair re-enters the skin causing inflammation in the form of a papule or pustule. This can result in darkening of the skin, which is discussed next.

PIGMENTATION ISSUES

Darkening of the skin, known as postinflammatory hyperpigmentation, is a reaction to injury in persons with darker skin tones, such as males of Mediterranean, Oriental, Indian, or African descent. The injury can be from acne, sunburn, skin disease, irritant contact dermatitis, allergic contact dermatitis, or a traumatic scratch. Since melanocytes are felt to be an important part of the immune system, it is postulated that this hyperpigmentation is an immune response to skin injury, but the exact reason for this reaction is largely unknown. Thus, products designed for male skin of color must be carefully formulated to minimize any skin irritation, since postinflammatory hyperpigmentation is the inevitable result. It may take six months to one year to return the skin to normal color after the injury, which accounts for the tremendous skin lightening product focus in cultures with darker complected individuals. In order for the skin to return to proper color, the extra melanin produced must be phagocytized or consumed by white blood cells and then removed from the skin.

Men typically need emollients to smooth facial skin scale after shaving rather than true moisturizers.

MOISTURIZERS

Shaving is usually the final male grooming activity, which is different from those of women who usually apply a facial moisturizer after cleansing. Why do most men not apply a moisturizer? This is because male facial sebum production is typically high, obviating the need to moisturize. Most men do not need to retard transepidermal water loss because they do not expose their skin to a number of products used by women, they do not engage in multiple barrier damaging procedures, and their rapid sebum replacement is adequate. Men typically

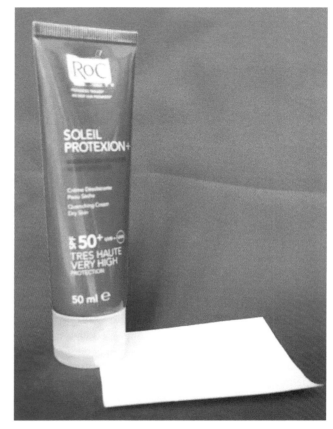

Figure 8.1 More aesthetic, high-SPF (sun protection factor) sunscreens have been developed with new formulation technology to appeal more to men.

need emollients, rather than moisturizers, unless skin disease is present, which smooth down the desquamating corneocytes by filling in the intercellular spaces where lipids may have been removed from over aggressive cleansing. The most popular emollient is dimethicone, which may be delivered to the skin surface in the form of a toner, aftershave lotion, skin bracer, etc. This is a key difference in products developed for men and women.

Female moisturizers are typically more occlusive to increase skin hydration and minimize periorbital wrinkling due to dehydration. These fine periorbital wrinkles are seen as signs of aging in women, but appear to contribute to character in men. Thus, antiaging moisturizers have been slow to catch on in the male skin care market. While young women are eager to purchase wrinkle creams, men are not. They value their rugged, tough look as a sign of masculinity and maturity. The thicker male skin is also not as responsive to beneficial effects of moisturization as female skin, especially on the hair-bearing upper cheeks. Wrinkle creams simply do not appeal to men as they do to women due to their perceived lack of need and poor immediate efficacy.

Some of the resistance of male skin to aging is due to the photoprotection afforded by facial hair.

PHOTOPROTECTION

Some of the resistance of male skin to aging is due to the photoprotection afforded by facial hair. The hair follicles also increase the skin thickness, decreasing the penetration of UVA radiation into male skin. This allows women to age more rapidly than men, a phenomenon magnified by the media preference for younger leading women paired with older leading men. Thus, men do not see the need for the application of sun protection to same degree as their female counterparts, although the incidence of skin cancer is higher in men than women (Fig. 8.1). A thorough discussion of sunscreens is found in the photoprotection and sunscreen chapter.

SUMMARY

Male skin care is similar, but different, from female skin care. The presence of the facial beard provides photoprotection and resistance to facial wrinkling, but hair removal can be challenging. Shaving can improve skin texture and minimize acne, but poor shaving techniques can cause razor burn and aggravate pseudofolliculitis barbae. The unique male biofilm, composed of apocrine sweat and sebum, requires different hygiene needs. It is not enough to package male skin care products in blue bottles and female skin care products in pink bottles. The material inside the bottle must cater to the unique skin needs of the different sexes.

9   Facial photoprotection

No one knows what encouraged the desire for tanned skin. Some believe that during prohibition, alcoholic beverages were readily available on the offshore islands of the U.S.A. and the affluent visited these islands to drink and tan. From this point forward, tanning became synonymous with wealth and tanned facial skin continues to be desirable to this day. The facial skin is constantly bombarded with photons of light during the day and shows the effects of excess UV radiation more readily than any other body area. The skin both absorbs and scatters these energetic photons. Photons that are scattered are reflected back to the eye and create the perception of beautiful skin that can be enhanced or adorned by cosmetics. The photons that are absorbed are converted into energy, which damages the collagen and promotes photoaging.

> The solar radiation, also known as the electromagnetic spectrum, comprises about 5% ultraviolet rays, 35% visible light, and 60% infrared rays.

The radiation that is emitted by the sun, also known as the electromagnetic spectrum, is about 5% ultraviolet (UV), 35% visible, and 60% infrared rays of light (Fig. 9.1). UV radiation in the form of UVB, in the range of 280–320 nm, and UVA, in the range of 320 to 380 nm, is invisible to the eye. Proteins, including DNA, absorb most of the UV rays and the amount absorbed is known as the dose calculated as intensity multiplied by time. High-intensity UV for a short period can be very damaging, which is the issue with artificial tanning booth radiation. These bulbs emit a predetermined number of watts per square centimeter with UVB possessing 1000 times the energy of UVA.

> The stratum corneum is the first line of defense functioning to reflect and scatter the damaging radiation and minimize penetration.

The stratum corneum is the first line of UV defense mechanism to reflect and scatter the damaging radiation and minimize penetration. It is for this reason that facial exfoliants, containing glycolic acid, lactic acid, and salicylic acid, should be followed by sunscreen application, since they decrease endogenous skin photoprotection. The sun rays are further absorbed by melanin, which is a physiochemical defense absorbing both UV and visible radiation. It is the oxidation of melanin that results in a tanned facial appearance not synonymous with health, but rather an oxidative damage. Radiation wavelengths of less than 320 nm are absorbed by the stratum corneum and epidermis, while wavelengths greater than 320 nm enter the dermis. Penetration into the dermis can be enhanced by wetting the stratum corneum and altering the refractive index. This is why applying baby oil to the face, which contains primarily mineral oil, increases the tanning response by decreasing endogenous facial photoprotection.

The target of UVA and UVB damage is DNA, cell membrane lipids, structural proteins, and enzymes. These breakdown products incite an inflammatory response designed to initiate skin repair, but may result in further skin damage. Cells that have been damaged by UV activate the p53 gene that determines whether the damage is fatal and the cell should be destroyed, a process known as apoptosis, or whether a DNA repair should be initiated. Apoptosis is the systematic destruction of the nucleus and cytoskeleton that results in a protein shell formation. Since its pink amorphous structure on H&E staining, it is also called a sunburn cell. They contain clumped filaments, melanin granules, and intact lysosomes amid a pink nucleus and cytoplasm. While UV damage can activate apoptosis and prevent abnormal cells from reproducing, it can also deactivate the p53 gene allowing genetically damaged cells to divide, which leads to neoplasia and skin cancer formation over time.

The initial symptom of sun damage is skin erythema produced by vasodilation in response to cellular damage. Erythema appears two to six hours after sun damage, also known as sunburn, and may peak up to 12 to 20 hours later depending on the amount of radiation received. It is this sunburn response that accounts for the minimal erythemal dose (MED) that is used to determine the sun protection factor (SPF) for sunscreens. The SPF, discussed again in detail in the body photoprotection chapter, indicates the increase in time afforded by a sunscreen to receive a dose of UV that induces erythema. Following the appearance of erythema, tanning occurs due to photo-oxidation of melanin, which is the immediate pigment darkening effect. Further pigment production occurs two to three days after sunburn when melanogenesis is initiated on the basis of the skin type (Table 9.1).

Over time, this cumulative skin damage manifests as photoaging. Histologically, the epidermis possesses a flattened dermal–epidermal junction and thinning of the spinous layer. The papillary dermis is thinned with dilated blood vessels and an amorphous, fragmented, fibrotic material representing solar elastosis accumulates in the reticular dermis. Facial photoprotection attempts to prevent such effects. This chapter examines the topic facial photoprotection in detail, but this should be read in conjunction with the body photoprotection chapter for a complete overview.

SUNSCREEN FILTER CLASSIFICATION

The first sunscreen was marketed in the United States in 1928 and consisted of an emulsion of benzyl salicylate and benzyl cinnamate. Para-aminobenzoic acid was introduced in 1943, which paved the way for many new sunscreen formulations. Physical agents, such as red petrolatum, were used by the military during World War II (1). In 1978, the FDA reclassified sunscreens from cosmetics to over-the-counter drugs designed to protect "the structure and function of the human integument

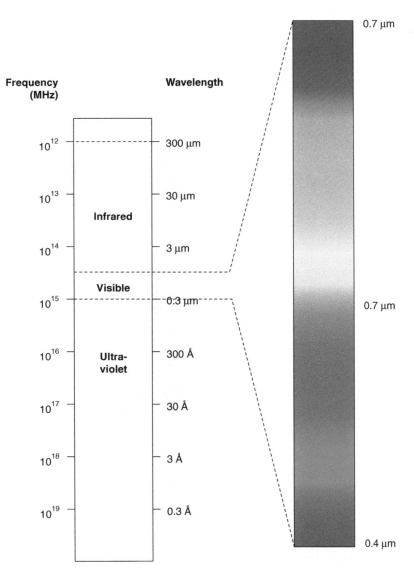

Figure 9.1 The electromagnetic spectrum.

Table 9.1 Skin Type Classifications

Fitzpatrick skin type	Description
I	Extremely fair skin, always burns, never tans
II	Fair skin, always burns, sometimes tans
III	Medium skin, sometimes burns, always tans
IV	Olive skin, rarely burns, always tans
V	Moderately pigmented brown skin, never burns, always tans
VI	Markedly pigmented black skin, never burns, always tans

against actinic damage" (2). From that point forward, many sunscreen formulations have been introduced providing better and better photoprotection.

Sunscreen filters are the active ingredients providing photoprotection (Table 9.2). Active ingredients can be classified into two major categories, organic and inorganic. Organic filters undergo a chemical transformation, known as resonance delocalization, to absorb UV radiation and transform it to heat (3). They are generally aromatic compounds based on the benzene ring's ability to transform high-energy ultraviolet radiation into harmless long-wave radiation above the 380 nm range. They are used up in the process of photoprotection and must be frequently reapplied to maintain proper protection from the sun. Inorganic filters, in contrast, are usually ground particulates that reflect or scatter UV radiation, absorbing relatively little of the energy. They are not used up and therefore, they stay and act longer on the skin surface, a property known as photostability.

Sunscreen filters can be classified as organic and inorganic filters.

Table 9.2 Sunscreen Filter Concentrations Allowed in the United States (FDA-OTC Panel)

	(%)
UVB filters	
Aminobenzoic acid	5–15
Amyl dimethyl PABA	1–5
2-ethoxyethyl p-methoxycinnamate	1–3
Diethanolamine p-methoxycinnamate	8–10
Digalloyl trioleate	2–5
Ethyl 4-bis (hydroxypropyl) aminobenzoate	1–5
2-ethylhexyl-2-cyano-3,3-diphenyl-acrylate	7–10
Ethylhexyl p-methoxycinnamate	2–7.5
2-ethylhexyl salicylate	3–5
Glyceryl aminobenzoate	2–3
Homomenthyl salicylate	4–25
Octyl dimethyl PABA	1.4–8
2-penylbenzimidazole-5-sulfonic acid	1.4
Triethanolamine salicylate	5–12
UVA filters	
Oxybenzone	2–6
Sulisobenzone	5–10
Dioxybenzone	3
Menthyl anthranilate	3.5–5
Organic filters	
Red petrolatum	3–100
Titanium dioxide	2–25

Abbreviations: FDA-OTC, Food and Drug Administration-over-the-counter; PABA, para-aminobenzoic acid.

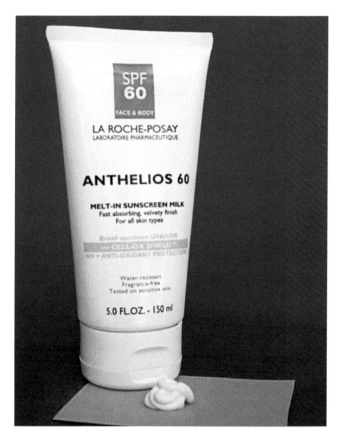

Figure 9.2 An avobenzone formulation stabilized with octocrylene to achieve a high sun protection factor rating.

Sunscreen filters can be divided into the following three groups:

- UVA absorbers: 320 to 360 nm (benzophenones, avobenzone, and anthranilates)
- UVB absorbers: 290 to 320 nm [para-amino benzoic acid (PABA) derivatives, salicylates, and cinnamates]
- UVB/UVA blocks: reflect or scatter UVA and UVB (titanium dioxide and zinc oxide)

The FDA has rated the chemicals listed in Table 9.2 as safe, effective sunscreen filters as described in the Sunscreen Monograph (4,5).

UVA ORGANIC SUNSCREEN FILTERS
There are three main families of UVA organic sunscreen filters. These are the benzophenones, avobenzone, and anthranilates. Each of these filters undergoes a chemical reaction when a photon of UV is absorbed with the energy released from the skin surface as heat. Their different aesthetic and photoprotective properties are used by the sunscreen formulator to develop a product that protects the skin, yet is pleasant to use.

Benzophenones
There are three sunscreens in the benzophenone family: oxybenzone, dioxybenzone, and sulisobenzone. Oxybenzone is approved for use in the U.S.A. and provides weak UVA photoprotection below 320 nm. Dioxybenzone and sulisobenzone are unapproved. With the increasing push for UVA photoprotection, the use of oxybenzone has increased dramatically resulting in increased reports of allergic contact dermatitis. Oxybenzone is also used in conjunction with avobenzone,

discussed next, to enhance photostability of sunscreen formulations. Oxybenzone is commonly used as a secondary sunscreen because it is an oily liquid making the sunscreen sticky if used in too high a concentration.

Oxybenzone and avobenzone are two commonly used organic UVA sunscreen filters.

Avobenzone
Avobenzone, also known as Parsol 1789, was an important step forward in UVA photoprotection. It is the most recently monographed sunscreen ingredient. Unfortunately, it is highly photounstable with 36% of the avobenzone destroyed shortly after sun exposure. It is estimated that all of the avobenzone is gone from a sunscreen after five hours or 50 Joules of exposure, necessitating frequent reapplication. Avobenzone is also chemically incompatible with other commonly used physical sunscreens, such as zinc oxide and titanium dioxide. However, avobenzone can now be stabilized by adding oxybenzone and other ingredients, such as 2-6-diethylhexylnaphthalate or octocrylene (Fig. 9.2). These ingredients absorb the photon of energy from avobenzone allowing avobenzone to return to a ground state and not undergo photodegradation. Since 2-6-diethylhexylnaphthalate is photostable, it radiates off the energy as heat or phosphorescence. Octocrylene, also an organic sunscreen, is photostable and can absorb the photon of energy without undergoing degradation (Fig. 9.3). This relatively new concept of photostabilization is important to ensure the longevity of sunscreens on the skin. Combining

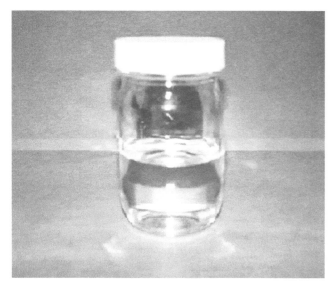

Figure 9.3 Octocrylene is a sticky thick liquid in the raw material form.

photounstable avobenzone with other photostable substances was a novel advance in photoprotection.

Anthranilates

There are several anthranilates available for sunscreen formulation, but only menthyl anthranilate is used in the U.S.A. Menthyl anthranilate, also known as meradimate, has its peak absorption at 336 nm and is used as a secondary sunscreen because it too is a clear thick sticky oil that can only be used in low concentration in formulations meant for aesthetic reasons. It has an excellent safety profile and low allergenicity. It is very stable in formulation without the photodegradation issues discussed in the case of avobenzone.

> Menthyl anthranilate, a clear sticky oil, is a secondary UVA organic filter, because in high concentration it makes the sunscreen sticky.

UVB ORGANIC SUNSCREEN INGREDIENTS

UVB organic sunscreen ingredients also undergo a chemical reaction radiating off the UV rays as heat. The chemical families that function in UVB photoprotection are the PABA derivatives, salicylates, and cinnamates. Each are briefly discussed in relation to current sunscreen formulations.

> PABA derivatives, salicylates, and cinnamates are the major UVB organic sunscreen filters.

PABA Derivatives

For all practical purposes, the PABA derivatives are rarely used in modern sunscreen formulations. A recent review of marketplace showed that as few as 2% of sunscreens use PABA derivatives because of allergenicity concerns. PABA derivatives can also stain clothing. Octyl dimethyl PABA, also known as Padimate O, is the most commonly PABA used with a maximal absorption at 296 nm. It has average photostability with about

15.5% lost with UV exposure. There have been some popular press articles questioning the cancer causing potential of pure PABA. This is not a relevant concern, since pure PABA is not used in any of the modern sunscreens.

Salicylates

The salicylates are an important class of UVB photoprotectants. This class includes octyl salicylate (octisalate), homomenthyl salicylate (homosalate), and trolamine salicylate. The internal hydrogen bonding of the salicylates provides for UVB absorption at 300 to 310 nm. Approximately 56% of the sunscreens in the current marketplace use the salicylates as a secondary active sunscreen agent since they have an excellent safety record with minimal reports of allergic reactions.

Cinnamates

The cinnamates are the most popular sunscreen category currently used in sunscreens, sunscreen-containing moisturizers, and facial foundations; 86% of products with an SPF rating contain octyl methoxycinnamate, also known as Octinoxate, which has maximal absorption at 305 nm. Octyl methoxycinnamate has excellent photostability with only 4.5% degradation after UVB exposure. For this reason, octyl methoxycinnamate is a popular primary sunscreen. Primary sunscreen means that it is used in highest concentration and is listed first under the active ingredient disclosure on the back of the sunscreen box. All sunscreens must have an active ingredient disclosure required by law as they are classified as OTC drugs. The secondary sunscreen is listed second and is next highest in concentration followed the by the tertiary and quaternary sunscreens. Most sunscreen formulations contain several sunscreen filters to provide broad-spectrum photoprotection by mixing filters with different absorptive wavelengths while balancing aesthetic qualities.

UVA/UVB INORGANIC SUNSCREEN FILTERS

The inorganic UVA/UVB sunscreen filters are titanium dioxide and zinc oxide. These are the main inorganic filters, but a complete list of the monographed ingredients is found in Table 9.3. Titanium dioxide is usually micronized to contain particles of various sizes to provide optimal UV scattering abilities (Fig. 9.4). Unfortunately, it leaves a white film on the skin and is used mainly for beach wear products. Zinc oxide is usually available in a microfine form meaning it contains small particles of one size making it appropriate for day wear (Fig. 9.5). Titanium dioxide and zinc oxide are known as inorganic filters because they do not undergo a chemical reaction when struck by a photon of UV energy. They are inherently photostable. These particulates reflect most of the energy, but a small amount may be absorbed. The absorbed energy may result in the formation of secondary oxygen radicals; therefore, most titanium dioxide and zinc oxide sunscreen powders are now coated with dimethicone to quench the secondary oxygen radicals (Fig. 9.6).

> Zinc oxide and titanium dioxide are the two broad-spectrum inorganic sunscreen filters.

A newly introduced colorless zinc oxide with extremely small particles is finding its way into many cosmetics and

Table 9.3 Inorganic Sunscreen Filters

Kaolin
Magnesium silicate
Magnesium oxide
Red petrolatum
Titanium dioxide
Iron oxide
Zinc oxide
Red veterinary petrolatum

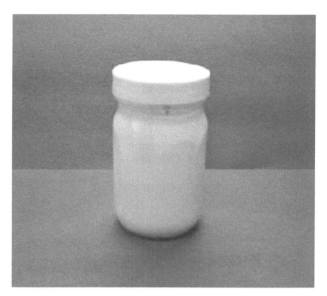

Figure 9.6 Dimethicone-coated zinc oxide is used to decrease secondary oxygen radical formation in sunscreens.

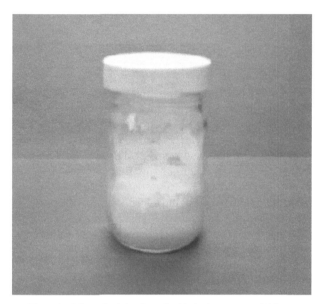

Figure 9.4 Micronized titanium dioxide in the raw material form.

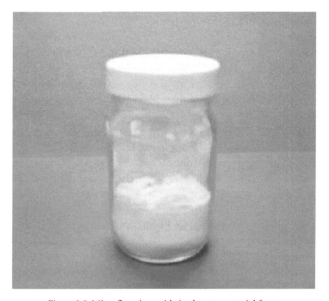

Figure 9.5 Microfine zinc oxide in the raw material form.

NANOPARTICLE SUNSCREENS

There is a growing concern over the presence of nanoparticles in the environment. These particles with size less than 100 nm are invisible to the human eye and can penetrate the skin and lung tissues, gaining access to the lymphatics and blood circulation. From there, these particles can be widely distributed throughout the body. Once these particles enter the body, they cannot be removed because their small size escapes detection. Concern has been voiced in the medical community that nanoparticles of metals might be responsible for neurologic diseases. Others have wondered whether the chronic inflammation induced by nanoparticles might not cause other degenerative diseases.

The biggest present concern in the skin care industry is the use of nanoparticle zinc oxide and titanium dioxide. These white particles become invisible when manufactured in a nanoparticle size making them suitable for all skin types. Otherwise, persons of Fitzpatrick skin types III to VI cannot use these inorganic sunscreens. These highly effective, nanoparticle sunscreens are poised to dominate the market, but environmental concerns arise when the disposition of nanoparticles in the environment is considered. After a day at the beach, the sunscreen is rinsed into the ocean water and finally completely removed in the shower. These zinc oxide nanoparticles find their way into the water columns of the world. Nanoparticle zinc is antibacterial, another possible use for this technology, but it is also toxic to plankton, the first line of the aquatic food chain. Imagine the consequences of large-scale aquatic organism death due to invisible nanoparticles. It is for this reason that many countries are taking a regulatory stance on nanoparticle use.

The cosmetic industry in the U.S.A. has called for a voluntary halt on widespread nanoparticle use until more information can be obtained. No reputable manufacturer wants to put nanoparticle products in the marketplace with long-term adverse health implications, even though there is no governmental organization forbidding its use in the United States. This is not the case in Europe. Sweden has banned the use of

moisturizers. Some of the particles are so small that they are known as nanoparticles, which are less than 100 μm in size. These particles are controversial because their small size may allow them to penetrate the skin, but they escape body removal by macrophage phagocytosis. Nanoparticle sunscreens are the next topic of discussion.

nanoparticle formulations and the European Union has asked that all presently marketed nanoparticle-containing products have the term "nano" on the packaging. Further, all products marketed with nanoparticles after 2013 must be registered with the government. The U.S. FDA convened a taskforce to examine nanoparticles, but no documents have been produced.

The penetration of nanoparticles into the skin is perhaps the biggest immediate health concern. However, it is impossible to generalize. The skin barrier composed of protein-rich corneocytes and intervening covalently bound lipid layers is extremely effective at keeping out substances deleterious to the body. Larger nanoparticles of size 14 to 100 nm do not penetrate the skin, but smaller nanoparticles 13 nm and less can penetrate the skin. These extremely small nanoparticles in the range of 10 nm are labeled as quantum dots. Quantum dots are a specialized form of nanoparticle with unique electrical and magnetic properties. Quantum dots are currently being investigated for their use in computing for the next generation of microcomputers.

> Nanoparticles less than 13 nm in size can penetrate the skin.

So, the answer to the question of nanoparticle penetration is it is theoretically less if they are smaller than 13 nm. However, in reality, nanoparticles do not remain as nanoparticles in skin care and sunscreen formulations. Nanoparticles can be sprinkled into an emulsion and put into a zinc oxide sunscreen, but they do not remain nanoparticles. Nanoparticles like to aggregate, meaning that they stick together. A clump of 15 10 nm nanoparticles is no longer a nanoparticle, since their cumulative size of 150 nm is larger than 100 nm, the upper limit for nanoparticles. Further, nanoparticles placed in emulsions, which are the basis for the lotion that suspends the nanoparticles in sunscreens, tend to agglomerate. This means that the clumps of nanoparticles stick together even further when placed in an oil–in-water mixture. Ten clumps of 150 nm aggregated nanoparticles become 1500 nm, well above the nanoparticle limit. In theory, nanoparticles could exist singly and penetrate the skin, but in actuality the aggregation and agglomeration of particles found in nature protects both the body and the environment from deleterious effects. This is not to say, however, that further research is not needed to evaluate the behavior and safety of nanoparticles.

> The tendency of nanoparticles to aggregate and agglomerate prevents them from penetrating the skin when used in sunscreen formulations.

SUNSCREEN FORMULATION

Sunscreens are typically made from combinations of the ingredients previously discussed. Usually, sun filters with different areas of UV protection are combined to yield a sunscreen with the broadest protection possible. Oily ingredients are usually used in low concentration to prevent a sticky feel, but may be required to achieve the desired SPF. Sunscreen formulation is definitely an art, yet the question remains as to why sunscreens do not provide optimal protection. Careful formulation is only

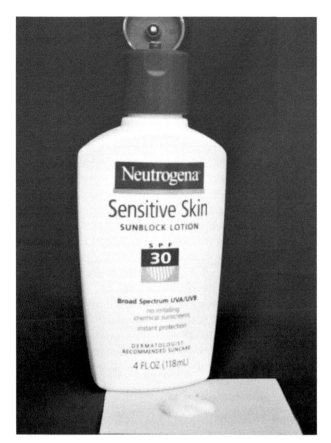

Figure 9.7 A sun protection factor rating of 30 or higher is indicative of some degree of UVA photoprotection.

a part of the success of a sunscreen. The ability of the sunscreen to be applied in an even thin film that will not separate or move is important. Sunscreens combine with sebum, sweat, topical medications, and cosmetics, which can interrupt or destroy the film. Furthermore, most sunscreens are tested in a laboratory under ideal wearing conditions. For practical purposes, it can be assumed that most sunscreens perform at half of their rated SPF.

The SPF is calculated as follows:

$$\frac{\text{UV energy required to produce an MED on protected skin}}{\text{UV energy required to produce an MED on unprotected skin}}$$

Thus, a patient who experiences reddening of the skin in 10 minutes of sun exposure without protection would be able to stay in the sun 60 minutes before the same degree of erythema developed while wearing a sunscreen with an SPF of 6. Many dermatologists feel that patients should wear a sunscreen with an SPF of 15 or higher to obtain adequate sun protection. Unfortunately, SPF is an evaluation of the UVB protective skin effects and does not account for UVA photoprotection. Methods have been proposed to define a protection factor for UVA protection factor, but no final rating system as been released as of this writing (6). Given the current SPF rating system, patients probably need to use a sunscreen with an SPF of 30 or higher to receive some degree of UVA photoprotection, especially important on the face for photoaging and skin prevention (Fig. 9.7).

> The performance of a sunscreen depends on the concentration of the sunscreen filter and its ability to remain on the skin.

The performance of a sunscreen depends on the concentration of the filters and the ability to remain on the skin. Increasing the concentration of a sunscreen filter can increase the SPF, for example 3% octyl dimethyl PABA has an SPF of 4 while 4% octyl dimethyl PABA has an SPF of 5. A better performance can be obtained with the octyl dimethyl ester of PABA since it is less water soluble than PABA accounting for its use in waterproof sunscreens and superior performance under humid conditions. Environmental factors such as heat, wind, humidity, perspiration, and thickness of sunscreen film application are also important in sunscreen performance, but these cannot be controlled (7). Higher SPF sunscreens are not necessarily more irritating than lower SPF varieties.

A superior sunscreen can also be produced by combining sunscreening agents. A sunscreen containing only 8% octyl dimethyl PABA has an SPF of 8 while a sunscreen combining 8% octyl dimethyl PABA with 3% oxybenzone has an SPF of 20. Most sunscreens will combine organic and inorganic filters for optimal photoprotection.

> Sunscreens are a more common source of irritant than allergic contact dermatitis.

Sunscreens are a more common source of irritant than allergic contact dermatitis, but distinguishing dermatitis from solar-induced phenomena can occasionally be difficult (8,9). Reports of contact urticaria have also been published, but again the reaction may be solar induced rather than sunscreen induced (10). PABA is a known sensitizer at a 5% concentration (11), but few presently marketed sunscreen formulations contain PABA. PABA esters, such as padimate A and padimate O, are used instead and possess a lower sensitization potential (12). The cinnamates are also sensitizers, even though they are commonly incorporated into hypoallergenic sunscreen formulations. Cinnamates interact with balsam of Peru, coca leaves, cinnamic acid, cinnamic aldehyde, and cinnamon oils (13). Both the salicylates (14) and anthranilates are rare sensitizers (15,16). Finally, photoallergic reactions have been reported with the benzophenones (17,18).

The organic filters are not sensitizers, but are occlusive and can produce miliaria. It has been reported that the inclusion of titanium dioxide in sunscreen formulations reduces the incidence of photoallergic contact dermatitis, possibly due to its ability to reflect ultraviolet radiation (10).

SUMMARY

Photoprotection of the face is an important dermatologic consideration. Most of the antiaging facial products based their claim on the inclusion of sunscreen filters. While no one has proven that sunscreens inhibit skin aging in humans, it is assumed that photoprotection is the key to beautiful skin for life. This chapter has discussed the types of ingredients that can be incorporated into sunscreens to provide photoprotection and sunless tanning products as a method for simulating tanned skin. The best solution to the problems associated with tanning is to change current fashion norms to rediscover the beauty of untanned naturally pigmented skin.

REFERENCES

1. Shaath NA. Evolution of modern chemical sunscreens. In: Lowe NJ, Shaath NA, eds. Sunscreens Development, Evaluation and Regulatory Aspects. New York: Marcel Dekker, Inc., 1990: 3–4.
2. Food and Drug Administration. Sunscreen drug products for over the counter human drugs: proposed safety, effective and labeling conditions. Fed Regist 1978; 43: 38206.
3. Shaath NA. The chemistry of sunscreens. In: Lowe NJ, Shaath NA, eds. Sunscreens Development, Evaluation and Regulatory Aspects. New York: Marcel Dekker, Inc., 1990: 223–5.
4. Murphy EG. Regulatory aspects of sunscreens in the United States. In: Lowe NJ, Shaath NA, eds. Sunscreens Development, Evaluation and Regulatory Aspects. New York: Marcel Dekker, Inc., 1990: 127–30.
5. Lowe NJ. Sun protection factors: comparative techniques and selection of ultraviolet sources. In: Lowe NJ, ed. Physician's Guide to Sunscreens. New York: Marcel Dekker, Inc., 1991: 161–5.
6. Ole C. Multicenter evaluation of sunscreen UVA protectiveness with the protection factor test method. J Am Acad Dermatol 1994; 30: 729–36.
7. Geiter F, Bilek PK, Doskoczil S. History of sunscreens and the rationale for their use. In: Frost P, Horwitz SN, eds. Principles of Cosmetics for the Dermatologist. St. Louis: CV Mosby Company, 1982: 187–206.
8. Freeman S, Frederiksen P. Sunscreen allergy. Am J Contact Dermatitis 1990; 1: 240.
9. Thompson G, Maibach HI, Epstein J. Allergic contact dermatitis from sunscreen preparations complicating photodermatitis. Arch Dermatol 1977; 113: 1252.
10. Dromgoole SH, Maibach HI. Sunscreening agent intolerance: contact and photocontact sensitization and contact urticaria. J Am Acad Dermatol 1990; 22: 1068–78.
11. Mathias CGT, Maibach HI, Epstein J. Allergic contact photodermatitis to para-aminobenzoic acid. Arch Dermatol 1978; 114: 1665–6.
12. Fisher AA. Sunscreen dermatitis: para-aminobenzoic acid and its derivatives. Cutis 1992; 50: 190–2.
13. Thune P. Contact and photocontact allergy to sunscreens. Photodermatology 1984; 1: 5–9.
14. Rietschel RL, Lewis CW. Contact dermatitis to homomenthyl salicylate. Arch Dermatol 1978; 114: 442–3.
15. Fisher AA. Sunscreen dermatitis: part IV the salicylates, the anthranilates and physical agents. Cutis 1992; 50: 397–8.
16. Menz J, Muller SA, Connolly SM. Photopatch testing: a six year experience. J Am Acad Dermatol 1988; 18: 1044–7.
17. Knobler E, Almeida L, Ruzkowski A, et al. Photoallergy to benzophenone. Arch Dermatol 1989; 125: 801–4.
18. Ramsay DL, Cohen HS, Baer RL. Allergic reaction to benzopenone. Arch Dermatol 1972; 105: 906–8.

SUGGESTED READING

Bennat C, Müller-Goymann CC. Skin penetration and stabilization of formulations containing microfine titanium dioxide as physical UV filter. Int J Cosmet Sci 2000; 22: 271–83.

Berneburg M, Plettenberg H, Krutmann J. Photoaging of human skin. Photodermatol Photoimmunol Photomed 2000; 16: 239–44.

Cross SE, Innes B, Roberts MS, et al. Human skin penetration of sunscreen nanoparticles: in-vitro assessment of a novel micronized zinc oxide formulation. Skin Pharmacol Physiol 2007; 20: 148–54.

Diffey BL. When should sunscreen be reapplied? J Acad Dermatol 2001; 45: 882–5.

Fisher GJ, Wang ZQ, Datta SC, et al. Pathophysiology of premature skin aging induced by ultraviolet light. N Engl J Med 1997; 337: 1419–28.

Giacomoni PU. Sunscreens, suntan and anti-sun-burn preparations today. J Appl Cosmetol 2002; 20: 129–36.

Gonzalez H. Percutaneous absorption with emphasis on sunscreens. Photochem Photobiol Sci 2010; 9: 482–8.

Green HA, Drake L. Aging, sun damage, and sunscreens. Clin Plast Surg 1993; 20: 1–8.

Harrison JA, Wlaker SL, Plastox SR, et al. Sunscreens with low sun protection factor inhibit ultraviolet B and A photoaging in the skin of the hairless albino mouse. Photodermal Photoimmunol Photomed 1991; 8: 12–20.

Klein K, Kollias N. Sunscreens (Chapter 20). In: Reiger MM, ed. Harry's Cosmeticology, 8th edn. Chemical Publishing Co., Inc., 2000: 415–36.

Klein K, Palefsky I. Formulating sunscreen products (Chapter 18). In: Shaath N, ed. Sunscreens, 3rd edn. Taylor & Francis Group, 2005: 354–83.

Kligman LH. Photoaging: manifestations, prevention, and treatment. Dermatol Clin 1986; 4: 517–28.

Kullavanijaya P, Lim H. Photoprotection. J Am Acad Deratol 2005; 52: 937–58.

Levy S. UV filters (Chapter 23). In: Paye M, Barel AO, Maibach HI, eds. Handbook of Cosmetic Science and Technology, 2nd edn. Informa Healthcare USA, Inc., 2007: 299–311.

Lintner K. Antiaging actives in sunscreens (Chapter 33). In: Shaath N, ed. Sunscreens, 3rd edn. Taylor & Francis Group, 2005: 673–95.

Maier H, Schauberger G, Brunnhofer K, Honigsmann H. Change of ultraviolet absorbance of sunscreens by exposure to solar-simulated radiation. J Invest Dermatol 2001; 117: 256–62.

Nohynek GJ, Dufour EK, Roberts MS. Nanotechnology, cosmetics and the skin: is there a health risk? Skin Pharmacol Physiol 2008; 21: 136–49.

Nohynek GJ, Lademann J, Ribaud C, Roberts MS. Grey goo on the skin? Nanotechnology, cosmetic and sunscreen safey. Crit Rev Toxical 2007; 37: 251–77.

Nole G, Johnson AW. An analysis of cumulative lifetime solar ultraviolet radiation exposure and the benefits of daily sun protection. Dermatol Ther 2004; 17: 57–62.

Palm MD, O'Donoghue MN. Update on photoprotection. Dermatol Ther 2007; 20: 360–76.

Rabe JH, Mamelak AJ, McElgunn JS, Morison WL, Sauder DN. Photoaging: mechanisms and repair. J Am Acad Dermatol 2006; 55: 1–19.

Scharffetter-Kochanek K, Brenneisen P, Wenk J, et al. Photoaging of the skin from phenotype to mechanisms. Exp Gerontol 2000; 35: 307–16.

Seite S, Fourtanier AM. The benefit of daily photoprotection. J Am Acad Dermatol 2008; 58 (5 Suppl 2): S160–6.

Shaath NA. The chemistry of ultraviolet filters (Chapter 13). In: Shaath N, ed. Sunscreens, 3rd edn. Taylor & Francis Group, 2005: 218–38.

Steinberg D. Sunscreens. Cosmet Toilet 2006; 121: 40–6.

Uitto J. The role of elastin and collagen in cutaneous aging: intrinsic aging versus photoexposure. J Drugs Dermatol 2008; 7 (2 Suppl): s12–16.

Wang SQ, Balagula Y, Osterwalder U. Photoprotection: a review of the current and future technologies. Dermatol Ther 2010; 23: 31–47.

Wissing AS, Müller RH. Solid lipid nanoparticles as carrier for sunscreens: in vitro release and in vivo skin penetration. J Control Release 2002; 81: 225–33.

Wlaschek M, Tantcheva-Poor I, Naderi L, et al. Solar UV irradiation and dermal photoaging. J Photochem Photobiol B 2001; 63: 41–51.

Wright MW, Wright ST, Wagner RF. Mechanisms of sunscreen failure. J Acad Dermatol 2001; 44: 781–4.

10 Lip cosmetic considerations

The lips are a site of great interest, since they are involved in phonation and eating. Also, they are an important part of personal appearance. Lips are formed from transitional epithelium wedged between traditional keratinized dry skin and moist mucosal skin, which is a portal of entry for bacteria, viruses, food, and medication (Fig. 10.1). They are an instrument of affection as delivered by a kiss and the focal point of the face. Much poetry has been written about beautiful ruby red lips through the ages. However, as the lips age, they begin to thin and lose their characteristic shape. This is due to loss of the fat that gives the lip substance. A profile view of a child will reveal lips that protrude from the face, while the profile of a 70-year-old woman will reveal lips that are flat and even depressed form the facial surface. Many of the new cosmetic fillers, such as hyaluronic acid, are designed to replace this lost fat. The loss of lip shape is also accentuated by loss of teeth and bony gum structures that give the lips their characteristic Cupid's bow shape. The lip muscles remain intact throughout life, but cannot make up for the loss of the underlying fat suspended over a bony frame.

Luscious lips are considered a sign of female beauty. While lip fashion may change over the time, the definition of beautiful lips is constant. Well-proportioned lips should begin at one pupil and extend to the opposite the pupil. Lipsticks can be used to elongate the lips and correct suboptimal proportions. They can also be used to add shine, attract attention, and coordinate colors. Lip cosmetics have been used since 7000 BC when the Sumerians adorned the lips of their male and female royalty. The art of lip adornment was passed on through generations from the Egyptians to the Syrians to the Babylonians to the Persians to the Greeks to the Romans to present day civilizations. Usually plant materials, such as hybrid saffron or brazilwood were used to obtain a reddish color. The earliest true lipsticks consisted of beeswax, tallow, and pigment. Modern lipstick was introduced in the 1920s when the "push-up" holder, still used today, was invented. Lipsticks can create or assist in the treatment of lip conditions (Table 10.1). This chapter focuses on the various types of lip cosmetics and their use in a variety of dermatologic situations.

LIPSTICK FORMULATION
Lipstick is an extruded rod of color dispersed in a blend of oils, waxes, and fats packaged in a roll-up tube (Fig. 10.2). The ratio of the oils and waxes is varied by the cosmetic chemist to arrive at the final attributes of the product. For example, a lipstick designed to camouflage lip imperfections must be long wearing. Elevating the wax concentration, reducing the oil concentration, and increasing the pigment concentration can increase the length of time the color remains on the lips. Lipsticks can also be used to treat non–actinic chelitis by providing higher lip emollience. This formulation would be composed of a low-wax and high-oil concentration to produce a smooth creamy lip feel.

Lipsticks can be used to treat non–actinic chelitis by providing higher lip emollience.

Waxes are used to facilitate the lip color adhere to the lip. The waxes commonly incorporated into lipstick formulations are white beeswax, candelilla wax, carnauba wax, ozokerite wax, lanolin wax, ceresin wax, and other synthetic waxes. Usually, lipsticks contain a combination of these waxes carefully selected and blended to achieve the desired melting point. Oils are then added to soften the wax and add shine to the lips. The oils that can be used include castor oil, white mineral oil, lanolin oil, hydrogenated vegetable oils, or oleyl alcohol. The oils are also necessary for the dispersion of the pigments.

Various types of coloring agents are used in lipsticks in addition to the waxes and oils previously discussed. Recently, the safety of these coloring agents has been questioned, since a consumer watchdog group announced that several red lipsticks possessed detectable lead levels. The colors used in all cosmetics, including lipsticks, must be approved by the Food and Drug Administration (FDA) (Table 10.2). The FDA divides certified colors into three groups: food, drug, and cosmetic (FD&C) colors, drug and cosmetic (D&C) colors, and external drug and cosmetic colors. Only the first two groups can be used in lipsticks. The external drug and cosmetic colors can only be used in locations where they are not likely to enter the mouth.

Companies that manufacture lip cosmetics purchase their individual ingredients from suppliers. The cosmetic company typically receives a certificate indicating that the purchased ingredient meets certain standards. On top of this safeguard, most companies also perform internal testing to ensure ingredient purity. There are many checks and balances to prevent the inadvertent contamination of cosmetics.

There are a variety of lipsticks designed for unique consumer needs. Since lipsticks can be used for camouflaging, moisturizing, and photoprotection, there are formulations designed specifically for each need (Fig. 10.3). An evaluation of these special needs products is important, as the dermatologist is likely to encounter patients who can supplement their lip therapy with proper lipstick selection.

LONG WEARING LIPSTICKS
Individuals who have a lip deformity or problems with lip bleeding due to upper and lower lip rhagades may find a long wearing lipstick helpful. Basically, the lipstick stays in place once applied and does not migrate because it stains the lip. These lipsticks should be used in persons who are undergoing lip filler enhancement where not all of the lines can be filled or when the lines cross from the perioral skin onto the vermillion.

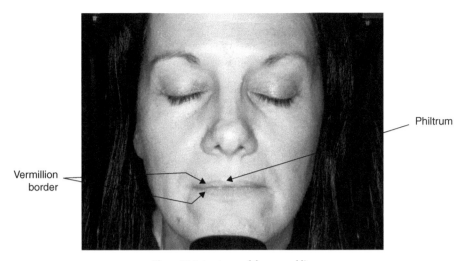

Figure 10.1 Anatomy of the normal lips.

Table 10.1 Lip Cosmetics

Lipsticks	Appearance	Coverage	Wearability	Main ingredients
Lipsticks				
Pigmented	Matte	Full	Moderate	Wax, oil, pigment
Frosted	Pearlescent	Full	Moderate	Wax, oil, pigment
Transparent	Shiny	Very sheer	Short	High percentage of oil, soluble dyes
Indelible	Matte	Moderate	Very long	Wax, oil, bromo acid dyes
Lip crayons	Pearlescent or matte	Full	Moderate	Wax, less oil lipstick, pigment
Lip liners	Matte	Not applicable	Long	Wax, pigment
Lip creams and gloss pots	Shiny	Sheer	Very short	Petrolatum, oil, pigment
Lip sealants	Matte	Not applicable	Long	Water, glycerin, wax, oil, dimethicone
Lip balm	Matte	None	Long	Wax, mineral oil, chemical sunscreen

Coverage: very sheer = transparent, sheer = semitransparent, moderate = translucent, heavy = semiopaque, full = opaque.
Wearability: very short = 2 hours, short = 3 hours, moderate = 4 hours, long = 8 hours.

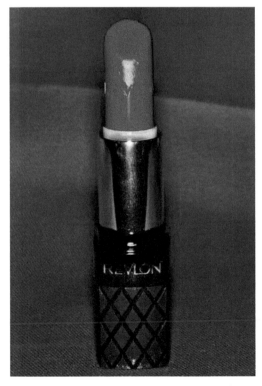

Figure 10.2 Lipstick is a creamy pigmented cosmetic dispensed from a roll-up tube to temporarily color the lips.

Table 10.2 Lipstick Colorants Permitted in the U.S.A.

FD&C or D&C Blue No. 1, Al Lake	D&C Red No. 11, Ca
FD&C or D&C Blue No. 2, Al Lake	D&C Red No. 12, Ba
FD&C or D&C Red No. 2, Al Lake	D&C Red No. 13, Sr
FD&C or D&C Red No. 3, Al Lake	D&C Red No. 19, Al Lake
FD&C Yellow No. 5, Al Lake	D&C Red No. 21
D&C Yellow No. 5, Zr-Al Lake	R&C Red No. 27
D&C Yellow No. 6, Al Lake	D&C Red No. 27, Al Lake
FD&C or D&C Yellow, No. 6, Al Lake	D&C Red No. 30D&C Red No. 36
D&C Orange No. 5	D&C Blue No. 1, Al Lake
D&C Orange No. 5, Al Lake	Iron oxide—all shades
D&C Orange No. 10	Carmine
D&C Orange No. 10, Al Lake	Bronze powder
D&C Orange No. 17, Ba Lake	Carbon black
D&C Red No. 3, Al Lake	Guanine
D&C Red No. 6, Na or Ba	Manganese violet
D&C Red No. 7, Ca	Mica
D&C Red No. 8, Na	Aluminum powder
D&C Red No. 9, Ba	Bismuth oxychloride
D&C Red No. 10, Na	Carotene

Source: Adapted from deNavarre MG. Lipstick. In: The Chemistry and Manufacture of Cosmetics. 2nd edn. Allured Publishing Corporation, Wheaton, IL: 1975: 778.

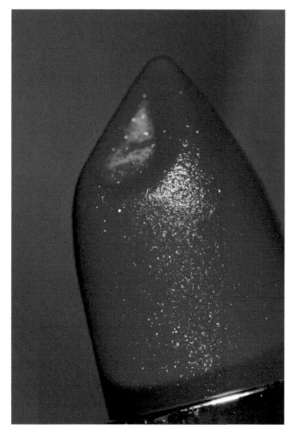

Figure 10.3 A moisturizing lipstick with a central core of lip moisturizer surrounded by an outer layer of pigmented lipstick.

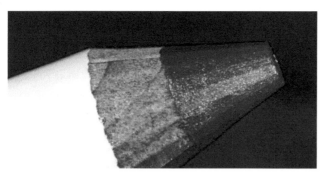

Figure 10.4 A long wearing lipstick in the form of a lip crayon.

Long wearing lipsticks employ indelible coloring agents to stain the lip. Indelible coloring agents include bromo acids, such as fluoresceins, halogenated fluoresceins, and related water-insoluble dyes. The most commonly used indelible coloring agent is acid eosin, a tetrabromo derivative of fluorescein. Acid eosin, also known as bromo acid or D&C Red No. 21, is naturally colored orange, but changes to a red salt at a pH of 4. Conditions present on the lip change the orange lipstick to a vivid red indelible stain that is long lasting. This accounts for the red color of all long wearing lipsticks (Fig. 10.4).

Long wearing lipsticks employ indelible coloring agents, most commonly eosin, to stain the lip.

The biggest problem with long wearing lipsticks is that they dry the lips and precipitate chelitis. For this reason, long wearing lipsticks should not be used in persons with dry lips, as the lip xerosis will worsen with continued use of a lip stain. It is also possible to develop an irritant contact dermatitis to bromo acid in lipsticks. In patients who have unexplained lip dryness and irritation, it may be worthwhile to recommend the discontinuation of long wearing lip products.

LIP BALMS

An important variant of the lipstick is the lip balm. Lip balms do not contain pigment and are not used for decoration of the lips, but rather to provide moisturization of the lips and protection from the sun and cold. These products form a moisture-resistant film over the lips and act as an occlusive moisturizer to prevent water loss from the transitional mucosa. They usually contain a mixture of mineral oil, wax, and dimethicone. Lip balms may also contain organic sunscreens. Most lip balms have a sun protection factor (SPF) in the 15 to 30 range. Higher SPF lip balms are difficult to develop because the organic filter concentration would need to be increased and these filters have a horrible bitter taste. Yet, lip balms remain an excellent source of photoprotection in persons with actinic chelitis, leukoplakia, or a history of photo-induced lip cancer.

Lip balms can provide both moisturization and photoprotection to the lips.

There is a great deal of information on the Internet about the "addictive" potential of lip balms. Some consumers claim that they are addicted to lip balm, carry a tube in their pocket at all times, and must reapply the lip balm several times an hour. I did some research into this phenomenon several years ago and determined that patients were not addicted to the lip balm, but rather the waxy feel of the lip balm on the lips. It was a sensory rather than a functional addiction. The lip balm did not precipitate further lip dryness, but created a warm moist feel immediately after application that disappeared as the product remained on the lips. This necessitated the frequent reapplication as the film dissolved.

LIP SEALANTS

Lip sealants are similar in function to eye shadow setting creams in that both products prepare the skin for increased cosmetic wearability. Lip sealants prevent movement of the product into the fine lines around the lips, encouraging the lip cosmetic to remain in place. They contain water, talc, glycerin, wax, mineral oil, and dimethicone. The cream is applied to the lips like lipstick or with a finger and allowed to dry before a pigmented lip cosmetic is applied. Facial foundation can also be applied to the lips as a sealant.

Lip sealants contain dimethicone; can fill in lip wrinkles and provide a base for the subsequent application of lipstick.

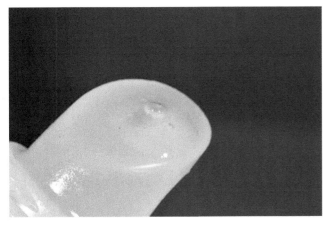

Figure 10.5 Lip gloss may be dispensed from a plastic tube and stroked over the lips with its angled application tip.

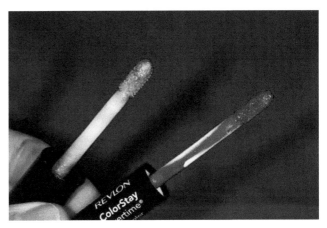

Figure 10.7 Angled brushes are used to stroke the colored polymer lip product over the lips.

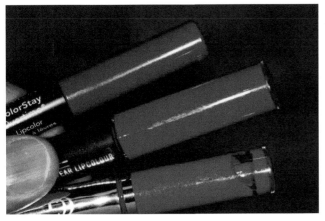

Figure 10.6 Tubes of various polymer lipstick colors that also contain a lip stain.

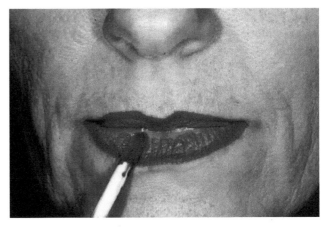

Figure 10.8 The artistic application of the lip polymer to the lips.

LIP GLOSS

Another popular product to moisturize the lips is lip gloss. Lip gloss is different from lip balm as it does not contain waxes, but only oils and dimethicone. Lip gloss is most popular among adolescents who may select lip gloss as their first cosmetic. It adds shine, smell, and taste to the lips, but not necessarily moisturization (Fig. 10.5). Lip gloss migrates rapidly off the lip and is not a good choice in mature individuals. Additionally, some of the oils may be comedogenic. The dermatologist should caution about the use of lip gloss in acne patients with refractory vermillion border comedones.

Lip gloss has seen a resurgence in the popularity of film-forming polymer lipsticks. The polymer dries to a hard pigmented film on the lips, but is extremely drying. To prevent chelitis and add shine, many polymer lip products are co-packaged with a lip gloss for frequent application, and this is the next topic of discussion.

POLYMER FILM LIPSTICKS

Another method for enhancing the ability of a lip color to remain on the lips is through the creation of polymer films. Polymer film lipsticks are the newest introduction into the lipstick market. These lip products are packaged as two-tube products where one end contains the lip color and the opposite end contains a lip gloss or balm. The pigmented polymer is applied first and allowed to dry followed by the moisturizing gloss or balm. These products stay on until peeled or rubbed off (Fig. 10.6).

For persons who need a long wearing lip product for camouflage purposes, the polymer film lipsticks are wonderful. They form an opaque film, which can cover pigmentation or vascular abnormalities of the lip. Another layer of camouflage can be added by putting a creamy opaque lipstick on top for moisturization and shine.

The polymer lip products can be used to artistically draw on the lips, if they are asymmetric or too small (Fig. 10.7). The polymer film sticks well to any skin surface, but the best results are obtained when combined with a lip liner. The lip liner forms an even edge that can be painted over with the polymer film applicator. As opposed to lipsticks that are rubbed from a waxy stick, polymer film lip products are stroked across the lips with an angled sponge brush. This requires a steady hand for successful application (Fig. 10.8).

To prevent chelitis and add shine, many polymer lip products are co-packaged with a lip gloss for frequent application.

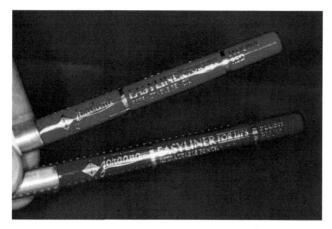

Figure 10.9 Pigmented lip liners in an automatic pencil-type holder.

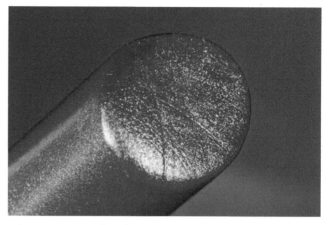

Figure 10.10 Opaque lipsticks provide excellent sun protection in women.

LIP LINERS

As mentioned previously, the new polymer lip products are best combined with a lip liner. Lip liners are thin extruded pigmented rods encased in wood or placed in an automatic pencil-type holder (Fig. 10.9). Their formulation is similar to lipsticks, except that stiffer waxes with higher melting points are used with minimal oil. This creates an extremely hard rod that applies a thick layer of pigment to the lips. Lip liners are used to define the outer edge of the lips and are valuable in reconstructing a normal lip contour. The thick wax layer applied around the lips also prevents creamier lip products from bleeding. Lip liner is usually selected one to two shades darker than the lipstick.

> Lip liners are used to define the outer edge of the lips and are valuable in reconstructing a normal lip contour.

Lip liners are indispensable in persons who require lip definition or lip enhancement. They can nicely aid in lip definition for women who have undergone lip augmentation with fillers. Lip liner can also be used to temporarily draw lip proportions prior to filler injections to make sure that the patient is comfortable with the proposed lip size.

OPAQUE LIPSTICKS

Opaque lip cosmetics can be used over polymer lip products to prevent inevitable lip dryness (Fig. 10.10). An opaque lip cosmetic is also preferred in patients who require lip camouflaging. The opaqueness is due to incorporation of high titanium dioxide levels in the lipstick. Titanium dioxide provides the best coverage of all the white pigments, including zinc oxide. It must be ground to a fine powder to enable smooth application of the lipstick. It also adds color brightness to lip cosmetics and is used to create pastel shades. Opaque lipsticks are the best lip protection for women with actinic chelitis. They can nicely protect the lip transitional mucosa after cryosurgery or lip advancement for reconstruction following lip cancer surgery.

> Opaque lipsticks are the best lip protection for women with actinic chelitis.

TOOTH WHITENING LIPSTICKS

Another new category of lipsticks is tooth whitening lipsticks. These are sold primarily in drug stores. The name may be misleading, however, since the lipstick does not actually whiten the teeth like the popular tooth whitening kits containing peroxide. These lipsticks have a bluish-red color that makes the teeth appear white due to the color contrast.

> Tooth whitening lipsticks have a bluish-red color that makes the teeth appear white due to the color contrast.

LIP COSMETICS AND ALLERGIC CONTACT DERMATITIS

Lipstick can be a cause of allergic contact dermatitis. The lipstick ingredients reported to cause allergic contact dermatitis include ricinoleic acid (1), benzoic acid (2), lithol rubine BCA (Pigment Red 57-1) (3), microcrystalline wax (4), oxybenzone (5), propyl gallate (6), and C18 aliphatic compounds (7).

> The most common cause of allergic contact dermatitis in lipstick is castor oil.

The castor oil in lipstick causes allergic contact dermatitis. Castor oil is found in all lipsticks. It is used to dissolve bromo acid dyes (8–10). However, the bromo acid dye eosin (D&C Red No. 21) is also a cause (11). If a patient has recurrent allergic contact dermatitis to different types and brands of lipstick, castor oil allergy is almost always the problem. Still, most women want to wear lipstick. An excellent alternative is one of the polymer lipsticks previously discussed. These products do not contain castor oil.

LIP TATTOOING

Definition of the vermillion border can be achieved temporarily with lip cosmetics, as previously discussed, or permanently enhanced through lip tattooing. Less conventional than the use of lip liners, this method is practiced by dermatologists and plastic surgeons. Lip tattooing is performed by inserting a red pigment such as cinnabar, a red dye containing mercuric sulfide, into the upper dermis along the vermilion border through punctures created by a specially designed needle. The normal lip contour can be followed, resulting in the appearance of permanent lipstick, or the pigment can be placed to reshape malformed lips. Lip tattooing can also be used to reconstruct the vermilion border in patients with treated actinic cheilitis or leukoplakia. It is possible to develop a tattoo granuloma since cinnabar is the most allergenic of the tattoo pigments.

> Lip tattoo granulomas may occur from cinnabar, the red pigment used for permanently tattooed lipstick.

This technique is not recommended for women, except in cases of extreme surgical deformity, since fashion dictates the desirable lip appearance and the patient will not be able to wear lighter lipstick shades in pink or peach. However, the permanence of lip color may be more desirable in male patients, who do not require fashion flexibility. Patients should recognize that there is some fading of the pigment color with time and the movement of the pigment within the dermis occurs due to macrophage phagocytosis.

Lip cosmetics are used by many individuals, some of whom may have special dermatologic needs. The discussion now turns to the special lip needs of acne patients, mature patients, and individuals who require the assistance of corrective lip cosmetics.

LIP COSMETICS FOR ACNE PATIENTS

Lip cosmetics are used by acne patients, but must be carefully selected to avoid worsening of the acne. Acne patients should select lip cosmetics with low oil content to minimize the formation of comedones around the vermilion border and perioral acne. Lip creams and gloss pots contain mostly oil and should be avoided in favor of lip crayons and lipsticks. Lip cosmetics with a higher oil content have a creamy feel and a glossy shine on application. Acne patients with oily complexions will also notice the movement of the lip cosmetic away from the lips as sebum combines with the cosmetic. Lip crayons and lip liners will provide the longest wear in these patients. The use of a lip stain may also be considered.

> Acne patients should select lip cosmetics with low oil content to minimize the formation of comedones around the vermilion border and perioral acne.

LIP COSMETICS FOR MATURE PATIENTS

Lip cosmetics are important to mature patients also, not only to pigment and enlarge the important facial landmark, that is the lips, but also to assist in the prevention and treatment of lip disease. With maturity, the lip architecture changes giving rise to a biofilm disease of the lips known as perleche. Perleche arising as the collection of saliva in the folds of the corners of the mouth creates maceration providing a perfect environment for the growth of yeast. The yeast causes further tissue breakdown and painful cracked skin that is best treated by a combination of topical low-potency topical corticosteroids

and topical antifungal/anti-yeast creams. Perleche can actually be prevented by the use of an occlusive lip balm that does not support the yeast growth and protects the lip corners from moisture contact.

> Perleche can be prevented by using an occlusive lip balm that does not support yeast growth and protects the lip corners from moisture contact.

In addition to biofilm diseases, the lips can also be subject to dryness in mature patients. Abundant oil glands can be visualized lining the vermillion of the lips, but the production of these glands decreases with advancing age. Dryness of the lips, known as chelitis, leads to cracking and peeling of the lips. Chelitis can be accentuated by heat exposure from smoking or actinic damage. Lip balms, lip moisturizers, or lipsticks can be used to aid in the treatment of chelitis. Good occlusion is typically required to allow these conditions to resolve, achieved with oily substances, such as petrolatum, waxes, and silicones. Some elderly individuals may appear to have chronic chelitis due to the continual presence of peeling skin over the lips. This may be due to dryness, but may also be due to insufficient exfoliation of the lip surface. The use of a stiff lip balm with high drag over the lips when applied may be helpful in this condition, as well.

Lip balms can be further adapted to provide both lip moisturization and sun protection. A quality lip balm used on a daily basis with an SPF of at least 15 can prevent actinic chelitis. A sunscreen-containing lip balm is also the best way to prevent the recurrence of a herpes simplex fever blister, since the virus is photo reactivated. Lastly, sunscreen-containing lip balms can prevent skin cancer of the lip, a serious medical condition in mature individuals.

Finally, color can be added to a pale mature face quickly with lip cosmetics. In addition, only a minimal application skill is required and the steady hand necessary for eye cosmetic application is not needed. These characteristics make lip cosmetics popular among mature patients. The most common complaint in this age group is the movement, or "bleeding," of lip cosmetics into the fine wrinkles that develop on the upper and lower lips from elastic tissue degeneration or gingival bone resorption. Often mature persons with dry lips select a moisturizing lipstick and subsequently experience lipstick bleeding. Lip cosmetic bleeding can be minimized by preparing the lips first with a lip sealant or facial foundation, using a stiff lip liner, and avoiding creamy lipsticks or lip creams in favor of lip crayons. All lipsticks are moisturizers to some extent. Stiff lip balms or sticks cannot be applied as moisturizers under lipsticks since this will encourage lipstick bleeding.

Mature patients may wish to use a lip cosmetic to cover lentigines, venous lakes, or actinic cheilitis. Darker lipstick colors provide better coverage than lighter colors. Lipsticks that contain titanium dioxide are superior to lip crayons or lip creams. Application to the lips of a facial foundation containing titanium dioxide adds additional coverage. A bluish-red lipstick will have the added advantage of seeming to whiten the discolored teeth.

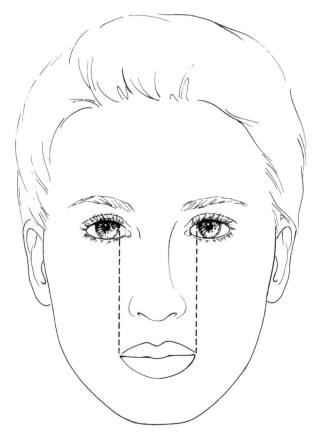

Figure 10.11 The length of the closed, relaxed mouth should equal the distance between the medial aspect of the irises in a well-proportioned face.

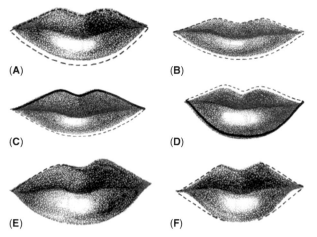

Figure 10.12 Contouring of the lips: (**A**) to enlarge small lips, (**B**) to thicken thin lips, (**C**) to thicken a thin lower lip, (**D**) to thicken a thin upper lip, (**E**) to decrease the size of thick lips, (**F**) to correct crooked lips, (**G**) to correct bow lips, and (**H**) to correct downturned lips.

CORRECTIVE LIP COSMETICS

Abnormal lip shape due to congenital causes or surgery can be masked by an effective application of lip cosmetics. A well-proportioned mouth in a closed, relaxed state should be positioned between the medial aspect of the irises (Fig. 10.11) (12). Lips that do not extend this distance are perceived as small. Small lips can be enlarged by using a lip liner to draw the lip boundary on the outer edge of the vermilion and then filling

in with a deeply pigmented, matte finish lipstick (Fig. 10.12A). Uniformly thin lips (Fig. 10.12B), a thin lower lip possibly due to lip advancement surgery, (Fig. 10.12C), or a thin upper lip (Fig. 10.12D) can be thickened by also lining outside the vermilion where required and selecting a lighter, frosted finish lipstick. Conversely, thick lips possibly due to a congenital hemangioma are lined inside the vermilion (Fig. 10.12E). Figure 10.12 also demonstrates the lip lining technique with a dashed line for crooked (Fig. 10.12F), bow (Fig. 10.12G), and downturned lips (Fig. 10.12H). The lip liner should be one shade darker than the lipstick for optimal effect.

> Abnormal lip shape due to congenital causes or surgery can be masked by effective application of lip cosmetics.

SUMMARY

Lipsticks are useful for cosmetic adornment, but can also be used by the dermatologist to facilitate the healing of a variety of lip conditions. For example, actinic chelitis can be minimized by using a sunscreen-containing lip balm or an opaque lipstick. Remember that an opaque lipstick has an unlimited SPF, since the transitional lip mucosa is completely protected. Lip abnormalities can be minimized by selecting a polymer lip product combined with a lip liner. Finally, patients who experience problems such as lip swelling with the use of lipsticks may be allergic to castor oil. Lipsticks and lip balms are to the lips what hand cream is to the hands. Both are important therapeutic adjuvants in the treatment of dermatologic disease.

REFERENCES

1. Sai S. Lipstick dermatitis caused by ricinoleic acid. Contact Dermatitis 1983; 9: 524.
2. Calnan CD. Amyldimethylamino benzoic acid causing lipstick dermatitis. Contact Dermatitis 1980; 6: 233.
3. Hayakawa R, Fujimoto Y, Kaniwa M. Allergic pigmented lip dermatitis from lithol rubine BCA. Am J Contact Dermatitis 1994; 5: 34–7.
4. Darko E, Osmundsen PE. Allergic contact dermatitis to Lipcare lipstick. Contact Dermatitis 1984; 11: 46.
5. Aguirre A, Izu R, Gardeazabal J, et al. Allergic contact cheilitis from a lipstick containing oxybenzone. Contact Dermatitis 1992; 27: 267–8.
6. Cronin E. Lipstick dermatitis due to propyl gallate. Contact Dermatitis 1980; 6: 213–14.
7. Hayakawa R, Matsunaga K, Suzuki M, et al. Lipstick dermatitis due to C18 aliphatic compounds. Contact Dermatitis 1987; 16: 215–19.
8. Sai S. Lipstick dermatitis caused by castor oil. Contact Dermatitis 1983; 9: 75.
9. Brandle I, Boujnah-Khouadja A, Foussereau J. Allergy to castor oil. Contact Dermatitis 1983; 9: 424–5.
10. Andersen KE, Neilsen R. Lipstick dermatitis related to castor oil. Contact Dermatitis 1984; 11: 253–4.
11. Calan CD. Allergic sensitivity to eosin. Acta Allergol 1959; 13: 493–9.
12. Powell N, Humphreys B. Proportions of the aesthetic face. New York: Thieme-Stratton Inc, 1984: 32–4.

SUGGESTED READING

Angelini E, Marinaro C, Carrozzo AM, et al. Allergic contact dermatitis of the lip margins from para-tertiary-butylphenol in a lip liner. Contact Dermatitis 1993; 28: 146–8.
Duke D, Urioste SS, Dover JS, Anderson RR. A reaction to a red lip cosmetic tattoo. J Am Acad Dermatol 1998; 39: 488–90.

Engasser PG. Lip cosmetics. Dermatol Clin 2000; 18: 641–9.

Ha JH, Kim HO, Lee JY, Kim CW. Allergic contact cheilitis from D&C Red no 7 in lipstick. Contact Dermatitis 2003; 48: 231.

Le Coz CJ, Ball C. Recurrent allergic contact dermatitis and cheilitis due to castor oil. Contact Dermatitis 2000; 42: 114–15.

Leveque JL, Goubanova E. Influence of age on the lips and perioral skin. Dermatology 2004; 208: 307–13.

Ryu JS, Park SG, Kwak TJ, et al. Improving lip wrinkles: lipstick-related image analysis. Skin Res Technol 2005; 11: 157–64.

Sai S. Lipstick dermatitis caused by castor oil. Contact Dermatitis 1983; 9: 75.

Schena D, Antuzzi F, Girolomoni G. Contact allergy in chronic eczematous lip dermatitis. Eur J Dermatol 2008; 18: 688–92.

Schram SE, Glesne LA, Warshaw EM. Allergic contact cheilitis from benzophenone-3 I lip balm and fragrance/flavorings. Dermatitis 2007; 18: 221–4.

Wilson AG, White IR, Kirby JD. Allergic contact dermatitis from propyl gallate in a lip balm. Contact Dermatitis 1989; 20: 145–6.

Zug KA, Kornik R, Belsito DV, et al. Patch-testing North America lip dermatitis patients: data from the North American Contact Dermatitis Group, 2001 to 2004. Dermatitis 2008; 19: 202–8.

11 Eyes

Eyes, more than any other body part, express a person's inner thoughts and emotions. For this reason, the eyes are elaborately adorned, but the anatomy of the eyelid area also makes the eyes a common site of irritation, dermatitis, and infection. Eyelid cosmetic use dates back to antiquity, recorded as early as 4000 BC. Green powder made from malachite was heavily applied to both the upper and lower eyelids accompanied by dark kohl eyeliner paste composed of powdered antimony, burnt almonds, black copper oxide, and brown clay ocher. The eyeliner paste was stored in a pot and moistened with saliva prior to application. Eyelid glitter from ground beetle shells was used for additional effect (1).

This chapter examines eyelid cosmetics, eyelash cosmetics, and eyelid skin issues. It assesses the unique needs of the eyelid skin and the impact of colored adornments in the form of eye shadow, eyeliner, mascara, and eyebrow pencil as it relates to dermatology. Our discussion opens with a discussion of the eye area skin and then segue ways to the world of colored eye cosmetics.

EYELID CONSIDERATIONS

The eyelid skin is one of the most interesting areas on the body (Fig. 11.1). It moves constantly as the eyes open and close, thus it must possess unique mechanical properties. It must be thin enough for rapid movement, yet strong enough to protect the tender eye tissues. Eyelid tissue shows the state of health and age of an individual more rapidly than any other skin of the body. When others comment on a tired appearance, they are usually assessing the appearance of the eyes and the eyelid tissue. When others comment on a sickly appearance, they are also assessing the appearance of the eyes and the eyelid tissue. The eyelid skin appears to age quickly resulting in the presence of redundant upper eyelid tissue and lower eyelid bags. The redundant upper eyelid tissue is due to loss of facial fat, cumulative collagen loss in the eyelid skin from UV exposure, and the effect of gravity pulling down the upper eyelid skin. Lower eyelid bags are also formed due to the effect UV damage and gravity, but edema or swelling may also contribute. This edema may be due to retained body fluids or the release of histamine from inhaled allergens. All of these factors contribute to the complexity of the eyelid skin.

> The eyelids are the most common site for irritant and allergic contact dermatitis from cosmetics and skin care products.

The eyelids are the thinnest skin on the body; hence, the eyelids are the most common site for irritant contact dermatitis and allergic contact dermatitis, either from products that are directly applied to the eyelids or from products transferred to the eyelids by the hands. The eyelid skin also has a paucity of sebaceous glands, making it a common area of skin dryness. While there are no hairs on the eyelids themselves, the eyelashes form an interesting transition between the keratinized eyelid skin and the cartilage of the tarsal plate giving structure to the edge of the eyelid. Tearing from the eye impacts the skin of the eyelid, since wetting and drying of the eyelid tissues can predispose to dermatitis.

The eyelids are also a common source of symptoms induced by allergies. These symptoms can be itching, stinging, and/or burning. Most persons with these symptoms respond by vigorously rubbing the eyelids. This can cause a mechanical damage to the eyelid skin from a minor trauma resulting in sloughing of portions of the protective stratum corneum to a major trauma resulting in small tears in the skin. Most of the skin on the body responds by thickening or callousing when rubbed. Eyelid skin will also thicken, but this predisposes to decreased functioning and worsening of the symptoms.

The eyelid bridges the transitional area between the well-keratinized skin of the face and the moist tissue of the conjunctiva that lines the inner eyelid and the eyeball. The moisture from tearing wets the eyelid skin and enhances irritant and allergen penetration. It can also help dissolve any allergen or irritant, possibly enhancing the adverse reaction. The eyes are also uniquely designed to sense substances that might cause vision damage and thus the eyelids have a heightened immune response. Swelling induced by topical, inhaled, or ingested allergens are frequently seen initially in the eyelids. The thin nature of the skin also allows the swelling, due to tissue edema, to appear more dramatic than on other body areas where the skin is thicker and less mobile.

In addition to irritant and allergic contact dermatitis involving the eyelid skin, the eyelids can also be the site of biofilm diseases. Ocular rosacea and styes are basically acne of the glands in the eyelid resulting from alterations in the tear biofilm. Overgrowth of bacteria can precipitate the problem. Fungal overgrowth in the eye area results in seborrheic blepharitis.

The eyelid skin is also uniquely affected by the immune status of the individual. Most persons with inhaled allergies to pollen, fragrance, dust, etc. will complain not only of a runny nose but also of itchy eyes. The eyelids and the nose both represent areas possessing transitional skin bridging the wet mucosa with the traditional dry keratinized skin. Since the wet mucosa is devoid of a skin barrier to allergens and infection, the immune system is particularly fortified in these locations. For this reason, hyperimmune states that affect the overall body skin are keenly present in the eyelid area. For example, persons with atopic dermatitis will demonstrate an additional skin fold on the lower eyelid, an accurate marker for the diagnosis. They represent a unique population of sensitive eyelid persons who have problems with many eye area cosmetics and skin care products.

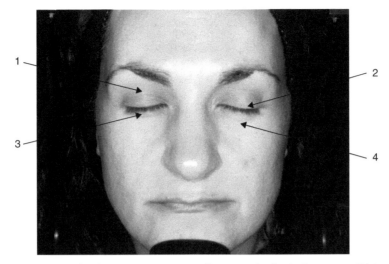

Figure 11.1 The eyelids are of considerable medical and cosmetic concern: 1, puffiness may develop in the upper eyelid; 2, extra skin in the upper eyelid may obscure the natural fold and impair vision; 3, extra skin in the lower eyelid may cause fine wrinkles; 4, bags or dark circles can develop under the lower eyelid.

By far the most common dermatologic disease to afflict the eyelid is eczema. Since the eyelid is relatively poor in oil glands, dry eyelid skin is frequently seen due to overaggressive removal of lipids. This may be due to the use of a strong cleanser or products designed to solubilize oil-based waterproof cosmetics, such as mascara and eyeliner. Anything that damages the intercellular lipids or the corneocytes will result in eyelid eczema. Thus, eyelid hygiene must strike a careful balance between the removal of excess sebum and old cosmetics to prevent from eyelash infections and seborrheic blepharitis, while preventing any damage to the intercellular lipids and ensuing eyelid eczema. Moisturizers for the eye area should contain occlusive substances that have minimal chance for allergenicity or irritancy, reduced ability to enter the eye, and excellent moisturization properties.

The thinness of the eyelid skin also makes the use of sunscreens important. UVA radiation can easily penetrate to the dermis of the thin eyelid skin, causing premature wrinkling. The eyelids are also a common site for UVB-induced sunburn. Eyelid sunscreens must be carefully formulated to avoid allergic and irritant contact dermatitis, prevent stinging and burning should the product enter the eye, and provide superior photoprotection.

There are more color cosmetics for the eyelid area than any other body area such as mascara, eyeliner, eye shadow, and eyebrow pencil.

Finally, eyelids are also a common site for cosmetic adornment. The eyelid area has more separate color cosmetics than any other body area like mascara, eyeliner, eye shadow, and eyebrow pencil. These cosmetics and the products used to remove them can be a source of both allergic and irritant contact dermatitis. Modern, color cosmetics for eyelids became popular between 1959 and 1962 (2). This chapter will now focus on eye cosmetics and discuss the subject for the dermatologist.

EYE SHADOWS

Eye shadows are applied to the upper eyelid to add color to the face and accentuate the emotionally expressive eyes. Eye shadows are available in several forms: pressed powders, anhydrous

Table 11.1 Eyelid-Approved Pigments

Iron oxides
Titanium dioxide (alone or combined with mica)
Copper, aluminum, and silver powder
Ultramarine blue, violet, and pink
Manganese violet
Carmine
Chrome oxide and hydrate
Iron blue
Bismuth oxychloride (alone, or on mica or talc)
Mica

creams, emulsions, sticks, and pencils. Color variety is extensive, but coal tar derivatives cannot be used in the eye area. Only purified, natural colors or inorganic pigments can be used in the United States as a result of the Food, Drug and Cosmetic Act of 1938 (Table 11.1) (3).

No coal tar derivatives for pigments can be used in the eye area, only approved purified natural colors or inorganic pigments can be used.

Variations in eye shadow surface texture can range from dull to a pearly shine to an iridescent finish. Titanium dioxide (TiO_2) is used in pastel matte (dull) finish eye shadows to improve coverage. However, it is not found in frosted (pearled shine) finish eye shadows since it tends to mask the desired pearled effect. Bismuth oxychloride (BiOCl), mica, and fish scale essence are the standard materials used to produce a pearly shine. A metallic (iridescent) finish is provided by copper, brass, aluminum, gold, or silver powders (Fig. 11.2).

Eye shadows are used to adorn the eyelid with a rainbow of colors for personal expression.

Pressed powder eye shadows are the most popular formulation and are applied to the eyelid by lightly stroking a soft sponge-tipped applicator across the skin (Fig. 11.3). They are

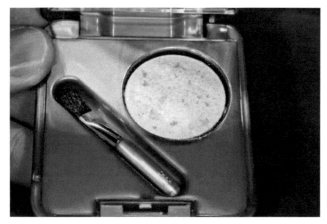

Figure 11.2 An iridescent eye shadow with a glittery shine draws attention to the eyelid, but can cause irritation in persons with sensitive eyes.

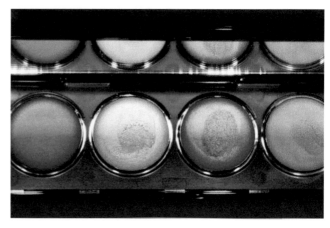

Figure 11.5 Cream eye shadows tend to migrate into the eyelid folds in mature patients, but are more water resistant than powder varieties.

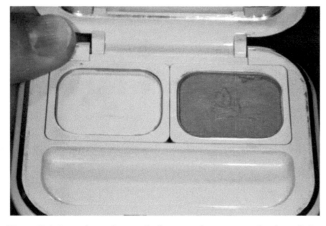

Figure 11.3 Pressed powder eye shadows are the most popular formulation and are packaged in compacts with various color combinations to create dramatic upper eyelid fashion statements.

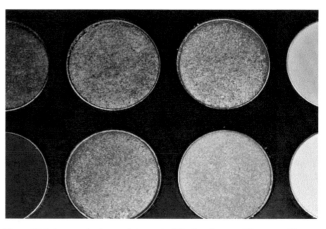

Figure 11.6 An eye shadow palate created for hazel eyes with tones of brown and green.

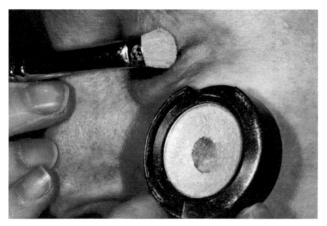

Figure 11.4 A brush is used to apply the powder eye shadow to the eyelid.

predominantly talc with pigments and zinc or magnesium stearate used as a binder. Kaolin or chalk may be added to improve oil absorption and increase wearability. A water or oily binder system may also be used, with oily binder systems such as mineral oil, beeswax, or lanolin is predominating. Powder eye shadows that are labeled "creamy" or "enriched" contain increased amounts of the oily binder (Fig. 11.4).

Anhydrous, or water-free, cream eye shadows contain pigments in petrolatum, cocoa butter, or lanolin (Fig. 11.5). These formulations are waterproof, but have a short wearing time due to their tendency to migrate into the eyelid folds, especially in patients with oily complexions or redundant eyelid skin. The product is applied with the finger and gently rubbed across the eyelid skin. Anhydrous cream eye shadows have also been formulated as an emulsion applied with a sponge-tipped applicator or wand withdrawn from a cylindrical tube and stroked across the eyelid. These products, known as automatic eye shadows, are also waterproof, with increased wear duration over the creams. They contain beeswax, cyclomethicone, and pigments in a volatile petroleum distillate vehicle.

The most popular anhydrous eye shadows are eye shadow sticks and pencils. They are composed of pigments in petrolatum, but have added waxes, such as paraffin, carnauba, or ozokerite wax, to allow extrusion of the product into a rod. Eye shadow sticks come in roll-up tubes and must be creamy to prevent drag as they are rubbed across the eyelid skin. For this reason, eye shadow sticks tend to migrate into eyelid creases in oily-complected patients or those with redundant eyelid skin. A more modern packaging is to encase the rod in wood, thus forming an eye shadow pencil that is rubbed across the eyelid. The pencil form is not as creamy as the eye shadow stick.

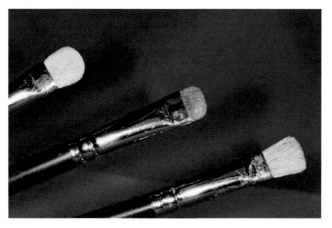

Figure 11.7 Eye shadows are applied with a variety of brushes, similar to paint brushes, to create living temporary art on the female eyelid.

Eye shadows are stroked or rubbed across the eyelid, depending on the type of formulation. Selection of eye shadow color is a matter of personal preference and fashion, although colors complementary to the natural color of the iris are most attractive (Figs. 11.6 and 11.7).

EYE SHADOW SETTING CREAMS

Eye shadow setting creams are unpigmented and designed to provide an adherent base over which the pigmented eye shadow can be applied. They increase the wearability of eye shadows and are most useful in oily-complected patients or those with redundant eyelid skin who experience migration of eye shadow into eyelid creases. The setting cream is composed of beeswax, talc, and cyclomethicone. Beeswax seals the eyelid skin while the talc provides an increased adherence for the eye shadow pigment. Some of the newer cream eye shadows incorporate a setting cream for a longer wear.

> Eye shadow setting creams are useful in patients with redundant upper eyelid skin to prevent migration of makeup materials into the folds.

EYELID COSMETIC REMOVERS

Waterproof eye shadows must be removed with special removal products containing surfactants, such as cocamidopropyl betaine. These products may be oil based or oil free and can be designed to remove all eye cosmetics, including eyeliner and mascara. Incidence of allergic contact dermatitis has been reported with the use of these eye cosmetic removers (4).

EYELID CONTACT DERMATITIS

The eyelid skin is the thinnest on the body and frequently affected by both irritant and allergic contact dermatitis (5, 6). The North American Contact Dermatitis Group has determined that 12% of cosmetic reactions occur on the eyelid, but only 4% could be linked to eye makeup use (7). Furthermore, it may be difficult to determine the etiology of the eyelid dermatitis with routine patch testing (8). Many substances can be transferred to the eye area by the hands, such as nail polish, complicating dermatologic evaluation (9).

Table 11.2 Causes of Upper Eyelid Dermatitis Syndrome

Mechanical rubbing
Irritant contact dermatitis
Allergic contact dermatitis
Infection
Photoirritation
Contact urticaria
Atopic dermatitis
Psoriasis
Collagen vascular disease
Conjunctivitis
Seborrheic blepharitis
Idiopathic causes

Table 11.3 Cosmetic Ingredients that Cause Allergic Contact Dermatitis in Eyelids

Preservatives (12)
    Parabens
    Phenyl mercuric acetate
    Imidazolidinyl urea
    Quaternium-15
    Potassium sorbate
Antioxidants
    Butylated hydroxyanisole (13)
    Butylated hydroxytoluene (13)
    Di-tert-butyl-hydroquinone (14)
Resins
    Colophony (15)
Pearlescent additives
    Bismuth oxychloride (16)
Emollients
    Lanolin (17)
    Propylene glycol (18)
Fragrances (19)
Pigment contaminants
    Nickel (20)

> The North American Contact Dermatitis Group has determined that 12% of cosmetic reactions occur on the eyelid, but only 4% could be linked to eye makeup use.

A thorough evaluation of eyelid dermatitis requires consideration of a variety of entities. Maibach and Engasser have developed the concept of upper eyelid dermatitis syndrome (Table 11.2) (10,11).

Once it has been determined that eye cosmetics are the source of the dermatitis, the distinction between irritant and allergic contact dermatitis must be made. Irritant contact dermatitis is more common than allergic contact dermatitis. Eye cosmetic ingredients associated with allergic contact dermatitis are listed in Table 11.3 (21,22).

Open or closed patch testing can be performed "as is" with eye cosmetics, but automatic emulsions, such as mascara, should be allowed to thoroughly dry prior to occlusion (23). Use testing is recommended, however, for eye cosmetics: the product is placed at the corner of the eye for five consecutive nights and evaluated for allergic or irritant contact dermatitis.

EYELID COSMETICS FOR SPECIAL POPULATIONS
Eyelid Cosmetics for Sensitive Skin Patients and Contact Lens Wearers

Patients with sensitive skin and multiple allergies frequently have difficulty finding an eye shadow product that does not burn or itch upon application. Certainly, any eye shadow applied over a broken or inflamed skin will cause discomfort. Patients with these problems should avoid all eye cosmetics until they heal. The patients should also be evaluated for Upper Eyelid Dermatitis Syndrome, as previously discussed.

In order to minimize the recurrence of dermatitis, allergic patients should avoid shiny, frosted, or iridescent eye shadows; the bismuth oxychloride, mica, metal powders, or fish scale essence may contribute to an irritant contact dermatitis. These substances may have sharp edged particles that can produce pruritus. Matte finish eye shadows are therefore recommended for sensitive skin patients (Fig. 11.8).

Some patients also experience more irritation with darker eye shadow colors, such as deep purple, forest green, or navy blue. Selection of a lighter shade product in peach, pink, or tan may resolve the irritancy.

> Patients with sensitive upper eyelid skin should select matte finish eye shadows without shine or iridescence.

Creams, sticks, and pencils may cause irritation as the product is rubbed on the eyelid. The friction from this rubbing may cause tears to develop in the eyelid skin, increasing the probability of irritation. Automatic eye shadows containing volatile vehicles, emulsifiers, and surfactants that may also be irritating. Thus, matte finish, pressed powder eye shadows applied gently with a sponge applicator have the least potential for irritation (24).

Matte finish eye shadows are also recommended for contact lens wearers because the mica, metal powders, or fish scale essence in frosted finish eye shadows may lodge under the contact lens causing irritation or possibly corneal abrasion. It is advisable to insert the contact lens prior to application of an appropriate eye shadow and to take the lens out prior to cosmetic removal.

Eyelid Cosmetics for Acne Patients

Cream, stick, and pencil eye shadows do not perform well on acne patients with oily complexions. Since these products are oil based, the patient's sebum mixes with the eye shadow, encouraging migration into folds. Placing an unpigmented eye shadow setting cream beneath the colored eye shadow may improve wearability slightly, but the oil-based eye shadow product may exacerbate acne or increase follicular irritation. Pressed powder eye shadows are recommended for acne patients since the talc base has oil-control qualities and does not place additional oils on the face. For extended wear, the powder eye shadow can be applied with a moistened sponge applicator.

> Cream, stick, and pencil eye shadows do not perform well on acne patients with oily complexions.

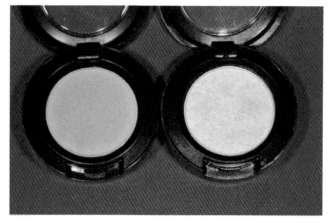

Figure 11.8 The matte finish eye shadow on the left will cause less irritant contact dermatitis than the frosted shiny finish eye shadow on the right.

Eyelid Cosmetics for Mature Patients

Mature patients should select eyelid cosmetics that minimize the appearance of redundant skin on the upper eyelid. Redundant skin encourages migration of cream, stick, and pencil eye shadows into the folds, drawing attention to the creases. Pressed powder eye shadows are recommended, even though patients may think that rich creamy eye shadows aid in moisturizing dry eyelids. Frosted finish and iridescent eye shadows also draw attention to the crepe texture of the redundant skin. Therefore, matte finish or light shine eye shadows are recommended. All eye shadows should be placed over an eye shadow setting cream in mature patients. Mature patients can also extend the wearing time of powder eye shadow by applying it with a moistened sponge applicator.

The mature skin on the upper eyelid may also demonstrate dyspigmentation from lentigines or telangiectasias. Mature patients may be tempted to select vivid, dark eye shadow colors to cover the undesirable eyelid skin color. However, vivid colors draw attention to the upper eyelid and should be avoided in favor of pastels and muted colors (pink, bluish gray, mauve, tan, and peach). Dyspigmentation can be covered by applying a facial foundation to the upper eyelid followed by a pressed powder eye shadow. Applying facial foundation to the upper eyelid improves the eye shadow wearability also.

> Dyspigmentation of the upper eyelid in mature patients can be camouflaged by applying a facial foundation to the upper eyelid followed by a pressed powder eye shadow.

Eye Cosmetic Camouflage Techniques

Eye cosmetics can be used to correct the appearance of eye defects arising from surgery, congenital anomalies, or dermatoheliosis. The correction is effected by carefully selecting eye shadow colors and placing them appropriately on the eyelids.

The eyes on a well-proportioned face are placed in such a way that the inner canthal distance is equal to the width of one eye (Fig. 11.9). If the eyes are closer together, the patient appears hypoteloric; if the eyes are further apart, the patient appears hyperteloric. Abnormal intercanthal distance is congenital and may or may not be associated with other anomalies. A more pleasing appearance can be imparted to

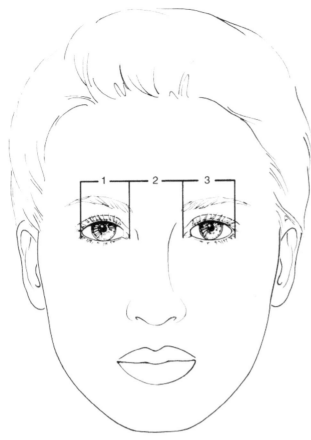

Figure 11.9 The intercanthal distance should equal the width of one eye in a well-proportioned face.

hypoteloric eyes by sweeping deeply colored eye shadow up and out from the center to outer corners of the lid (Fig. 11.10A). Hyperteloric eyes are de-emphasized by placing deeply colored eye shadow from the inner canthus to the central eyelid (Fig. 11.10B). The color draws any attention away from the abnormality (25).

> The eyes should be placed on the face in a way that the inner canthal distance is equal to the width of one eye.

Deeply colored eye shadows can also be effectively used to correct the size of the eyes. Female patients who have had skin cancer on the eyelid margin may appear to have smaller eyes due to wedge resection. The eyes can be made to appear larger if deeply colored eye shadow is placed along the lateral orbital ridge and eyebrow with a small amount placed beneath the lateral lower lash line (Fig. 11.10C). A light colored eye shadow should be placed medially beneath the eyebrow. Large eyes in a female patient with exophthalmos due to hyperthyroidism can be made to appear smaller by applying a dark eye shadow only in the crease and on the lateral eyelid (Fig. 11.10D). A light eye shadow is then placed on the medial eyelid (26).

Probably the most common cosmetic eye problem seen in female patients is blepharochalasis, commonly known as drooping or hooded eyelids. A drooping eyelid can be cosmetically corrected by covering the entire eyelid from the lash line to the crease with a light matte finish eye shadow (Fig. 11.10E). A complementary matte finish eye shadow two to three shades

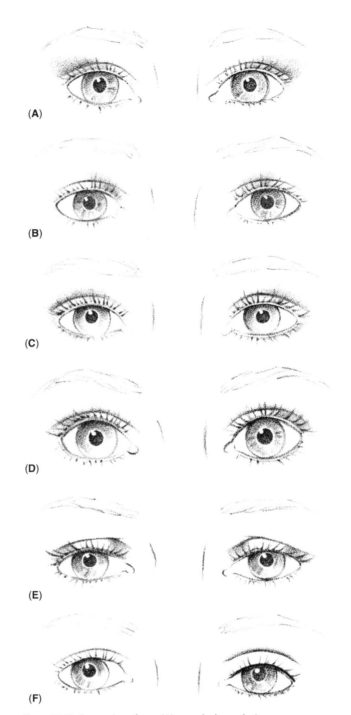

Figure 11.10 Contouring of eyes (**A**) to make hypoteloric eyes appear more widely set, (**B**) to make hyperteloric eyes appear more closely set, (**C**) to enlarge small eyes, (**D**) to decrease large eyes, (**E**) to de-emphasize bilateral blepharochalasis, and (**F**) to de-emphasize unilateral ptosis.

darker should be applied on the medial and lateral eyelids, leaving the area above the iris in a lighter color. Sometimes unilateral ptosis develops following Bell's palsy or surgery. Normally, the upper eyelid should touch the superior border of the iris and the lower eyelid should touch the inferior border of the iris. More dramatic eye makeup should be applied to the drooping eyelid. Both eyes should be initially colored as illustrated in Figure 11.10E; however, a brown eye shadow crayon should be used on the dropping eyelid to apply a line in the crease and above the lash line (Fig. 11.10F).

Unfortunately, none of these suggestions for eye recontouring can restore the eye to its normal appearance. The intention is to provide the physician with some suggestions to share with female patients who are distraught about their appearance following surgery or as a result of the process of aging.

EYELASH COSMETICS

Eyelash cosmetics include mascaras, eyeliners, eyelash dyes, and artificial eyelashes (Table 11.4). Our discussion begins with mascara, the most commonly used eyelash cosmetic, whose application dates to Biblical times. Its purpose is to darken, thicken, and lengthen the eyelashes. Since the eyelashes form a frame for the eye, luxuriant eyelashes can attract attention to this expressive facial feature. Most women consider long eyelashes a prerequisite to being attractive.

The original mascara worn by women of many ancient civilizations was kohl, which was based on antimony trisulfide. Mascara was subsequently refined into a cake comprising sodium stearate soaps and lampblack. The product was mixed with water and stroked from the cake with a brush and applied to the eyelashes. This formulation produced eye irritation on contact and the reason was sodium stearate; and it was reformulated with triethanolamine stearate. Beeswax was subsequently added to allow the product to be somewhat water resistant (27).

Mascaras must be carefully formulated to allow easy and even application without smudging, irritancy, or toxicity. Coal tar colors are prohibited by the U.S. Food, Drug and Cosmetic Act for use on the eyelashes. Therefore, mascara colorants must be selected from vegetable colors or inorganic pigments and lakes. Colors employed include iron oxide to produce black, ultramarine blue to create navy, and umber (brown ochre) or burnt sienna (a mixture of hydrated ferric oxide with manganic oxide) or synthetic brown oxide to create brown (28).

Modern liquid mascaras, available in tubes with a multitufted applicator brush, have virtually replaced cake- and cream-type mascaras (Fig. 11.11). The applicator is inserted into the tube between uses, providing numerous opportunities to inoculate bacteria into the mascara. The most dangerous of these bacteria is *Pseudomonas aeruginosa*. Even though mascaras contain antibacterials, it is still wise to discard all mascara tubes after three months and not allow multiple persons to use the same mascara tube (29). Persons susceptible to infection, or known bacterial carriers should select solvent-based or disposable mascaras.

> It is still wise to discard all mascara tubes after three months and not allow multiple persons to use the same mascara tube to prevent serious eye infections.

Mascaras are available in a variety of formulas to coordinate with current color and fashion styles. Color selection is wide, with various shades of blacks and browns most commonly seen, but pinks, greens, yellows, purples, and blues are also available. Even unpigmented mascara is available for those who wish to lengthen but not darken lashes.

Mascara styles, dictated by fashion, are based on the type of applicator brush employed. If thick eyelashes are fashionable,

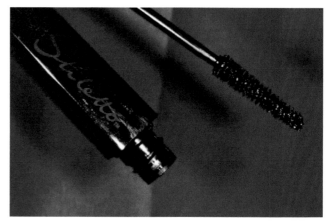

Figure 11.11 Mascara is removed from a tube on a tufted applicator to darken the eyelashes.

Table 11.4 Eyelash Cosmetics

Eyelash cosmetics	Main ingredients	Function	Adverse reactions
Cake mascara	Soap and pigments	Darken and thicken eyelashes	Irritation due to soaps
Cream mascara	Vanishing base and pigments	Darken and thicken eyelashes	Irritant contact dermatitis
Water-based liquid mascara	Waxes, pigments, and resins	Darken and thicken eyelashes	Irritant and allergic contact dermatitis
Solvent-based liquid mascara	Petroleum distillates, pigments, and waxes	Darken and thicken eyelashes	Irritant and allergic contact dermatitis
Water/solvent mascara	Water-in-oil or oil-in-water emulsions	Darken and thicken eyelashes	Irritant and allergic contact dermatitis
Cake eyeliner	Talc, pigment, and binders	Define eyelash line	Minimal
Liquid eyeliner	Latex or other polymers and pigments	Define eyelash line	Irritant contact dermatitis
Pencil eyeliner	Waxes and pigment	Define eyelash line	Minimal
Eyeliner tattooing	Tattoo pigments	Permanently define lash line	Minimal
Eyelash dyes	See chart under hair dyes (page)	Darken eyelashes	Irritant and allergic contact dermatitis
Artificial eyelashes	Human or synthetic hair fibers	Thicken eyelashes	Irritant contact dermatitis to lashes, allergic contact dermatitis to glue

lash-thickening mascaras are used with a larger, longer bristle brush applicator to apply mascara generously. If long eyelashes are fashionable, lash-lengthening mascaras with a short bristle brush are used to apply successive thin mascara coats and increase lash separation (Fig. 11.12).

Mascaras are available in several modern formulations: cake, cream, and liquid. The liquid mascaras can be further divided into water-based, solvent-based, and a water/solvent hybrid.

Cake Mascara

Cake mascara consists of soap and pigments compressed into a cake. The cake is stroked with a water-moistened brush and applied to the eyelashes (Fig. 11.13). Unfortunately, this form is not water-resistant and smudges with tears, perspiration, or rain. Furthermore, the soaps are somewhat irritating to the eye. Less irritating soaps, such as triethanolamine stearate, and waxes have been subsequently added to make the mascara less irritating and more water-resistant.

Cake mascaras remained popular until the 1960s when cream and liquid preparations were introduced, which provided a greater ease of application. Cake mascaras are still available and may be appropriate for patients who have developed eyelid or conjunctival irritation to the newer formulations.

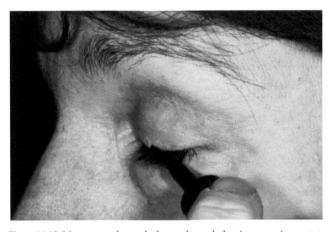

Figure 11.12 Mascara can be stroked over the eyelashes in successive coats to thicken and lengthen the eyelashes.

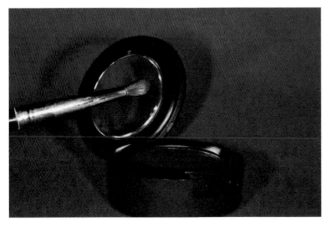

Figure 11.13 Cake mascaras are moistened and then stroked over the eyelashes.

Cream Mascara

Cream mascaras developed after cake mascaras, were quickly becoming popular due to their lesser propensity to run with moisture contact. Additionally, they did not clump or cake as easily on the eyelashes. The product consisted of a pigment suspended in a vanishing cream base that was brushed from a tube onto the eyelashes.

Liquid Mascara

Liquid mascara has largely replaced cake and thicker cream mascaras since the development of the automatic mascara tube. This invention consists of a tube into which a round brush is inserted through a small aperture to remove a metered amount of the product. There are water-based, solvent-based, and hybrid mascaras, which are discussed next.

Water-based Mascaras

Water-based mascaras are so named because they are formulated of waxes (beeswax, carnauba wax, and synthetic waxes), in addition to pigments (iron oxides, chrome oxides, ultramarine blue, carmine, and titanium dioxide) and resins dissolved in water. They are classified as oil-in-water emulsions. The water evaporates readily, creating a fast-drying product that thickens and darkens the lashes. The product is water soluble, allowing for easy removal, but unfortunately smudges with perspiration and tearing. Some water-based mascaras are labeled "water-resistant" if they contain an increased amount of wax or a polymer to improve adherence of pigment to the lashes.

Water-based mascaras are easily contaminated with bacteria, which readily grow in water, and must include preservatives, usually parabens. Thus, these products may potentially cause an allergic reaction in paraben-sensitive individuals; however, water-based mascaras are generally the least sensitizing of the mascara types. Some patients may experience a contact irritation from the emulsifiers required to maintain the pigment in solution.

> Water-based mascaras are easily contaminated with bacteria, which readily grow in water, and must include preservatives, usually parabens.

Specialty additives can be incorporated into the formulation to enhance the cosmetic appearance of the lashes. These substances include hydrolyzed animal protein to condition lashes, nylon or rayon fibers to elongate lashes and polyvinylpyrrolidone resins to decrease smudging.

Solvent-based Mascara

Solvent-based mascaras are formulated with petroleum distillates to which pigments (iron oxides, chrome oxides, ultramarine blue, carmine, and titanium dioxide) and waxes (candelilla wax, carnauba wax, ozokerite, and hydrogenated castor oil) are added, thus making them waterproof. As a result, the product performs well with perspiration and tearing, but the removal of which is difficult and requires an oil-based lotion or cream. Deposits may form on the lashes if the product is not removed completely. Care must be taken to avoid smudging the product immediately after application, as solvent-based mascaras have a prolonged drying time.

Preservatives are still added, but microbial contamination is not a great problem since the petroleum-based solvent is antibacterial. Some products also contain talc or kaolin to improve lash thickening and nylon or rayon fibers to lengthen lashes. Solvent-based mascaras can be an eye irritant.

Water/Solvent Hybrid Mascaras

Some of the mascaras combine both solvent-based and water-based systems to form either a water-in-oil or oil-in-water emulsion. The idea is to create an optimal product that thickens with a short drying time like the water-based mascaras, but provides waterproof lash separation like a solvent-based mascara. The water in the formulation requires incorporation of a good preservative system.

EYELASH COSMETIC SAFETY ISSUES

The most feared adverse reaction to mascaras is that of infection, particularly *P. aeruginosa* corneal infections which can permanently destroy visual acuity (30,31). *Staphylococcus epidermidis* and *S. aureus* organisms may also proliferate in contaminated mascaras (32). Infections are more common if the eyeball is traumatized with the infected mascara. As mentioned previously, individuals with recurrent bacterial infections due to colonization should probably select solvent-based mascaras (33).

Fungal organisms can also contaminate mascaras and result in eye infection (34). This is rarer and usually only found in patients who are immunocompromised or wear contact lenses.

The pigment contained within mascaras can result in conjunctival pigmentation if the mascara is washed into the conjunctival sac by lacrimal fluid (35). This colored particulate matter can be observed on the upper margin of the tarsal conjunctiva. Histologically, the pigment is seen within macrophages and extracellularly with varying degrees of lymphocytic infiltrates. Electron microscopy suggests that ferritin, carbon, and iron oxides are present within the tissues (36). Unfortunately, there is no treatment for the condition, which fortunately is usually asymptomatic.

> The pigment contained within mascaras can result in conjunctival pigmentation if the mascara is washed into the conjunctival sac by lacrimal fluid.

Allergic contact dermatitis has been reported of rosin (colophony) (37) and dihydroabietyl alcohol (Abitol, Eastman Chemical Company) (38,39) contained in some mascaras. But waterproof eye cosmetic removal products (discussed on page), used to remove solvent-based mascaras, can also be a source of eyelid dermatitis (4). Mascaras can be open or closed patch tested "as is," but should be allowed to thoroughly dry prior to closed patch testing to avoid an irritant reaction from the volatile vehicle.

EYELINER

Eyeliner defines the margins of the eye. It is placed immediately outside and sometimes inside the lash line. The color and placement of eyeliner are dictated by fashion. In the 1960s, a well-defined, thin black line drawn outside the upper and lower lash line was considered appropriate; however, the 1980s look was

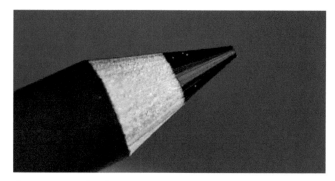

Figure 11.14 Pencil eyeliners are rubbed on the eyelash line and leave behind a wax pigmented film.

to use a subdued gray or deep blue smudged thick line outside the lower lash line only. The look of the 1990s was a thick sharp black line surrounding the entire eye with extension beyond the lateral canthus, a look sometimes termed as "cat eye."

> Eyeliner defines the margins of the eye and can be placed outside or inside the lash line.

Eyeliner is available in cake, liquid, and pencil forms. Cake eyeliner has the same composition as eye shadow, except for the addition of surfactants promoting formation of a paste when the powder is mixed with water. Cake eyeliner has largely been replaced by liquid eyeliner, which contains the same pigments premixed in a water-soluble latex base. Latex-based liquid eyeliners contain water, cellulose gum, thickeners (magnesium aluminum silicate), and styrene-butadiene latex. These products are packaged as marking pens or in the same form as mascaras, with a cylindrical tube and unitufted applicator brush. Automatic eyeliners are based on polymers, such as an ammonium acrylate copolymer, which leave a pigmented film after drying (40).

Pencil type eyeliners are popular due to their application ease (Fig. 11.14). Automatic liquid eyeliners create a defined line that requires a steady artistic hand for application, but pencil eyeliners give a smudged look and require less application skill. Pencil eyeliners contain natural and synthetic waxes combined with pigments, mineral or vegetable oils, and lanolin derivatives that are extruded into rods and encased in wood. The pencil is then sharpened to the desired tip, which can be thin or broad depending on the patient's preference. Resharpening also removes the exposed part of the eyeliner, thus decreasing contamination.

The application method used for eyeliners depends largely on fashion. The cake, liquid, or pencil is stroked across the upper and/or lower eyelid in the amount and position desired (Fig. 11.15).

Eyeliners are subject to the same bacterial and fungal contamination seen with mascaras, especially if the liquid form is chosen. But the main adverse reaction is the possibility of conjunctival pigmentation, also seen with mascaras (41). This problem is more commonly associated with eyeliner when it is applied within the lower lid margin. Usually, blue eyeliner is used in this location to create the appearance of a whiter sclera. This practice is unsafe.

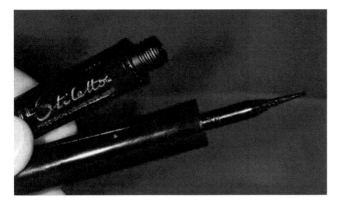

Figure 11.15 Liquid eyeliners are frequently stroked outside the eyelash line and leave behind a pigmented polymer film.

Open and closed patch testing can be performed "as is," but liquid eyeliner should be allowed to dry prior to occlusion.

EYELINER TATTOOING

Eyeliner tattooing, practiced by ophthalmologists, dermatologists, plastic surgeons, and some beauty operators, involves the intradermal insertion of black pigment, or other colored pigments such as brown or navy blue, on or outside of the upper and lower eyelash line. The pigment is inserted into the upper dermis at a constant depth by punctures created with a specially designed needle. The black, brown, green, or navy blue pigments are of low allergenic potential, accounting for the rare incidence of side effects.

Permanent eyeliner is a black tattoo artistically placed to highlight the eyelash margin.

Eyeliner tattooing has gained popularity among entertainment personalities, both male and female; however, for the average patient, a permanent eyeliner does not allow the fashion versatility that most people desire. Patients with permanent eyelash loss may wish to consider eyeliner tattooing, which can be applied as outlined under corrective eyelash cosmetics. The tattooing should be done in a thin line so that the patient can apply a colored eyeliner pencil, if desired, to conform to fashion trends.

Patients who elect eyeliner tattooing should recognize that the color will fade with time and some migration of the pigment is possible. The decision should be considered carefully prior to tattooing as the pigment is exceedingly difficult to remove once inserted into the dermis.

EYELASH DYES

Eyelash dyes are used by those persons who have light-colored eyelashes due to canities, natural hair color, or dermatoses such as vitiligo. No over-the-counter eyelash dyes are available, due to the risk of eye damage. The U.S. FDA is currently attempting to outlaw the use of eyelash dyes. Some dyeing products are imported illegally from Europe, and other salons use products intended for scalp hair on the eyelashes. Products used by professional cosmetologists may contain either paraphenylenediamine dyes or metallic dyes. A further discussion of these products is included in the chapter on hair coloring.

Eyelash dyes are not available for home use.

Eyelash dyes should not be used more than every three weeks since they are extremely irritating to the eye and can cause an irritant or allergic contact dermatitis. They are patch tested in the same manner as hair dyes.

Light-colored eyelashes can be darkened nicely by a repeated application of black or brown waterproof mascara containing talc or kaolin for lash thickening.

ARTIFICIAL EYELASHES

Artificial eyelashes are most popular among those in the entertainment industry, although they can be effectively used by patients who have thin or absent eyelashes. Human hair and synthetic nylon lashes are available in varying colors and lengths with costs ranging from $1 to $20. The lashes are attached to existing lashes on the upper or lower eyelids with a clear or pigmented methacrylate-based glue.

Artificial eyelashes are available as singlets, demilashes, and complete eyelashes to camouflage eyelash loss.

Artificial eyelashes are available as lash singlets, demilashes, and complete eyelashes. If lash singlets are used, several artificial lashes are glued to the patient's existing natural eyelashes. Demilashes, which are sparse artificial lashes, and complete lashes, which are dense artificial lashes, are glued immediately above the existing lash line. The eyelashes are removed with a solvent specially designed to remove the adhesive.

Lash singlets are difficult for the novice to apply, but can be used effectively at the lateral upper lash line to minimize the appearance of overhanging eyelids. Complete lashes are only appropriate for patients who have total loss of their own eyelashes. Demilashes are appropriate for the patient with short, thinned, or partially absent lashes. Demilashes are routinely worn by television personalities and can be quite natural appearing if the length is not exaggerated. Artificial eyelashes can be easily trimmed and customized with scissors.

Artificial eyelashes may be difficult to wear since the eyelashes themselves can irritate the eye, tarsal plate, and eyelid. Both irritant and allergic contact dermatitis can develop in response to the attachment glue and removal solvent. The most adherent eyelash glues are methacrylate based, which is a known sensitizer.

EYELASH COSMETICS FOR SPECIAL NEEDS

Certain patients within a physician's practice may require careful selection of eyelash cosmetics. These are patients with allergies and/or contact lenses, as well as patients undergoing treatment for acne. Mature patients may require special eyelash cosmetic consultation to achieve an optimal appearance.

Eyelash Cosmetics for Sensitive Patients and/or Contact Lens Wearers

Eyelash cosmetics are commonly a source of irritant or allergic contact dermatitis. Most cases represent irritant dermatitis, since the FDA closely regulates the chemicals, preservatives, and pigments used in eyelash cosmetics. Many sensitive skin patients find mascaras extremely irritating to their eyes and should be advised to wear a product specifically designed for allergic patients or a water-based mascara. Unpigmented mascaras seem to cause less irritation in some patients.

Application techniques can also minimize problems. Mascara can be applied in several coats only to the eyelash tips. This emphasizes the lashes while limiting mascara contact with the eye and skin. All waterproof mascaras should be avoided since the removal solvent and the rubbing required to remove the mascara may produce irritation. Artificial eyelashes and eyelash dyeing should also be avoided.

Pencil-type eyeliners are better tolerated by some sensitive skin patients, but the eyeliner should never be placed inside the lower lid margin where it will be removed by tearing and washed into the eye. This is not advisable as the pigment may tattoo the conjunctiva and possibly the lower palpebral sac.

Some contact lens wearers are bothered by mascaras that cake on the lashes and flake into the eye. Water-based mascaras are more likely to cake than solvent-based mascaras. Patients wearing soft contact lenses, with a high water content, may prefer waterproof solvent-based mascaras since these are less likely to bind to the lens. The pigment in mascaras and eyeliners can actually stain water- and gas-permeable contact lenses.

Eyelash Cosmetics for Acne and/or Oily-Complected Patients

Many dermatologists recommend water-based cosmetics for their acne patients as a general rule, including water-based mascaras. Acne patients who have oily complexions may find that water-based mascaras become easily wet by sebum, causing running and smudging. Solvent-based mascaras should be recommended for oily-complected patients. The solvent-based mascaras can smudge if not adequately allowed to dry between coats but, once dry, they are resistant to smudging.

Patients with oily complexions may also notice that pencil-type eyeliners wear poorly and smudge. This is due to poor adhesion between the cosmetic and skin caused by sebum. The pencil-type eyeliner will wear longer if a foundation covered by a loose powder is placed on the eyelid prior to eyeliner application. A polymer eyeliner could also be selected as an alternative.

Eyelash Cosmetics for Mature Patients

Eyelash cosmetics are important in the mature patient. Mascara can darken lashes lightened by canities and should be applied from the base of the lash to the tips in long strokes to cover the lashes completely with pigment. However, black mascara should be avoided in patients with recessed eyes since it will only darken the already shadowed eyes. Brown or navy blue mascara is more appropriate.

> Eyelash length and thickness decrease in mature patients and can be camouflaged with mascara.

Eyelash length and thickness also tend to decrease in the mature patient. Eyelash length can be maximized by using a lengthening mascara that contains nylon or rayon fibers. Each successive coat should dry completely to maximize lash length. Thickening mascaras containing talc or kaolin can increase lash size with repeated applications to the tips only.

The appearance of blepharochalasis can be minimized by lengthening the eyelashes, since some of the eyelash length is covered by redundant skin. An appearance of lengthened eyelashes can be created by curling the eyelashes with an eyelash curler immediately after mascara application. The eyelashes are placed in a rubber padded holder that bends them upward at a more acute angle. This decreases the natural curl of the eyelashes, making them appear longer, but can also promote eyelash breakage. Demilashes slightly longer than the patient's natural lashes can also be used to create the appearance of longer eyelashes.

CORRECTIVE EYELASH COSMETICS

Eyelashes function cosmetically as a frame for the eye. Unfortunately, they may thin due to age, alopecia areata or eyelid scarring secondary to surgery, or infections such as herpes zoster. Thinned or absent eyelashes result in nondescript eyes and loss of the main focal point for the face.

Eyeliner, mascara, and loose transparent face powder can be used to cosmetically compensate for thinned eyelashes. The first step is to use a liquid eyeliner to dot the upper and lower eyelid (Fig. 11.16A) creating the illusion of eyelashes. A light application of dark brown or black fibered mascara should then be applied to the remaining lashes. A powder brush is then dipped in loose powder and dusted on the wet mascara with the eye closed to prevent powder from entering the eye. Another layer of mascara is then applied and the process is repeated until the remaining lashes have been thickened to the desired degree. This technique is useful only in patients who have generalized eyelash thinning or focal areas of complete loss.

It is more difficult to reconstruct the lash line in patients who have large areas of eyelash loss or total eyelash loss. In these female patients, a brown or black liquid or pencil eyeliner should be used to rim the entire eye, except for one-quarter

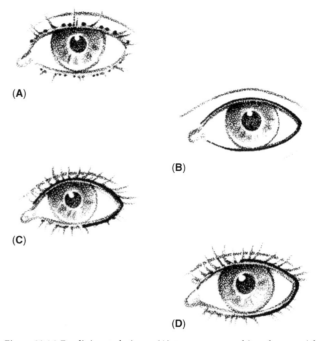

(A)

(B)

(C)

(D)

Figure 11.16 Eye lining techniques (**A**) to reconstruct thinned or partially absent eyelashes, (**B**) to reconstruct totally absent eyelashes, (**C**) to enlarge small eyes, and (**D**) to widen hypoteloric eyes.

inch around the inner canthus on the upper and lower eyelids (Fig. 11.16B). On the normal eye, terminal hairs do not grow around the inner canthus. For female patients with more extensive loss, artificial demilashes can be applied at this point or, in patients with total eyelash loss, complete artificial eyelashes can be applied.

Eyeliner can also be used to contour the eyes while simultaneously reconstructing a lash line. Small eyes can be enlarged by lining the entire upper lash line and the lateral half of the lower lash line (Fig. 11.16C). Hypoteloric eyes can be widened by lining the lateral half of both the upper and lower lash lines (Fig. 11.16D).

EYEBROW COSMETICS

The accepted shape and width of the eyebrows are subject to fashion trends. Eyebrows were almost completely plucked in the 1950s with a thin pencil line drawn to connect the few remaining hairs. Unfortunately, many women who are now in their 60s and 70s can no longer grow eyebrow hairs as a result of overplucking during their younger years. This is in direct contrast to the eyebrow look of the 1960s, which was totally natural and ungroomed. The 1990s have compromised with thick eyebrows considered attractive, but stray hairs beneath the brow line are plucked to give a groomed appearance.

There are several eyebrow cosmetics: pencils, sealers, dyes, and artificial eyebrows (Table 11.5).

Eyebrow Pencil

Eyebrow pencils are used to darken light or gray eyebrows, fill in sparse or absent eyebrow hairs, and reconstruct malformed or misshapen eyebrows. Eyebrow pencils are formed by mixing pigments, petrolatum, lanolin, and synthetic or natural waxes (Fig. 11.17). This formulation is similar to that of lipstick products, but differs in one aspect that higher melting point waxes are used to yield a firmer product. Formulations may be encased in wood to form a pencil, or extruded into rods placed in a plastic holder.

Pencils are available in a variety of colors from grays to browns to blacks. Inert, mainly inorganic, pigments are used since the Federal Food, Drug and Cosmetic Act prohibits the use of coal tar colors in the eye area. They are stroked over the skin in the eyebrow region to actually color the skin and eyebrow hairs (42).

Contact dermatitis to eyebrow pencils is rare. The product can be open or closed patch tested "as is."

Eyebrow Sealer

Eyebrow sealers are intended as a grooming agent for unruly eyebrows and a glossing agent to add shine to eyebrow hairs. Originally, white petroleum jelly was used for this purpose, but now cosmetic companies market a more elegant product. The sealer is essentially a liquid hair spray containing polymer-holding agents packaged in a mascara-type tube. A brush is used to stroke the product over the eyebrow hairs.

> Eyebrow sealers can be used to groom unruly eyebrows in mature individuals.

Eyebrow sealers can be used by persons with bushy eyebrows to hold the hairs closer to the orbital ridge or by those with multidirectional eyebrow hairs who wish to hold the hairs in a more cosmetically acceptable line. The sealer can also be pigmented to darken graying eyebrows. The product is easily removed with soap and water.

Eyebrow sealers could be a source of irritant contact dermatitis due to the incorporation of volatile vehicles. The product can be patch tested "as is," but should thoroughly dry prior to occlusion.

Eyebrow Dye

Eyebrow hair can be dyed in the same manner as scalp hair. This service is offered by many professional salons; however, hair dye packaging specifically states the dyestuff is not to be used in the eye area and contains the following warning: "Caution: This product contains ingredients which may cause skin irritation on certain individuals and a preliminary test according to accompanying directions should first be made.

Table 11.5 Eyebrow Cosmetics

Eyebrow cosmetic	Main ingredients	Function	Adverse reactions
Eyebrow pencil	Pigment, wax, petrolatum, lanolin	Darken and thicken eyebrows	Minimal
Eyebrow sealer	Synthetic polymer	Eyebrow hair grooming agent	Minimal
Eyebrow dye	Metallic dyes, stains, or permanent dyes	To darken eyebrow hairs	May be illegal, blindness, contact dermatitis
Artificial eyebrows	Human, synthetic, or wool hair	Replace missing eyebrow hair	Irritant contact dermatitis to hair, allergic contact dermatitis to adhesive
Eyebrow tattooing	Tattoo pigments	Replace missing eyebrows	Allergic contact dermatitis to tattoo pigment

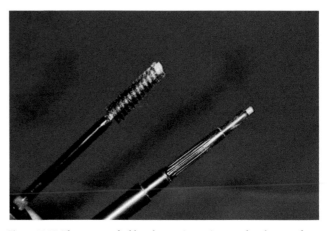

Figure 11.17 The upper tufted brush contains a pigmented eyebrow sealer to groom and darken the eyebrows. The lower stick is an eyebrow pencil dispensed from a plastic tube and stroked across the eyebrow to darken and thicken the brow appearance.

This product must not be used for dyeing the eyelashes or eyebrows; to do so may cause blindness." The U.S. FDA has engaged unsuccessfully in several law suits to remove eye area dyes from the market (43).

Eyebrow dyes that are present in some salons are of the metallic type, stains, or permanent hair dyes. The metallic dyes, containing lead or silver, are applied over a period of weeks and cause gradual darkening of the hairs due to the formation of metallic oxides and sulfides on the hair shaft, imparting a yellow brown to black color. Some salons use professional stains that are specifically manufactured for eyebrow dyeing. The stain is applied with a toothpick only to the eyebrow hairs as skin contact will result in staining. A special product is used to remove stain from the skin. Other salons use the same dye that is applied to the scalp for dyeing the eyebrows, taking care to keep material from entering the eye.

> The U.S. FDA considers eyebrow dye products illegal.

It should be reemphasized that the U.S. FDA considers all the eyebrow dyeing products that have been previously discussed dangerous and illegal.

Artificial Eyebrows

Artificial eyebrows are available for individuals who have permanently lost a substantial amount of their natural eyebrow hair. Synthetic or natural human hair can be knotted onto a thin netting in the appropriate amount and shape for a patient's face. The netting is then glued on the superior orbital ridge with a waterproof adhesive. Salons specializing in hair replacement can provide patient assistance.

The use of crepe hair is an eyebrow replacement technique, adapted from the theater, which is more appropriate for the patient who has temporarily lost substantial eyebrow hair (44). Crepe hair is made from wool and available as braids in a variety of colors. The braided fibers are separated, straightened, and cut to the desired length. Adhesive is then used to glue the fibers directly to the skin. New fibers must be prepared and glued for each application.

Possible adverse reactions include irritant contact dermatitis to the eyebrow prosthesis and/or allergic contact dermatitis to the adhesive, which may contain methacrylate.

Eyebrow Tattooing

Eyebrows can be reconstructed or thickened with the use of a tattoo pigment. Brown, black, gray, yellow, or orange pigments can be blended and placed within the superficial dermis to add color to the eyebrow area. Certainly, this must be done by a trained individual under hygienic conditions. Unfortunately, eyebrow tattooing is less than optimal since the overlying skin has a rather unnatural shiny appearance. Allergic contact dermatitis is possible to some of the pigments.

Corrective Eyebrow Cosmetics

The structure of the eyebrows can be abnormal due to congenital deformity, surgical procedures, or acquired loss from alopecia universalis, hypothyroidism, leprosy, traumatic scarring, and other conditions. Before cosmetic reconstruction can begin, it is important to identify the proper location of the

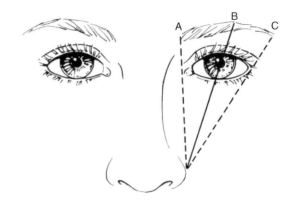

Figure 11.18 A well-proportioned eyebrow should begin at point A, maximally arch at point B, and end at point C.

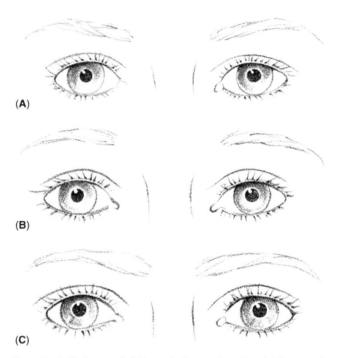

Figure 11.19 The intercanthal distance is the same in **A**, **B**, and **C**; however, the distance between the medial eyebrows has been changed. Note the resultant illusion of hypertelorism in **B** and hypotelorism in **C**.

eyebrow on the face (Fig. 11.18). The medial aspect of the eyebrow should begin at a point defined by a straight line drawn from the lateral nose upward. The eyebrow should maximally arch at a point defined by a line drawn from the lateral nose through the pupil. The eyebrow should end at a point defined by a line drawn from the lateral nose through the lateral aspect of the eyeball. Any hair removal to improve eyebrow appearance should be from the inferior aspect of the eyebrow. Hairs should never be removed from the superior border; this will disturb the natural eyebrow contour.

> Improper placement of the eyebrows can alter facial expression and the appearance of the eyes.

Improper placement of the eyebrows can alter facial expression and the appearance of the eyes while normal placement gives an aesthetically pleasing appearance (Fig. 11.19A).

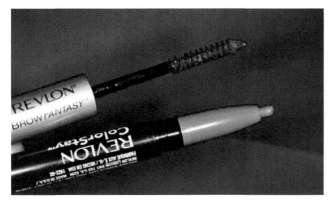

Figure 11.20 An eyebrow crayon can be used to draw in absent hairs, shown at the bottom of the image, with further darkening provided with pigment on a tufted brush, shown in the upper image.

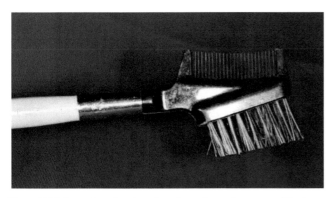

Figure 11.21 An eyebrow brush and comb can be used to groom thinning or absent eyebrows.

Eyebrows that are placed too far apart give the impression of surprise and can make the patient appear hyperteloric (Fig. 11.19B) while eyebrows that are too close together give an angry, intense look and impart hypotelorism (Fig. 11.19C). If the eyes are improperly placed on the face, these concepts can be used to alter eyebrow position to create the illusion of properly spaced eyes.

> Eyebrow pencil can be used to camouflage thinning eyebrows.

An eyebrow pencil or a crayon can be used to draw absent hairs (Fig. 11.20). A more natural appearance is created if the pencil is used in short strokes rather than to draw one straight line (45). The eyebrow pencil will adhere better if the skin is first covered with a facial foundation. A brush can also be used to push the eyebrows into place to cover areas of thinning or loss (Fig. 11.21).

SUMMARY
Eye cosmetics can be used to both adorn and camouflage. They can minimize the appearance of eyelash loss seen in several dermatologic conditions while also serving as a source of contact dermatitis and infection. This chapter has presented the formulation of eye cosmetics for the lid and eyelashes to help the dermatologist understand the important considerations for this class of popular cosmetics.

REFERENCES
1. Panati C. Extraordinary origins of everyday things. New York: Harper & Row Publishers, 1987: 223.
2. Wells FV, Lubowe II. Rouge and eye make-up. In: Cosmetics and the Skin. New York: Reinhold Publishing Corporation, 1964: 173–4.
3. Lanzet M. Modern formulations of coloring agents: facial and eye. In: Frost P, Horowitz SN, eds. Principles of Cosmetics for the Dermatologist. St. Louis: C. V. Mosby Company, 1982: 138–9.
4. Ross JS, White IR. Eyelid dermatitis due to cocamidopropyl betaine in an eye make-up remover. Contact Dermatitis 1991; 25: 64.
5. Fisher AA. Cosmetic dermatitis of the eyelids. Cutis 1984; 34: 216–21.
6. Valsecchi R, Imberti G, Martino D, Cainelli T. Eyelid dermatitis: an evaluation of 150 patients. Contact Dermatitis 1992; 27: 143–7.
7. Adams RM, Maibach HI. A five-year study of cosmetic reactions. J Am Acad Dermatol 1985; 13:1062–9.
8. Wolf R, Perluk H. Failure of routine patch test results to detect eyelid dermatitis. Cutis 1992; 49: 133–4.
9. Nethercott JR, Nield G, Linn Holness. D. A review of 79 cases of eyelid dermatitis. J Am Acad Dermatol 1989; 21: 223–30.
10. Maibach HI, Engasser PG. Dermatitis due to cosmetics. In: Fisher AA, ed. Contact Dermatitis, 3rd edn. Philadelphia: Lea & Febiger, 1986: 378–9.
11. Maibach HI, Engasser P, Ostler B. Upper eyelid dermatitis syndrome. Dermatol Clin 1992; 10: 549–54.
12. Marks JG, DeLeo VA. Preservatives and vehicles. In: Contact and Occupational Dermatology. St. Louis: CV Mosby, 1992: 107–33.
13. White IR, Lovell CR, Cronin E. Antioxidants in cosmetics. Contact Dermatitis 1984; 11: 265–7.
14. Calnan CD. Ditertiary butylhydroquinone in eye shadow. Contact Dermatitis Newsl 1973; 14: 402.
15. Fisher AA. Allergic contact dermatitis due to rosin (colophony) in eyeshadow and mascara. Cutis 1988; 42: 505–8.
16. Eiermann HJ, Larsen W, Maibach HI, Taylor JS. Prospective study of cosmetic reactions: 1977-1980. J Am Acad Dermatol 1982; 6: 909–17.
17. Schorr WF. Lip gloss and gloss-type cosmetics. Contact Dermatitis Newsl 1973; 14: 408.
18. Hannuksela M, Pirila V, Salo OP. Skin reactions to propylene glycol. Contact Dermatitis 1975; 1: 112–16.
19. Larsen WG. Cosmetic dermatitis due to a perfume. Contact Dermatitis 1975; 1: 142–5.
20. Goh CL, Ng SK, Kwok SF. Allergic contact dermatitis from nickel in eyeshadow. Contact Dermatitis 1989; 20: 380–1.
21. deGroot AC, Weyland JW, Nater JP. Face cosmetics. In: Unwanted Effects of Cosmetics and Drugs Used in Dermatology. Amsterdam: Elsevier, 1994: 513.
22. Pascher F. Adverse reactions to eye area cosmetics and their management. J Soc Cosmet Chem 1982; 33: 249–58.
23. Van Ketel WG. Patch testing with eye cosmetics. Contact Dermatitis 1979; 5: 402.
24. Draelos ZK. Eye cosmetics. Dermatol Clin 1991; 9: 1–5.
25. Greene A, Pomerance M. The successful face. New York: Summit Books, 1985: 67–73.
26. Arpel A. 851 Fast Beauty Fixes and Facts. New York: GP Putnam's Sons, 1985: 97–100.
27. Rutkin P. Eye make-up. In: deNavarre MG, ed. The Chemistry and Manufacture of Cosmetics. Allured Publishing Corp, 1988: 712–17.
28. Wilkinson JB, Moore RJ. Harry's Cosmeticology, 7th edn. New York: Chemical Publishing, 1982: 341–7.
29. Bhadauria B, Ahearn DG. Loss of effectiveness of preservative systems of mascaras with age. Appl Environ Microbiol 1980; 39: 665–7.
30. Wilson LA, Ahern DG. Pseudomonas-induced corneal ulcer associated with contaminated eye mascaras. Am J Ophthalmol 1977; 84: 112–19.
31. MMWR Reports: Pseudomonas aeruginosa corneal infection related to mascara applicator trauma. Arch Dermatol 1990; 126: 734.
32. Ahearn DG, Wilson, LA. Microflora of the outer eye and eye area cosmetics. Dev Ind Microiol 1976; 17: 23–8.
33. Ahern DG, Wilson LA, Julian AJ, et al. Microbial growth in eye cosmetics: contamination during use. Dev Ind Microbiol 1974; 15: 211–16.
34. Kuehne JW, Ahearn DG. Incidence and characterization of fungi in eye cosmetics. Dev Ind Microbiol 1971; 12: 1973–7.
35. Jervey JH. Mascara pigmentation of the conjunctiva. Arch Opthalmol 1969; 81: 124–5.

36. Platia EV, AMichaels RG, Green WR. Eye cosmetic-induced conjunctival pigmentation. Ann Ophthalamol 1978; 10: 501–4.
37. Fisher AA. Allergic contact dermatitis due to rosin (colophony) in eyeshadow and mascara. Cutis 1988; 42: 507–8.
38. Rapaport MJ. Sensitization to abitol. Contact Dermatitis 1980; 6: 137–8.
39. Dooms-Goosens A, Degreef J, Luytens E. Dihydroabietyl alcohol (Abitol), a sensitizer in mascara. Contact Dermatitis 1979; 5: 350–3.
40. Lanzet M. Modern formulations of coloring agents: facial and eye. In: Frost P, Horwitz SN, eds. Principles of Cosmetics for the Dermatolgist. St. Louis: CV Mosby, 1982: 143–4.
41. Stewart CR. Conjunctival absorption of pigment from eye make-up. Am J Optom 1973; 50: 571–4.
42. Klarmann EG. Cosmetic Chemistry for the Dermatologist. Springfield, IL: Charles C Thomas, 1962: 53–4.
43. Draelos ZK. Caution: eyebrow dyeing may be illegal. Cosmet Dermatol 1990; 3: 39–40.
44. Rayner V. Clinical cosmetology: a medical approach to esthetics procedures. Albany, New York: Milady Publishing Company, 1993: 143–5.
45. Allsworth J. Skin Camouflage. Cheltenham, England: Stanley Thornes Ltd, 1985: 41–2.

SUGGESTED READING

Bielory L. Contact dermatitis of the eye. Immunol Allergy Clin N Am 1997; 17: 131–8.
Cuyper CD. Permanent makeup: indications and complications. Clin Dermatol 2008; 26: 30–4.
Draelos ZD. Special considerations in eye cosmetics. Clin Dermatol 2001; 19: 424–30.
Draelos ZK. Eye cosmetics. Dermatol Clin 1991; 9: 1–7.
Draelos ZK, Yeatts RP. Eyebrow loss, eyelash loss, and dermatochalasis. Dermatol Clin 1992; 10: 793–8.
Gallardo MJ, Bradley J. Ocular argyrosis after long-term self-application of eyelash tint. Am J Ophthalmol 2006; 141: 198–200.
Goh CL, Ng SK, Kwok SF. Allergic contact dermatitis from nickel in eyeshadow. Contact Dermatitis 1989; 20: 380–1.
Goldstein N. Tattoos defined. Clin Dermatol 2007; 25: 417–20.
Goossens A. Contact allergic reactions on the eyes and eyelids. Bull Soc Beige Ophtalmol 2004; 292: 11–17.
Guin JD. Eyelid dermatitis: experience in 203 cases. J Am Acad Dermatol 2002; 47: 755–65.
Kaiserman I. Servere allergic blepharoconjunctivitis induced by a dye for eyelashes and eyebrows. Ocul Immunol Inflamm 2003; 11: 149–51.
Karlberg AT, Liden C, Ehrin E. Colophony in mascara as a cause of eyelid dermatitis. Acta Dermatol Venereol 1991; 71: 445–7.
Lee IW, Ahn SK, Choi EH, Whang KK, Lee SH. Complications of eyelash and eyebrow tattooing: report of 2 cases of pigment fanning. Cutis 2001; 68: 53–5.
Loden M, Wessman C. Mascaras may cause irritant contact dermatitis. Int J Cosmet Sci 2002; 24: 281–5.
Loginova Y, Shah V, Allen G, Macchio R, Farer A. Approaches to polymer selection for mascara formulation. J Cosmet Sci 2009; 60: 125–33.
Meinik JD. Eye cosmetics for wearers of contact lenses. Cutis 1987; 39: 549–50.
O'Donoghue MN. Eye cosmetics. Dermatol Clin 2000; 18: 633–9.
Pack LD, Wickham MG, Enloe RA, Hill DN. Microbial contamination associated with mascara use. Optometry 2008; 79: 587–93.
Peralego B, Beltrni V. Dermatologic and allergic conditions of the eyelid. Immunol Allergy Clin N Am 2008; 28: 137–68.
Ross JS, White IR. Eyelid dermatitis due to cocamidopropyl betaine in an eye make-up remover. Contact Dermatitis 1991; 25: 64.
Saxena M, Warshaw E, Ahmed DD. Eyelid allergic contact dermatitis to black iron oxide. Am J Contact Dermatitis 2001; 12: 38–9.
Sher MA. Contact dermatitis of the eyelids. S Afr Med J 1979; 55: 511–13.
Vagefi MR, Dragan L, Hughes S, et al. Adverse reactions to permanent eyeliner tattoo. Ophthalmic Plast Reconstr Surg 2006; 22: 48–51.
Van Ketel WG, Liem DH. Eyelid dermatitis from nickel contaminated cosmetics. Contact Dermatitis 1981; 7: 217.
Wachsmuth R, Wilkinson M. Loss of eyelashes after use of a tinting mascara containing PPD. Contact Dermatitis 2006; 54: 169–70.

12 Postsurgical cosmetics

Postsurgical cosmetics are important in dermatology to aid the patient in proper wound healing while attending to the appearance and emotional needs of the patient. Cosmetics assume medical importance when used in the postsurgical patient to facilitate return to normal daily activities and improve emotional well-being (1,2). This chapter discusses the proper use and selection of cosmetics and skin care products in the postsurgical period.

Cosmetic selection criteria in the postsurgical patient depend upon the type of wound created. Incisional wounds, closed by sutures, expose only a small amount of unhealed skin to topical cosmetics while large surface area wounds, such as those created by shave excisions, dermabrasions, and chemical peels, are allowed to heal by secondary intention exposing large unhealed skin areas to topical cosmetics.

WOUND HEALING AND COSMETICS

Wounds created in dermatology heal by both primary and secondary intention. Incisional wounds, closed by sutures that remain in place for 5 to 14 days, heal by primary intention and require a clean surgical site free of foreign bodies. Therefore, cosmetics should not be applied to the wound until the sutures are removed. Facial foundations should be avoided over sutured areas as they contain finely ground titanium dioxide particles that could act as foreign bodies and impeding wound healing through initiation of an inflammatory response or by inciting milia formation. Facial foundation pigments, such as iron oxide, can also become imbedded in the dermis during healing resulting in permanent tattooing of the skin. Once the sutures have been removed the skin barrier has returned and cosmetics of all types can be safety used.

Large surface area wounds healing by secondary intention are devoid of the protective stratum corneum making postsurgical cosmetic selection important. No cosmetics should be applied to the wound until serous drainage has stopped (Fig. 12.1). This is generally not a problem for patients, since cosmetics will not adhere to the skin until an epithelial barrier has been reestablished. Premature application of cosmetics can create the same foreign body problem and pigment tattoos discussed under incisional wounds. Individuals who attempt to apply facial foundation too soon following chemical peeling or dermabrasion may also encourage milia formation, a common side effect of both the procedures. Bland moisturizers to impede transepidermal water loss, such as purified petroleum jelly, are recommended; however, until re-epithelialization has occurred.

Cosmetics should not be worn over an incision until the sutures have been removed.

COLOR COSMETIC SELECTION

Following re-epithelialization or suture removal, patient may wish to use color cosmetics to camouflage the postsurgical erythema. The application of color cosmetics to the face is important for the patient to re-establish social and emotional well-being following surgery. New cosmetics may need to be selected on a temporary or permanent basis following surgery.

Facial Foundations

Facial foundation is the most important cosmetic used in the postsurgical patient. It can camouflage redness and scarring while providing photoprotection (3). The foundation selected should be easily applied and removed while containing a paucity of ingredients. Cream or cream/powder formulations are recommended. Cream foundations are dipped from a jar or squeezed from a tube while cream/powder foundations are wiped from a compact with a dry sponge (powder) or a moistened sponge (cream) (4). These foundations are more difficult to bacterially contaminate than liquid foundations due to their low water content. The cream also provides a good barrier to transepidermal water loss and smoothes easily around any remaining desquamating stratum corneum (Fig. 12.2). They cause less stinging and burning as compared with liquid varieties. A loose powder can be applied over the facial foundation to improve coverage and impart better rub resistant characteristics (Fig. 12.3).

Cream or cream/powder foundations are the best choice in the postsurgical period.

In addition, the patient may need to alter facial foundation color selection in the immediate postoperative period. The color of the foundation may need to contain more reddish hues; however, most patients can return to their pre-surgery foundation formulation four to six weeks postoperatively.

Undercover Foundations

Some patients with pronounced, long-lasting redness or bruising following surgery may wish to use a product known as an undercover foundation or a color corrector foundation. These products are designed to mask undesirable tones present in the skin using a complementary color combination rather than a heavy-coverage, surgical facial foundation (5). Coverage refers to the ability of the facial foundation to obscure the view of the underlying skin and is related to the opaqueness of the cosmetic. Use of color correctors allows the patient to wear a moderate-coverage foundation, which appears more natural and may be more acceptable to the patient. For example, redness of the face common after dermabrasion, chemical

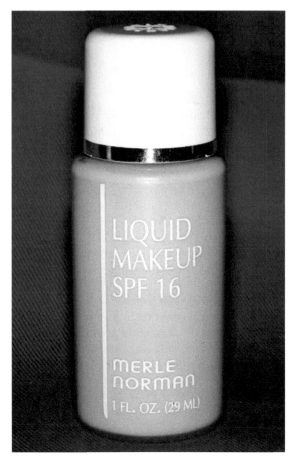

Figure 12.1 Pigmented facial foundations should be avoided until re-epithelialization has occurred.

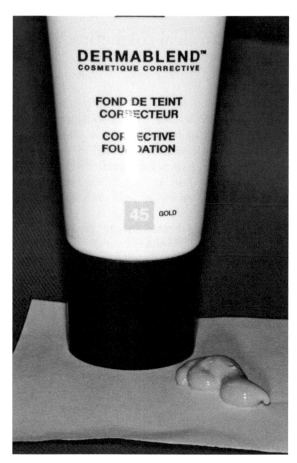

Figure 12.2 Higher-coverage facial foundations are useful for camouflaging in postsurgical patients while waiting for the erythema to resolve, especially in post–laser resurfacing patients.

peeling, and laser resurfacing procedures can be minimized with a green color corrector. Green is the complementary color to red and the combination of both colors yields brown. A green cream or liquid cosmetic applied over a red scar allows camouflaging with a facial foundation that is less opaque and provides less coverage. Less opaque facial foundations appear more natural and are easier to apply and wear.

> Green color correctors are the complementary color to red and may assist in camouflaging red scars.

Color correctors are available in other colors besides green for camouflaging other unwanted skin colors. For example, yellow facial tones can be masked by the complementary color purple. Yellow and purple when mixed yield brown. The sallowness of photoaging or the yellow hemosiderin deposits of bruising can be masked by applying a purple cream or liquid color corrector. Conversely, purple bruising commonly seen after facial surgery can be camouflaged with a yellow color corrector (6). Standard brown concealers can also be used (Fig. 12.4).

> Purple is the complementary color to yellow and purple color correctors can be used to camouflage the final yellow stage of ecchymosis resolution.

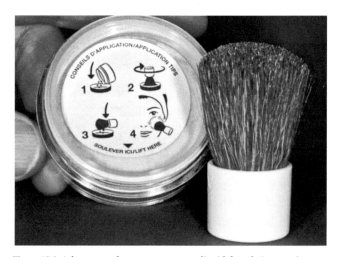

Figure 12.3 A loose powder over a cream or liquid foundation can improve rub-resistant characteristics.

Powders and Blushes

Facial powders and blushes are applied alone or on top of a facial foundation. Generally, their use should not be resumed until the face has healed to the point where facial foundations can be worn, as discussed previously. Powders without ground particulate matter, such as nutshells or mica, should be selected to avoid damaging the follicular ostia, which can lead to milia

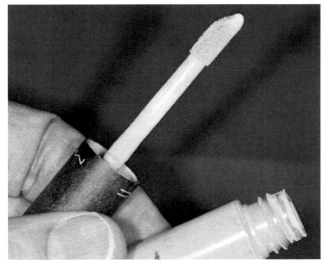

Figure 12.4 An example of a liquid brown concealer with an automatic applicator brush that can be dabbed over healing surgical scars.

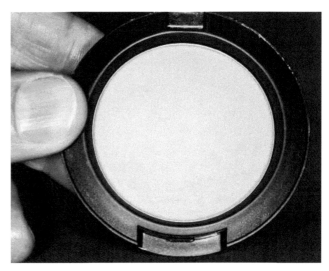

Figure 12.5 A blush can help redefine the cheeks after applying a full-coverage more opaque facial foundation in postsurgical patients.

and closed comedone formation. Thus, powders with a dull or matte finish are preferred (Fig. 12.5).

Matte finish powders and blushes without iridescent particles are the best choice after surgery.

Facial blushes are colored powders designed to add color to the cheeks and face. These products are extremely useful in postsurgical patients to:

1. restore facial landmarks, such as cheekbones, in patients who are wearing a high-coverage foundation;
2. camouflage facial redness by applying the blush to the upper cheeks, central forehead, nasal tip, and central chin;
3. add color to impart the appearance of health.

As with facial powders, blushes should be selected with a matte finish, meaning a dull finish, to avoid the light reflective particulate matter. The particulates can cause itching in an unhealed or early healed surgical wound.

Eye Cosmetics

Most patients can resume wearing selected eye cosmetics immediately following surgery, unless the surgery involves the eye area (i.e., eyelid tumor, blepharoplasty, eyelid resurfacing, etc.). Mascara, applied to darken, lengthen, and thicken the eyelashes may be immediately resumed. However, water-soluble varieties are recommended since the solvents required to remove waterproof varieties may cause stinging. Water-soluble eyeliners may also be resumed to highlight and cosmetically enlarge the eye. Eye shadows, on the other hand, represent a pigmented powder cosmetic and should not be worn until facial foundation use is resumed.

Water-removable mascara and eyeliner should be used in the postsurgical period.

Lip Cosmetics

Lip cosmetics may also be resumed immediately following surgery, unless the surgical site involves the lips (i.e. lip tumor removal, lip advancement flap, upper lip dermabrasion, etc.). Lip cosmetics are highly recommended as they represent a quick way to add color to the face and restore an acceptable cosmetic appearance.

All cosmetics should be removed from the face before bed.

REMOVAL OF COSMETICS

Postsurgical patients should wear cosmetics only when necessary and thoroughly remove them as soon as possible. They should remove all cosmetics before going to bed. Ideally, the cosmetic should be removed with mild soap and water; however, the waterproof camouflaging foundations require a special removal product. Waterproof cosmetics should be avoided until healing is complete as the solvents required to remove cosmetics can sting and burn. With new rub-resistant polymer-based mascaras and eyeliners, it is no longer necessary to use waterproof cosmetics. Removal of the cosmetics is necessary to prevent infection and other complications in the postsurgical period.

REFERENCES

1. Theberge L, Kernaleguen A. Importance of cosmetics related to aspects of self. Precept Mot Skills 1979; 48: 827.
2. Cash TF, Cash DW. Women's use of cosmetics: psychosocial correlates and consequences. Int J Cosmet Sci 1982; 4: 1.
3. Brauer EW. Coloring and corrective make-up preparations. Clin Dermatol 1988; 6: 62–7.
4. Schlossman ML, Feldman AJ. Fluid foundation and blush make-up. In: deNavarre MG, ed. The Chemistry and Manufacture of Cosmetics. Wheaton IL: Allured Publishing Corp, 1988: 748–51.
5. Draelos ZK. Cosmetic camouflaging techniques. Cutis 1993; 52: 362.
6. Draelos ZK. Use of cover cosmetics for pigment abnormalities. Cosmet Dermatol 1989; 5: 14.

SUGGESTED READING

Arpey CJ, Whitaker DC. Post surgical wound management. Dermatol Clin 2001; 19: 787–97.

Draelos ZD. Camouflaging techniques and dermatologic surgery. Dermatol Surg 1996; 22: 1023–7.

Draelos ZD. Cosmetics, skin care products, and the dermatologic surgeon. post-surgical selection of cleansing products. Dermatol Surg 1998; 24: 543–6.

Draelos ZK. Cosmetics in the postsurgical patient. Dermatol Clin 1995; 13: 461–5.

Karagoz H, Yuksel F, Ulkur E, Evinc R. Comparison of efficacy of silicone gel, silicone gel sheeting, and topical onion extract including heparin and allantoin for the treatment of postburn hypertrophic scars. Burns 2009; 35: 1097–103.

Morganroth P, Wilmot AC, Miller C. Over-the-counter scar products for postsurgical patients: disparities between online advertised benefits and evidence regarding efficacy. J Am Acad Dermatol 2009; 61: e31–47.

13 Facial adornment

Facial adornment is the use of colored facial cosmetics to improve appearance. These cosmetics serve little use for functional purpose, but can de-emphasize facial defects and accentuate attractive facial features. The basic facial cosmetics for adornment are powders, blushes, bronzing gels, cover sticks, and undercover creams.

FACIAL POWDERS

Facial powders provide coverage of complexion imperfections, oil control, a matte finish, and tactile smoothness to the skin. Originally, facial powder was applied over a moisturizer to function as a type of powder foundation. Liquid foundations have largely replaced the powder foundation, but for patients who wish sheer coverage with excellent oil control, a powder foundation performs excellently. An appropriate moisturizer for the patient's skin type is first applied and allowed to set or dry, followed by application of a full-coverage, translucent powder.

> Facial powders provide coverage of complexion imperfections, oil control, a matte finish, and tactile smoothness to the skin.

Full coverage powders contain predominantly talc, also known as hydrated magnesium silicate, and increased amounts of covering pigments. The covering pigments used in face powder are listed in order of increasing opaqueness: titanium dioxide, kaolin, magnesium carbonate, magnesium stearate, zinc stearate, prepared chalk, zinc oxide, rice starch, precipitated chalk, and talc. It is generally accepted that the optimum opacity is achieved with a particle size of 0.25 µm. Magnesium carbonate can also be used to improve oil blotting, keep the powder fluffy, and absorb any added perfume. Kaolin (hydrated aluminum silicate) may also function to absorb oil and perspiration. Full-coverage face powders are usually packaged in a compact and applied to the face with a puff (Fig. 13.1) (1).

Transparent facial powders are more popular today to add coverage and improve oil blotting abilities of a previously applied liquid foundation. Transparent powders have the same formulation as full-coverage powders except they contain less talc, titanium dioxide, or zinc oxide, since coverage is not a priority. Transparent facial powders commonly have a light shine, produced by nacreous pigments, such as bismuth oxychloride, mica, titanium-dioxide-coated mica, or crystalline calcium carbonate.

Facial powder usually uses iron oxides as the main pigment, but other inorganic pigments such as ultramarines, chrome oxide, and chrome hydrate may also be used. These powders are designed to augment the underlying skin and foundation tones, thus transparent powders can be used by patients who have difficulty finding an appropriately tinted facial foundation. Transparent powders may also be selected in complementary colors, such as a pale bluish-green, to decrease facial erythema in rosacea, psoriasis, and systemic lupus patients (see for further details chap. 2 and Table 13.1).

> Facial powder usually uses iron oxides as the main pigment, but other inorganic pigments such as ultramarines, chrome oxide, and chrome hydrate may also be used.

Specialty additives to some transparent powders include partially hydrolyzed ground raw silk to improve absorbency and impart a velvety matte finish; corn silk also to impart a velvety matte finish; and treated starch and synthetic resins for increased oil absorption. Most transparent powders are packaged loose and come with an applicator brush or puff.

Facial powders are removed from a compact with a puff or dusted loosely from a container with a brush. They impart a matte finish to the face. Patients who desire a shiny or moist semimatte facial appearance should avoid powder since it will absorb the oil in the foundation, thus destroying the "dewy" look. Patients with dry complexions may also wish to avoid facial powder since it can further dry the skin. However, the oil-absorbing abilities of facial powder are extremely valuable in a patient with an oily complexion prone to develop a facial shine.

The incidence of allergic contact dermatitis to facial powder itself is low; however, added fragrances may pose a problem. A more common problem with facial powders is irritant contact dermatitis due to coarse particulate matter, such as nacreous pigments, in the formulation. Inhalation of the powders may cause problems in patients with asthma or vasomotor rhinitis. Facial powder may be open or closed patch tested "as is."

FACIAL BLUSHES

Facial blushes, also known as rouges, are designed to enhance rosy cheek color. In many cases, rosy cheeks simply indicate vasomotor instability or fine telangiectatic mats from actinic damage; however, cheek color remains fashionable.

> Facial blushes are designed to enhance rosy cheek color.

Blush and rouge are actually synonyms for a cosmetic designed to add color to the cheeks, but to many consumers blush denotes a powdered product while rouge denotes a cream product. Powdered blushes are more popular and are formulated identically to compact face powder, except more vivid pigments are added (Fig. 13.2). Since color rather than coverage is desired, powdered blushes do not contain much zinc oxide. Cream rouges are formulated like anhydrous foundations which contain light esters, waxes, mineral oil, titanium dioxide, and pigments (2). Some patients use lipstick on the

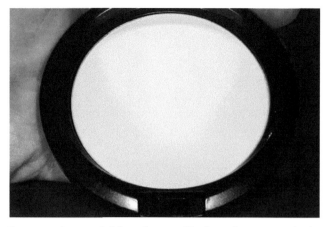

Figure 13.1 Compact facial powder can add color and coverage to the face while assisting with oil control.

cheeks as a form of cream rouge. Lipstick-type formulations used as cream rouge are known as facial gleamers. Powdered blushes can be easily brushed over any foundation formulation, but cream rouges will remove and smudge oil-free and low-oil-content foundations. Cream rouges also do not perform well if the face is powdered.

For a natural appearance, cheek color should be applied beginning at a point directly beneath the pupil on the fleshy part of the cheek, sweeping upward beyond the lateral eye (Fig. 13.3) (3). This placement is designed to create or accentuate high cheek bones, which are a desired quality among women (4).

The adverse reaction concerns with blushes and rouges are identical to those for facial powders. The products can be open or closed patch tested "as is."

Table 13.1 The Color Chart Showing Cosmetics for Different Skin Colors

Cosmetic	Light skin	Medium skin	Dark skin
(A) Caucasian skin			
Facial foundation	Light beige, pale ivory, light pink	Medium beige, ivory, medium pink, peach	Beige, tan, dark peach
Blush and lipstick	Rose pink, true red	Deep pink, blue red, cherry red, coral	Deep red, cinnamon, burgundy
Eyebrow pencil and mascara	Charcoal gray, dark brown, brown black	Dark brown	Dark brown
Eyeliner	Charcoal gray, brown black	Dark brown	Black
Eye shadow	Light green, purple, pink, light brown, light blue	Deep green, brown, blue	Muted green, brown, muted blue
(B) Black skin			
Facial foundation	Rose, medium beige, medium peach	Medium beige, bronze	Sun bronze, taupe
Blush and lipstick	Medium coral, medium pink, orange red	Deep coral, rose, translucent red	Cinnamon, deep translucent rose, true translucent red
Eyebrow pencil and mascara	Dark brown, charcoal, black	Charcoal, black	Black
Eyeliner	Beige, charcoal, black	Beige, charcoal, black	Beige, charcoal, black
Eye shadow	Beige, lavender, aqua, light blue	Beige, deep lavender, medium blue	Deep violet, deep sea green
(C) Oriental skin			
Facial foundation	Light pink, peach, beige	Medium pink, deep peach, medium beige	Dark pink, dark beige
Blush and lipstick	Light pink, orange	Rose, light red	Rose, red
Eyebrow pencil and mascara	Black, charcoal	Black, charcoal	Black
Eyeliner	Black, charcoal	Black, charcoal	Black
Eye shadow	Beige, pink, violet, blue	Turquoise, aqua, lavender, deep blue, green	Deep violet, deep pink, vivid blue, vivid green
(D) American indian skin			
Facial foundation	Light beige	Medium beige	Dark beige
Blush and lipstick	Pink, light red	Peach, pink, light red	Deep rose, cranberry red
Eyebrow pencil and mascara	Charcoal, dark brown, black	Black, charcoal	Black
Eyeliner	Black, charcoal	Black, charcoal	Black
Eye shadow	Beige, cool turquoise, green, aqua	Medium beige, turquoise, aqua, green, deep blue	Beige, deep green, deep blue
(E) Asian skin			
Facial foundation	Beige, rose beige	Medium beige, rose beige	Beige, light taupe
Blush and lipstick	Peach, pale orange, rose	Red, rose, pink, coral	Deep red, deep rose, orange
Eyebrow pencil and mascara	Dark brown, charcoal	Black, charcoal	Black
Eyeliner	Black, charcoal	Black, charcoal	Black
Eye shadow	Pink, lavender, blue, turquoise, sea green	Deep violet, deep beige, deep pink	Violet, purple, blue

FACIAL BRONZING GELS

Facial bronzing gels are alternative products available to add facial color. If the product is intended to add color only to the cheeks, it is called a gel rouge, but if the product is designed to provide overall facial color, it is known as a bronzing gel. Gel rouge is available in shades of red and orange while bronzing gels, as the name suggests, are intended to give a tanned appearance (5). Both products stain the skin and provide no coverage. They contain light esters, propylene glycol, alcohol, and water-soluble organic colors in a neutral aqueous gel. They must be applied and spread quickly as the volatile vehicle yields a short playtime. Staining of the fingertips and clothing during application is a common problem.

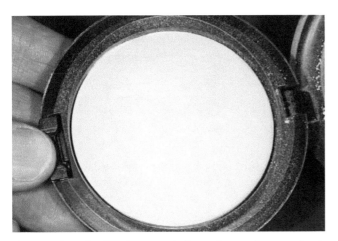

Figure 13.2 A powdered blush appears similar to a face powder except that the product is pigmented more vividly to create the appearance of rosy cheeks, considered a sign of general health.

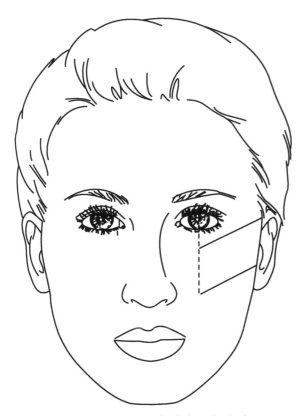

Figure 13.3 Placement of a blush on the cheek.

> Bronzing gels add color to the face usually simulating a tan.

Another product that provides facial color without coverage is a color wash. Color washes are liquid foundations with pigment but no titanium dioxide, frequently containing some pearl additive, such as bismuth oxychloride or mica. Color washes can be worn alone or under a sheer foundation. They may not be applied over a foundation or on a powdered face. Color washes are more appropriate for patients with dry skin, while bronzing gels are more appropriate for patients with oily skin.

FACIAL BUFFERS AND HIGHLIGHTERS

Facial buffers and highlighters are formulated exactly like powdered facial blushes except that the color and amount of pearl may vary. Facial blushes are usually of an intense color, ranging from red to orange for accentuating the upper cheeks. Facial buffers, on the other hand, are usually a light pink or peach with a moderate amount of pearl. Their purpose is to blend other facial cosmetics. For example, after the blush is applied to the cheek, a border forms where the color stops. Applying a facial buffer over the blush blends the edges of color into the natural skin tones. Facial buffers can also be used to blend eye shadows into the upper eyelid.

Facial highlighters are more intensely pigmented than facial blushes. They are available in deep burgundy, bronze, or brown and function to color and contour the face (Fig. 13.4). For example, a bronze facial highlighter can be applied to the central forehead, nasal tip, and central chin to create the appearance of a tan, since these three protuberant areas of the face generally are more deeply pigmented in a patient with recent sun exposure. Facial buffers and highlighters can be artfully used by the patient with facial defects to improve facial contour.

FACIAL COVER STICKS

Facial cover sticks are intended for use under a facial foundation to cover imperfections. Facial cover sticks, also known as under eye concealers, are matched to the skin color and applied to cover an abnormal skin color, such as the redness of an acne

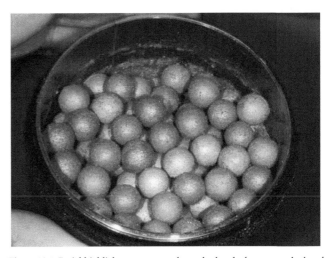

Figure 13.4 Facial highlighter compressed powder beads that are stroked and blended with a brush to obtain the desired color blend prior to brushing over the face and body.

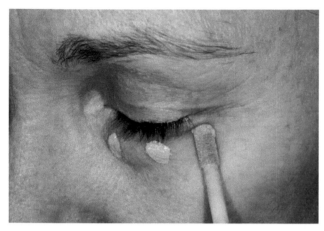

Figure 13.5 A skin colored cream is dabbed and blended under the eyes to camouflage under eye circles.

lesion or the darkness of under eye circles (6) (Fig. 13.5). These are maximum coverage products with high amounts of titanium dioxide. Other ingredients include mineral oil, waxes, pigments, and kaolin or talc. Formulations available in a roll-up stick contain more wax than cream formulations, which contain more oil. A popular packaging of the cream formulation is in a cylindrical tube with an insertable sponge tip applicator. The long wearing, high coverage characteristics of facial cover sticks require pigment suspended in an oil base. There are some products labeled as "oil-free," however they contain silicone oils.

> Facial cover sticks are intended for use under a facial foundation to cover imperfections.

FACIAL UNDERCOVER CREAMS
Facial undercover creams are designed to mask undesirable skin tones. They are formulated like cream foundations with oils, waxes, talc, and pigment. Undercover creams come in a variety of complementary colors and are intended for application under a full-coverage facial foundation. Green undercover creams are used to camouflage a reddish complexion created by such dermatologic conditions as rosacea, psoriasis, lupus, acne, or a facial nevus flammeus. The application of a green cover over underlying red skin produces a net result of brown under a foundation since green mixed with red pigments produces a brown tone. A light purple undercover can be used by patients with a yellow complexion due to renal failure or Oriental background to yield a pink skin tone. A peach colored undercover can be used to mask the bluish tones of bruised skin. If the patient chooses to use an undercover cream, she must also commit herself to wearing a full line of facial cosmetics since the cream by itself does not cover the defect.

> Facial undercover creams come in a variety of complementary colors for camouflage purposes and are intended for application under a full-coverage facial foundation.

Another undercover product, known as a white pearlized undercover, is an oil-based liquid makeup that contains increased amounts of titanium dioxide without any pigment. This undercover is designed for the patient with actinically damaged skin characterized by fine wrinkling, telangiectasia, and mottled pigmentation. The increased amount of titanium dioxide whitens the discolored skin and the pearl created by bismuth oxychloride or mica minimizes the fine wrinkling.

BRONZING POWDERS AND TINTED MOISTURIZERS
Bronzing powders and tinted moisturizers are used to add temporary color the face and body, generally trying to simulate a tan. Bronzing powders are identical in formulation to face powders except for the addition of different pigments. The powder is stroked from a compact with a powder sponge or puff and applied to the body. The product is usually dusted down the central face, neck, and shoulders to simulate a tan (7). The powder is easily removed by rubbing and provides slight physical sun protection due to the titanium dioxide in most formulations.

> Bronzing powders and tinted moisturizers are used to add temporary color to the face and body to simulate a tan.

Tinted moisturizers are liquids, as opposed to the previously discussed bronzing powders, and they contain a brown pigment that provides a sheer tanned appearance in addition to possessing emollient qualities. Technically, it is impossible to separate a tinted moisturizer from a sheer, moisturizing facial foundation. Usually, a facial foundation contains titanium dioxide to provide coverage to underlying cutaneous pigment defects whereas a tinted moisturizer does not, but the distinction is slight.

FACIAL COSMETICS FOR ACNE PATIENTS
Facial cosmetics selection for acne patients poses a challenge for the dermatologist. Acne patients are generally self-conscious about the blemishes on their complexion and anxious to apply cosmetics that will completely mask the erythema, papules, and nodules that characterize acne. They will generally select the facial foundation with the longest wear and highest amount of coverage. These products are inevitably oil based and extremely occlusive, resulting in additional facial oil and follicular irritation that may aggravate the underlying acne, necessitating further cosmetic application. High-coverage foundations also create a need to use blush, lipstick, and eye shadow since they cover not only the acne lesions but all facial contours. Unfortunately, there is no optimal solution to this problem.

> Facial powder can aid in oil control in the acne patient.

Facial powder can be extremely valuable for the acne patient. It can absorb oil, thus increasing the wear of oil-free facial foundations that will rub off or separate when mixed with sebum. Powder can also increase the coverage of an oil-free foundation. In order to obtain maximum benefits from powder and eliminate a "floured" facial appearance, the powder must be properly selected and applied. A loose transparent powder is best. Transparent powders come in tones of pink, yellow, or brown and the patient should select the tone that best matches her underlying complexion and foundation. The fingertips are then dipped in the loose powder and it is massaged into the foundation over the entire face. Rubbing the powder into the foundation is superior to dusting the powder onto the face, since it adheres more closely to the foundation, resulting in an increased foundation wearability and better oil control. Rubbing also eliminates the "floured" facial look and imparts a smooth feel. A fluffy brush is then used to dust away excess powder. The technique may be repeated if oily breakthrough occurs. Oily breakthrough occurs when the foundation has absorbed as much oil as possible, resulting in the development of a facial shine due to oil seeping through the layer of foundation.

Powder can also be used to increase the coverage of oil-free foundations in acne blemish areas. Foundation is dabbed onto the acne lesions with the fingertips and allowed to dry. Loose transparent powder is then massaged into the area. Another layer of foundation is then applied and the process is repeated until the desired coverage is achieved. Foundation is then applied to the entire face and finished with a facial powder rub as previously described.

Loose powders usually contain less oil than pressed compact powders and are therefore recommended for the acne patient. Most of the loose talc-based powders will work well, except for those that contain ground particulate matter, such as walnut shell powder. These products tend to encourage the formation of closed comedones and milia. Perhaps this is due to sharp-edged particles occluding the follicle, forming closed comedones, or causing epidermal damage resulting in milia.

Acne patients should also select powdered and gel facial cosmetic formulations over oily creams. This means that powdered blush should be selected over cream rouge and bronzing gels should be selected over color washes. Powdered blush can be used effectively by acne patients to absorb oil and provide a reddish color to the upper cheeks, which may aid in blending acne blemishes. For light-skinned acne patients, bronzing gels can effectively add facial color without worsening acne or creating the need to wear a full line of facial cosmetics.

FACIAL COSMETICS FOR MATURE PATIENTS
Mature patients generally have dry skin with wrinkling and other effects of actinic damage. In the presence of dry skin, oil-absorbing products such as powders should be avoided. If a powder is desired, it should be low in magnesium carbonate and zinc oxide, since these two substances have an astringent or drying effect on the face. Powder also tends to migrate into the creases accentuating wrinkling. However, powdered blushes are still recommended over cream rouges. Cream rouge does not spread well when applied over a foundation of any type. Facial bronzing gels are also difficult to apply over a furrowed skin. If increased facial color is desired, a color wash used alone or under an oil-containing foundation is preferable.

Powders should be avoided in mature patients with dry skin.

Cream undercover cosmetics perform well on mature skin because their oil base can replace a facial moisturizer. Green undercover on the upper cheeks is especially useful in the mature patient with fine facial telangiectasias. The green undercover must be covered with an oil-containing foundation. Powder blush applied to the upper cheeks will also help to blend the telangiectasias. White pearlized undercover can be used beneath a foundation to minimize wrinkling and improve uneven facial pigmentation.

FACIAL COSMETICS FOR MEN
Facial color cosmetics for men have been slowly gaining acceptance, but they remain unpopular (8,9). Men in the entertainment industry use cosmetics designed for women and apply the cosmetics in the same manner as women to accentuate facial color (10). For average daily use, facial cosmetics are impractical for men. The beard precludes even application of facial foundations, since the pigment tends to adhere to the hair shafts and prominent follicular structures. The coarse texture of male skin also is accentuated. If total facial color is required, facial foundations should be avoided in favor of bronzing gels. This product stains the skin, thus providing color, but does not provide coverage. If coverage is required, men should select opaque cover cosmetics discussed in the chapter on facial scarring. Color can be effectively added to the cheeks, forehead, nose, and chin with powdered facial blushes, buffers, or highlighters. A transparent facial powder dusted over the entire face can minimize the appearance of large pore structures and the "five o'clock shadow" created on the cheeks by the regrowth of dark facial hair after early morning shaving. No nationally distributed color cosmetic line developed especially for men is currently available.

FACIAL COSMETICS FOR CHILDREN
Color facial cosmetics are available for young girls to adorn the face and cheeks. Most preadolescent and early adolescent girls do not want to "look like they wear makeup," but still want to go through the motions of applying cosmetics to their face. Popular facial cosmetics in this age group include transparent facial color gels and rouges. Transparent facial color gels and teenage rouges are similar in formulation except that color gels are more lightly colored for all over application to the face while the rouge is brightly colored and only applied to the upper cheeks. They contain light esters, propylene glycol, alcohol, and water-soluble organic colors in a neutral aqueous gel. The product must be applied evenly and quickly to avoid streaking and stains everything it contacts, including fingertips.

CORRECTIVE FACIAL COSMETICS
Corrective cosmetics for facial lesions are based on the principle that dark colors make the lesions appear smaller and to recede while light colors make the lesions look larger and appear to come forward. This concept is illustrated in Figure 13.6 where the black oval appears recessed and smaller compared with the white oval. Powdered blush-type products are best suited for this purpose. Areas of the face that need to be lightened should be brushed with a light pink or peach pearled blush or buffer. Areas of the face that need to be darkened should be brushed with a deep plum or bronze matte finish blush or highlighter.

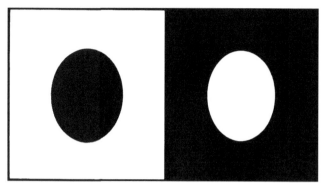

Figure 13.6 The two fundamental rules of facial contouring: dark contours look smaller and appear to recede; light contours look larger and appear to come forward.

Corrective facial cosmetics are based on the principle that dark colors make the lesions appear smaller and to recede while light colors make the lesions look larger and appear to come forward.

Cosmetic facial sculpting is most successful for optimizing the shape of the face, the size of the forehead and chin, or the contour of the nose. The perfect facial shape is oval and symmetrical about the midline, as this form is most pleasing to the eye. An oval face is one and one-half times as long as it is wide and should taper gradually from its widest dimension at the forehead to its smallest dimension at the chin. The face should be divided into equal thirds from superior to inferior: forehead to the glabella, glabella to the subnasale, and subnasale to the base of the chin. The face should divide equally into fifths from ear to ear with each fifth being the width of one eye (11).

The ideal face should be divided into three equal parts from superior to inferior: forehead to the glabella, glabella to the subnasale, and subnasale to the base of the chin.

Other facial shapes are round, where the facial length is short; oblong, where the facial length is long; square, where the jaw is wide; diamond, where the forehead is small; triangular, where the cheeks are wide; and inverted triangular, where the jaw is narrow. By appropriately shading the face, the less optimal shapes described can more closely approximate a perfect oval.

For example, a round face should be shaded with a dark color along the lateral margins to de-emphasize the increased width, whereas an oblong face should be shaded along the forehead and chin to de-emphasize the increased length. A square face should be darkened bilaterally at the jaws. Both diamond and triangular faces should be lightened at the forehead for emphasis and an inverted triangular face should be lightened at the chin (12).

This same shading technique can also be used to correct a poorly formed forehead and chin. Low-set foreheads should have a light blush applied beneath the hairline while high foreheads should have a dark blush applied here. A receding chin should have a light blush applied at the tip and sides. A double

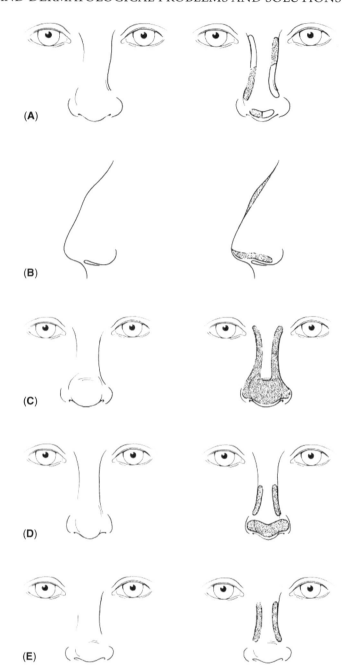

Figure 13.7 Contouring of the nose. (**A**) Crooked nose. (**B**) Hook or aquiline nose. (**C**) Bulbous nose. (**D**) Long nose. (**E**) Short nose.

chin should be shaded with a dark blush under the entire jawbone (13).

Facial recontouring is most useful on the nose, where hair, jewelry, or glasses cannot hide the abnormality. Figure 13.7 illustrates the shading techniques. Areas to be darkened are cross-hatched and areas to be lightened are outlined. Figure 13.7A demonstrates a broken nose that has healed crookedly with a deviation to the patient's left. The prominent upper left side of the nose is darkened, along with the lower right side and right tip. The opposite sides are lightened. A hook nose or aquiline nose (Fig. 13.7B) can also be minimized by darkening the hook along with the lateral nasal tips. A bulbous nose can be improved by shading the entire bulb on the tip and the lateral margins to the nasal root (Fig. 13.7C). Shading for long and short noses is shown in Figure 13.7D and E, respectively (14).

Corrective facial cosmetics are no substitute for a perfect face, and in some cases patients should be advised to consider surgical revision. These suggestions may be offered to the patient who is awaiting surgery or the patient who has not previously considered cosmetics as a way of creating the illusion of a more perfect face.

ADVISING THE PATIENT ON COSMETIC SELECTION

The dermatologist is called upon with increasing frequency to give advice on cosmetic selection. Patients are searching for cosmetics that improve skin quality while offering value. Dermatologists, with their understanding of skin physiology and disease, are best suited to render opinions in this area; however, unfamiliarity with available cosmetics and their use may make physicians unable to give valuable, concrete advice. This text is intended to serve as a basic guide for formulating individual patient recommendations. I now outline my approach to advising the patient on cosmetic selection.

The first step in making cosmetic selection recommendations is to determine where the patient purchases her cosmetics. This is important because the point of purchase is related to the cost of the product. It is wise to keep cost in mind when making patient recommendations. Cosmetic manufacturers intentionally produce products to reach consumers through a variety of markets. Some cosmetics are sold in mass merchandisers, such as grocery stores, drug stores, and discount stores. Cosmetics sold through these vendors generally range in price from $2 to $15. Other cosmetics are sold exclusively through cosmetic counters in department stores. Even within the department store market there are products designed for lower price point department stores and higher price point department stores. Lower price-point department stores market cosmetics that sell for $8 to $20 as compared to higher price-point department store cosmetics that sell for $20 to $60. The most expensive cosmetics are sold through boutiques and spas. These products range from $25 to $90. Interestingly enough, some of these exclusive products are manufactured by the same companies that produce cosmetics under a different label for sale in mass merchandisers. Generally, boutique lines have more attractive, elaborate packaging accompanied by a greater color selection, more expensive fragrances, and innovative specialty additives.

Another route for cosmetics purchase is through household parties and individuals who sell door-to-door in their neighborhood. These products generally are in the $8 to $25 range. Lastly, private cosmetics are produced on a contract basis, generally through small manufacturers. Cosmetics can be customized to the needs of the business or simply a standard formulation with a customized label. The price variation in this market is tremendous. It is worthwhile noting that cosmetics sold in these manners, which are produced and marketed for intrastate use, do not fall under the guideline of the U.S. Food and Drug Administration. Furthermore, smaller cosmetic manufacturers do not have the capital or the facilities to undertake extensive premarketing and postmarketing consumer research. However, there are several large cosmetic companies that market quality products worldwide who reach the consumer through these routes.

The second step is to determine the patient's skin type: very oily, oily, combination, normal, dry, very dry, etc. Moisturizer and facial foundation recommendations must be carefully chosen with the skin type in mind. Interestingly enough, many patients do not know their skin type or have been erroneously assigned a skin type by a salesperson at a cosmetic counter. In my opinion, skin type can be most easily assigned by asking the patient about the amount of sebum production on her/his nose throughout the day following morning washing. Sebum production can be assessed by having the patient run her/his finger down the nose at various times during the day. If the patient has flaking skin on the nose all day and no sebum from morning until 5 PM, they have very dry skin. If the patient has no flaking, but no sebum on their nose at 5 PM, they have dry skin. If the patient has minimal sebum on the nose at 5 PM, they have normal skin. If the patient has sebum on the nose at noon, they have oily skin. Moreover, if the patient has sebum on the nose one hour following morning washing, they have very oily skin. Combination skin, the most common skin type in both women and men, can be assessed by comparing the amount of sebum present on the nose at 5 PM with the amount present on the cheeks. This is a simplistic, but fairly accurate, method of determining the skin type.

Thirdly, once the skin type has been determined, appropriate sections within this text can be consulted for specific cosmetic product recommendations. Some patients, however, also wish to know what color cosmetics should be selected to enhance the appearance of their skin and facial features. This advice may be beyond the realm of what most dermatologists can provide and questions of this nature may be more appropriately handled by cosmetologists. Nevertheless, for the physician with an interest in this area, color charts based on skin pigmentation have been provided to coordinate facial foundation, blush, lipstick, eyebrow pencil, mascara, and eye shadow color with skin tones (Table 13.1) (15,16).

Finally, there is no doubt that a personal visit to a mass merchandiser cosmetic display or the department store cosmetic counter can provide valuable first-hand experience. Smelling, touching, and applying cosmetics can provide a wealth of information that cannot be fully described in a text.

REFERENCES

1. Wetterhahn J. Loose and compact face powder. In: deNavarre MG, ed. The Chemistry and Manufacture of Cosmetics. Vol. 4. 2nd edn. Wheaton, IL: Allured Publishing Corportation, 1988: 921–46.
2. Lanzet M. Modern formulations of coloring agents: facial and eye. In: Frost P, Horwitz SN, eds. Cosmetics for the Dermatologist. St. Louis: CV Mosby, 1982: 133–51.
3. Begoun P. Blue eyeshadow should be illegal. Seattle, WA: Beginning Press, 1986: 62–4.
4. Soldo BL, Drahos M. The Inside-Out Beauty Book. Old Tappan, New Jersey: Fleming H. Revell Company, 1978: 78–9.
5. Jackson EM. Tanning without the sun: accelerators, promoters, pills, bronzing gels, and self-tanning lotions. Am J Contact Dermatitis 1994; 5: 38–40.
6. Wesley-Hosford Z. Face value. Toronto: Bantam Books, 1986: 148–50.
7. Draelos ZD. Cosmetics to imitate a summer tan. Cosmet Dermatol 1990; 3: 8–10.
8. Dichter P, Fils VM. The men's product explosion. Cosmet Toilet 1985: 75–6.
9. Kavaliunas DR, Nacht S, Bogardus RE. Men's skin care needs. Cosmet Toilet 1985: 29–32.
10. Draelos ZD. Cosmetics designed for men. Cosmet Dermatol 1992; 5: 14–16.
11. Powell N, Humphreys B. Proportions of the aesthetic face. New York: Thieme-Stratton Inc, 1984: 1–13.
12. Taylor P. Milady's makeup techniques. Albany, New York: Milady Publishing Company, 1994: 18–23.

13. Miller C. 8 minute makeovers. Washington, DC: Acropolis Books Ltd.,
     1884: 166–7.
14. Newman A, Ebenstein RS. Adrian Arpel's 851 Fast Beauty Fixes and Facts.
     New York: G. P. Putnam's Sons, 1985: 47.
15. Soldo BL, Drahos M. The Inside-Out Beauty Book. Old Tappan, NJ:
     Fleming H. Revell Company, 1978: 85–100.
16. Bruce J, Cohen SS. About face. New York: G. P. Putnam's Sons, 1984: 94–6.

SUGGESTED READING

Draelos ZD. Colored facial cosmetics. Dermatol Clin 2000; 18: 621–31.
Hollenberg J. Color cosmetics (Chapter 26). In: Rieger MM, ed. Harry's
     Cosmeticology, 8th edn. Chemical Publishing Co., Inc., 2000: 523–72.
Levy SB. Cosmetics that Imitate a Tan. Dermatol Ther 2001; 14: 215–19.

Palma DD. Looking younger: cosmetics and clothing to look more vibrant.
     Clin Dermatol 2008; 26: 648–51.
Schlossman ML. Decorative products (Chapter 54). In: Barel AO, Paye M,
     Maibach HI, eds. Handbook of Cosmetic Science and Technology. Marcel
     Dekker, Inc., 2001: 649–83.
Sun JZ, Erickson MCE, Parr JW. Refractive index matching: principles and
     cosmetic application. C & T magazine.
Tedeschi A, Dall'Oglio F, Micali G, Schwartz RA, Janniger CK. Corrective
     camouflage in pediatric dermatology. Cutis 2007; 79: 110–12.
Weisz A, Milstein SRT, Scher AL. Colouring agents in cosmetic products
     (excluding hair dyes): regulatory aspects and analytical methods. Anal
     Cosmet Prod 2007: 153–89.
Westmore MG. Camouflage and makeup preparations. Clin Dermatol 2001;
     19: 406–12.

14 Troubleshooting problematic ingredients

Cosmetic formulation involves the careful selection of ingredients to produce a safe, elegant, efficacious product suitable for patient purchase (1). There are many substances that must be combined to produce such a cosmetic, and consideration must be given to factors, such as moisture barrier effects, pH, lubricating action, soothing effects, osmotic effects, emollience, and percutaneous absorption (2). This chapter discusses the dermatologic concerns of key ingredients found in many cosmetic formulations, which are preservatives, color additives, biologic additives, herbal additives, vitamin additives, and liposomes.

PRESERVATIVES

Preservatives have received their share of bad press as of late, being accused of everything from breast cancer to environmental damage. While preservatives are not terribly appealing ingredients they are a necessary part of every cosmetic and skin care formulation. Without a preservative, the lipids in most formulations would rapidly oxidize rendering the cream rancid, or the bacterial contamination would render the product unsafe. Preservatives are the second most common allergenic group of substances beyond fragrances (3). However, the number of cases of irritant and allergic contact dermatitis is indeed small compared with the two necessary functions preservatives perform in cosmetics: spoilage prevention prior to purchase and prevention of contamination after purchase (4,5). In short, preservatives reduce the likelihood of infection from cosmetics use. An independent survey of 250 cosmetics covering a wide range of products revealed a 24.4% contamination rate in unused products, primarily by *Pseudomonas* species and other gram-negative rods in 1969 (6). The most frequently contaminated products were hand and body lotions and liquid eyeliners. The development of new and better preservatives has improved cosmetic preservation tremendously.

Preservatives are the second most common allergenic group of substances beyond fragrances.

Unfortunately, the ideal preservative does not exist (7). Valuable qualities in a cosmetic preservative include those listed in Table 14.1(8). An important function of the cosmetic chemist and the microbiologist is to select the preservative that most closely meets all of the aforementioned needs in a given product. Additionally, the preservative must undergo rigorous dermatologic testing to ensure that it is safe for use on human skin (9,10). Some Internet watchdog groups have singled out preservatives as bad or unnatural ingredients that are unsafe for human use. Much of the data they cite is from the animal ingestion of large quantities of preservatives. The preservatives used in skin care products are not intended for consumption and the concentration of preservatives in skin care products is small, evidenced by the fact that they are listed at the end of the ingredient disclosure. Preservatives are necessary to ensure a long shelf life and prevent infection.

All cosmetics and skin care products contain preservatives.

There is no such thing as a product is designed without preservation considerations. All products use some type of preservation technique either in packaging, such as an oxygen-free dispenser with a one-way valve, or in formulation, such as incorporating spice extracts as fragrances and natural preservatives. Key to stability of any skin care product on the shelf is consumer safety. The concept that the elimination of preservatives is beneficial for the consumer is not necessarily true.

Numerous preservatives are available for incorporation into cosmetics. Table 14.2 lists some of the preservative substances organized into chemical classes. Each of these chemicals has certain advantages and disadvantages which are summarized in Table 14.3. There is no perfect preservative substance for cosmetics on the market. Some of the more popular preservatives in use today, due to their relatively low irritancy and allergenicity, include paraben esters, imidazolidinyl urea, phenoxyethanol, Quaternium-15, and Kathon CG (11). The most commonly used preservative in cosmetics in the United States are the paraben esters followed by imidazolidinyl urea (12).

The most commonly used preservative in U.S. cosmetics and skin care products is paraben ester followed by imidazolidinyl urea.

There has been a move as of late to eliminate paraben preservatives from some skin care products. Consumer groups have linked parabens with breast cancer on their websites encouraging manufacturers to use other preservatives. One of the more popular preservatives substituted for parabens is Kathon-CG, but this preservative is a much greater source of contact dermatitis than parabens and in many respects more problematic. Some of the "natural" skin care products use essential oils and fragrances with antimicrobial capabilities, such as oil of clove, cinnamon, eucalyptus, rose, lavender, lemon, thyme, rosemary, and sandalwood (13). Products that claim to be preservative-free may actually incorporate one of these aromatic preservatives accompanied by special packaging (Fig. 14.1).

The complexity of cosmetic formulations requires a preservative to function under a variety of conditions. Microorganisms tend to proliferate in the aqueous phase of cosmetics. Under these circumstances the preservative selected must have a high water solubility and low oil solubility to

Table 14.1 Characteristics of an Ideal Cosmetic Preservative

1. Lack of irritation
2. Lack of sensitization
3. Stable at a wide range of temperatures and pH
4. Stable for extended periods of time
5. Compatible with numerous ingredients and packaging materials
6. Effective against numerous microorganisms
7. No odor or color

Table 14.2 Some Preservatives Used in Cosmetics

Organic acids
    Benzoic acid
    Sorbic acid
    Monochloroacetic acid
    Formic acid
    Salicylic acid
    Boric acid
    Propionic acid
    Sulfurous acid
    Citric acid
    Dehydroacetic acid
Parabens
    Methyl p-hydroxybenzoate
    Ethyl p-hydroxybenzoate
    Propyl p-hydroxybenzoate
    Butyl p-hydroxybenzoate
    Benzyl p-hydroxybenzoate
Mercurial compounds
    Phenyl mercury acetate
    Phenyl mercury borate
    Phenyl mercury nitrate
Essential oils
    Eucalyptus
    Origanum
    Thyme
    Savory
    Lemongrass oil
Aldehydes
    Formaldehyde
Alcohols
    b-Phenoxy ethyl alcohol
    b-p-Chlorophenoxy ethyl alcohol
    b-Phenoxy propyl alcohol
    Benzyl alcohol
    Isopropyl alcohol
    Ethyl alcohol
Phenolic compounds
    Phenol
    o-Phenylphenol
    Chlorothymol
    Methyl cholorthymol
    Dichlorophene
    Hexachlorophene
Quaternary ammonium compounds
    Benzethonium chloride
    Benzalkonium chloride
    Cetyl trimethyl ammonium bromide
    Cetylpyridinium chloride

(Continued)

Table 14.2 (*Continued*) Some Preservatives Used in Cosmetics

Miscellaneous
    5-Bromo-5-nitro-1,3-dioxan (Dioxin)
    2-Bromo-2-nitropropane-1,3-diol (Bronopol)
    Imidazolidinyl urea (Germall 115)
    Trichlorosalicylanilide
    Trichlorocarbanilide
    5-Chloro-2-methyl-4-isothiazolin-3-one and 2-methyl-4-isothiazolin-3-one (Kathon CG)

Source: Adapted from Harry's Cosmetology. In: Wilkinson JB, Moore RJ, eds. 7th edn. New York: Chemical Publishing, 1982: 673–706.

function. Furthermore, care must be taken to ensure that other ingredients in the formulation do not inactivate the preservative either by binding to active sites or altering the effective pH range. Some solid substances such as talc, kaolin, titanium dioxide, and zinc oxide actually adsorb the preservative, thus lowering its effective concentration (14).

Organisms that frequently contaminate cosmetics include gram-positive bacteria (*Staphylococcus aureus, Streptococcus* species), gram-negative bacteria (*Pseudomonas aeruginosa, Escherichia coli, Enterobacter aerogenes*), fungi (*Asperigillus niger, Penicillium* species, *Alternaria* species), and yeasts (*Candida* species) (15). The necessity of preservatives cannot be denied, but infrequently adverse reactions to cosmetic and skin care preservatives can occur. Paraben esters are the most popular preservatives used in cosmetics as their sensitization potential is low and they infrequently cause irritancy when applied to healthy skin (16). They are usually found in concentrations of 0.5% or less in the United States, but concentrations up to 5% have been shown to produce minimal irritation. Some individuals who are allergic to parabens may actually tolerate cosmetics containing them, a phenomenon known as the "paraben paradox" (17). Tolerance is related to application site, concentration, duration, and the status of the skin (18). Since they are most effective against gram-positive organisms and fungi, paraben esters are sometimes used in combination with phenoxyethanol to provide better gram-negative coverage (19). Parabens and imidazolidinyl urea (Germall 115) or diazolidinyl urea (Germall II) also act synergistically (20).

Some preservatives, such as imidazolidinyl urea (Germall 115), 2-bromo-2 nitropropane-1,3-diol (Bronopol) (21,22), Quaternium-15 (Dowicil 200) (23), and dimethylol dimethyl hydantoin (Glydant) are formaldehyde releasers. This means that free formaldehyde is produced in the presence of water. However, the concentration of formaldehyde is usually too low to cause irritancy or allergenicity. Nevertheless, patients who are allergic to formaldehyde may have difficulty with these preservatives (24).

Kathon-CG, the CG standing for cosmetic grade, is a relatively new preservative to the United States (25). It is a source of sensitization and recommended for use in products that are rinsed off the skin, such as hair conditioners and shampoos, in concentrations of less than 5 ppm (26,27). It is used, however, in some leave-on products, such as hand creams, in low concentration. Kathon-CG and quaternium-15 were

Table 14.3 A Comparison of Preservatives

Preservative	Advantage	Disadvantage
Alcohols	Broad coverage, inexpensive	Volatile, high concentration required
Quaternium-15 (Dowicil 200)	Broad coverage (bacteria, yeasts, molds)	Ineffective against some *Pseudomonas* species, formaldehyde releaser
Formaldehyde	Broad coverage (fungicide and bactericide)	Irritant, allergen, concentration-regulated unpleasant odor
Quaternary ammonium compounds	Mainly gram-positive bacteria, some gram negative	Incompatible with anionics and proteins
Parabens	Moderate coverage (fungi, gram positive bacteria), low allergenicity, low irritancy	Poor against gram-negative bacteria, incompatible with nonionics and cationics, effective only at acidic pH
Organic mercurials	Broad coverage	High toxicity, high irritancy
Phenolics	Broad coverage, effective over wide pH range	High irritancy, volatile
2-Bromo-2-nitropropane-1,3-diol (Bronopol)	Moderate coverage (bacteria)	Formaldehyde releaser, least effective against yeast and fungi
Methylisothiazolinone and methylchloroisothiazolinone (Kathon CG)	Broad coverage (bacteria, yeasts, fungi)	Allergenicity, irritancy, inactivated at high pH
Imidazolidinyl urea (Germall 115)	Moderate coverage (gram-negative bacteria)	Best used combined with parabens and antifungals to obtain a broader coverage
Diazolidinyl urea (Germall II)	Moderate coverage (gram-negative bacteria, *Pseudomonas* species)	Best used combined with parabens and antifungals to obtain a broader coverage
Organic acids	Broad coverage (bacteria, yeasts)	Irritating, effective only at acidic pH
Dimethyloldimethyl hydantoin (Glydant)	Broad coverage, effective over wide pH range	Less active against yeasts

Source: Adapted from Harry's Cosmeticology. In: Wilkinson JB, Moore RJ, eds. 7th edn. New York: Chemical Publishing, 1982: 673–707.

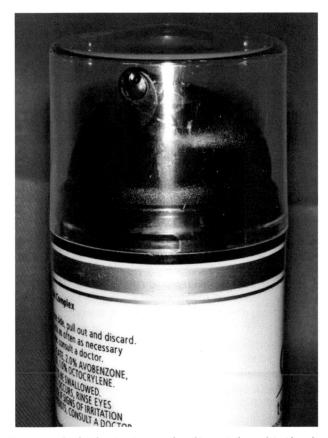

Figure 14.1 This facial moisturizer is packaged in an air-free sack inside a plastic container dispensed through a one-way valve. This prevents oxygen from contacting the moisturizer and aids in product preservation.

found to be the most allergic preservatives in a patch testing study (28).

Parabens are being replaced by Kathon-CG in many cosmetic formulations, but Kathon-CG is a source of allergic contact dermatitis.

Some patients may also develop allergic contact dermatitis or contact urticaria to sorbic acid, but this a less frequently used preservative in cosmetics (29). It is patch tested at a 2% concentration in petrolatum (30).

Preservatives can be difficult to patch test due to their inherent irritancy. Excellent articles discussing patch testing methods and concentrations are available (31). Table 14.4 lists the patch test concentrations of some of the more commonly used preservatives and their typical concentration in cosmetic formulations. It is interesting to note that there is some variability in recommended patch concentrations depending on the reference used (32,33).

COLOR ADDITIVES

The other problematic groups of ingredients from a media standpoint, besides preservatives, are color additives. Color additives are indispensable in colored cosmetics and account for the perceived benefits of other cosmetic preparations. The use of synthetic organic colors for cosmetic purposes has been regulated since 1938 (34) (Fig. 14.2). The coloring agents most frequently used in cosmetics are listed in Table 14.5 (35).

Table 14.4 Patch Test and Use Concentrations

Preservative	Use concentration	Patch test concentration
Quaternium-15 (Dowicil 200)	0.02–0.3%	2% in petrolatum
Formaldehyde	0.05–0.2%	1% aqueous
Parabens	0.1–0.8%	3% in petrolatum if tested individually, otherwise use 12% in petrolatum of paraben mixture[a]
2-Bromo-2-nitropropane-1,3-diol (Bronopol)	0.01–0.1%	0.5% in petrolatum
Methylisothiazolinone and methylchloroisothiazolinone (Kathon CG)	3–15 PPM	100 PPM aqueous
Imidazolidinyl (Germall 115)	0.05–0.5%	1% in petrolatum or aqueous
Diazolidinyl urea (Germall II)	0.1–0.5%	1% aqueous
Dimethylol dimethyl hydantoin (Glydant)	0.15–0.4%	1–3% aqueous

[a]Paraben mixture contains 3% each of methyl-, ethyl-, propyl-, and butyl paraben.

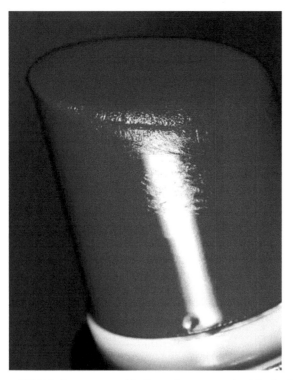

Figure 14.2 Coloring agents used in lip products are regulated by the U.S. government.

There are 116 permitted certified colors available for the cosmetic chemist to combine into three classes:

1. FD&C colorants are permitted for use in food, drugs, and cosmetics.
2. D&C colorants are permitted for use in drugs and cosmetics.

Table 14.5 Frequency of Cosmetic Color Additive Use (in Order of Decreasing Frequency)

Titanium dioxide
Iron oxides
Mica
FD&C Yellow No. 5
Ultramarine blue
FD&C Blue No. 1
D&C Red No. 7 calcium lake
Bismuth oxychloride
FD&C Red No. 4
FD&C Yellow No. 6

3. External D&C colorants are permitted for use in externally applied drugs and cosmetics, but the lips and any body surface area covered by mucous membranes are excluded.

The use of synthetic organic colors for cosmetic purposes has been regulated since 1938.

Color additives can be divided into those that are soluble and insoluble (36). Soluble colors may be soluble in a variety of substances which include water, alcohol, and oil. These colors are almost all synthetic organic dyestuffs that impart color only when in solution. These soluble synthetic dyestuffs can be further divided into acid dyes, mordant dyes, basic dyes, vat dyes, solvent dyes, and xanthene dyes. Acid dyes are used in the dyeing of many items, such as cosmetics, textiles, food, inks, wood stains, and varnishes. The dyestuffs of this category used in cosmetics are FD&C Blue No. 1,2; FD&C Green No. 1,2,3; FD&C Red No. 2,3,4; FD&C Violet No. 1, FD&C Yellow No. 5,6; D&C Blue No. 4; D&C Green No. 5; D&C Orange No. 4,11; D&C Red No. 22,23,28,33; D&C Yellow No.7,10 and Ext. D&C Yellow No. 7. Mordant dyes, basic dyes, and vat dyes are not generally used in cosmetics. Solvent dyes listed for use are D&C Green No. 6; D&C Red No. 17, 37; D&C Violet No. 2 and D&C Yellow No. 11. Xanthene dyes, such as fluorescein, are used in the coloring of lipsticks. Dyes of this group approved for use are the acid forms of D&C Orange No. 5,6,7,10 and D&C Red No. 21,27 and D&C Yellow No. 7. These xanthene dyes are used in their water-soluble form: FD&C Red No. 3; D&C Orange No. 11,12 and D&C Red No. 22,23,28.

Insoluble colors consist of inorganic and organic substances. The organic materials are lakes of soluble dyes and pigments while the inorganic materials are largely oxides and metals. The lakes are soluble dyestuffs that are rendered insoluble by precipitation onto a base. Pigments are usually dyes of the azo type. Oxide pigments that are naturally occurring include iron oxides known as ochre, raw and burnt siennas, red oxides, and raw and burnt umbers. Synthetic oxides and ochres are also available to yield shades of red and yellow. Blues are produced as ultramarines, greens formed from chrome oxide, and Guignet's green while blacks are available as carbon black, vegetable black, bone black, and black oxide of iron. Metallic colors include aluminum powders and bronze powders. This is a quick, but useful, overview of the many colorants use in cosmetics and skin care products.

Other popular colorants that do not fit into the above classification include pearl essences, formed from fish scale or bismuth oxychloride, and manganese violet. Color additives are rarely a cause of dermatitis in cosmetics, but reports of dermatitis to coal tar dyes exist (37). Additionally, the D&C Red dyes have been shown to be comedogenic (38).

BIOLOGIC ADDITIVES

Another controversial area of product formulation is the use of biologic additives, or substances that are animal derived. Some cosmetic companies advertise that none of their products contain animal materials, which may be of more value from a marketing, than formulation, standpoint. Biologic additives are derived from the extracts and hydrolysates of glands and tissues of animals of different species. Animal organ extracts can be formulated as aqueous, hydroglyceric, hydroalcoholic, hydroglycolic, and oily. Examples of biologic additives are collagen, elastin, hyaluronic acid, keratin, placenta, amniotic fluid, pancreas, egg extract, blood derivatives, and extracts of the brain and aorta.

> Biologic additives are derived from animal products.

Topically applied biologic additives, also known as biofactors, are thought by the cosmetic community to function as active ingredients due to the presence of "intrinsic factors" (39). Intrinsic factors are as of yet unidentified chemicals that have physiologic effects on the human body. These animal-derived materials are briefly examined.

Collagen

Collagen is a biologic additive found in moisturizers, hair conditioners, hair shampoos, and nail polishes. It is also available in a form suitable for cutaneous and subcutaneous injection. Collagen is a large molecule composed of three twisted alpha helical peptide chains. It is usually obtained from shredded calf skin that is carefully handled to eliminate denaturation. Injectable collagen is processed to separate the chains through hydrolysis. The nonhelical end of the chains, known as the telopeptide, is also removed since it is responsible for the antigenicity of bovine collagen experienced in humans (39).

Injectable bovine and porcine collagen used to be marketed as a filler substance to cosmetically improve facial depressions due to scarring or wrinkling, but it was recently removed. Topical collagen, on the other hand, can be used in its microfibrillar form for hemostasis or in its hydrolyzed form as a protein humectant in moisturizers. Collagen can absorb up to 30 times its weight in water. Hydrolyzed collagen protein can also be used in hair products, especially instant conditioners, as it can reversibly penetrate chemically treated or damaged hair. Hydrolyzed collagen is still widely used in many modern formulations even though its use decreased during the mad cow scare.

Elastin

Elastin is a structural component of the dermis responsible for the ability of the skin to regain its original configuration following stretching and other deformations. The elastin used topically in cosmetic preparations is obtained from bovine neck ligaments, but most preparations contain some collagen contamination. The elastin is usually added in the form of a hydrolysate consisting of a clear yellow liquid with a pronounced odor. It is added for its ability to function as a humectant; however, collagen has a greater water-binding capacity than elastin.

Hyaluronic Acid

Hyaluronic acid is a component of the dermis that has a great cosmetic potential for water retention. In other words, hyaluronic acid can function as a humectant when topically applied. It also can facilitate penetration of other substances through the stratum corneum since a hydrated epidermis is more permeable. For this reason, hyaluronic acid has been termed a "transdermal delivery system" by some cosmetic manufacturers.

Hyaluronic acid is a glycosaminoglycan as are chitin, chondroitin sulfate, and heparin. It falls into the broad category of mucopolysaccharides which are hexosamine-containing polysaccharides of animal origin occurring in their pure state or as protein salts. Hyaluronic acid is obtained from animal sources such as avian combs, calf connective tissue, umbilical cord, and synovia. The hyaluronic acid that is used as a filler for injection is NASHA, which is human hyaluronic acid manufactured by bacteria to eliminate any animal components. This form of hyaluronic acid is not widely used in topical skin care preparations due to cost.

Keratin

Keratin, a protein component of the stratum corneum, is used in cosmetics as a humectant moisturizer and to deposit a thin film on the hair and nails. It allows longer curl retention in hair-setting products and can minimally penetrate chemically treated or damaged hair to temporarily replace removed hair proteins. Several salon lines use keratin as their major "hero" ingredient for marketing purposes. One line uses heat-denatured human hair keratin for its hair-strengthening products. Keratin is also found in nail polishes to improve nail hardness. Keratin is a scleroprotein and typically obtained from hydrolyzed bovine horn, horse hair, and boar bristles. It is a brown powder that can be readily added to gels, solutions, and emulsions thus facilitating its addition to many cosmetic products.

> Keratin obtained from heated denatured human hair is a high priced cosmetic additive in many hair care products.

Placenta

Placenta, as used in cosmetic preparations, is a complex mixture of proteins and enzymes such as alkaline phosphatase, lactate dehydrogenase, malate dehydrogenase, glutamate oxaloacetate transaminase, and glutamate pyruvate transaminase. The number of substances present within the extract depends upon the care with which the placenta was handled. Human and animal placentas are used as sources. In general, the placenta is frozen, ground, and rinsed with sterile deionized water to remove any blood products. The cells are then lysed. The preparation can be treated further depending on the needs of the cosmetic chemist. In the cosmetic literature, placenta extract is thought to accelerate cellular mitosis, enhance blood circulation, and stimulate cellular metabolism (39). It is used in a variety of cosmetics from facial moisturizing creams to hair conditioners.

Amniotic Fluid

Amniotic fluid is used in cosmetics as a moisturizer and a purported "epidermal growth enhancer." It is found in facial and body moisturizers, bust creams, hair lotions, and scalp treatments. Amniotic fluid is formed by the secretions of the amnion and the vascular transudate. The origin of the fluid used for cosmetic purposes is pregnant cows at three to six months' gestation. The fluid is withdrawn from the amniotic sac through a hollow needle. It is a sterile yellow liquid of pH 7 that can be supplied as a water-soluble additive or a sterile powder. At present, the use of placenta in skin care formulations is minimal.

Egg Extract

The whole egg extract and the egg yolk extract are used in shampoos, face masks, hair conditioners, and moisturizers. Egg extract is obtained from chicken eggs in the form of a hydrolyzed transparent yellow liquid. An extract can also be prepared from the egg yolk alone. This extract is viscous, opalescent, gold liquid containing fats, lecithin, and sterols.

Blood Derivatives

There are several cosmetic extracts obtained from bovine blood: blood extract, serum albumin, fetuin, and fibronectin. Pure bovine blood extract is obtained by treating the blood to remove unwanted substances, histamines, and pyrogens. The remaining product is then dried to yield a water-soluble yellow powder. It is thought that this extract stimulates oxygen absorption and is therefore used in shampoos, conditioners, revitalizing creams, and after shave products.

Bovine serum albumin is the fluid that remains after the fibrin and blood cells have been removed. It is available as a liquid and freeze dried powder. Since bovine serum albumin is used as a growth factor in cultured skin cells, it is thought to increase epidermal cell renewal rate. It is a common additive in creams that "revitalize" the skin.

HERBAL ADDITIVES

Herbal additives are currently more popular than biologic additives as plants are felt to be more "pure" and less problematic, even though many herbals are contaminated with herbicides and heavy metals. The list of cosmetic plant materials is almost endless and can only be appreciated by reading chemical company advertisements in cosmetics and toiletries trade journals. Most cosmetic manufacturers do not formulate their own additives, but rather buy them in bulk from wholesalers. Table 14.6 contains a few of the many herbal additives and their purported benefit (40).

The area of plant additives is made more confusing by the centuries of mystique that have surrounded herbal medicine, still actively practiced, and herbal aestheticians, who are making a resurgence with aromatology and herbology. There is no doubt that many of the plant additives impart a pleasing smell and color to the cosmetic (41). Plant additives can be obtained as hydroglycolic extracts, essential oils, and whole plant extracts (42). Hydroglycolic extracts are a combination of

Table 14.6 Herbal Additives

Plant derivative	Purported function
Allantoin	Anti-irritating
Almond oil	Emollient
Aloe vera	Skin soother, moisturizer
Avocado oil	Skin soother
Camomile (bisabolol)	Skin soother
Camphor	Skin refresher
Cypress	Skin refresher
Elder	Skin toner
Geranium	Skin softener
Hawthorne	Astringent
Hazelnut oil	Emollient
Horse tail	Skin toner
Hypericum	Skin refresher
Jojoba	Humectant, moisturizer
Licorice	Skin soother, softener
Linden flower	Skin soother
Lotus	Skin soother, softener
Marigold	Decrease skin edema
Marjoram	Skin toner
Myrrh	Nail strengthener
Sage	Skin toner
Seaweed	Skin soother
Sesame oil	Emollient
Shea butter	Moisturizer
Wheat germ oil	Emollient
Witch hazel	Astringent

propylene glycol and water, which yield the water-soluble plant constituents, but not the oil-soluble aromatic fragrances. These extracts are formulated into finished cosmetics in a 3–10% concentration. Essential oils, extensively discussed under fragrance chapter, yield the volatile nonaqueous constituents but no tannins, flavonoids, carotenoids, or polysaccharides. These extracts are formulated into cosmetics in a 2–5% concentration. Lastly, whole plant extracts, also known as aromaphytes, are produced by double extraction and contain all the constituents of the plant. They are used at a 5–20% concentration in cosmetic formulations.

Plant additives impart a pleasing smell and color to cosmetics.

Some of the currently popular herbal additives include aloe, avocado oil, sesame oil, and tea tree oil. Aloe is derived as a gelatinous substance squeezed from the leaf of the *Aloe arborescens* Miller (43). It is thought to be of benefit in healing burns and enhancing skin repair, although no published wound-healing studies have confirmed this belief (44). However, it has been shown to induce capillary vasodilation and act as an antimicrobial in concentrations greater than 70% (45). Avocado, sesame, and tea tree oil are used in moisturizers as emollients. But tea tree oil, also known as melaleuca oil, is derived from the *Melaleuca alternifolia* Cheel and thought to be effective in the treatment of furuncles, psoriasis, and fungal infections. These claims have not been proven, but cases of allergic contact dermatitis to d-limonene, a constituent of tea tree oil, have been documented (46).

Table 14.7 Vitamin Additives

Vitamin	Purported function
Beta-carotene	Antioxidant
Biotin	Improve fat metabolism
Panthenol	Hair conditioner
Riboflavin	Maintain healthy skin
Vitamin A	Promote skin elasticity, smoothness
Vitamin C	Antioxidant
Vitamin E	Antioxidant
Vitamin F (essential fatty acids)	Skin nourishing

Other plant additives, such as witch hazel, are well-established astringents while allantoin and alpha-bisabolol, a chamomile extract, have been used for years in cosmetics designed for sensitive skin due to anti-inflammatory properties. There is no doubt that many of the original dermatologic medications had their origin as herbal derivatives.

VITAMIN ADDITIVES
Vitamin additives have become popular due to the recognition that beta-carotene, vitamin C, and vitamin E can act as antioxidants. Table 14.7 summarizes some of the currently used vitamins and their purported cosmetic value.

Further study is required before it can be stated that topical vitamin C, vitamin E, and beta-carotene can function as antioxidants, quenching oxygen radicals that can damage structures within the dermis (47). Nevertheless, some interesting preliminary work has been published in this area. Vitamin C is a hydrophilic substance that can function as an antioxidant, or as an oxidant if combined with iron. It has been shown to protect porcine skin from UVB- and UVA-induced phototoxic reactions when topically applied (48). Thus, it may act as a broad-spectrum photoprotectant by enhancing cutaneous levels of vitamin C (49). Studies have demonstrated the value of alpha-tocopherol, also known as vitamin E, as a lipid-soluble chain-breaking antioxidant in erythrocyte membranes (50). Topically applied alpha-tocopherol has also been shown to inhibit UVB-induced edema and erythema conferring a sun protection factor (SPF) of 3 (51). This is thought to be due to its ability to marginally absorb light and function as a free radical quenching, lipid-soluble antioxidant (52). Carotenoids, of which beta-carotene is an example, have been shown to function as antioxidants in hydrophobic compartments not accessible to tocopherols due to their unique solubility properties (53).

> Vitamin additives are commonly used as topical antioxidants, although their oral efficacy is higher.

LIPOSOMES AND NIOSOMES
Liposomes and niosomes are not individual ingredients, but rather a formulation technique used to deliver materials to the skin. Nanoparticles are another delivery method, but this discussion is found in the sunscreen chapter. Liposomes and niosomes were initially discovered in the 1960s and reported by AD Bangham in 1965 in the Journal of Molecular Biology.

His discovery centered on the observation that phospholipids could be dispersed in an aqueous solution to spontaneously form hollow vesicles, or liposomes, containing the dispersing medium (54). This observation received immediate attention from the pharmaceutical industry who theorized that liposomes could be used as a delivery system for aqueous solutions of active agents. Later, the cosmetics industry adapted the technology for the delivery of nonprescription items to the skin.

> Liposomes are spherical vesicles with diameters between 25 and 5000 nm formed from membranes which consist of a bilayer of amphiphilic molecules space (55).

Amphiphilic refers to the fact that the molecules have both polar and nonpolar ends. Both the polar heads are directed toward the inside of the vesicle and to its outer surface. The nonpolar, or lipophilic tails, are directed toward the middle of the bilayer. This unique structure thus allows the sustained release of water-soluble chemicals from the liposome structure. Liposomes may be one double layered (unilamellar), two to four double layered (oligolamellar), or multilayered (multilamellar) vesicles.

The bilayer that forms the liposome and separates its interior compartment from the external environment is remarkably similar to the cell membrane of mammalian cells. This membrane structure has been highly conserved through evolutionary change. Advocates of liposomes argue that this allows biocompatibility with cells, minimizing adverse reactions (56).

The primary substances used to form liposomes are phospholipids such as phosphatidylcholine. Other minor components may include phosphatidylethanolamine, phosphatidylinositol, and phosphatidic acid. Vegetable phospholipids are also used because of their high concentration of the essential fatty acids, linoleic and linolenic acid. Parameters that influence the function of liposomes in topical preparations include chemical composition, vesicle size, shape, surface charge, lamellarity, and homogeneity. Liposome function is also dependent upon where the active agent is trapped (inside the vesicles, in the membrane, or on the outer surface of the vesicle) and the chemical nature of the active agent (hydrophilic, amphiphilic, or lipophilic).

Niosomes are a specialized form of liposome composed of non-ionic surfactants. Their main components are ethoxylated fatty alcohols and synthetic polyglycerol ethers (polyoxyethylene alkyl ester, polyoxyethylene alkyl ether).

> Niosomes are a specialized form of liposome composed of non-ionic surfactants.

Theoretically, liposomes offer the cosmetic chemist new formulations with new physical properties, a new transport system for active agents and possibly increased efficacy of active agents. Liposomes, however, are somewhat unstable as they are readily deformed and possibly lysed by the weight of a glass cover slip when viewed under the microscope. They are also subject to fusion, aggregation and precipitation. The vesicular structure can be stabilized by cholesterol and incorporation of an ionic charge, but they remain fragile.

The mechanism of action of liposomes and niosomes on the skin remains controversial. Many articles in cosmetic trade publications have tried to use radiolabeled substances and freeze fracture electron microscopy to observe their interaction with the stratum corneum and papillary dermis. It is unlikely that liposomes and niosomes are able to diffuse intact intercellularly across the stratum corneum. The corneocytes are imbedded in lipids, such as ceramides, glycosylceramides, cholesterol, and fatty acids, which are structurally different from the phospholipids and non-ionic surfactants (57). It is possible that they may enter the skin through appendageal structures, but this accounts for only a small proportion of the skin surface area. Thus, absorption through this route is small.

There is evidence, however, that the components of liposomes and niosomes are able to interact with skin lipids, even if they are not in an intact vesicular form (58). They may be able to reduce transepidermal water loss by supplementing missing substances within the skin lipid barrier. Furthermore, liposomes and niosomes can form chemical associations with keratin proteins.

Liposomes can also be incorporated into cosmetics, bath products, moisturizers, and sunscreens. Empty liposomes have possibilities as bath oils, emollients and wound healing aids due to their rich concentration of phospholipids. Loaded liposomes can be devised to release their contents at specific temperatures or specific pH levels, a concept known as "triggering." These liposomes can be loaded with sunscreens to enhance distribution within the stratum corneum or moisturizers to reduce transepidermal water loss. The liposome concentration in such formulations is usually 1% to 10%.

SUMMARY

This chapter has discussed some of the problematic ingredients in cosmetic formulations. Certainly, preservatives and color additives lead the list. Recently, there was some media discussion that lipsticks contained lead and could be a source of lead poisoning. As with all media reports, there is some truth to the concern. Many red lipstick pigments contain very small amounts of lead, but their safety is excellent due to the extremely small amount and the fact that lipstick is not eaten 500 tubes at a time. It must be remembered that no ingredient is 100% safe in all individuals. This realization is important, as the dermatologist must listen carefully to patients who note difficulty with certain ingredients in order to troubleshoot the problem and to arrive at acceptable formulations for patient use.

REFERENCES

1. Kabara JJ. Cosmetic preservation. In: Kabara JJ, ed. Cosmetic and Drug Preservation. New York: Marcel Dekker, Inc, 1984: 3–5.
2. Van Abbe NJ, Spearman RIC, Jarrett A. Pharmaceutical and Cosmetic Products for Topical Administration. London: William Heinemann Medical Books Ltd, 1969: 91–105.
3. Adams RM, Maibach HI. A five-year study of cosmetic reactions. J Am Acad Dermatol 1985; 13: 1062–9.
4. Orth DS. Handbook of Cosmetic Microbiology. New York: Marcel Dekker, Inc., 1993: 75–99.
5. Parsons T. A microbiology primer. Cosmet Toilet 1990; 105: 73–7.
6. Wolven A, Levenstein I. TGA. Cosmet J 1969; 1: 34.
7. Smith WP. Cosmetic preservation: a survey. Cosmet Toilet 1993; 108: 67–75.
8. Wells FV, Lubowe II. Cosmetics and the skin. New York: Reinhold Publishing Corporation, 1964: 586.
9. Bronaugh RL, Maibach HI. Safety evaluation of cosmetic preservatives. In: Kabara JJ, ed. Cosmetic and Drug Preservation. New York: Marcel Dekker, Inc, 1984: 503–27.
10. Eiermann HJ. Cosmetic product preservation: safety and reulatory issues. In: Kabara JJ, ed. Cosmetic and Drug Preservation. New York: Marcel Dekker, Inc, 1984: 559–69.
11. Steinberg DC. Cosmetic preservation: current international trends. Cosmet Toilet 1992: 77–82.
12. Frequency of preservative use in cosmetic formulas as disclosed to the FDA-1990. Cosmet Toilet 1990; 105: 45–7.
13. Kabara JJ. Aroma preservatives: essential oils and fragrances as antimicrobial agents. In: Kabara JJ, ed. Cosmetic and Drug Preservation. New York: Marcel Dekker, Inc, 1984: 237–70.
14. McCarthy TJ. Formulated factors affecting the activity of preservatives. In: Kabara JJ, ed. Cosmetic and Drug Preservation. New York: Marcel Dekker, Inc, 1984: 359–86.
15. Wilkinson JB, Moore RJ. Harry's Cosmeticology. 7th edn. New York: Chemical Publishing, 1982: 673–706.
16. Schorr WF, Mohajerin AH. Paraben sensitivity. Arch Dermatol 1966; 93: 721–3.
17. Fisher AA. The paraben paradoxes. Cutis 1973; 12: 830.
18. Fisher AA. The parabens: paradoxical preservatives. Cutis 1993; 51: 405–6.
19. Hall AL. Cosmetically acceptable phenoxyethanol. In: Kabara JJ, ed. Cosmetic and Drug Preservation. New York: Marcel Dekker, Inc, 1984: 79–107.
20. Rosen WE, Berke PA. Germall 115: a safe and effective preservative. In: Kabara JJ, ed. Cosmetic and Drug Preservation. New York: Marcel Dekker, Inc, 1984: 191–203.
21. Croshaw B, Holland VR. Chemical preservatives: use of Bronopol as a cosmetic preservative. In: Kabara JJ, ed. Cosmetic and Drug Preservation. New York: Marcel Dekker, Inc, 1984: 31–59.
22. Frosch PJ, White IR, Rycroft RJG, et al. Contact allergy to Bronopol. Contact Dermatitis 1990; 22: 24–6.
23. Marouchoc SR. Dowicil 200 preservative. In: Kabara JJ, ed. Cosmetic and Drug Preservation. New York: Marcel Dekker, Inc, 1984: 143–59.
24. Fransway AF. The problem of preservation in the 1990s. Am J Contact Dermatitis 1991; 2: 6–23.
25. DeGroot AC, Weyland JW. Kathon CG: a review. J Am Acad Dermatol 1988; 18: 350–8.
26. Law AB, Moss JN, Lashen ES. Kathon CG: a new single-component, broad-spectrum preservative system for cosmetics and toiletries. In: Kabara JJ, ed. Cosmetic and Drug Preservation. New York: Marcel Dekker, Inc, 1984: 29–141.
27. DeGroot AC, Liem DH, Weyland JW. Kathon CG: cosmetic allergy and patch test sensitization. Contact Dermatitis 1985; 12: 76–80.
28. DeGroot AC, Liem DH, Nater JP, Van Ketel WG. Patch tests with fragrance materials and preservatives. Contact Dermatitis 1985; 12: 87–92.
29. Luck E, Remmert IK. Sorbic acid the preservation of cosmetic products. Cosmet Toilet 1993; 108: 65–70.
30. Marks JG, DeLeo VA. Contact and occupational dermatology. St. Louis: Mosby Yearbook, 1992: 119–20.
31. Andersen KE, Rycroft RJG. Recommended patch test concentrations for preservatives, biocides and antimicrobials. Contact Dermatitis 1991; 25: 1–18.
32. DeGroot AC, Weyland JW, Nater JP. Unwanted effects of cosmetics and drugs used in dermatology, 3rd edn. Amsterdam: Elsevier, 1994: 57–65.
33. Fisher AA. Contact dermatitis. 3rd edn. Philadelphia: Lea & Febiger, 1986: 238–57.
34. Berdick M. Color additives in cosmetics and toiletries. Cutis 1978; 21: 743–7.
35. US Food and Drug Administration: cosmetic color additives: frequency of use. Cosmet Toilet 1989; 104: 39–40.
36. Anstead DF. Cosmetic colours. In: Hibbott HW, ed. Handbook of Cosmetic Science. New York: The Macmillan Company, 1963: 101–18.
37. Sugai T, Takahashi Y, Tagaki T. Pigmented cosmetic dermatitis and coal tar dyes. Contact Dermatitis 1977; 3: 249–56.

38. Fulton JE, Pay SR, Fulton JE. Comedogenicity of current therapeutic products, cosmetics, and ingredients in the rabbit ear. J Am Acad Dermatol 1984; 10: 96–105.

39. Hermitte R. Formulating with selected biological extracts. Cosmet Toilet 1991; 106: 53–60.

40. Dweck AC, Black P. Natural extracts and herbal oils: concentrated benefits for the skin. Cosmet Toilet 1992; 107: 89–98.

41. Purohit P, Kapsner TR. Natural essential oils. Cosmet Toilet 1994; 109: 51–5.

42. Bishop MA. Botanicals in bath care. Cosmet Toilet 1989; 104: 65–9.

43. McKeown E. Aloe vera. Cosmet Toilet 1987; 102: 64–5.

44. Jackson EM. Natural ingredients in cosmetics. Am J Contact Dermatitis 1994; 5: 106–9.

45. Waller T. Aloe vera in personal care products. Cosmet Toilet 1992; 107: 53–4.

46. Knight TE, Hausen BM. Melaleuca oil dermatitis. J Am Acad Dermatol 1994; 30: 423–7.

47. Rieger MM. Oxidative reactions in and on skin: mechanism and prevention. Cosmet Toilet 1993; 108: 43–56.

48. Darr D, Combs S, Dunston S, et al. Topical vitamin C protects porcine skin from ultraviolet radiation-induced damage. Br J Dermatol 1992; 127: 247–53.

49. Rackett SC, Rothe MJ, Grant-Kels JM. Diet and dermatology. J Am Acad Dermatol 1993; 29: 447–61.

50. Burton GW, Joyce A, Ingold KU. Is vitamin E the only lipid-soluble, chain-breaking antioxidant in human blood plasma and erythrocyte membranes? Arch Biochem Biophys 1983; 221: 281–90.

51. Idson B. Vitamins and the skin. Cosmet Toilet 1993; 108: 79–92.

52. Mayer P, Pittermann W, Wallat S. The effects of vitamin E on the skin. Cosmet Toilet 1993; 108: 99–109.

53. Sies H. Oxidative stress: from basic research to clinical applications. Am J Med 1991; 91: 31S–38S.

54. Lautenschlager H. Liposomes in dermatological preparations, Part 1. Cosmet Toilet 1990; 105: 89–96.

55. Junginger HE, Hofland HEJ, Bouwstra JA. Liposomes and niosomes: interactions human skin. Cosmet Toilet 1991; 106: 45–50.

56. Hayward JA. Potential of liposomes in cosmetic science. Cosmet Toilet 1990; 105: 47–54.

57. Elias PM. Structure of function of the stratum corneum permeability barrier. Drug Dev Res 1988; 13: 97.

58. Mahjour M, Mauser B, Rashidbaigi Z, Fawzi MB. Effect on egg yolk lecithins and commercial soybean lecithins on in vitro skin permeation of drugs. J Control Release 1990; 14: 243–52.

SUGGESTED READING

Albrecht J, Begby M. The meaning of "safe and effective". J Am Acad Dermatol 2003; 48: 144–7.

Bergfeld WF, Belsito DV, Marks JG, Andersen FA. Safety of ingredients used in cosmetics. J Am Acad Dermatol 2005; 52: 125–31.

Fox C. Skin and skin care. Cosmet Toilet 2001; 116.

Fox C. Ceramides and other topics. Cosmet Toilet Magazine 2002; 117: 37–42.

Matts PJ, Oblong JE, Bissett DL. A review of the range of effects of niacinamide in human skin. IFSCC Magazine 2002; 5: 2–6.

Rangarajan M, Zatz JL. Effect of Formulation on the topical delivery of alpha-tocopherol. J Cosmet Sci 2003; 54: 161–74.

Facial cosmetic dermatology: Summary

This section of the book discusses color cosmetics and skin care products for the face with special reference to the incorporation of these products into the practice of dermatology. Cosmetics are useful for camouflaging and for presenting a more polished, youthful facial appearance. They can supplement the treatment of facial dermatoses with skin care products that can maintain facial skin health. However, sometimes a patient will present who has undergone a major life change and requests cosmetic assistance to achieve a better self-image. The dermatologist should be prepared to counsel this patient in an organized meaningful manner.

The first step in providing a cosmetic consultation is to identify the area of concern. A hand-held mirror in the hand of the patient is indispensable when asking them to point to the exact features they wish to address. Once the patient has identified the area that has to be improved cosmetically and a realistic goal has been established, the dermatologist can proceed with counseling. The second step is to evaluate whether the defect should be corrected surgically or cosmetically; sometimes a combination of both is optimal. The following discussion will focus on a patient who has completed surgery or needs only cosmetic correction in keeping with the scope of this book.

The third step is to determine whether the defect should be covered or de-emphasized. Discrete defects are generally best covered. A forehead scar can be covered with bangs, a dark congenital nevus on the cheek can be covered with an opaque facial foundation, psoriatic nails can be covered with sculptured nails, ophiasis can be covered with a hair piece, etc. If the defect is not discrete, it may not be possible to cover it appropriately. For example, the appearance of actinically wrinkled facial skin will not improve with use of a thick foundation. On the contrary, the thick foundation will only accentuate the wrinkling. This situation demands that the defect be de-emphasized.

De-emphasizing a defect involves drawing attention away from the negative feature and directing it toward positive features. For example, upper eyelid blepharochalasis cannot be improved by thick application of colored eye shadow. Rather, a patient with intact eyelashes can de-emphasize the blepharochalasis by using fibered lash lengthening mascara followed by curling the thickened, elongated eyelashes. A thin, subdued eye shadow can then be applied to the upper lid. Learning how to de-emphasize negative features is part of the art of using cosmetics.

The fourth step is to encourage the patient to practice and experiment. A proper cosmetic application is not easy. Fortunately, a bad result can be removed in a matter of minutes. Even though the patient may choose not to purchase cosmetic counter products, most clerks are more than happy to assist the patient in the use of sample cosmetics. Some physicians may wish to have sample products in their office for demonstration.

The fifth and final step is to have the patient evaluate the success of the cosmetic result. The patient should check the appearance under the lighting conditions present where the cosmetic will be worn. A patient who works in an office should look at the appearance under bright office lighting, while a cosmetic for evening wear should be evaluated under subdued incandescent lighting. A makeup mirror that simulates various lighting conditions is valuable since color is perceived as reflected light. Subtle changes in lighting may change an attractive cosmetic application into a theatrical result. Patients should be advised that department and drug store lighting is extremely bright and most cosmetics will appear lighter than under natural sunlight. This means that when selecting cosmetics for purchase, a sample should be placed on the skin and then evaluated under natural sunlight.

The physician can optimize patient satisfaction by taking a systematic approach when advising the patient with cosmetic problems. This section on facial cosmetics has provided the background information required to provide an effective cosmetic consultation.

II Cosmetics in dermatology of the body: Introduction

The body encompasses the largest area of skin including the neck, back, chest, arms, and legs. Unique cosmetic products are available for the adornment and treatment of all these body areas to meet the needs of odor management, hair growth, and sebum removal. This customization of products has given rise to a multitude of bottles on the store shelf, yet each must have a need, since products that do not sell are quickly removed. Let us begin our discussion with the neck and move down the body to examine how skin care products can be used in the treatment and maintenance of this large body surface area.

The neck is an interesting area of a highly mobile skin that provides a transition between the thin skin of the face and the thicker skin of the upper chest and back. It contains fully mature hairs in men and thin vellus hairs in women. It is an important area from a cosmetic standpoint since it is an area affected by shaving in men, fragrance application in women, and photodamage in both sexes. Poikiloderma is one of the most common visible cosmetic problems of the neck resulting from photoaging that results in the loss of dermal collagen, visible sebaceous glands, damaged elastin, mottled pigmentation, and telangiectasia. The neck is also the site where women and men apply fragrance, which can be a cause of allergic or irritant contact dermatitis. Finally, the neck in men is a transition area for hair growth between the beard of the face and the body hair of the chest. For this reason, the hair exits the skin in many different directions, which predisposes to inflammation of the hair follicular ostia, more commonly known as razor burn. Severe razor burn accompanied by ingrown hairs in African American men, known as pseudofolliculitis barbae, occurs when the curved hair shafts re-enter the skin causing inflammation and infection. Thus, the neck requires careful cosmetic consideration.

The next area moving down the body is the back and chest. These areas contain the thickest skin of the body required to sustain pulling and twisting movements from arm motion. This thick skin does not heal well and is a common site of unsightly hypertrophic or keloidal scars. In addition, the chest and back have fewer sebaceous glands than the face, yet receive abundant hot water from the shower head, predisposing to eczematous conditions and the need for mild cleansing and superb moisturization.

Tucked away between the chest and the back are the underarms, representing a unique intertriginous body area. Other intertriginous sites on the body that have the same hygiene and skin care needs include the ones beneath the female breasts, between the upper inner thighs, and in persons who are obese, beneath the abdomen. Intertriginous sites are characterized by moisture retention, skin movement, and warmth. This environment is perfect for the growth of fungus, yeast, and bacteria, thus the intertriginous sites are frequent sites of dermatologic disease. These areas combine hair with abundant eccrine and apocrine sweat glands. Eccrine sweat glands produce a clear odorless sweat designed to cool the body and prevent overheating. Apocrine sweat glands do not participate in thermoregulation, but rather produce a yellowish scented sweat that provides a perfect growth media for odor-producing bacteria and yeast. Controlling the sweat prevents body odor, skin barrier damage, infection, and emotionally disturbing wetness. This is the realm of deodorants and antiperspirants. Further, hair removal is challenging in the armpit due the concavity.

Similar challenges for hair removal exist on the arms and legs of both men and women. Shaving these large body surfaces can result in irritation from razor trauma while depilatories and waxing can traumatize the follicular ostia. These areas also receive excess bathing resulting in eczematous disease that can be minimized by proper cleanser selection and the use of moisturizers.

Perhaps one of the most interesting aspects of cosmetics in dermatology is the difference between the skin structure, biochemistry, and functionality of men versus women as it may explain the gender aspects of dermatologic disease. While obvious differences exist between men and women concerning hair growth patterns, the other subtle aspects of skin structure uniqueness may not be so apparent (Table II.1). For example, male skin is more deeply pigmented than female skin, perhaps accounting for the saying that women are the "fairer" of the species. Male skin is also thicker and thus contains more collagen. This may explain why women appear to age more quickly than men, as both genders experience the same rate of collagen loss, but women begin with a lower baseline and loose, proportionately more collagen. Women, on the other hand, possess more subcutaneous fat, which predisposes to cellulite and creates less muscle definition. Gender-specific fat also distributes in different body areas, with men depositing truncal fat while women deposit more gluteal and femoral fat. Men also appear to age more slowly than women, not only due to increased skin thickness but also due to the presence of facial hair. As the collagen is degraded with intrinsic and extrinsic aging, the terminal hair bulbs on the male face take up more of the space preventing the fine cigarette paper wrinkling on female cheeks.

Structural skin differences can be visibly appreciated, but skin biochemical differences are equally important (Table II.2). Male skin secretes more sebum than female skin throughout life. While female sebum production dramatically decreases after menopause, male sebum secretion continues. This reduction is sebum is also accompanied by a reduction in stratum corneum lipids in women, which may be attributed to a reduction in estrogen with advancing age. This sebum reduction may explain why mature men have a higher incidence of seborrheic dermatitis than mature women.

There are also differences in the ability of female versus male fibroblasts to proliferate. Female fibroblasts proliferate at a 16% higher rate than male fibroblasts at age 30. This may

Table II.1 Gender Differences in Skin Structure

Attribute	Female	Male
Skin color	Lighter	Darker
Red skin tones	Lower	Higher
Yellow skin tones	Higher	Lower
Skin thickness	Thinner	Thicker
Amount of collagen	Less	More
Rate of collagen loss	Same	Same
Subcutaneous fat	More	Less
Fat distribution	Gluteal and femoral	Truncal
Cellulite	More	Less
Appearance of aging	Faster	Slower

Table II. 2 Gender Differences in Skin Biochemistry

Attribute	Female	Male
Sebum production	Less	More
Fibroblast proliferation	More	Less
Sweat production	Less	More
Sweat evaporation rate	Higher	Lower
Transcutaneous oxygen level	Higher	Lower
Body skin pH	Higher	Lower
Axilla skin pH	Same	Same

explain why women tend to heal better than men, especially after facial surgery. Another explanation for superior healing may also be the reduced thickness of female facial skin.

While differences exist in skin structure between men and women, there are also differences in the substances that are present on the skin surface. Men tend to sweat more than women, creating an environment more conducive to bacteria growth resulting in odor production. Male sweat also remains on the skin longer. In addition, men possess more body hair, which increases the body surface area for bacterial colonization. This may be due to the increased popularity of antibacterial soaps among men. The presence of sweat may also contribute to differing skin pH measurements between men and women. Women have a higher more alkaline pH, while men have a relatively lower pH, but the pH of the axilla is identical in both sexes.

Finally, women have a higher transcutaneous oxygen level than men. The exact significance of this is not known, but may be explained by the thinner epidermis.

Table III. 3 Gender Differences in Skin Functionality

Attribute	Female	Male
Transepidermal water loss rate	Lower	Higher
Skin blistering times	Longer	Shorter
Skin elasticity	Same	Same
Stratum corneum stiffness	Higher	Lower
Tape stripping removal of stratum corneum	Same	Same
Skin temperature	Cooler	Hotter
Fingertip temperature	28C	33C
Heat-induced vasodilatation temperature	Lower	Higher
Sympathetic tone	Increased	Decreased
Irritant contact dermatitis incidence	Higher	Lower
Facial lactic acid stinging	Higher	Lower
Minimal erythema dose	Higher	Lower

In addition to skin biochemical differences, there are also differences in skin functionality (Table II.3). These functional differences can impact how skin care products perform on the skin and may dictate product formulation specifics. It is interesting to note that transepidermal water loss is lower in women than in men, even though women feel that their skin is drier when polled. Women also generally feel that their skin sags more than that of men, but skin elasticity is identical between the sexes. The increased impression of sagging may be due to thinning collagen rather than decreased skin elasticity.

Female skin is more functionally responsive than male skin. This is manifested by the lower temperature at which heat induces vasodilatation. It also presents as an increase in irritant contact dermatitis and increased sympathetic tone. This may explain why women exhibit increased redness and irritation to skin care products, sometimes referred to as "tender" skin, over men, who are characterized as having "tough" skin.

The differences between male and female skin structure, biochemistry, and functionality and the differences in skin of various body areas of create opportunities for skin care and cosmetic product development. This section of the book will examine products for skin care of the body from moisturizers to cleansers, sunless tanners to sunscreens, and cellulite to stretch mark creams to encompass the entire category of body cosmetics in dermatology.

15 Personal hygiene, cleansers, and xerosis

Optimal personal hygiene has come to mean bathing daily with lots of soap lather and abundant hot water, as hot as the skin can stand. Furthermore, many patients bathe in the morning to "wake up" and bathe in the evening to "go to sleep." Others bathe a third time after finishing a workout at the gym. Certainly, these personal hygiene habits require lots of cleansers and may result in xerosis and ultimately xerotic eczema. Cleansing the body has become an essential part of personal hygiene and the desire to bathe daily has created a demand for cleansing products that simply do not cleanse as well. This chapter examines cleanser formulations for the body and how cleanser selection can aid the patient in maintaining their self-perceived personal hygiene standards without creating dermatologic problems.

CLEANSER TYPES

Selecting a good cleanser can be a challenge for any patient. The shelves are full of body cleansing products in every color of the rainbow, each with a unique skin-enhancing ingredient like vitamin E, shea butter, jojoba oil, emu oil, cleansing cream, lavender, chamomile, ginger, glycerin, panthenol, and collagen. Every scent imaginable can be found including kiwi, pineapple, pear, vanilla, raspberry, apple, lemon, sage, rosemary, and mango to name a few. Every scent can also be found in combination with every other scent to create stores selling nothing but hundreds of cleansers each with a different color and scent combination, but all accomplishing the same end of removing sebum, perspiration, environmental dirt, cosmetics, and medications from the skin surface.

> Selecting the proper cleanser is key to maintaining the skin acid mantle and preserving skin health.

Cleansers come in many different formulations for body cleansing including bars, liquids, and scrubs all trying to achieve the optimal clean and fresh feel. There are foaming and nonfoaming cleansers customized to each and every body area. There are scented and unscented cleansers with some labeled as appropriate for sensitive skin. There are cleansers for women and separate formulations for men. However, in reality, there are some basic categories of cleansers upon which many variations have been manufactured.

> The three basic cleansing types are true soaps, syndets, and combars.

SOAPS

Soap is the most basic of cleansers and has been a cleansing staple for 4000 years, ever since the Hittites of Asia Minor cleaned their hands with the ash of the soapwort plant suspended in water and the Sumerians of Ur produced alkali solutions for washing. Neither of these products, however, is chemically similar to soap as it is known today. The actual modern soap preparation was developed about 600 BC by the Phoenicians who first saponified goat fat, water, and potassium carbonate-rich ash into a solid, waxy product. The popularity of soap has waxed and waned over the years. During the Middle Ages, soap was outlawed by the Christian Church who believed that exposing the flesh, even to bathe, was evil. Later, when the idea of bacteria-induced infection surfaced, the sale of soap soared.

The first widely marketed soap was developed by Harley Procter in 1878, who decided that his father's soap and candle factory should produce a delicately scented, creamy white soap to compete with imported European products. He accomplished this feat with the help of his cousin chemist, James Gamble, who made a richly lathering product called "White Soap." By accident, they discovered that whipping air into the soap solution prior to molding resulted in a floating soap that could not be lost in the bathe (1). This resulted in a product known as "Ivory" soap, still manufactured today.

Soap functions by employing a surfactant to lower the inter-skin tension between the nonpolar soil and the rinsing water, which floats away the dirt in the lather. The manufacturing stages in a typical bar soap are listed in Table 15.1 (2).

In basic chemical terms, soap is a reaction between a fat and an alkali resulting in a fatty acid salt with detergent properties (3). Modern refinements have attempted to adjust its alkaline pH, possibly resulting in less skin irritation (4), and incorporate substances to prevent precipitation of calcium fatty acid salts in hard water, known as "soap scum" (5). Nevertheless, modern soap is basically a blend of tallow and nut oil, or the fatty acids derived from these products, in a ratio of 4:1. Increasing this ratio results in "superfatted" soaps designed to leave an oily film behind on the skin. Bar soaps can be divided into three different cleanser types as listed in Table 15.2.

> Soap is a reaction between a fat and an alkali resulting in a fatty acid salt with detergent properties.

Soap is a common term used by many as synonymous with cleanser. However, soap is a specific cleanser with a definite chemical composition. Soap is defined as a chemical reaction between a fat and an alkali resulting in a fatty acid salt with detergent properties (7). The simplest soaps are manufactured in the bar form. There are currently three different types of bar cleansers on the market, all called "soap" by consumers, but with very different skin effects. There are the true soaps, which are composed of long-chain fatty acid alkali salts, with a pH between 9 and 10 (8). This is the original soap formulation developed that revolutionized health care in the United States. Perhaps soap, more than any other invention, has improved

Table 15.1 Steps in Soap Manufacture

1. Saponification of natural fats and preparation of milling chips
2. Blending of soap chips with other ingredients
3. Milling and shredding
4. Extrusion into long strips, known as billets, and cutting into appropriate lengths
5. Stamping into the final shape
6. Ageing and packaging

Table 15.2 Types of Cleansers

1. True soaps composed of long-chain fatty acid alkali salts, pH 9–10
2. Syndets composed of synthetic detergents and fillers, which contain less than 10% soap, pH adjusted to 5.5–7.0 (6)
3. Combars composed of alkaline soaps to which surface active agents have been added, pH 9–10

the quality of human life by preventing the spread of disease. This is the type of soap that grandma cooked in her backyard from ash and animal fat. The high pH of these cleansers is excellent at thoroughly removing sebum, but can also damage the intercellular lipids in diseased or sensitive skin. This formulation also experiences difficulty when used with hard water. The alkali chemically combines with calcium and other minerals in the water to form what is commonly termed "soap scum." Soap scum decreases the ability of the soap to rinse cleanly from the skin, causing irritant contact dermatitis in susceptible individuals. The only major brand of true soap left on the market today is Ivory soap (Procter & Gamble, Cincinnati, Ohio), as previously mentioned.

SYNDETS
Following the development of true soaps, came the invention of synthetic detergents. Synthetic detergents are known as syndets and contain less than 10% real "soap." Rather than possessing a highly alkaline pH, these products can be made with a pH adjusted to 5.5 to 7. This more neutral pH is similar to the normal acid mantle pH of the skin causing less irritation. The tightness that is experienced following cleansing is actually the perception of altered skin pH. This is not a problem in normal complected individuals, but can be a source of concern in persons with eczema or atopic dermatitis. Unfortunately, many associate the tight feeling with cleanliness and it can be a challenge to convince a patient that the tight feeling is possibly an indicator of impending skin disease. Most syndet cleansers leave the skin with a smooth, sometimes slimy, feel that indicates that the intercellular lipids have not been removed and the skin barrier is intact. Syndet cleansers, sometimes known as beauty bars, are the most popular cleansers in use today. They offer milder, yet thorough, cleansing of all body areas.

Syndets are made from synthetic detergents, most commonly sodium cocoyl isethionate, and provide the most gentle cleansing.

The purpose in developing new synthetic detergents over traditional soaps was to provide a product less irritating to the skin. Commonly used detergents in bar type cleansers are sodium cocoate, sodium tallowate, sodium palm kernelate, sodium stearate, sodium palmitate, triethanolamine stearate, sodium cocoyl isethionate, sodium isethionate, sodium dodecyl bezene sulfonate, and sodium coco glyceryl ether sulfonate. Detergents in liquid formulations are sodium laureth sulfate, cocoamido propyl betaine, lauramide diethanolamine, sodium cocoyl isethionate, and disodium laureth sulfosuccinate. The normal pH of the skin is acidic, between 4.5 and 6.5. Applying alkali soap theoretically raises the pH of the skin allowing it to feel dry and uncomfortable (9). However, healthy skin rapidly regains its acidic pH (10). The effects and measurement of surfactant-induced irritation remains a controversial area under investigation (11).

COMBARS
The third form of cleanser is combination bar (combar). Combars combine true alkaline soaps with syndets to create a bar with greater cleansing abilities, but less intercellular lipid damage (12). The majority of the bars in this category are also known as deodorant bars. They contain triclosan, a commonly used topical antibacterial, to decrease body odor caused by bacteria, especially in the armpits and groin.

Combars contain soap and synthetic detergents to provide moderate cleansing and are most commonly formulated as deodorant soaps with triclosan.

Selecting the proper type of "soap" may be tricky for the physician, but once the three categories of cleansers are identified the task becomes much easier. In general, all beauty bars, mild cleansing bars, and sensitive skin bars are of the syndet variety (Oil of Olay, Dove, and Cetaphil). Most deodorant bars or highly fragranced bars are of the combar variety (Dial, Coast, and Irish Spring), and very few true soaps are currently on the market (Ivory).

CLEANSER ADDITIVES
Special additives added to the previously discussed formulations allow the tremendous variety of soaps marketed today (Table 15.3). Lanolin and paraffin may be added to a moisturizing syndet soap to create a superfatted soap while sucrose and glycerin can be added to create a transparent bar. Adding olive oil instead of another form of fat distinguishes a castile soap. Medicated soaps may contain benzoyl peroxide, sulfur, resorcinol, or salicylic acid. Deodorant bars have an added antibacterial, such as triclocarban or triclosan. Triclocarban is excellent at eradicating gram-positive organisms, but triclosan eliminates both gram-positive and gram-negative bacteria. These soaps have a pH between 9 and 10 and may cause skin irritation. Moisturizing syndet bar soaps contain sodium lauryl isethionate with a pH adjusted to between 5 and 7 by lactic or citric acid. These products are less irritating to the skin and are sometimes labeled beauty bars.

Additives to soap are also responsible for a characteristic appearance, feel, and smell. Titanium dioxide is added in concentrations up to 0.3% to opacify the bar and increase its optical whiteness. Pigments, such as aluminum lakes, can color the bar without producing colored foam, a characteristic

Table 15.3 Specialty Soap Formulations

Type of soap	Unique ingredients
Superfatted soap	Increased oil and fat; fat ratio up to 10%
Castile soap	Olive oil used as main fat
Deodorant soap	Antibacterial agents
French milled soap	Additives to reduce alkalinity
Floating soap	Extra air trapped during mixing process
Oatmeal soap	Ground oatmeal added (coarsely ground to produce abrasive soap, finely ground for gentle cleanser)
Acne soap	Sulfur, resorcinol, benzoyl peroxide, or salicylic acid added
Facial soap	Smaller bar size, no special ingredients
Bath soap	Larger bar size, no special ingredients
Aloe vera soap	Aloe vera added to soap, no special skin benefit
Vitamin E soap	Vitamin E added, no special skin benefit
Cocoa butter soap	Coca butter used as major fat
Nut or fruit oil soap	Nut or fruit oils used as major fat
Transparent soap	Glycerin and sucrose added
Abrasive soap	Pumice, coarse oatmeal, maize meal, ground nut kernels, dried herbs, or flowers added
Soap-free soap	Contains synthetic detergents (syndet bar)

considered undesirable. Foam builders, such as sodium carboxymethyl cellulose and other cellulose derivatives, can make the lather feel creamy. Lastly, perfume in concentrations of 2% or more can be added to ensure that the soap bar retains its scent until completely used (2).

ASSESSING CLEANSER IRRITANCY

Several methods are used to evaluate the effect of various soap and detergent formulations on the skin. One method of measuring the effects of cleansers on the skin is the soap chamber test developed by Frosch and Kligman (13). An 8% soap solution is applied under occlusion to the volar surface of the forearm in human volunteers. The site is evaluated for scaling and erythema several days later (14). This technique has been expanded to include measurements of transepidermal water loss (TEWL). As expected, soaps induce more transepidermal water loss than the synthetic detergents listed previously. A modified chamber test is also used where a 5% solution of the soap or detergent is applied to the forearm and covered with an aluminum chamber for 18 hours. These tests exaggerate the cleanser's contact with the skin, thus an actual use is required. This is accomplished by having human volunteers wash their forearms for two-minute duration four times per day for a week. Visual and transepidermal water loss assessments are used to evaluate the skin effect.

One of the most important aspects of cleanser interaction with the skin is the ability of the cleanser to thoroughly rinse from the skin surface. Excellent rinsing ensures minimal irritation, but the ability of soap to rinse from the skin depends on the mineral content of the water. As mentioned previously, calcium in the water can interact with soap to form a sticky white film that can adhere to the sink, tub, and even the skin. Soap scum has an alkaline pH that breaks down the skin acid mantle

and cause barrier damage. Mild soaps with minimal irritancy must rinse clean from the skin with water to avoid this problem. Thus, tests are commonly performed to assess the rinsability of cleansers under various pH values and water conditions. Most soap manufacturers have a laboratory where they can adjust the pH, hardness, and temperature of the water to simulate washing under various conditions that exist throughout the world. Excellent cleansers with minimal irritancy perform superbly under a wide variety of cleansing environments.

LIPID-FREE LOW FOAMING CLEANSERS

In addition to soaps, syndets, and combars, there is another category of cleanser that produces minimal foam specially designed for persons with limited sebum production. These cleansers are known as lipid-free low-foaming cleansers. Lipid-free cleansers are liquid products that clean without fats, a point which distinguishes them from the cleansers previously discussed. They are applied to dry or moistened skin, rubbed to produce minimal lather, and rinsed or wiped away (Cetaphil cleanser, Aquanil cleanser, and CeraVe cleanser).

Lipid-free low-foaming cleansers may contain water, glycerin, cetyl alcohol, stearyl alcohol, sodium laurel sulfate, and occasionally propylene glycol. They leave behind a thin moisturizing film and can be used effectively in persons with excessively dry, sensitive, or dermatitic skin. They do not have strong antibacterial properties, however, and may not remove odor from the armpits or groin. They also are not good at removing excessive environmental dirt or sebum. Lipid-free cleansers are best used where minimal cleansing is desired, but can be used to remove face and eye cosmetics in persons with sensitive skin.

Lipid-free low-foaming cleansers are excellent for dry, sensitive skin and effective at removing eye cosmetics.

BODY SCRUBS

Another form of body cleansing combines sebum removal with exfoliation, the removal of the desquamating corneocytes. With advancing age, the ability of the corneocytes to slough is decreased. The retained corneocytes give the skin a rough texture and yellowish appearance. Exfoliation removes the corneocytes, smoothes the skin surface, and restores a pinker skin color. Many antiaging cleansers are abrasive scrubs because the exfoliated skin may have a younger appearance. However, an aggressive frequent use of an abrasive scrub can remove too much stratum corneum resulting in sensitive skin and can even provoke eczema.

Body scrubs produce cleansing and exfoliation simultaneously.

Abrasive scrubs use a particulate material rubbed over the skin surface with the hands to mechanically remove the corneocytes. Abrasive scrubs incorporate polyethylene beads, aluminum oxide, ground fruit pits, or sodium tetraborate decahydrate granules to induce various degrees of exfoliation (15). The most abrasive scrub is produced by aluminum oxide particles and ground fruit pits. In general, products containing these rough edged particulates are not appropriate for sensitive skin patients, eczema patients, or atopic dermatitis patients. Polyethylene beads are the most common particle used in body scrubs and produce mild exfoliation without damaging the skin due to the round bead. Recently, concern has arisen about the safety of polyethylene beads in the environment as the beads remain in the water columns for years without degrading. The beads can act as a nidus for the growth of bacteria and may be toxic to some marine life forms. This concern has increased the popularity of dissolving scrubs using sodium tetraborate decahydrate granules.

The main problem with abrasive scrub products for exfoliation is the tendency for overuse by the patient. The harder and longer the patient rubs, the more that the stratum corneum will be removed. Too much stratum corneum abrasion will result in self-induced sensitive skin. One of the best uses of body scrubs is on the anterior shins of patients with ichthyosis vulgaris. The occurrence of ichthyosis vulgaris increases with advancing age due to a desquamatory failure resulting in the appearance of dry skin. Moisturizers can improve the appearance by smoothing down the edges of the desquamating corneocytes, but the effect is cosmetic and temporary. Body scrubs can dislodge the corneocytes revealing the well-hydrated skin beneath. Lactic acid and other hydroxy acid moisturizers have been recommended to chemically exfoliate the skin, but the body scrub is the most efficient way to improve the appearance of ichthyosis vulgaris.

BODY WASHES

A variation on the soap, syndet, and combar detergents discussed earlier is the body wash. Body washes are liquid cleansers with a unique emulsion. The emulsion is characterized as a two-phase liquid with a hydrophobic phase and a hydrophilic phase held together by an emulsifier. The surfactant cleanser is in the hydrophilic phase and binds to the dirt, which is washed down the drain. Vegetable oils, humectants, dimethicone, and petrolatum are in the hydrophobic phase, which bind to the skin surface decreasing transepidermal water loss and providing an environment optimal for barrier repair. This is the mechanism of action body washes claiming to both cleanse and moisturize. These products are of use in atopic patients who either wish to bathe more frequently or those with severe disease.

The key question is how does the body wash know whether to cleanse away sebum or deposit the moisturizer? This is accomplished by varying the water concentration between the two skin care events, one being cleansing and the other being moisturizing. During the first phase of washing, the body wash is placed on a puff, to increase the amount of air and water in the emulsion, followed by rubbing it over the body (Fig. 15.1). At this time, the concentration of water is very low and the concentration of body wash is very high, and cleansing occurs. During the rinse phase, the water concentration is very high and the body wash concentration is very low. It is during the rinse phase that the moisturizing ingredients are deposited on the skin surface.

Body washes are available for extra dry, dry, and normal skin. These products can deposit different amounts of moisturizer based on the construction of the emulsion (Fig. 15.2). Large moisturizing ingredient droplets within the emulsion,

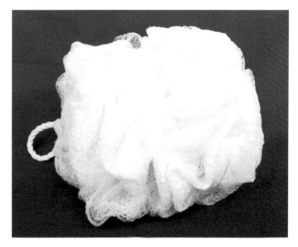

Figure 15.1 An example of a puff that is necessary to introduce air and water into the body wash emulsion.

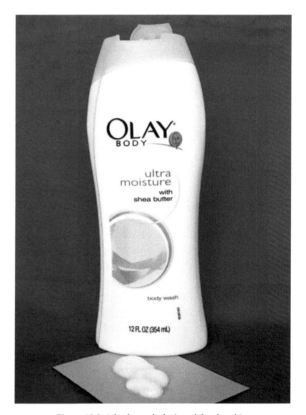

Figure 15.2 A body wash designed for dry skin.

containing petrolatum, soybean oil, and dimethicone, create a high depositing body wash. During the rinse phase, these droplets are left behind on the skin surface. A product for normal skin might be a medium depositing product with smaller droplets leaving behind a lesser amount of moisturizing ingredients. The dry skin body washes are most appropriate for atopic patients because they leave behind a lot of skin protectant ingredients. Thus, the size of the oil droplets in the emulsion determine the amount of moisturizing ingredient left behind on the skin during the rinse phase of body wash use (Fig. 15.3).

It is possible to measure the efficacy of body wash products by examining TEWL measurements in patients with atopic

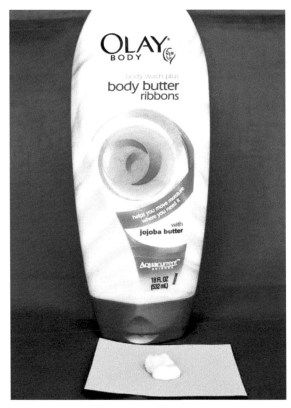

Figure 15.3 An example of a body wash with two phases for extra dry skin.

dermatitis. TEWL measurements are made with an evaporimeter, which consists of two humidity meters placed at a known distance from the skin surface. The distance between the two humidity meters is also known, as well as how much water vapor is going into the probe, allowing the calculation of water loss from the skin surface in terms of grams of water loss per meter square per hour. This water vapor loss is an indirect measurement of the degree of barrier damage, which directly correlates with the skin injury caused by cleansing. Patients with atopic dermatitis have an increased TEWL based on their disease and defective barrier function. The improvement in barrier function following the use of a body wash can be measured by assessing TEWL before and after bathing. Good cleansers for patients with dermatologic disease will not increase TEWL with repeated use.

Body washes can both clean and moisturize the skin on the basis of sophisticated emulsion technology.

MOISTURINSES
A variant of the body wash is known as a moisturinse. Body washes are comparable in formulation to 2-in-1 hair shampoos and moisturinses are comparable to hair conditioners. After the cleansing has occurred with the body wash, a moisturinse can be applied. The moisturinse is nonfoaming and rubbed over the entire body followed by rinsing. It has a very small amount of surfactant and a large amount of dimethicone and other oils. This is in contrast to the body wash that has a large amount of surfactant and a small amount of the skin conditioning agents, dimethicone, and other oils. The moisturinse deposits moisturizing ingredients on the skin during the rinse phase and increases the amount of moisturizer left on the skin during bathing. The goal is to remove sebum, perspiration, and environmental dirt, but replace the lost skin lipids with synthetic and natural oils to decrease the barrier damage.

Moisturinses are of use in patients who insist on bathing frequently despite problems with recurrence eczema. It is possible that the moisturinse will allow daily bathing in some patients assisting in compliance and minimizing the use of prescription medications, such as topical corticosteroids. Moisturinses also can be used as cleanser in atopic dermatitis patients who need minimal cleansing and maximal moisturization.

Moisturinses are similar in formulation to hair conditioners and can leave a thin moisturizing film on dry skin.

REFERENCES
1. Panati C. Extraordinary Origins of Everyday Things. New York: Perennial Library, Harper & Row Publishers, 1987: 217–19.
2. Van Abbe NJ, Spearman RIC, Jarrett A. Pharmaceutical and Cosmetic Products for Topical Administration. London: William Heinemann Medical Books Ltd, 1969: 136–9.
3. Willcox MJ, Crichton WP. The soap market. Cosmet Toilet 1989; 104: 61–3.
4. Wortzman MS. Evaluation of mild skin cleansers. Dermatol Clin 1991; 9: 35–44.
5. Jackson EM. Soap: a complex category of products. Am J Contact Dermatitis 1994; 5: 173–5.
6. Wortzman MS, Scott RA, Wong PS, et al. Soap and detergent bar rinsability. J Soc Cosmet Chem 1986; 37: 89–97.
7. Willcox MJ, Crichton WP. The soap market. Cosmet Toilet 1989; 104: 61–3.
8. Wortzman MS. Evaluation of mild skin cleansers. Dermatol Clin 1991; 9: 35–44.
9. Prottey C, Ferguson T. Factors which determine the skin irritation potential of soap and detergents. J Soc Cosmet Cem 1975; 26: 29.
10. Wickett RR, Trobaugh CM. Personal care products. Cosmet Toilet 1990; 105: 41–6.
11. Wilhelm KP, Freitag G, Wolff HH. Surfactant-induced skin irritation and skin repair. J Am Acad Dermatol 1994; 30: 944–99.
12. Wortzman MS, Scott RA, Wong PS, et al. Soap and detergent bar rinsability. J Soc Cosmet Chem 1986; 37: 89–97.
13. Frosch PJ, Kligman AM. The soap chamber test. A new method for assessing the irritancy of soaps. J Am Acad Dermatol 1979; 1: 35.
14. Frosch PJ. Irritancy of soaps and detergents. In: Frost P, Horwitz SN, eds. Principles of Cosmetics for the Dermtologist. St. Louis: CV Mosby Company, 1982: 5–12.
15. Mills OH, Kligman AM. Evaluation of abrasives in acne therapy. Cutis 1979; 23: 704–5.

SUGGESTED READING
Abbas S, Goldberg JW, Massaro M. Personal cleanser technology and clinical performance. Dermatol Ther 2004; 17(Suppl 1): 35–42.
Ananthapadmanabhan KP, Moore DJ, Subramanyan K, Misra M, Meyer F. Cleansing without compromise: the impact of cleansers on the skin barrier and the technology of mild cleansing. Dermatol Ther 2004; 17 (Suppl 1): 16–25.
Ananthapadmanabhan KP, Subramanyan K, Nole G. Moisturizing cleansers (Chapter 31). In: Loden M, Maibach HI, eds. Dry Skin and Moisturizers: Chemistry and Function, 2nd edn. Taylor & Francis Group, Ltd., 2006: 405–28.

Bikowski J. The use of cleansers as therapeutic concomitants in various dermatologic disorders. Cutis 2001; 68(5 Suppl): 12–19.

Boonchai W, Iamtharachai P. The pH of commonly available soaps, liquid cleansers, detergents, and alcohol gels. Dermatitis 2010; 21: 154–6.

Draelos ZD. Cosmeceuticals off the face in body rejuvenation (Part 7). New York: Springer, 2010: 227–32.

Ertel E. Personal cleansing products: properties and use (Chapter 4). In: Draelos ZD, Thaman LA, eds. Cosmetic Formulation of Skin Care Products. Vol. 30. Taylor & Francis Group, LLC., 2006: 40–8.

Ertel K. Modern skin cleansers. Dermatol Clin 2000; 18: 561–75.

Fox C. Skin cleanser review. Cosmet Toilet Magazine 2001; 116: 61–70.

Friedman M, Wolf R. Chemistry of soups and detergents: various types of commercial products and their ingredients. Clin Dermatol 1996; 14: 7–13.

Ghaim JB, Volz ED. Skin cleansing bars (Chapter 39). In: Paye M, Barel AO, Maibach HI, eds. Handbook of Cosmetic Science and Technology, 2nd edn. Informa Healthcare USA, Inc., 2007: 479–503.

Kanko D, Sakamoto K. Skin cleansing liquids (Chapter 40). In: Paye M, Barel AO, Maibach HI, eds. Handbook of Cosmetic Science and Technology, 2nd edn. Informa Healthcare USA, Inc., 2007: 493–503.

Kersner RS, Froelich CW. Soaps and detergents: understanding their composition and effect. Ostomy Wound Manage 1998; 44(3A Suppl): 62S–9S; discussion 70S.

Kuehl BL, Shear NH. Cutaneous cleansers. Skin Ther Lett 2003; 8: 1–4.

Story DC, Simion FA. Formulation and assessment of moisturizing cleansers (Chapter 26). In: Leyden JJ, Rawlings AV, eds. Skin Moisturization. Vol. 25. Marcel Dekker, Inc., 2002: 585–95.

Subramanyan K. Role of mild cleansing in the management of patient skin. Dermatol Ther 2004; 17(Suppl 1): 26–34.

Suero M, Miller D, Walsh S, Wallo W. Evaluating the effects of a lipid-enriched body cleanser on dry skin. J Am Acad Dermatol 2009; 60(3 Suppl 1): AB87.

Tan L, Nielsen MH, Young DC, Trizna Z. Use of antimicrobial agents in consumer products. Arch Dermatol 2002; 138: 1082–8.

16 Body xerosis and moisturization

The body is particularly prone to xerosis due to aggressive frequent bathing habits and the decrease in sebaceous gland concentration. Current beliefs regarding hygiene have created the need for bathing followed by moisturization, which may seem paradoxical since cleansers remove the intercellular lipids from the body skin that are then temporarily and artificially replaced by moisturizers. Problems arise because cleansers cannot distinguish between sebum, which has to be removed for hygiene reasons, and intercellular lipids, which should not be removed to maintain a healthy skin barrier. The skin barrier is an essential element of health, separating the body from the external world. Without this barrier, human life cannot exist. Protection is necessary from infectious organisms that might enter the body causing a serious disease and possibly death. A means of regulating electrolyte balance, body temperature, and sensation is also part of this barrier. While the barrier is self-maintaining, with replacement on a 14-day cycle, disease states may perturb the barrier delaying repair or altering repair kinetics. This chapter examines body xerosis and the role of moisturizers.

THE BODY SKIN BARRIER

The skin barrier is formed by the protein-rich cells of the stratum corneum with intervening intercellular lipids. In the viable epidermis, the nucleated cells possess tight, gap, and adherens junctions with desmosomes and cytoskeletal elements that contribute to the barrier. Moisturizers attempt to mimic the intercellular lipids that are synthesized in the keratinocytes during epidermal differentiation and then extruded into the extracellular domains. These lipids are composed of ceramides, free fatty acids, and cholesterol, which covalently bind to the cornified envelope proteins. It is changes in these intercellular lipids and alterations in epidermal differentiation that lead to barrier defects and ultimately skin disease.

Moisturizers do not moisturize the body. This is a misnomer. The water that is listed as the first ingredient in body lotions does not increase the water content of the skin, since the skin cannot be moisturized externally unless the ambient humidity exceeds 70%. Most controlled indoor spaces maintain humidity below 30%, meaning that there is continuous water loss to the environment. Only the protein-rich corneocytes and intercellular lipids prevent the entire body from dehydration. Water that is orally consumed or topically sprayed on the body does not increase skin's water content. Moisturizers work by preventing evaporation in the short term and providing an environment for barrier repair in the long term. They are composed of oily substances that lower transepidermal water loss (TEWL), the technical term for skin water evaporation, allowing barrier repair to proceed. Only when the skin barrier is intact is TEWL normalized and healthy skin achieved.

Moisturizers do not moisturize the body. They create an environment for barrier repair.

BODY MOISTURIZER INGREDIENTS

Even though the number of moisturizers available for purchase is astounding, most body moisturizers use the same basic ingredients as the formulation backbone to achieve efficacy. The three main ingredients in most of the modern body moisturizers are petrolatum, dimethicone, and glycerin. These are the substances that provide the barrier repair environment for the healing of body dermatoses that can be characterized by xerosis.

Petrolatum

The most commonly used active agent in skin care products, after water, is petrolatum.

Petrolatum is a semisolid mixture of hydrocarbons obtained through the dewaxing of heavy mineral oils. Pure cosmetic grade petrolatum is practically odorless and tasteless appearing in the U.S. Pharmacopoeia in 1880. It is interesting that it has never been duplicated synthetically.

Petrolatum is the most effective moisturizing ingredient on the market today, reducing TEWL by 99% (1). It functions as an occlusive to create an oily barrier through which water cannot pass. Thus, it maintains cutaneous water content until barrier repair can occur. Petrolatum is able to penetrate into the upper layers of the stratum corneum and aid in the restoration of the barrier, which is initiated through the production of intercellular lipids, such as sphingolipids, free sterols, and free fatty acids (2). Products containing petrolatum increase the rapidity with which these lipids are synthesized.

Petrolatum impacts all phases of skin remoisturization, the first step toward barrier repair and wound healing. Petrolatum allows the water content of the skin to rise by decreasing evaporative losses, which creates the moist environment necessary for fibroblast migration leading to wound healing and eventual barrier restoration. Furthermore, it is hypoallergenic, noncomedogenic, and nonacnegenic.

Petrolatum also decreases the appearance of fine lines on the face and body due to dehydration. It functions to reduce itching and mild pain by creating a protective film over exposed lower epidermal and dermal nerve endings. It acts as an emollient by entering the space between the rough edges of desquamating corneocytes, restoring a smooth skin surface. It can also function as an exfoliant by loosening desquamating corneocytes, which are physically removed as the petrolatum is rubbed into the skin. Petrolatum is also an important component of many other cosmeceutical formulations that contain additional actives.

Petrolatum is the occlusive moisturizing substance most like the intercellular lipids.

Dimethicone

The major drawback with pure petrolatum as a moisturizer is its greasiness, which most patients find unaesthetic. This can be minimized by lowering the petrolatum concentration and adding dimethicone, known as an astringent moisturizer, to improve product aesthetics. Dimethicone is the second most common active agent in moisturizers today because it too is hypoallergenic, noncomedogenic, and nonacnegenic (3). Dimethicone is one of a family of silicones that form the basis of all oil-free moisturizers and facial foundations.

Silicone originates from silica, which is found in sand, quartz, and granite. It derives its properties from the alternating silica and oxygen bonds, known as siloxane bonds, which are exceedingly strong. These strong bonds account for the tremendous thermal and oxidizing stability of silicone. Silicone is resistant to decomposition from ultraviolet radiation, acids, alkalis, ozone, and electrical discharges. The silicone used in topical preparations is an odorless, colorless, nontoxic liquid. It is soluble in aromatic and halocarbon solvents, but poorly soluble in polar and aliphatic solutes. Because silicone is immiscible and insoluble in water, it is used as an active agent in products designed to be water resistant. To date there is no report of toxicity from the use of topical silicone.

Dimethicone cannot replace petrolatum, however, as a moisturizer for decreasing fine facial lines of dehydration or for creating an environment optimal for healing skin (4). While dimethicone is insoluble in water, it is permeable to water vapor. Thus, if the skin barrier is wounded, dimethicone will not reduce transepidermal water loss. However, this water vapor permeability is important in the manufacture of facial foundations and sunscreens, since perspiration must evaporate or the product will contribute to miliaria and leave the skin feeling warm and heavy.

Dimethicone can provide many other skin benefits as an active agent besides moisturization. It can function as an emollient, making the skin smooth and soft to the touch by filling in spaces between the desquamating corneocytes. It can also smooth skin scale from the use of drying acne medications, such as benzoyl peroxide or tretinoin, without creating a greasy shine undesirable in oily-complected patients. Dimethicone also does not easily mix with facial sebum, allowing other ingredients in the formulation to remain in place on the face. This is valuable in sunscreens and facial cosmetics.

Dimethicone is a popular body moisturizer ingredient because it leaves the skin smooth without a greasy feeling.

Glycerin

Glycerin is a commonly used humectant in skin moisturizers. Humectants are substances that attract water from the dermis and viable epidermis into the dehydrated stratum corneum (5). However, if the skin barrier is damaged, the water will immediately evaporate into the lower humidity environment. For this reason, humectants are always combined with occlusive moisturizers that retard water loss, such as the previously discussed petrolatum and dimethicone. Glycerin, petrolatum, and dimethicone form the backbone of most skin care products to which other novel agents are added.

Glycerin offers some unique skin benefits. It is one of the few moisturizers, in addition to petrolatum, that is able form a reservoir effect on the skin. In other words, the effect of glycerin appears to persist long after the glycerin is no longer present. Previously, this effect was thought to be due to glycerin affecting the intercellular lipids. It is now recognized that glycerin is capable of modulating water channels in the skin, known as aquaporins.

Aquaporins are highly conserved water channels present in plants, bacteria, and human skin composed of integral membrane proteins from a larger family of major intrinsic proteins (6). The 2003 Nobel Prize in Chemistry was awarded to Peter Agre and Roderick MacKinnon for their research on aquaporins and ion channels. These channels conduct water in and out of the cell while preventing the passage of ions and some solutes. They are composed of a six transmembrane alpha helical structures arranged in a right-handed bundle. Aquaporins form tetramers in the cell membrane and control the transport of water as well as glycerin, carbon dioxide, ammonia, and urea. Different aquaporins contain different peptide sequences controlling the size of the molecules that are able to pass; however, aquaporins are impermeable to charged molecules, such as protons. Typically, molecules can only pass a single file through the channel.

The primary aquaporin in the epidermis is aquaporin-3. It is found in the basal and suprabasal layers of the epidermis, but not in the stratum corneum. Aquaporin-3 expression is also increased in human skin diseases with elevated transepidermal water loss. Thus, glycerin is being rediscovered as a moisturizing ingredient with the potential to dramatically affect skin water balance. Since facial lines of dehydration are the easiest sign of aging to rapidly correct, skin care products based on glycerin, petrolatum, and dimethicone are commonly used to rapidly hydrate the skin and improve appearance. However, petrolatum, dimethicone, and glycerin are also present in the vehicle of most facial skin care creams and lotions. The vehicle not only is responsible for improving skin condition but also delivers other active agents to the skin surface.

Glycerin is a time-tested body moisturizer that modulates cell osmotic balance through aquaporin channels.

SPECIALTY MOISTURIZING INGREDIENTS

Many substances can be added to moisturizers to enhance their marketing claims and possibly their efficacy, which can be characterized as specialty moisturizing ingredients. These ingredients provide for a tremendous variety of body moisturizers available for consumer purchase. This section evaluates the scientific data published regarding the utility of the most popular moisturizer specialty additives.

Ceramides

Ceramides are an important component of the intercellular lipids. The initiating step in barrier repair is ceramide synthesis. Many body moisturizers contain ceramides as a specialty ingredient theorizing that externally applied ceramides may somehow facilitate barrier repair. There are nine different ceramides that have been identified and three are synthetically available to the cosmetic chemist. Ceramides are oily substances and it is unclear whether their efficacy is derived from their incorporation into the intercellular lipids or their effect as an occlusive moisturizer. The location of ceramides in the skin has been studied through tape stripping where the corneocytes are removed layer by layer with an adhesive tape for 20 tape strippings. My research has shown that externally applied ceramides can be retrieved in the first 5 to 8 corneocyte layers.

One commercially available body lotion formulation combines ceramides in a multivesicular emulsion, also known as an MVE (Fig. 16.1). MVEs are physically constructed by rapid stirring to create a moisturizing entity known as a liposome. Liposomes are discussed more fully under the chapter on facial moisturization, but are briefly spheres composed of phospholipids containing moisturizing ingredients in their interior. MVEs are a liposome within a liposome within a liposome. The multiple vesicles can time-release moisturizing ingredients onto the skin surface, one layer at a time to create a physical sustained delivery system for moisturizers. MVEs are manufactured using a cationic quaternary amine salt emulsifier, such as behentrimonium methosulfate. The active agents, such as ceramides which may be combined with other moisturizing ingredients (hyaluronic acid, phospholipids, and dimethicone) are mixed into either the oil or water phase, depending on the compatibility. High-shear mixing of the active agents with the emulsifier produces an MVE.

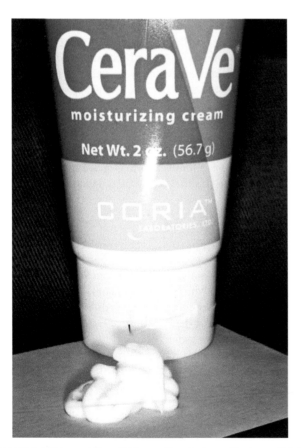

Figure 16.1 A commercially available over-the-counter moisturizer containing ceramides.

Behentrimonium methosulfate is the unique emulsifier allowing formation of the multilamellar concentric spheres of oil and water that trap the active agents in either the alternating lamellar lipid layers or within the aqueous sphere compartment.

Ceramides are found along with petrolatum, dimethicone, and glycerin in many higher priced body moisturizers in the mass and prestige markets. As more of the naturally produced ceramides are available synthetically, more ceramide containing products will appear in the marketplace. Most newly synthesized moisturizing ingredients are first used in department store and spa moisturizers that sell for a premium price. As the novelty of the ingredient wears off and manufacturing costs drop, new moisturizing ingredients find their way into products sold at department stores and boutiques. Finally, when the ingredient can be synthesized in mass quantities, it can be found in drug store and mass merchandiser lines. This is the natural history of most cosmetic ingredients, which are affected by fashion trends and marketing efforts.

> Synthetic ceramides are found in body moisturizers with the intent to stimulate barrier repair by providing a substance found in the intercellular lipids.

Essential Fatty Acids

In addition to ceramides, another component of the intercellular lipids is essential fatty acids, such as unsaturated linoleic and linolenic acid. In the body moisturizing vernacular, these fatty acids are sometimes referred to as vitamin F. The rationale for topical application is to supplement the skin with fatty acids to drive production of the intercellular lipids, though this fact has never been proven. It is known that fatty-acid-deficient rodents present with skin that resembles xerotic eczema. The topical application of sunflower oil, a rich source of essential fatty acids, on these rodents normalizes the condition (7). It is rare to find fatty-acid-deficient humans and it is uncertain whether increased fatty acids make for improved skin. Much of the problem with the topical supplementation in body moisturizers is the questionable penetration of the ingredient into the skin and its ability to improve "normal" skin beyond its healthy state.

Vitamins

Vitamins are also a common body moisturizer additive. Their popularity is due to their safety, low cost, and consumer popularity. It seems natural that you should be able to "feed" the skin from the outside. Most consumers understand the need to "eat a healthy diet for healthy skin" so it seems a natural extension that topical vitamins might also be beneficial. Pantothenic acid or vitamin B complex is commonly used in many chemical forms: panthenol, pantethine, or pangamic acid. Many body moisturizers contain bee pollen and jelly, naturally high sources of vitamin B that have a "natural" appeal. Panthenol, also known as vitamin B5, is the most commonly used synthetic form of vitamin B and functions as a humectant to draw water from the dermis and viable epidermis to the stratum corneum. The water must of course be trapped in the skin with either an intact skin barrier or occlusive agents, such as petrolatum or dimethicone, as previously discussed.

Niacinamide, also known as the amide form of vitamin B3, is found in body moisturizers for its purported ability to increase cell turnover and lighten skin pigmentation by interfering with melanin transfer. Since niacin is part of the nicotinamide adenine dinucleotide phosphate (NADP) and NADPH energy production pathway in the mitochondria, some believe that niacinamide can make older skin cells behave more youthfully. These are very ingenious consumer appealing concepts, but cosmetic companies can only make appearance claims, such as niacinamide "improves the appearance of aging skin." This claim does not imply functionality. If niacinamide were claimed to decrease skin pigmentation, it would be considered a drug not allowed in the cosmetic market. It is this approach to cosmetic development that has limited the ability of manufacturers to more scientifically validate their claims.

Perhaps the most popular vitamin in a body moisturizer is vitamin E. Vitamin E is a fat-soluble antioxidant vitamin that is easily mixed with the occlusive lipids to retard TEWL in body moisturizers. It is inexpensive and widely available. In actuality, vitamin E functions as an emollient to smooth down the desquamating corneocytes making the skin feel smooth and soft. Vitamin E is also said to enhance percutaneous absorption of other oil-soluble substances. Sometimes body moisturizers will contain a cocktail of fat-soluble vitamins including vitamins E, A, and D which are added, but the usefulness of topical vitamins is dubious. Vitamins must be in a water-soluble form to have any chance of penetrating the stratum corneum, and thus oil-soluble preparations are of little value (8). Oral administration of vitamins is far superior to cutaneous administration for the treatment of vitamin deficiencies. It is thought, however, that some vitamins can act as humectants thus enhancing the efficacy of the moisturizing product.

Vitamin E is the most commonly used vitamin in body moisturizers because it functions as an emollient to make the skin smooth and soft.

Natural Moisturizing Factor
A group of substances reported to regulate the moisture content of the stratum corneum is known collectively as the natural moisturizing factor (NMF). The NMF consists of a mixture of amino acids, derivatives of amino acids, and salts. More specifically it contains amino acids, pyrrolidone carboxylic acid, lactate, urea, ammonia, uric acid, glucosamine, creatinine, citrate, sodium, potassium, calcium, magnesium, phosphate, chlorine, sugar, organic acids, and peptides (9). Ten percent of the dry weight of the stratum corneum cells is composed of NMF. Skin that cannot produce NMF is dry and cracked (10). More recently, it has been discovered that fillaggrin breaks down to become the NMF of the skin. It is theorized that abnormalities in fillaggrin breakdown may account for the dry skin associated with atopic dermatitis.

A synthetic NMF has been created for use in body moisturizer formulations.

Sodium PCA
Sodium PCA is a sodium salt of 2-pyrrolidone-5-carboxylic acid and has been termed one of the NMFs, along with urea and lactic acid. Experimentally, it has been shown to be a better moisturizer than glycerol (11). Sodium PCA is used as a humectant in many cosmetics in concentrations of 2% or greater. It can prevent a body lotion from desiccating on the store shelf, but also draw water to the stratum corneum. Many of the spray body moisturizers contain water and sodium PCA. It is best to use a body moisturizer that contains both humectants, such as sodium PCA, and occlusive substances, such as petrolatum, mineral oil, or dimethicone. The more mechanisms of moisturization that are employed, the more successful the body moisturizer will be in promoting an environment for barrier repair.

Urea
Another way to increase water in the stratum corneum is to use a substance that can create water binding sites on the protein-rich desquamating corneocytes. Urea is such a substance. It digests keratin and allows water to bind, thus hydrating and softening the rigid corneocyte protein shells. It is for this reason that urea is commonly used in dermatology for the treatment of calluses and cracked heels. Only when the skin is hydrated can the enzymes that promote desquamation function. Thus, urea diffuses into the outer layers of the stratum corneum and disrupts hydrogen bonding, which exposes the water-binding sites on the corneocytes. Urea also promotes desquamation by dissolving the intercellular cementing substance between the corneocytes. In this manner, it can also promote the absorption of other topically applied drugs, functioning as a penetration enhancer (12). However, urea is a challenge to formulate, since it must be kept at an acidic pH in formulation or it will decompose to the malodorous ammonia. Problems with irritancy have been somewhat overcome by adsorbing the urea onto talc prior to dispersion into the emulsion. Urea is an important therapeutic ingredient in many body moisturizers.

Urea functions as a humectant to increase water binding sites on corneocytes that are not desquamating properly.

Lactic Acid
Lactic acid, or sodium lactate, is also considered a NMF in that it enhances water uptake better than glycerin. It is found in many therapeutic moisturizers as it can increase the water-binding capacity of the stratum corneum. Additionally, it can increase stratum corneum pliability in direct proportion to the amount of lactic acid that is absorbed (13). Lactic acid, in the form of ammonium lactate, is found in many body moisturizers recommended for improvement in the feel of keratosis pilaris, a condition where there is retained stratum corneum around the hair as it exits the follicular ostia. Lactic acid is a hydroxy acid and can also enhance desquamation in mature individuals, thus providing treatment for ichthyosis vulgaris when placed in a body moisturizer. Many a time urea and lactic acid have been combined for optimal therapeutic benefit in body moisturizers designed to encourage desquamation.

BODY MOISTURIZER FORMULATIONS

Body moisturizers come in a variety of preparations including lotion, cream, mousse, and ointment. Lotions are the most popular formulation because they are easy to spread, but lotions typically contain more water and offer less moisturization. Creams and ointments can be used on the body, but are more difficult to spread, especially in hair-bearing areas. Female patients desire a nongreasy body lotion with a rich texture; however, a rich texture does not necessarily identify a superior moisturizer. Richness can be added to a thin lotion with water-soluble gums that impart a silky feel to the skin but do not provide improved moisture retention. Patients should be careful not to equate body moisturizer viscosity with efficacy.

Body lotions are generally oil-in-water emulsions containing 10–15% oil phase, 5–10% humectant, and 75–85% water phase. More specifically, they are composed of water, mineral oil, propylene glycol, stearic acid, and petrolatum or lanolin. Most also contain an emulsifier such as triethanolamine stearate. Humectants such as glycerin or sorbitol may also be used along with other vitamin additives, such as vitamins A, D, and E, and soothing agents, such as aloe and allantoin that are anti-inflammatories. Most body lotions contain some "hero" ingredient or a patented combination of ingredients to allow for expanded consumer claims and distinction in the marketplace.

> Body lotions are generally oil-in-water emulsions containing 10–15% oil phase, 5–10% humectant, and 75–85% water phase.

The basic recipe for a body moisturizer is water, lipids, emulsifiers, preservatives, fragrance, color, and specialty additives. Interestingly enough, water accounts for 60–80% of any moisturizer, however, externally applied water does not remoisturize the skin. In fact, the rate of water passage through the skin increases with increased hydration (14). The water functions as a diluent and evaporates leaving the active agents behind. Emulsifiers are generally soaps in concentrations of 0.5% or less and function to keep the water and lipids in one continuous phase. Parabens, the most commonly used preservatives in moisturizers, are combined with one of the formaldehyde donor preservatives to prevent bacteria from growing in the water phase of the body moisturizer (15). All body lotions must contain some type of a preservative to prevent contamination. The idea of a preservative-free body lotion is an illusion.

A marketable body moisturizer formulation must fulfill three criteria: it must increase the water content of the skin (moisturization), it must make the skin feel smooth and soft (emollience), and it must protect injured or exposed skin from harmful or annoying stimuli (skin protectant). The formulation designed by the cosmetic chemist must fulfill these three needs to be successful in producing skin appearance improvement. The dermatologist should keep these concepts in mind when assessing body moisturizer efficacy.

> The basic recipe for a body moisturizer comprises water, lipids, emulsifiers, preservatives, fragrance, color, and specialty additives.

PRESCRIPTION BODY MOISTURIZERS

The prior discussion has focused on body moisturizers in the over-the-counter (OTC) realm. However, the invention of prescription body moisturizers, known as barrier creams, has changed the moisturizer category. Recently, moisturizers have been developed and approved as medical devices by the U.S. Food and Drug Administration (FDA) through the 510K approval route, which requires the demonstration of safety, but does not require the rigid clinical testing required for pharmaceuticals. The use of occlusive, humectant, and anti-inflammatory ingredients in 510K barrier devices provides an alternative to the more traditional topical corticosteroids used in dermatologic therapy. The barrier repair creams can be used as steroid-sparing aids or to maintain barrier health once the prescription drugs have been discontinued. The main question is whether these more expensive 510K barrier devices provide anything that is currently not available in the OTC body moisturizing market. All of the ingredients that are used in the device creams are found in cosmetic formulations. These barrier devices are not drugs; they are simply devices that must be obtained with a prescription.

Prescription barrier repair moisturizers possess many of the same ingredients found in the OTC body moisturizing market, yet these creams are different because the FDA has approved them as a 510K device. The 510K device approval process was originally developed to ensure the safety of equipment with an on/off switch. Lasers, light devices, cardiac pacemakers, and insulin pumps represent equipment requiring this type of approval. While creams are not traditionally thought of as "devices," they received approval because they induce a physical change in the skin. This physical change was documented as an increase in skin hydration resulting from a decrease in water loss to the environment, known as TEWL.

> Prescription moisturizers, known as barrier creams, are 510K-approved medical devices that function to decrease TEWL.

Barrier repair products place a water impervious film over the skin surface, which decreases TEWL. TEWL is elevated when the skin barrier is damaged, representing the physiologic signal for barrier repair initiated by ceramide synthesis. There are a variety of different formulations that presently have 510K approval producing barrier repair by different mechanisms based on a key ingredient. The key ingredients in the prescription moisturizers are all available in the OTC body moisturizer market; however, their value in barrier repair is discussed.

THE SKIN BARRIER AND CERAMIDE REPLACEMENT

As mentioned previously, ceramide synthesis is the first step in barrier repair. This recognition has led to a variety of OTC creams based on ceramide technology (CeraVe, Valeant; Curel, Kao Corporation). Nine different ceramides have been identified and synthetically duplicated for inclusion in moisturizer formulations (16). The ceramides are distinguished by their polar head group architecture, as well as by their hydrocarbon chain properties (17). A ceramide-dominant, triple-lipid barrier repair formulation (EpiCeram,

Promius Pharma) was designed to correct the lipid-biochemical abnormalities in atopic dermatitis. It contains capric acid, cholesterol, and conjugated linolenic acid. In addition candelilla in the past and petrolatum are included to decrease TEWL. It received FDA approval in April 2006 for use as a nonsteriodal lipid barrier emulsion to manage the symptoms of dry skin associated with a variety of dermatologic diseases (18). It was compared with fluticasone cream in 121 patients with moderate to severe atopic dermatitis for 28 days. The researchers found that the ceramide device reduced SCORAD (SCORing Atopic Dermatitis) scores, decreased pruritus, and improved sleep habits; however, a faster improvement was seen with the topical corticosteroid at day 14 (19). The unique aspect of this cream is that the patented ratio of the triple lipid combination mimics that of physiologic lipids.

OTC ceramide formulations contain similar ceramides to prescription formulations, but do not utilize the patented ratio. To do so, they would have to purchase a license for use of the patent from the inventor. It is unknown how important the ratio is versus the presence of ceramides. While it is possible to demonstrate penetration of ceramides into the stratum corneum by analyzing the tape stripping of the skin following application, it is hard to know exactly how these externally applied ceramides affect skin physiology. Since the skin heals itself eventually, with or without the external application of moisturizers, it is difficult to study the subtleties of moisturizer that expedited healing. OTC moisturizers cannot make the same claims as barrier repair device moisturizers, but their ingredient disclosure and effect on the skin are similar.

NATURAL HYALURONIC ACID HUMECTANCY AND BARRIER REPAIR

Maintaining proper water balance in the skin is key to human life for surviving in a hostile environment. The skin must have some capacity to hold water or desiccation would occur immediately. The natural water-holding material in the dermis is primarily hyaluronic acid, which is the same material used for injection as a cosmetic filler (Juvaderm, Allergan; Restylane, Medicis). These injectable hyaluronic acids are approved as devices and so are some prescription moisturizers based on hyaluronic acid. Topically, hyaluronic acid is known as a humectant, which is the technical name for substances that attract and hold water. Prescription hyaluronic acid moisturizers are available as high concentration foams combined with glycerin, dimethicone, and petrolatum (Hylatopic, Onset Therapeutics) and liquids in combination with glycerol and sorbitol (Bionect, JSJ Pharmaceuticals).

Does the inclusion of hyaluronic acid make a product a prescription? Not necessarily. Several high-end OTC cosmetic moisturizers contain hyaluronic acid. Is hyaluronic acid the only humectant in the marketplace? No. Glycerin, proteins, vitamins, propylene glycol, and polyethylene glycol are more commonly used, less expensive humectants. Humectant ingredients are included in all highly effective OTC moisturizers. The difference is that prescription moisturizers have submitted a 510K application based on the humectancy of hyaluronic acid while the OTC moisturizers have not.

FATTY ACIDS, LIPID TRILAYERS, AND BARRIER REPAIR

A different approach to skin moisturization is the use of free fatty acids. Free fatty acids are found in the intercellular lipids that reside between corneocytes to create a waterproof, moderately impermeable barrier. Scanning electron micrographs show the intercellular lipid bands as trilayer entities with a dimension of 3.3 nm. These bands usually occur in groups of 6 or 9 and are again essential for human life. It is estimated that the lipid layer has a total thickness of 13 nm and accounts for the inability of particles larger than 13 nm to penetrate the skin. Indeed, nanoparticles smaller than 13 nm can penetrate causing the health concerns currently debated.

It is theorized that supplementing the skin with free fatty acids can lead to barrier repair. One such 510K-approved barrier cream contains palmitamide monoethanolamine (PEA) and olive oil, glycerin, and vegetable oil (Mimyx, Stiefel a GSK Company). PEA is a fatty acid that is said to be deficient in atopic skin and it is theorized that replacing this fatty acid can hasten disease resolution (20). It is also thought that PEA, an analogue of cannabis, the active agent in marijuana, may also affect the itch pathways.

In an open label study of 2456 patients, the intensity of erythema, pruritus, excoriation, scaling, lichenification, and dryness were significantly reduced with a combined score reduction of 58.6% when subjects applied the PEA-based barrier cream (21). However, there was no placebo in this uncontrolled prospective cohort study. This always presents challenges in data interpretation. Is it the olive oil and glycerin that are the active agents or the PEA? Olive oil has been touted to have many healing properties in the homeopathic literature. It is rich in essential fatty acids, perhaps accounting for its reputation as healthy heart cooking oil, which have also been shown to reduce signs of atopic dermatitis when topically applied to rodents. Certainly, animals that feed essential fatty-acid-deficient diets experience a skin condition similar to atopic dermatitis, but oral consumption is preferable to topical application. Olive oil is also on the list of facial comedogens, being the culprit in pomade acne. While the final formulation has unique effects, it can be difficult to determine which ingredient really works. This is easy to do with prescription dermatologics where the main drug is identified, followed by the other inactive constituents. This type of disclosure is not required of prescription device barrier creams.

BARRIER REPAIR WITH ANTI-INFLAMMATORY AGENTS

One of the earliest signs of barrier damage is the onset of inflammation, accounting for the redness and itching characteristic of dermatoses manifesting barrier issues. To alleviate symptoms, many barrier repair products incorporate anti-inflammatory agents derived from botanical sources. These anti-inflammatory agents are found in both OTC and prescription moisturizers. One currently marketed prescription barrier cream contains glycyrrhetinic acid and *Vitis vinifera* extracts (Atopiclair, Graceway). In addition, it contains allantoin, alpha-bisabolol, hyaluronic acid, and shea butter. Glycyrrhetinic acid is a licorice extract that was reported to be safe by the Cosmetic Ingredient Review. It has the ability to block gap junction intracellular communication; however, it is cytotoxic at high concentrations. It is mainly used in moisturizer formulations as an anti-inflammatory agent (22). In an open label multicenter study, the product was shown to reduce the median visual analogue scale (VAS) rating for itching in atopic dermatitis from 48.5 mm to 34.1 mm after three weeks of treatment with a further reduction to 24.6 mm after six weeks of treatment (23). In a second study of 142 pediatric patients at ages 6 months to 12 years, the same formulation was compared to a vehicle cream and found to be statistically more effective in reducing the symptoms of mild to moderate atopic dermatitis (24).

Licorice derivatives are also found in OTC moisturizers, especially those targeted for redness reduction in rosacea patients (Eucerin, Beiersdorf). One formulation contains an extract of *Glycyrrhiza inflata*. There are many different species of licorice extracts, not all of which possess the same cutaneous effects. Some licorice extracts are used for skin-lightening purposes and not primarily as anti-inflammatories. Again, is the licorice extract anti-inflammatory the active agent in the barrier repair cream? Does it function like a naturally occurring topical corticosteroid to reduce the signs and symptoms of atopic dermatitis? Or, is it the hyaluronic acid humectant that is attracting water, which is trapped in the skin by the shea butter occlusive moisturizer? In reality, it may be hard to tell what is really working unless each of the "active agents" is tested separately in the same vehicle. Even then, it may be hard to separate the vehicle arm from the vehicle plus single ingredient arms. This is the challenge in designing clinical studies to validate the efficacy of barrier creams.

> Licorice extract is a popular anti-inflammatory agent in OTC and prescription body moisturizers.

BODY MOISTURIZER EFFICACY

The efficacy of moisturizers can be difficult to assess, but all formulations should be clinically tested for both efficacy and tolerability. The major part of this assessment involves the trained eye and hands of the investigator to assess skin barrier improvement and better tactile qualities. Subjective assessments from the study participants can be used to evaluate the alleviation of noxious sensory stimuli, such as itching, stinging, burning, and tingling. Yet, this objective and subjective data requires the addition of instrumentation to assess the functioning of the skin in real time. A good body moisturizer should yield excellent results with all three assessment methods. The use of instrumentation to study the skin uses probes that noninvasively assessed water leaving the skin and water in the skin. Several methods are commonly used including regression analysis, profilometry, squametry, twistometry, corneometry, and evaporimetry (25).

Regression analysis is a method of evaluating the moisturizer efficacy under clinical conditions. Here patients are selected and treated by an objective observer with moisturizers applied at a predetermined test site for two weeks. The test site is evaluated on days 7 and 14. If an improvement is noted, the moisturizer application is discontinued and the test site is evaluated daily for two weeks, or until the baseline pathology has reappeared (26). This method is particularly valuable since the efficacy of all moisturizers is excellent immediately following application, but the true effectiveness can only be assessed with the passage of time (27).

Profilometry involves an analysis of silicone rubber (Silflo) replicas of the skin surface. These silicone replicas are then cast into plastic positives, which are then measured with a computerized stylus instrument that provides a contour tracing of the surface. Thus, a two- or three-dimensional topogram is created. Unfortunately, this method can be inaccurate since the silicone application to the skin surface tends to flatten and disturb the desquamating skin scale (28). This method is best to assess the skin around the eyes for improvement in wrinkles of dehydration.

Squametry involves an analysis of skin squames harvested by pressing a sticky tape against the skin known as a D-squame. The outermost, loosely adherent skin scale is then removed. The tape provides a specimen that retains the topographical relationships of the skin surface and the pattern of desquamation. Image processing is then used to evaluate the scaliness of the skin (29). This evaluation is helpful in assessing the amount of exfoliation induced by a body moisturizer. The skin scale can also be removed from the tape and various lipid fractions are extracted to determine the composition of the intercellular lipids and the presence of various body moisturizer ingredients in the skin scale. Thus, squametry can be used to assess the extent of moisturizer penetration in a noninvasive manner without skin biopsy.

Several other noninvasive skin assessment methods deserve a quick mention including twistometry, corneometry, and evaporimetry. The twistometer uses torsion to measure in vivo the influence of stratum corneum hydration on skin extensibility. A weak torque is applied to a rotating disk that is placed in contact with the skin. It has been shown that dry skin is much less extensible than well-hydrated skin (30). Skin impedance can also be evaluated through a method known as corneometry. Here a dry electrode consisting of two concentric brass cylinders separated by a phenolic insulator operating at 3.5 MHz is applied to the skin (31). The impedance drops as the skin is better hydrated. This technique can evaluate the efficacy and the duration of effect of moisturizers by measuring the amount of water in the skin with a device known as a corneometer (32). Lastly, evaporimetry can be used to measure the cutaneous TEWL (33). More occlusive substances would be expected to lower water loss while some humectants, such as glycerin, actually increase water loss (34,35). Evaporimetry measures the water leaving the skin while corneometry measures the water in the skin. All of these measurements can be used to noninvasively assess the efficacy of a body moisturizer.

Even though these sophisticated noninvasive methods of cutaneous evaluation sound appealing, there is no substitute for the opinion of a trained unbiased observer when evaluating moisturizer effectiveness. Mechanistic evaluation can be easily biased to produce data that serve the best interest of the manufacturer. Computers cannot yet accurately synthesize all the tactile and visual information that can be obtained with human evaluation. The noninvasive techniques simply present another tool for assessing moisturizer function (36).

Noninvasive assessments can be used to better characterize the behavior of skin before and after application of a body moisturizer.

ADVERSE REACTIONS OF BODY MOISTURIZERS

Many patients with dry skin will claim that they are "allergic" to most moisturizers as a result of skin stinging experienced following application. This may represent an irritant contact dermatitis rather than a true allergic contact dermatitis (37). These patients should avoid moisturizers containing propylene glycol which may cause burning upon application to damaged skin. Other substances found in facial moisturizers that cause stinging include benzoic acid, cinnamic acid compounds, lactic acid, urea, emulsifiers, formaldehyde, and sorbic acid.

Moisturizing ointments, creams, lotions, and gels should be patch tested "as is." If an irritant reaction is experienced with closed patch testing, the product should be retested with open patch testing and provocative use testing (38).

REFERENCES

1. Friberg SE, Ma Z. Stratum corneum lipids, petrolatum and white oils. Cosmet Toilet 1993; 107: 55–9.
2. Grubauer G, Feingold KR, Elias PM. Relationship of epidermal lipogenesis to cutaneous barrier function. J Lip Res 1987; 28: 746–52.
3. Nair B. Final report on the safety assessment of dimethicone. Cosmetic Ingredient Review Expert Panel. Int J Toxicol 2003; 22(Suppl 2): 11–35.
4. Short RW, Chan JL, Choi JM, et al. Effects of moisturization on epidermal homeostasis and differentiation. Clin Exp dermatol 2007; 32: 88–90.
5. Spencer TS. Dry skin and skin moisturizers. Clin Dermatol 1988; 6: 24–8.
6. Hara-Chikuma M, Verkman AS. Aquaporin-3 functions as a glycerol transporter in mammalian skin. Bio Cell 2005; 97: 479–86.
7. Elias PM, Brown BE, Ziboh VA. The permeability barrier in essential fatty acid deficiency: evidence for a direct role for linoleic acid in barrier function. J Invest Dermatol 1980; 75: 230–3.
8. Wilkinson JB, Moore RJ. Harry's Cosmeticology, 7th edn. New York: Chemical Publishing, 1982: 61.
9. Wehr RF, Krochmal L. Considerations in selecting a moisturizer. Cutis 1987; 39: 512–15.
10. Rawlings AV, Scott IR, Harding CR, Bowser PA. Stratum corneum moisturization at the molecular level. Prog Dermatol 1994; 28: 1–12.
11. Wilkinson JB, Moore RJ: Harry's Cosmeticology, 7th edn. New York: Chemical Publishing, 1982: 62–4.
12. Raab WP. Uses of urea in cosmetology. Cosmet Toilet 1990; 105: 97–102.
13. Idson B. Dry skin: moisturizing and emolliency. Cosmet Toilet 1992; 107: 69–78.
14. Warner RR, Myers MC, Taylor DA. Electron probe analysis of human skin: determination of the water concentration profile. J Invest Dermatol 1988; 90: 218–24.
15. Jackson EM. Moisturizers: what's in them? How do they work? Am J Contact Dermatitis 1992; 3: 162–8.
16. Novotny J, Hrabalek A, Vavrova K. Synthesis and structure-activity relationships of skin Ceramides. Curr Med Chem 2010 May; (Epub ahead of print).
17. Garidel P, Fölting B, Schaller I, Kerth A, The microstructure of the stratum corneum lipid barrier: mid-infrared spectroscopic studies of hydrated ceramide: palmitic acid: cholesterol model systems. Biophys Chem 2010; 150: 144–56.
18. Madaan A. Epiceram for the treatment of atopic dermatitis. Drugs Today (Barc) 2008; 44: 751–5.
19. Sugarman JL, Parish LC. Efficacy of a lipid-based barrier repair formulation in moderate-to-severe pediatric atopic dermatitis. J Drugs Dermatol 2009; 8: 1106–11.
20. Amado A, Taylor JS, Murray DA, Reynolds JS. Contact dermatitis to pentylene glycol in a prescription cream for atopic dermatitis. Arch Deratmol 2008; 144: 810–12.
21. Cosmetic Ingredient Review Expert Panel, Final Report on the Safety Assessment of Glycyrrhetinic Acid, Potassium Glycyrrhetinate, Disodium Succinoyl Glycyrrhetinate, Glyceryl Glycyrrhetinate, Glycyrrhetinyl Stearate, Stearyl Glycyrrhetinate, Glycyrrhizic Acid, Ammonium Glycyrrhizate, Dipotassium Glyvyrrhizate, Disodium Glycyrrhizate, Trisodium Glycyrrhizate, Methyl Glycyrrhizate, and Potassium Glycyrrhizinate. Int J Toxicol 2007; 26(Suppl 2): 79–112.
22. Eberlein B, Eicke C, Reinhardt H-W, Ring J. Adjuvant treatment of atopic eczema: assessment of an emollient containing N-Palmitoylethanolamine (ATOPA Study). J Eur Acad Dermatol Venereol 2008; 22: 73–82.
23. Veraldi S, De Micheli P, Schianchi R, Lunardon L. Treatment of pruritus in mild-to-moderate atopic dermatitis with a topical non-steroidal agent. J Drugs Dermatol 2009; 8: 537–9.
24. Boguniewicz M, Zeichner JA, Eichenfield LF, et al. MAS063DP is effective monotherapy for mild to moderate atopic dermatitis in infants and children: a multicenter, randomized, vehicle-controlled study. J Pediatr 2008; 152: 854–9.
25. Grove GL. Noninvasive methods for assessing moisturizers. In: Waggoner WC, ed. Clinical Safety and Efficacy Testing of Cosmetics. New York: Marcel Dekker, Inc, 1990, 121–48.
26. Kligman AM. Regression method for assessing the efficacy of moisturizers. Cosmet Toilet 1978; 93: 27–35.
27. Lazar AP, Lazar P. Dry skin, water, and lubrication. Dermatol Clin 1991; 9: 45–51.
28. Grove GL, Grove MJ. Objective methods for assessing skin surface topography noninvasively. In: Leveque JL, ed. Cutaneous Investigation in Health and Disease. New York: Marcel Dekker, 1988: 1–32.
29. Grove GL. Dermatological applications of the Magiscan image analysing computer. In: Marks R, Payne PA, eds. Bioengineering and the Skin. Lancaster, England: MTP Press, 1981: 173–82.
30. de Rigal J, Leveque JL. In vivo measurements of the stratum corneum elasticity. Bioeng Skin 1985; 1: 13–23.
31. Tagami H. Electrical measurement of the water content of the skin surface. Cosmet Toilet 1982; 97: 39–47.
32. Grove GL. The effect of moisturizers on skin surface hydration as measured in vivo by electrical conductivity. Curr Ther Res 1991; 50: 712–19.
33. Idson B. In vivo measurement of transdermal water loss. J Soc Cosmet Chem 1976; 29: 573–80.
34. Rietschel RL. A method to evaluate skin moisturizers in vivo. J Invest Dermatol 1978; 70: 152–5.
35. Rietschel RL. A skin moisturization assay. J Soc Cosmet Chem 1979; 30: 360–73.
36. Grove GL. Design of studies to measure skin care product performance. Bioeng Skin 1987; 3: 359–73.
37. Lazar PM. The toxicology of moisturizers. J Toxicol-Cut Ocul Toxicol 1992; 11: 185–191.
38. Maibach HI, Engasser PG. Dermatitis due to cosmetics. In: Fisher AA, Contact Dermatitis, 3rd edn. Phildelphia: Lea & Febiger, 1986: 371.

SUGGESTED READING

Altemus M, Rao B, Dhabhar F, Ding W, Granstein R. Stress-induced changes in skin barrier function in healthy women. J Invest Dermatol 2001; 117: 309–17.

Ananthapadmanabhan KP, Subramanyan K, Rattinger GB. Moisturizing cleansers (Chapter 20). In: Leyden JJ, Rawlings AV, eds. Skin Moisturization. Vol. 25. Marcel Dekker, Inc., 2002: 405–32.

Arct J, Gronwald M, Kasiura K. Possibilities for the prediction of an active substance penetration through epidermis. IFSCC Magazine 2001; 4: 179–183.

Atrux-Tallau N, Romagny C, Padois K, et al. Effects of glycerol on human skin damaged by acute sodium lauryl sulphate treatment. Arch Dermatol Res 2009 December; [Epub ahead of print].

Barton S. Formulation of skin moisturizers (Chapter 25). In: Leyden JJ, Rawlings AV, eds. Skin Moisturization. Vol. 25. Marcel Dekker, Inc., 2002: 547–75.

Bikowski J. The use of therapeutic moisturizers in various dermatologic disorders. Cutis 2001; 68(5 Suppl): 3–11.

Bissonnette R, Maari C, Provost N, et al. A double-blind study of tolerance and efficacy of a new urea-containing moisturizer in patients with atopic dermatitis. J Cosmet Dermatol 2010; 9: 16–21.

Buraczewska I, Berne B, Lindberg M, et al. Changes in skin barrier function following long-term treatment with moisturizers, a randomized controlled trial. Br J Dermatol 2007; 156: 492–8.

Chamlin SL, Kao J, Frieden IJ, et al. Ceramide-dominant barrier repair lipids alleviate childhood atopic dermatitis: change in barrier function provide a sensitive indicator of disease activity. J Am Acad Dermatol 2002; 47: 198–208.

Coderch L, Lopez O, de la Maza A, Parra JL. Ceramides and skin function. Am J Clin Dermat 2003; 4: 107–29.

Crowther JM, Sieg A, Clenkiron P, et al. Measuring the effects of topical moisturizers on changes in stratum corneaim thickness, water gradients and hydration in vivo. Br J Dermatol 2008; 159: 567–77.

Denda M, Kumazawa N. Negative electric potential induces alteration of ion gradient and lamellar body secretion in the epidermis, and accelerates skin barrier recovery after barrier disruption. J Invest Dermatol 2002; 118: 65–72.

Draelos ZD. Botanicals as topical agents. Clin Dermatol 2001; 19: 474–7.

Draelos ZD, Ertel K, Berge C. Niacinamide-containing facial moisturizer improves skin barrier and benefits subjects with rosacea. Cutis 2005; 76: 135–41.

Draelos ZD. Therapeutic moisturizers. Dermatol Clin 2000; 18: 597–607.

Draelos ZD. Concepts in skin care maintenance. Cutis 2005; 76(6 Suppl): 19–25.

Draelos ZD. The ability of onion extract gel to improve the cosmetic appearance of postsurgical scars. J Cosmet Dermatol 2008; 7: 101–4.

Draelos ZD. Therapeutic moisturizers. Dermatol Clin 2000; 18: 597–607.

Endo K, Suzuki N, Yoshida O, et al. Two factors governing transepidermal water loss: barrier and driving force components. IFSCC Magazine 2003; 6: 9–13.

Fluhr J, Holleran WM, Berardesca E. Clinical effects of emollients on skin (Chapter 12). In: Leyden JJ, Rawlings AV, eds. Skin Moisturization. Vol. 25. New York: Marcel Dekker, Inc., 2002: 223–43.

Fluhr JW, Bornkessel A, Berardesca E. Glycerol—just a moisturizer? Biological and biophysical effects (Chapter 20). In: Loden M, Maibach HI, eds. Dry Skin and Moisturizers, 2nd edn. Taylor & Francis Group, LLC 2006: 227–43.

Ghali FE. Improved clinical outcomes with moisturization in dermatologic disease. Cutis 2005; 76(6 Suppl): 13–18.

Giusti F, Martella A, Bertoni L, Seidenari S. Skin barrier, hydration, and pH of the skin of infants under 2 years of age. Pediatr Dermatol 2001; 18: 93–6.

Hannuksela A, Kinnunen T. Moisturizers prevent irritant dermatitis. Acta Derm Venereol 1992; 72: 42–4.

Hannuksela M. Moisturizers in the prevention of contact dermatitis. Curr Probl Dermatol 1996; 25: 214–20.

Harding CR, Rawlings AV. Effects of natural moisturizing factor and lactic acid isomers on skin function (Chapter 18). In: Loden M, Maibach HI, eds. Dry Skin and Moisturizers, 2nd edn. Taylor & Francis Group, LLC 2006: 187–209.

Harding, CR. The stratum corneum: structure and function in health and disease. Derm Ther 2004; 17: 6–15.

Hawkins SS, Subramanyan K, Liu D, Bryk M. Cleansing, moisturizing, and sun-protection regimens for normal skin, self-perceived sensitive skin, and dermatologist- assessed sensitive skin. Derm Ther 2004; 17: 63–8.

Held E, Agner T. Effect of moisturizers on skin susceptibility to irritants. Acta Derm Venereol 2110; 81: 104–7.

Held E, Lund H, Agner T. Effect of different moisturizers of SLS-irritated human skin. Contact Dermatitis 2001; 44: 229–34.

Held E, Sveinsdottir S, Agner T. Effect of long-term use of moisturizer on skin hydration, barrier function and susceptibility to irritants. Acta Derm Venereol 1999; 79: 49–51.

Herman S. Lipid assets. GCI. 2001: 12–14.

Herman S. The new polymer frontier. GCI. 2002.

Jemec GB, Wulf HC. Correlation between the greasiness and the plasticizing effect of moisturizers. Acta Derm Venereol 1999; 79: 115–17.

Johnson, AW. Overview: fundamental skin care—protecting the barrier. Derm Ther 2004; 17: 1–5.

Kao JS, Garg A, mao-Qiang M, et al. Testosterone perturbs epidermal permeability barrier homeostasis. J Invest Dermatol 2001; 116: 443–50.

Kraft JN, Lynde CW. Moisturizers: what they are and a practical approach to product selection. Skin Therapy Lett 2005; 10: 1–8.

Lachapelle JM. Efficacy of protective creams and/or gels. Curr Probl Dermatol 1996; 25: 182–92.

Le Fur I, Reinberg A, Lopez S, et al. Analysis of circadian and ultradian rhythms of skin surface properties of face and forearm of healthy women. J Invest Dermatol 2001; 117: 718–24.

Lebwohl M, Herrmann LG. Impaired skin barrier function in dermatologic disease and repair with moisturization. Cutis 2005; 76(6 Suppl): 7–12.

Leyden JJ, Rawlings AV. Humectants (Chapter 13). In: Leyden JJ, Rawlings AV, eds. Skin Moisturization. Vol. 25. New York: Marcel Dekker, Inc., 2002: 245–66.

Lipozencic J, Pastar Z, Marinovic-Kulisic S. Moisturizers. Acta Dermatovenerol Croat 2006; 14: 104–8.

Loden M, Andersson AC, Lindberg M. Improvement in skin barrier function in patients with atopic dermatitis after treatment with a moisturizing cream (Canoderm). Br J Dermatol 1999; 140: 264–7.

Loden M. Role of topical emollients and moisturizers in the treatment of dry skin barrier disorders. Am J Clin Dermatol 2003; 4: 771–88.

Loden M. Barrier recovery and influence of irritant stimuli in skin treated with a moisturizing cream. Contact Dermatitis 1997; 36; 256–60.

Loden M. Do moisturizers work? J Cosmet Dermatol 2003; 2: 141–9.

Loden M. Hydrating substances (Chapter 20). In: Paye M, Barel AO, Maibach HI, eds. Handbook of Cosmetic Science and Technology, 2nd edn. Informa Healthcare USA, Inc., 2007: 265–80.

Loden M. Role of topical emollients and moisturizers in the treatment of dry skin barrier disorders. Am J Clin Dermatol. 2003; 4: 771–88.

Loden M. Skin barrier function: effects of moisturzers. Cosmet Toilet 2001; 116: 31–40.

Loden M. The clinical benefit of moisturizers. J Eur Acad Dermatol Venereol 2005; 19: 672–88; quiz 686–7.

Loden M. Urea-containing moisturizers influence barrier properties of normal skin. Arch Dermatol Res 1996; 288: 103–7.

Lynde CW, Moisturizers: what they are and how they work. Skin Terapy Lett 2001; 6: 3–5.

Madison, KC. Barrier function of the skin: "La Raison d'Etre" of the epidermis. J Invest Dermatol 2003; 121: 231–41.

Maes DH, Marenus KD. Main finished products: moisturizing and cleansing creams (Chapter 10). In: Baran R, Maibach HI, eds. Textbook of Cosmetic Dermatology, 2nd edn. Martin Dunitz Ltd 1998; 113–24.

Mao-Qiang M, Feingold KR, Thornfeldt CR, Elias PM. Optimization of physiological lipid mixtures for barrier repair. J Invest Dermatol 1996; 106: 1096–101.

Mao-Qiang M, Feingold KR, Wang F, et al. A natural lipid mixture improves barrier function and hydration in human and murine skin. J Soc Cosmet Chem 1996; 47: 157–66.

Norlen L. Skin barrier formation: the membrane folding model. J Invest Dermatol 2001; 117: 823–36.

Prasch Th, Schlotmann K, Schmidt-fonk K, Forster Th. The influence of cosmetic products on the stratum corneum by infrared and spectroscopy. IFSCC Magazine 2001; 4: 201–3.

Rawlings AV, Canestrari DA, Dobkowski B. Moisturizer technology versus clinical performance. Dermatol Ther 2004; 17(Suppl 1): 49–56.

Rawlings AV, Harding CR. Moisturization and skin barrier function. Dermatol Ther 2004; 17: 43–8.

Rieger M. Moisturizers and humectants. In: Rieger MM, ed. Harry's Cosmeticology, 8th edn. Chemical Publishing Co., Inc, 2000.

Simion FA, Abrutyn ES, Draelos ZD. Ability of moisturizers to reduce dry skin and irritation and to prevent their return. J Cosmet Sci 2005; 56: 427–44.

Simion FA, Story DC. Hand and body lotions (Chapter 33). In: Baran R, Maibach HI, eds. Textbook of Cosmetic Dermatology, 4th edn. Informa Healthcare, 2011: 269–89.

17 Hand dermatitis and moisturization

The hand is an amazing organ providing the structures needed to write, draw, paint, dance, and express affection. It is frequently said that much can be said about a person from their handshake, which is an assessment of the skin, muscle, and bones that form the hand. The hand can express gender, occupation, and age. Female hands are small while male hands are large and muscular. People who work with their hands outdoors have a much different skin feel than persons who type on a computer for most of the day. Children have soft, doughy, padded hands while the elderly have thin, sinewy, bony, arthritic hands. Hands are what make humans unique from every other living thing on the earth.

Hands are particularly vulnerable to xerotic dermatitis because they sustain considerable chemical and physical trauma. They are washed more than any other body area, yet are completely devoid of oil glands on the palmar surface. While the stratum corneum of the palm is uniquely designed to withstand physical trauma, it is not designed to function optimally when wet or when dehydrated. Thus, adequate moisturization is important to hand health, but overhydration can be disastrous.

> Adequate hand moisturization is important to hand health, but overhydration can be disastrous.

The hand responds to trauma by forming a callus. Calluses are formed from retained layers of keratin that form a dead skin pad over the area subjected to repeated physical trauma. For example, the palm of the hand will callus to protect the small bones in persons who use a hammer. The finger will callus in the location where a pencil is held in both children and adults. While the body forms a callus to protect underlying tender tissues, the callus can also cause dermatologic problems. Since a callus is made of retained keratin, it is dehydrated and inflexible and will fissure readily with trauma. Such are the complexities of designing products designed for the hands.

HAND DERMATOSES
Dermatologic disease needs to be divided into conditions that affect the dorsum of the hand and those that affect the palm of the hand. This is an important distinction because the two skin surfaces are quite different. The dorsum of the hand is a thin skin that becomes increasingly thinner with age. After the face, the back of the hand is generally the most photoaged skin location. The skin of the hand loses its dermal strength early leading to decreased skin elasticity, which can be simply measured by pinching the skin on the back of the hand and watching for the amount of time it takes for the skin to rebound to its original conformation. Skin that takes a long time to return to normal configuration is more photoaged than youthful skin that bounces back energetically.

In addition to losing elasticity, photoaged skin also becomes irregularly pigmented leading to lentigines and idiopathic guttate hypomelanosis. This irregular pigmentation is also accompanied by skin that is easily injured exhibiting senile purpura, and tissue tears from minimal trauma, which heal with unattractive white scars.

The palm of the hand is affected uniquely by inflammatory conditions like eczema and palmar psoriasis. Because the palm is the surface that the body uses to pick and touch, it more commonly is affected by chemical and physical trauma. This trauma may manifest as hand eczema. Highly occlusive and emollient hand creams are necessary to rehydrate damaged keratin and create an optimal environment for barrier repair.

> Highly occlusive and emollient hand creams are necessary to rehydrate damaged keratin and create an optimal environment for barrier repair.

HAND HYGIENE NEEDS
The hands receive more cleansing than any other part of the body. The basic ritual of washing the hands before eating is an effective method of preventing disease transmission, but may take its toll on the physiologically sebum lacking skin of the palms. Excessive hand washing can even be considered a medical disease, especially in persons with obsessive-compulsive disorder. There are a variety of methods of washing the hands. Basic hand washing is usually performed with a bar or liquid soap followed by water rinsing. Regimented, timed hand washing routines are used to thoroughly remove all bacteria from the hands before surgery. Lastly, a variety of hand cleansing antibacterial gels have been introduced, usually based on triclosan, which can be used without water to clean the hands. In general, it is felt that the physical rubbing of the hands to lather the cleanser followed by rubbing in a running stream of water to rinse away the cleanser is important. Both the physical rubbing of the hands and the chemical interaction of the cleanser and water are necessary for optimal hand hygiene.

> Physical rubbing of the hands and the chemical interaction of the cleanser and water are necessary for optimal hand hygiene.

HAND SKIN CARE NEEDS
The skin care needs of the hands go beyond basic cleansing to moisturization, healing, photoprotection, and skin lightening. As mentioned previously, hand moisturization is very important due to frequent cleansing. Hand moisturizers should be designed to occlude the skin reducing transepidermal water

loss, rehydrate the skin through the use of humectants, alleviate itch and pain, and smooth the skin surface with emollients. Hand moisturizers with this type of construction can be used for simple dry skin, as well as providing healing qualities for the dermatologic conditions previously discussed.

In addition to moisturization, the hands also need photo-protection both during sports and while driving a car, since photoaging UVA radiation passes through the windshield of a car. Sun protection is a unique challenge for the hands because they are frequently aggressively washed removing the sunscreen. However, the need for sun protection is obvious when one considers the thin dyspigmented skin that characterizes mature hands. This means that the hands require aggressive antiaging therapy and skin lightening.

> Hand moisturizers should occlude the skin reducing transepidermal water loss, rehydrate the skin through the use of humectants, alleviate itch and pain, and smooth the skin surface with emollients.

HAND MOISTURIZER FORMULATION
The simplest hand ointment is petroleum jelly, but most patients find this too greasy. To improve cosmetic appeal, the petroleum jelly can be whipped with water, color, and fragrance to make a hand cream. Thus, hand creams are oil-in-water emulsions with 15–40% oil phase, 5–15% humectant, and 45–80% water phase (1). The addition of silicone derivatives can also render the hand cream water resistant through four to six washings. Some hand creams even include a sunscreen agent.

> Hand creams are oil-in-water emulsions with 15–40% oil phase, 5–15% humectant, and 45–80% water phase.

One of the most effective hand moisturizing ingredients is glycerin. Glycerin can attract water to dehydrated hand keratin and encourage exfoliation of callused skin around the fingertips. High-glycerin- containing hand creams, identified by glycerin being listed among the first five substances in the ingredient disclosure, are especially effective at night to restore hand moisture balance. Day use of glycerin hand creams is not popular among patients because the glycerin is sticky and can leave fingerprints on paper. Since the hands are rested at night, bedtime hand moisturization is the most effective.

Urea can also be effectively used on the hands for the treatment of calluses and enhanced hydration of hyperkeratotic palms. It digests keratin and can increase the binding of water to callused skin. Once the callus is hydrated, it becomes soft and can be easily scrapped away or peeled off. In addition, hydrated callus can begin the natural desquamatory process, since the enzymes involved in hand desquamation only function in a moist environment. Hand creams using 5–10% urea, combined with glycerin and petrolatum, are very effective in treating hyperkeratotic palms.

REFERENCE
1. Schmitt WH. Skin-care products. In: Williams DF, Schmitt WH, eds. Chemistry and Technology of the Cosmetics and Toiletries Industry. London: Blackie Academic & Professional, 1992: 121.

18 Hyperhidrosis and antiperspirants

The desire to smell pleasant seems to be a basic human need. Olfactory stimulation seems to be an important human input to determine positive or negative evaluations of others. Certainly, the cosmetics and skin care industry understands this well as careful attention is paid to scent. An area of social concern for odor is the underarms because this moist, dark, warm body area is perfect for the growth of odor-causing bacteria, fungi, and yeast. This chapter investigates the axillary hyperhidrosis and the efficacy of antiperspirants.

The original deodorant to control axillary odor appeared on the U.S. market in 1888. Later, in 1919, advertising first introduced the notion that body odor was offensive, thus creating a market for deodorants and antiperspirants. Present popularity of such products can be attributed to social consciousness of body odor, development of nonirritating germicides, and products that do not contribute to fabric deterioration (1). Most patients would consider themselves uncivilized if an odor control product was not applied to the armpits, thus dermatologists must understand the effect of antiperspirants on the skin and how they function to minimize hyperhidrosis.

AXILLARY ODOR

Axillary odor is caused by the action of bacteria on sterile eccrine and apocrine sweat. The apocrine sweat is responsible for a large part of the odor as it is rich in organic material ideal for bacterial growth. Eccrine sweat, on the other hand, is more dilute and does not provide a high concentration of bacterial nutrients (Fig. 18.1). However, eccrine sweat indirectly promotes odor by dispersing the apocrine sweat over a larger area and providing the moisture necessary for bacterial growth. Axillary hair also contributes to odor by acting as a collecting site for apocrine secretions and increasing the surface area suitable for bacterial proliferation (2).

Each person has a unique odor due to a combination of physiologic factors, including sebaceous gland secretions, the combined effect of the foods last eaten, and the physical or psychological state of the body. Once the source of axillary odor is understood, a list of mechanisms to reduce odor can be developed (Table 18.1). These are the goals of all antiperspirant/deodorant products.

ANTIPERSPIRANTS VS. DEODORANTS

The words antiperspirant and deodorant are sometimes used interchangeably in the common vernacular, but to the cosmetic chemist these are two very different personal care products. Antiperspirants contain ingredients to decrease sweating, while deodorants are used solely to manage axillary odor. For this reason, all antiperspirants can be considered deodorants, but not all deodorants are antiperspirants. Most products in the current marketplace are both antiperspirants and deodorants.

Antiperspirants contain ingredients to decrease sweating, while deodorants are used solely to manage axillary odor.

DEODORANTS

Deodorants function either by masking the axillary odor with a perfume or by decreasing axillary bacteria. Therefore, many deodorants contain antibacterials, such as quaternary ammonium compounds (benzethonium chloride) and cationic compounds (chlorhexidine, triclosan). *Staphylococcus aureus*, Corynebacteria, and *Aerobacter aerogenes* are some of the key odor-causing axillary bacteria whose growth can be inhibited simply by decreasing the axillary pH to 4.5 or less (3). Antiperspirants are different in that they physically reduce the amount of sweat in the axilla.

A popular additive of deodorants and deodorant soaps, hexachlorophene, was banned by the Food and drug administration (FDA) in all nonprescription products in September 1972. Many companies were forced to reformulate their deodorant products at that time since it had been shown that brain lesions were produced in test animals fed high doses of hexachlorophene (4). Recently, natural deodorant/antibacterials have made a comeback in organic products containing ethyl alcohol, thyme oil (thymol) and/or, clove oil (eugenol).

The effectiveness of a deodorant can be measured in two ways: bacterial culture plates and the sniff test. Application of a proposed deodorant formulation to a culture plate swabbed with human perspiration can determine the percent reduction of bacterial growth, but this is not the best method to evaluate the consumer acceptability of a deodorant product. Most companies retain several individuals with highly trained noses to "sniff" armpits before and after application of a deodorant. Perspiration is usually induced by placing the subject in a hot room and a cupped hand is waved across the armpit to bring the odor to the trained nose (5).

MECHANISM OF ACTION OF ANTIPERSPIRANTS

Antiperspirants attempt to accomplish the daunting task of preventing perspiration release onto the skin surface from 25,000 eccrine glands per axilla capable of secreting in response to heat and emotional stimuli. There are several chemical categories of effective antiperspirants listed in Table 18.2 (6). Antiperspirants are considered over-the-counter (OTC) drugs and must use ingredients in the amount specified on the monograph. For this reason, most antiperspirant formulations are similar with different physical appearances and fragrances.

The efficacy of these antiperspirants is based on an understanding of the mechanism of sweat production. Several theories have been advanced to explain the efficacy of metal salts, which are the primary antiperspirants used today. Papa and Kligman originally proposed that the metal salts damaged the

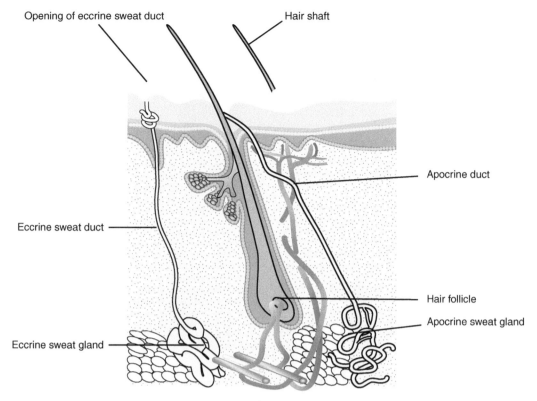

Figure 18.1 The anatomy of the apocrine and eccrine glands.

Table 18.1 Mechanisms for Axillary Odor Reduction

1. Reduce apocrine gland secretions
2. Reduce eccrine gland secretions
3. Remove apocrine and eccrine gland secretions from the axilla
4. Decrease axillary bacterial colonization

Table 18.2 Effective Antiperspirant Chemical Categories

1. Metal salts (aluminum chlorohydrate, aluminum zirconium chlorohydrate)
2. Anticholinergic drugs
3. Aldehydes (formaldehyde, glutaraldehyde)
4. Antiadrenergic drugs
5. Metabolic inhibitors
6. Botulinum toxin

sweat duct causing the secreted sweat to diffuse into the interstitial space (7), they have since retracted their theory. Shelley and Hurley proposed that the metal salts combine with intraductal keratin fibrils to cause eccrine duct closure and formation of a horny plug to obstruct sweat flow to the skin surface (8). A second paper by Holzle and Kligman also provided evidence that the metal salts cause a physical obstruction of the duct opening (9).

The most effective antiperspirants are metal salts that cause a physical obstruction of the eccrine duct opening.

Anticholinergic drugs are the most effective antiperspirant agents known. Blockage of the cholinergic innervation of the eccrine sweat glands effectively stops the sweating. Agents such as scopolamine and atropine have been studied in this regard; however, skin penetration is poor unless administered via injection or iontophoresis. Furthermore, their action is non-specific allowing for side affects such as dry mouth, urinary retention, and mydriasis. No antiperspirants containing anticholinergic drugs are available for OTC purchase in the U.S.A. at this time.

Aldehydes, such as formaldehyde and glutaraldehyde, can effectively decrease axillary sweating (10,11). It is believed that these chemicals also result in the blockage of the eccrine sweat duct. They are not popular at this time due to the sensitizing potential of formaldehyde and the brownish-yellow skin staining associated with glutaraldehyde. Both substances are toxic and are not in OTC use at this time.

Antiadrenergic drugs theoretically could also decrease sweating. Adrenergic neurotransmitters, such as epinephrine and norepinephrine, have been shown to decrease sweating in humans when they are injected intradermally. This is perhaps due to some adrenergic nerve fibers providing dual innervation to the sweat glands in addition to the cholinergic fibers. But this aspect of sweating is poorly understood. There are no commercially marketed antiperspirants of this type in the U.S.A. Lastly, metabolic inhibitors may decrease perspiration. Since the process of sweating is dependent upon a supply of energy, drugs that interrupt Na+/K+ - ATPase, such as ouabain, might also be effective. These substances are only of academic interest.

Perhaps the most promising antiperspirants are topical botulinum toxin formulations that interrupt nervous innervations of the sweat gland. It is unlikely that these formulations will enter the OTC market, however, making the metal salts the safest and most efficacious antiperspirants. The rest of our discussion will focus on these metal salts.

ANTIPERSPIRANT FORMULATION

Metal salts of aluminum, zirconium, zinc, iron, chromium, lead, and mercury have astringent properties on the skin. The only two metal salts that are presently used in antiperspirants are aluminum and zirconium (12). Zirconium salts, however, have had an interesting safety profile over the last 35 years. In 1955, sodium zirconyl lactate was used in deodorant sticks, but was found to cause axillary granuloma formation (13,14). In 1973, aerosol zirconium-based products were voluntarily removed from the market by several manufacturers who had received reports of skin irritation. Aerosol zirconium-based products were banned by the FDA in 1977, but no such products were left on the market at that time. Nonaerosol formulations at concentrations less than 20% are still allowed, but the incidence of axillary granulomas has greatly decreased (15,16).

The original antiperspirant formulation developed in 1914 was a 25% solution of aluminum chloride hexahydrate in distilled water (17). This solution was so effective that every second or third day application reduced axillary moisture. However, the solution was extremely irritating to skin and its high acidity damaging to clothing. Newer, less irritating aluminum formulations are more popular today, but they are also less effective. The FDA did express some concern in 1978 regarding long-term inhalation of aluminum-containing aerosol preparations (18).

Commonly used active agents in antiperspirants include aluminum chloride (concentration of 15% or less in an aqueous nonaerosol dosage form), aluminum chlorohydrate (concentration of 25% or less in an aerosol and nonaerosol dosage form), aluminum zirconium chlorohydrate (concentration of 20% or less or a nonaerosol dosage form), and buffered aluminum sulfate (concentration of 8% or less aluminum sulfate buffered with an 8% concentration of sodium aluminum lactate in a nonaerosol dosage form) (19). Other additives are employed to package the product as a stick, roll-on, or spray antiperspirant. Stick antiperspirants are packaged in a roll-up tube and consist of waxes, oils, volatile silicones, antibacterials, and aluminum or aluminum/zirconium complexes (Fig. 18.2). Roll-on products are an emulsion or clear liquid applied with a rolling ball mechanism to the armpits. These consist of aluminum chlorohydrate as the active ingredient in combination with gelling agents, emollients, and antibacterials. The spray antiperspirants are aluminum chlorohydrate complexes, oils, solvents, and antibacterials propelled by hydrocarbon gases (20,21).

ANTIPERSPIRANT EFFICACY

In order to be effective, an antiperspirant must reduce axillary sweating by 20% or more. Interestingly enough, antiperspirant effectiveness is dependent upon both the formulation and the form in which the product is applied, as demonstrated in Table 18.3. Efficacy is defined as the percentage reduction in the rate of sweating achieved after application of the antiperspirant product. The percentage sweating reduction can be determined gravimetrically, where a human volunteer holds an absorbent pad in the armpit while in a hot room, or hygrometrically, where the water content of dry gas sprayed in the

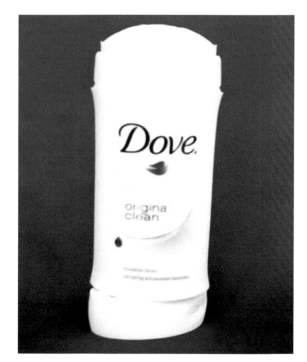

Figure 18.2 Stick products are presently the most popular in the marketplace.

Table 18.3 Antiperspirant Effectiveness by Form U.S. FDA OTC Antiperspirant Review Panel

Dosage form	Percent sweat reduction (%)
Aerosols	20–33
Creams	35–47
Roll-ons	14–70
Lotions	28–62
Liquids	15–54
Sticks	35–40

armpit of a human volunteer is measured and the rate of sweating calculated (22).

Antiperspirants are considered OTC drugs and thus must follow the rules set forth in the monograph covering their formulation. The types of materials that can be incorporated in antiperspirants and their concentration are carefully controlled by the FDA. This accounts for the similarity in formulation by a variety of manufacturers; however, the effectiveness of antiperspirants varies by formulation as demonstrated in Table 18.3.

Twice daily application of antiperspirants is the key to enhanced efficacy of clinical strength products.

A new category of antiperspirants introduced are labeled as "clinical strength" products. These products have a slightly higher concentration of active ingredients that must reduce sweat by 30% to substantiate the highly effective claim on package labeling, but are also recommended for twice daily use. The twice daily use is actually the key to their enhanced efficacy. The antiperspirant must remain the axillary vault long enough to form or maintain the plug in the acrosyringium. If heavy sweating is occurring during application, the antiperspirant is washed away and ineffective. Since the armpit is generally at rest at night, bedtime application of antiperspirants allows the ingredients to contact the skin longer and create a better plug that translates into enhanced efficacy. Increased efficacy can be achieved with any antiperspirant that is used morning and evening.

The most effective antiperspirants create a deep plug in the acrosyringium. The more superficial the plug, the less the sweat control obtained. Unfortunately, there is a direct connection between skin irritation and acrosyringial plug depth. Efficacious formulations must address both issues to create a skin friendly product. Some manufacturers are including skin protectant ingredients, such as dimethicone, in antiperspirant formulations to increase efficacy while counteracting the inherent possibility of irritant contact dermatitis.

PERSPIRATION CONTROL REQUIREMENTS
Antiperspirants reduce axillary moisture by employing aluminum salts to create a plug within the acrosyringium to occlude eccrine and apocrine ducts. Sometimes the aluminum is combined with zirconium to enhance efficacy. It takes about 10 days to create the plug, which physically blocks the transport of sweat from the gland on to the skin surface. Conversely, it takes 14 days for the plug to dissolve. It is for this reason that best results with antiperspirants are achieved with daily use to maintain the plug.

In order for the antiperspirant to work, it must physically contact every sweat duct. An even and thorough application to entire axillary vault is necessary for optimal results. Some antiperspirants have a grid to encourage even application and metered dosing administered through turning a knob at the bottom of the stick container. Using the amount of antiperspirant recommended on the packaging is important.

ADVERSE REACTIONS
The major drawback of aluminum and zirconium salt antiperspirants is their acidic pH (pH 1.8–4.2), which can irritate the skin, cause clothing discoloration, and weaken natural fabrics such as linen and cotton. Aluminum and zirconium chlorohydrates have the least skin irritancy. The sulfate forms are intermediate and chloride forms are the most irritating. Zinc oxide, magnesium oxide, aluminum hydroxide, and triethanolamine may be added to reduce irritancy in some products.

Many patients who develop underarm irritation to aerosol antiperspirants/deodorants find they can tolerate the roll-on type better or possibly need a product designed for sensitive skin in a cream or stick form. Certainly, these products are a common cause of irritant contact dermatitis in abraded underarm skin (23). A variety of different ingredients in antiperspirants and deodorants have been reported as causes of dermatitis: vitamin E (24), propantheline (25), quaternary ammonium compounds (26), etc. These products are open patch tested "as is." Stick antiperspirants that contain dimethicone appear to be the least irritating in consumer trials.

MAXIMIZING ANTIPERSPIRANT EFFICACY
Antiperspirants can and do fail to meet patient expectations for sweat control. As a matter of fact, most of the patients who enter a dermatologist's clinic for the purpose of discussing sweat control are antiperspirant failures. Following are a few

Table 18.4 Patient Recommendations for Optimal Antiperspirant Performance

1. Apply the antiperspirant to a dry armpit.
2. Do not shave the armpit aggressively.
3. Apply the recommended amount of antiperspirant.
4. Apply the antiperspirant daily.

easy tips that the dermatologist might wish to share with patients in need of assistance (Table 18.4):

1. Apply the antiperspirant to a dry armpit.

The antiperspirant must remain in physical contact with the acrosyringium long enough to create a plug. If the antiperspirant is applied to a wet armpit, wet either from showering or from perspiration, it will be diluted and not as effective. The armpit can be dried with a hair dryer before antiperspirant application, if necessary.

2. Do not shave the armpit aggressively.

The plugs created in the acrosyringium can be physically removed by shaving if they are located close to the skin surface. Persons who shave repeatedly over the armpit skin or shave multiple times daily may notice a decreased antiperspirant efficacy. It is best to shave the armpits weekly by dragging the razor once over the skin and avoid pulling the skin tight. This minimizes the chance of removing the sweat duct plug.

3. Apply the recommended amount of antiperspirant.

Many antiperspirants recommend twisting the knob at the bottom of the container three times and applying this amount in the axilla. This is the dose needed to obtain the optimal efficacy. Encourage patients to read the instructions and understand that just like medicines that do not work if enough is not ingested, antiperspirants also require the proper dose for optimal efficacy. The recommended amount should be thoroughly massaged throughout the armpit, especially over hair-bearing skin where the concentration of sweat glands is the greatest.

4. Apply the antiperspirant daily.

Compliance is the key to many things in medicine, including antiperspirant efficacy. As with any topical dermatologic, if you don't use it doesn't work. People who apply their antiperspirant sporadically will not get good sweat control. Daily application is necessary to efficacy, and twice daily application is even better, as previously discussed. Consecutive application for 10 days is necessary to determine the optimal benefit that can be achieved from a given antiperspirant formulation.

SUMMARY
Antiperspirants remain the most widely used method for controlling axillary perspiration. Proper application is the key to achieving the best results. The antiperspirant should be applied liberally to the entire axilla morning and evening to reduce sweating. In general, roll-on cream products offer the best efficacy, but care should be taken to apply the packaging recommended dose. Remember that shaving can decrease antiperspirant efficacy by physically removing the plug from the acrosyringium. For this reason, aggressive armpit shaving

by pulling the skin and shaving repeatedly over the skin should be avoided. Finally, compliance is important, as daily application is necessary to maintain the acrosyringial plug. The optimal effect for any antiperspirant can only be assessed after 10 consecutive days of use. Perhaps these are a few ideas that the dermatologist can share with patients in search of better topical axillary sweat control.

REFERENCES

1. Mueller WH, Quatrale RP. Antiperspirants and deodorants. In: deNavarre MG, ed. The Chemistry and Manufacture of Cosmetics. Wheaton, IL: Allured Publishing Corporation, 1975: 205–6.
2. Plechner S. Antiperspirants and deodorants. In: Balsam MD, Safarin E, eds. Cosmetics, Science and Technology. Vol. 2. 2nd edn. New York, NY: Wiley-Interscience, 1972: 373–415.
3. Chavkin L. Antiperspirants and deodorants. Cutis 1979; 23: 24–90.
4. Mueller WH, Quatrale RP. Antiperspirants and deodorants. In: deNavarre MG, ed. The Chemistry and Manufacture of Cosmetics. Wheaton, IL: Allured Publishing Corporation, 1975: 215–17.
5. Wilkinson JB, Moore RJ. Harry's Cosmeticology. 7th edn. New York, NY: Chemical Publishing, 1982: 133–4.
6. Quatrale RP. The mechanism of antiperspirant action in eccrine sweat glands. In: Laden K, Felger CB, eds. Antiperspirants and deodorants. New York: Marcel Dekker, Inc., 1988: 89–110.
7. Papa CM, Kligman AM. Mechanisms of eccrine anhidrosis: II. The antiperspirant effects of aluminium salts. J Invest Dermatol 1967; 49: 139–45.
8. Shelley WB, Hurley HJ Jr. Studies on topical antiperspirant control of axillary hyperhidrosis. Acta Dermatol Venereol 1975; 55: 241–60.
9. Holzle E, Kligman AM. Mechanism of antiperspirant action of aluminum salts. J Soc Cosmet Chem 1979; 30: 279–95.
10. Juhlin L. Topical glutaraldehyde for plantar hyperhidrosis. Arch Dermatol 1968; 97: 327–30.
11. Sato K, Dobson RL. Mechanism of the antiperspirant effect of topical glutaraldehyde. Arch Dermatol 1969; 100: 564–9.
12. Jass HE. Rationale of formulations of deodorants and antiperspirants. In: Frost P, Horwitz SN, eds. Principles of Cosmetics for the Dermatologist. St. Louis: CV Mosby Company, 1982: 98–104.
13. Rubin L, Slepyan H, Weber LF, et al. Granulomas of the axilla caused by deodorants. JAMA 1956; 162: 953–5.
14. Shelled WB, Hurley KJ. The allergic origin of zirconium deodorant granulomas. Br J Dermatol 1958; 70: 75–101.
15. Lisi DM. Availability of zirconium in topical antiperspirants. Arch Intern Med 1992; 152: 421–2.
16. Skelton HG, Smith KJ, Johnson FB, et al. Zirconium granuloma resulting from an aluminum zirconium complex. J Am Acad Dermatol 1993; 28: 874–6.
17. Emery IK. Antiperspirants and deodorants. Cutis 1987; 39: 531–2.
18. Klepak PB. Aluminum and health: a perspective. Cosmet Toilet 1990; 105: 53–6.
19. Morton JJP, Palazzolo MJ. Antiperspirants. In: Whittam JH, ed. Cosmetic Safety a Primer for Cosmetic Scientists. New York: Marcel Dekker, Inc, 1987: 221–63.
20. Calogero AV. Antiperspirant and deodorant formulation. Cosmet Toilet 1992; 107: 63–9
21. Walder D, Penneys NS. Antiperspirants and deodorizers. Clin Dermatol 1988; 6: 29–36.
22. Wilkinson JB, Moore RJ. Harry's Cosmeticology. 7th edn. New York, NY: Chemical Publishing, 1982: 130–2.
23. Mukin W, Cohen HJ, Frank SB. Contact dermatitis from deodorants. Arch Dermatol 1973; 107: 775.
24. Aeling JL, Panagotacos PJ, Andreozzi RJ. Allergic contact dermattis to vitamin E in aerosol deodorant. Arch Dermatol 1973; 108: 579.
25. Hannuksela M. Allergy to propantheline in an antiperspirant. Contact Dermatits 1975; 1: 244.
26. Shmunes E, Levy EJ. Quaternary ammonium compound contact dermatitis from a deodorant. Arch Dermatol 1972; 105: 91.

SUGGESTED READING

Benohanian A. Antiperspirants and deodorants. Clin Dermatol 2001; 19: 398–405.

Bowman JP, Wild JE, Shannon K, Browne J. A comparison of females and males for antiperspirant efficacy and sweat output. J Cosmet Sci 2009; 60: 1–5.

Burry JS, Evans RL, Rawlings AV, Shiu J. Effect of antiperspirants on whole body sweat rate and thermoregulation. Int J Cosmet Sci 2003; 25: 189–92.

Darrigrand A, Reynolds K, Jackson R, Hamlet M, Roberts D. Efficacy of antiperspirants on feet. Mil Med 1992; 157: 256–9.

Johansen JD, Rastogi SC, Bruze M, et al. Deodorants: a clinical provocation study in fragrance-sensitive individuals. Contact Dermatitis 1998; 39: 161–5.

McGee T, Rankin KM, Baydar A. The design principles of axilla deodorant fragrances. Ann NY Acad Sci 1998; 855: 841–6.

Minkin W, Cohen HJ, Frank SB. Contact dermatitis from deodorants. Arch Dermatol 1973; 107: 774–5.

Schreiber J. Antipersirants (Chapter 45). In: Barel AO, Paye M, Maibach HI, eds. Handbook of Cosmetic Science and Technology. 2nd edn. New York: Informa Healthcare USA, Inc., 2007.

Schreiber J. Deodorants (Chapter 63). In: Barel AO, Paye M, Maibach HI, eds. Handbook of Cosmetic Science and Technology. 3rd edn. New York: Informa Healthcare USA, Inc. 2009.

Taghipour K, Tatnall F, Orton D. Allergic axillary dermatitis due to hydrogenated castor oil in a deodorant. Contact Dermatitis 2008; 58: 168–9.

Uter W, Geier J, Schnuch A, Frosch PJ. Patch test results with patients' own perfumes, deodorants and shaving lotions: results of the IVDK 1998–2002. J Eur Acad Dermatol Venereol 2007; 21: 374–9.

19 Fragrances, dermatitis, and vasomotor rhinitis

Fragrance is an interesting part of any skin care, cosmetic, cosmeceutical, hair care, and nail care product. In many instances, the fragrance is the most expensive part of the formulation and accounts for much of the consumer enthusiasm regarding product use. While fragrance is often viewed as the most problematic part of any formulation from a contact dermatitis or vasomotor rhinitis standpoint, it is important to the consumer perception of beauty. Certainly, fragrance-free products have more dermatologic appeal, but many products without a scent fail in the marketplace even though they offer the same degree of efficacy as scented products. The ingredients used to construct a formulation have a chemical smell that may not be pleasant, thus fragrances are used to mask unappealing smells, to neutralize minimally noxious odors, and to heighten the consumer product experience. This chapter analyzes fragrances from a dermatologic perspective.

Perfumes and fragrances appeal to the most primordial part of the brain and can produce feelings of well being, lassitude, affection, disgust, etc. The use of fragrance to affect mood or induce relaxation is known as "aromatherapy" (1). Perfumery, the art of fragrance development, involves blending and mixing with more than 6000 possible ingredients to obtain a special scent.

Originally, perfume was used in the form of incense for religious purposes. The word itself is Latin for "through the smoke" (2). Incense was invented to mask the smell of burning flesh when an animal was sacrificed to the gods. The transition from incense to perfumes for adornment occurred about 6000 BC both in the Far East and the Middle East. By 3000 BC, the Sumerians and Egyptians were bathing in oils and alcohols of jasmine, iris, hyacinth, and honeysuckle. Cleopatra is said to have anointed her hands with an oil of roses, crocus, and violets and her feet with a lotion of almond oil, honey, cinnamon, orange blossoms, and tinting henna. Greek and Roman men both embraced perfumes considering a soldier unfit for battle unless he was duly anointed with fragrances.

The concept of cologne was introduced by an Italian barber, Jean-Baptiste Farina, who arrived in Cologne, Germany in 1709 to develop a fragrance trade. He concocted an alcoholic blend of lemon spirits, orange bitters, and mint oil from the bergamot fruit that became the first cologne. Soon perfume meant any mixture of ethyl alcohol with 25% or more essential fragrant oils; toilet water contained 5% essential oils and cologne contained 3% essential oils. These definitions are still used in the manufacture of modern fragrances.

> Perfume is any mixture of ethyl alcohol with 25% or more essential fragrant oils; toilet water contains 5% essential fragrant oils and cologne contains 3% essential oils.

While fragrances are powerful modulators of emotion and mental functioning, they also can cause problems such as allergic contact dermatitis, irritant contact dermatitis, and vasomotor rhinitis. The development of hypoallergenic fragrances has helped minimize contact dermatitis to some extent, but vasomotor rhinitis remains a problem. Modern fragrance trends are combinations of scents to produce complex mixtures, such as vanilla, lavender, pineapple, and kiwi. Further, fragrance has transcended body use and extended to candles, potpourri, air fresheners, jar oil wicks, soaps, shampoos, lipsticks, and hand lotions. Beauty products simply cannot be beautiful without a fragrance.

FRAGRANCE FORMULATION

The raw materials for perfume formulation fall into two categories: natural and synthetic. Natural components are of animal or plant origin while synthetic products are produced from a wide range of raw materials. The use of animal extracts in perfumery has declined due to animal rights issues; however, animal-derived products include musk from the musk deer, castoreum from the beaver, civet from the civet cat, and ambergris from the sperm whale. Most of these substances have been chemically analyzed and are now synthesized (3).

Plant products comprise the majority of substances used within perfumery. These extracts can be obtained through steam distillation, expression, and extraction. Distillation is the method used for removal of geranium, lavender, rose, and orange blossom scents. Expression is used to squeeze oil from the peel of bergamot, lemon, lime, and other citrus fruits. If the aromatic substance is unstable at the higher temperatures required for distillation or the yield of the oil minimal through expression, then extraction is employed.

Extraction can be accomplished by enfleurage, maceration, or the use of volatile solvents. Enfleurage involves the use of animal fats or vegetable oils to extract the scent at room temperature. The flower petals are sprinkled on glass plates encased in wooden frames that have been brushed with fats or oils. The wooden frames are then stacked to sandwich the petals between two glass plates. Fresh petals are added daily until the grease, known as pomade, absorbs a sufficient amount of perfume. This method is used for extracting the perfume of jasmine, orange blossom, jonquil, and lily (4). If heat is added, then the extraction technique is termed maceration. Here the flowers are mixed with hot liquid fats or oils at 60 to 70°C and stirred until the cells containing the fragrance rupture. The mixture is then poured on a screen allowing the scented grease to drain. Rose, acacia, and violet perfumes are obtained in this manner. Volatile solvents and percolators are used to extract the essential oils of mimosa, carnation, heliotrope, stock, and oakmoss (5).

Steam distillates are called "essential oils" while solvent extracts result in a nearly solid perfume wax referred to as "concretes." Ethanolic extractions of concretes yield "absolutes," but if raw materials are subjected to ethanolic extraction "tinctures" are produced. Organic solvent extraction yields

Table 19.1 Common Fragrance Materials

Fragrance material	Characteristics
Benzyl acetate	Light floral, slightly fruity
Benzyl salicylate	Warm, balsamic
Isobornyl acetate	Fresh, piney
p-t-Butyl cyclohexyl acetate	Soft, woody
Cedryl acetate	Sharp, woody
Citronellol	Rosy
Dihydro myrcenol	Citrus
Geraniol	Floral, rosy
Heliotropine	Sweet, floral, powdery
Hexyl cinnamic aldehyde	Light, delicate
Indole	Floral, animalic
Gamma-methyl ionone	Woody, floral
Musk ketone	Musky, animalic, warm
Phenyl ethyl alcohol	Floral
Vanillin	Sweet, powdery, vanilla

Source: Adapted from Ref. 7.

Table 19.2 Odor Descriptors

Odor	Description
Aldehydic	Sharp, fatty, or soapy
Amber	Sweet, warm
Animalic	Redolent of animal odors
Balsamic	Warm, sweet, and resinous
Camphoraceous	Medicated
Chemical	Harsh, aggressive, and basic
Citrus	Fresh, tangy, and zesty
Earthy	Green, rooty, and dank
Fatty	Odor of animal or vegetable oil
Floral	Odor of flowers
Fresh	Used subjectively
Fruity	Odor of natural fruit
Green	Odor of grass or leaves
Herbal	Odor of fresh plants
Leather	Phenolic, warm, and animalic
Light	Discrete
Medicinal	Pungent
Mossy	Earthy, mossy, phenolic, or green
Nutty	Odor of natural nuts
Pine	Odor or fine wood, needles, and resin
Powdery	Soft, gentle
Resinous	Warm, sweet, balsamic
Spicy	Pungent, hot, culinary
Sweet	Heavy, cloying
Warm	Ambery, animalic, sweet
Woody	Odor of natural wood

Source: Adapted from Ref. 7.

"resinoids," which can be further extracted with ethanol to yield "resin absolutes" (6). All parts of the plant, to include roots, fruits, leaves, flowers, bark, rind, etc., can be used in perfume production. Of the 250,000 species of flowering plants, only 2000 contain essential oils appropriate for fragrance production.

Synthetic fragrances are becoming more popular due to cost and inability to obtain natural animal and plant sources. Table 19.1 lists some of the more common aroma chemicals used in perfumery today (7).

FRAGRANCE CLASSIFICATION

A special vocabulary is used to describe the fragrances briefly outlined in Table 19.2. The perception of smell is very subjective accounting for the tremendous number of popular perfumes presently on the market. A successful formulation is a prized secret among fragrance manufacturers. Generally, perfumes fall into three categories:

1. simple notes representing naturally occurring aromas, such as fruits, herbs, spices, flowers, and animal smells;
2. complexes representing combinations of odors, such as green floral, spicy citrus, and fruity floral;
3. multicomplexes representing up to 12 identifiable fragrance themes.

Perfumes are further described by the manner in which their smell changes with time (8). The top note of a perfume refers to the rapidly evaporating oils that are discernible when the bottle is opened, but disappear shortly after skin application. The middle note is the smell of the dried perfume on the skin and the end note is the ability of the perfume to diffuse fragrance over time (9).

FRAGRANCE-INDUCED DERMATITIS

Irritant and allergic contact dermatitis to perfumes and fragrances is a well-known phenomenon (10–13). In fact, fragrances have been reported as the most common cause of cosmetic-related allergic contact dermatitis (14). The North American Contact Dermatitis Group reported that cinnamic

aldehyde, a fragrance material, was one of the 10 most common allergens on the standard dermatology patch test tray (15). Table 19.3 lists some of the more common fragrances and their irritancy potential as represented in the fragrance literature (16). Table 19.4 lists some of the common fragrances and their allergenic potential as represented in the dermatologic literature (17). The North American Contact Dermatitis Group found the following fragrance materials to be sources of allergic contact dermatitis in order of decreasing frequency: cinnamic alcohol, hydroxycitronellal, musk ambrette, isoeugenol, geraniol, cinnamic aldehyde, coumarin, and eugenol (18,19).

> The most allergenic fragrances are cinnamic alcohol, hydroxycitronellal, musk ambrette, isoeugenol, geraniol, cinnamic aldehyde, coumarin, and eugenol.

Fragrance sensitivities can be detected by patch testing with a fragrance mixture containing the most common fragrance allergens. It consists of a 2% concentration of cinnamic alcohol, cinnamic aldehyde, eugenol, isoeugenol, hydroxycitronellal, oakmoss absolute, geraniol, and alpha amyl cinnamic alcohol in petrolatum (20). Unfortunately, irritant reactions can occur (21). This mixture detects approximately 70–80% of fragrance sensitivities (17). Further evaluation of the allergic contact dermatitis needs to be carried out with individual fragrances (22). The patient's perfume can also be used for patch testing if diluted to a 10–30% concentration in alcohol or petrolatum. Interestingly enough, balsam of Peru, one of the standard substances on a patch test tray, serves as a marker

Table 19.3 Irritant Potential of Perfumes

Irritating perfumes
    Benzylidene acetone
    Methyl heptin carbonate
    Methyl octin carbonate
Moderately irritating perfumes
    Cyclamen aldehyde
    Ethyl methylphenyl glycinate
    Eugenols gamma-nonyl lactone
    Balsam of Peru
    Phenyl acetaldehyde
    Vanillin
Least irritating perfumes
    Benzaldehyde
    Benzoin resin
    Benzyl benzoate
    Cinnamic acid and cinnamates
    Citrus oils
    Cresol and methyl cresol
    Diethyl phthalate
    Heliotropin
    Higher aliphatic aldehydes
    Hydroxycitronellal
    Menthol
    Salicylates

Source: Adapted from Ref. 16.

Table 19.4 Allergic Potential of Perfumes

Perfume	Allergic potential	Patch test concentration in petrolatum (%)
Cinnamic alcohol	High	5
Cinnamic aldehyde	High	1
Hydroxycitronellal	High	4
Isoeugenol	High	5
Eugenol	High	5
Oakmoss absolute	High	5
Alpha amy cinnamic alcohol	Moderate	5
Geraniol	Moderate	5
Benzyl salicylate	Moderate	2
Sandalwood oil	Moderate	2
Anisyl alcohol	Moderate	5
Benzyl alcohol	Moderate	5
Coumarin	Moderate	5
Musk ambrette	Photoallergen	5

Source: Adapted from Ref. 17.

for fragrance sensitivity and is patch test positive in about 50% of cases of perfume allergy.

Determining the source of fragrance allergies can be quite complex (23). The average soap contains 50–150 fragrance ingredients, the average cosmetic contains 200–500 fragrance ingredients, and the average perfume contains 700 fragrance ingredients (24). The concentration of fragrance ingredients also varies. Fine perfumes contain 15–30% fragrance, colognes contain 5–8% fragrance, and scented cosmetics contain 0.1–1% fragrance, while masking fragrances are used at concentrations below 0.1% (25). Most of the cosmetic houses are able to provide fragrance products for testing (26).

FRAGRANCE AND VASOMOTOR RHINITIS

While patch testing is effective for the detection of contact dermatitis, it is not effective for the understanding of vasomotor rhinitis. Vasomotor rhinitis occurs when a fragrance is first perceived by a patient and consists of tearing, sneezing, a runny nose, nasal congestion, and headache. The symptoms appear to be autonomic, as the patient cannot control them. Problems can arise from fragrances found in perfumes, air fresheners, candles, laundry detergents, potpourri, etc. Sometimes the symptoms can be controlled with antihistamines, such as cetirizine, or nasal decongestants, such as oxymetazoline. Scent avoidance is the best treatment for this condition, which can be disabling for the patient. Vasomotor rhinitis does not appear to be related to asthma and is not found with increased incidence in patients with atopy. It occurs with many diverse fragrances that are different from those found on patch test trays. The phenomenon of vasomotor rhinitis has recently been identified by the fragrance industry and I am currently involved in a research to better understand this condition.

REFERENCES

1. Jackson EM. Aromatherapy. Am J Contact Dermatitis 1993; 4: 240–2.
2. Panati C. Extraordinary origins of everyday things. New York: Perennial Library, Harper & Row, Publishers, 1987: 238–43.
3. Launert E. Scent & Scent Bottles. London: Barrie & Jenkins, 1974: 29–32.
4. Guin JD. History, manufacture, and cutaneous reactions to perfumes. In: Frost P, Horwitz SN, eds. Prinicples of Cosmetics for the Dermatologist. St. Louis: CV Mosby Company, 1982: 111–29.
5. Ellis A. The Essence of Beauty. New York: The Macmillan Company, 1960: 132–42.
6. Balsam MS. Fragrance. In: Balsam MD, Gerson SD, Rieger MM, Sagarin E, Strianse SJ, eds. Cosmetics Science and Technology. 2nd edn. New York: Wiley-Interscience, 1972: 599–634.
7. Dallimore A. Perfumery. In: Williams DF, Schmitt WH, eds. Chemistry and Technology of the Cosmetics and Toiletries Industry. London: Blackie Academic & Professional, 1992: 258–74.
8. Jellinek JS. Evaporation and the odor quality of perfumes. J Soc Cosmet Chem 1961; 12: 168.
9. Poucher WA. A classification of odours and its uses. J Soc Cosmet Chem 1955; 6: 80.
10. Rothengorg HW, Hjorth N. Allergy to perfumes from toilet soaps and detergents in patients with dermatitis. Arch Dermatol 1968; 97: 417–21.
11. Maibach HI. Fragrance hypersensitivity. Cosmet Toilet 1991; 106: 25–6.
12. Maibach HI. Fragrance hypersensitivity, part II. Cosmet Toilet 1991; 106: 35–6.
13. Larsen WG, Maibach HI. Fragrance contact allergy. Semin Dermatol 1982; 1: 85–90.
14. Eiermann HJ, Larsen WG, Maibach HI, Taylor JS. Prospective study of cosmetic reactions; 1977-1980. J Am Acad Dermatol 1982; 6: 909–17.
15. Storrs FJ, Rosenthal LE, Adams RM, et al. Prevalence and relevance of allergic reactions in patients patch tested in North America. J Am Acad Dermatol 1989; 20: 1038–45.
16. Wells FV, Lubowe II. Cosmetics and the Skin. New York: Reinhold Publishing Corporation, 1964: 370–4.
17. Larsen WG. Perfume dermatitis. J Am Acad Dermatol 1985; 12: 1–9.
18. Adams RM, Maibach HI. A five-year study of cosmetic reactions. J Am Acad Dermatol 1985; 13: 1062–9.
19. Larsen WG. How to instruct patients sensitive to fragrances. J Am Acad Dermatol 1989; 21: 880–4.
20. Larsen WG. Perfume dermatitis: a study of 20 patients. Arch Dermatol 1977; 113: 623–6.
21. Calnan CD, Cronin E, Rycroft R. Allergy to perfume ingredients. Contact Dermatitis 1980; 6: 500–1.
22. Fisher AA. Patch testing with perfume ingredients. Contact Dermatitis 1975; 1: 166–8.

23. Larsen WG. Cosmetic dermatitis due to a perfume. Contact Dermatitis 1975; 1: 142–5.

24. Jackson EM. Substantiating the safety of fragrances and fragranced products. Cosmet Toilet 1993; 108: 43–6.

25. Marks JG, DeLeo VA. Contact and occupational dermatology. St. Louis: Mosby Yearbook, 1992: 145–7.

26. Yates RL. Analysis of perfumes and fragrances. In: Senzel AJ, ed. Newburger's Manual of Cosmetic Analysis. 2nd edn. Washington, DC: Published by the Association of Official Analytical Chemists, Inc, 1977: 126–31.

SUGGESTED READING

Cadby PA, Troy WR, Vey MGH. Consumer exposure to fragrance ingredients: providing estimates for safety evaluation. Regul Toxicol Pharmacol 2002; 36: 246–52.

de Groot AC. Adverse reactions to fragrances. Contact Dermatitis 1997; 36: 57–86.

Ellena C. Perfume formulation: words and chats. Chem Biodivers 2008; 5: 1147–53.

Frater G, Bajgrowicz JA, Kraft P. Fragrance chemistry. Tetrahedron 1998; 54: 7633–703.

Herman SJ. Odor reception: structure and mechanism. Cosmet Toilet 2002; 117: 83–93.

Larsen W, Nakayama H, Fischer T, et al. A study of new fragance mixtures. Am J Contact Dermatitis 1998; 9: 202–6.

Parekh JC. Axillary odor: its physiology, microbiology and chemistry. Cosmet Toilet 2002; 117: 53–60.

Teixeira MA, Rodriquez O, Mata VG, Rodrigues AE. The diffusion of perfume mixtures and the odor performance. Chem Eng Sci 2009; 64: 2570–89.

20 Body photoprotection

We live in an environment dependent on our sun, a third generation star from which all the elements on our earth and in our bodies arose. The sun provides energy that drives our solar system, but it also produces UVB and UVA radiation that damages our DNA and activates our collagenase. In order to maintain this delicate balance between the life-giving qualities of the sun and sun protection, our bodies have evolved an elaborate system of endogenous defenses. Sunscreens simply represent an extension and an amplification of these natural defense mechanisms. This chapter examines body photoprotection. Some of the basic principles of sunscreen formulation and use have already been discussed under facial sunscreens in chapter 9.

> Sunscreen formulations are based on the natural endogenous body protective mechanisms.

NATURAL PHOTOPROTECTIVE MECHANISMS
The natural protective mechanisms of the body begin at the stratum corneum and extend into the dermis. They are summarized in Table 20.1. In each layer of the skin, there are a variety of techniques used to reflect ultraviolet radiation, quench oxygen radicals, and repair the resultant cellular damage. Beginning at the outermost structure of the skin with the stratum corneum, ultraviolet radiation is scattered and reflected by the corneocytes. This is why the endogenous sun protection factor (SPF) of the skin is lower through procedures that induce exfoliation. The use of topical hydroxy acid body moisturizers also removes the corneocytes, further decreasing the SPF of the skin. This concept of light scattering is built upon by the inorganic sun filters, such as zinc oxide and titanium dioxide. Most currently marketed beach sunscreens for body application include an inorganic filter for this reason.

The next natural body defense mechanism against UV radiation is the melanin. Melanin performs numerous functions to act as a UV absorber and dissipate the heat byproduct. Melanin itself is a free radical scavenger and undergoes oxidation in the 300–360 nm range. It is this oxidation of melanin that results in the immediate pigment darkening phenomenon associated with the dermatologic use of therapeutic UVA exposure. In many ways, organic sun filters function like melanin, absorbing a photon of UV radiation and undergoing a chemical reaction to diffuse the energy and prevent collagen damage. The cinnamates, salicylates, oxybenzone, and avobenzone function in this manner.

> Melanin absorbs UV radiation and dissipates the energy as heat.

Finally, the body relies on antioxidants to prevent UV photodamage. Endogenous body antioxidants include the carotenoid pigments, urocanic acid, and superoxide dismutase, which quench oxygen radicals and stabilize cell membranes. No sunscreen can duplicate the protection of these endogenous substances. There are oral and topical supplements that claim to enhance this mechanism of photoprotection, but none have been proven effective. Two of the most important antioxidants in the body are vitamins C and E, but an increased dietary intake of these vitamins has not been shown to increase the antioxidant capacity of the skin. For this reason, clothing and sunscreens are important body photoprotection.

BODY PHOTOPROTECTION
Sunscreens for the face and body are very similar in composition. Table 20.2 lists the approved sunscreens for use in the U.S.A. and their maximum allowable concentration. There is no difference in the composition of sunscreens for different body areas, but the attributes of sunscreens for the body are different from those for the face. Body sunscreens may be selected with a higher SPF and it may also be desirable for the formulation to have some water- resistant capabilities. The reader is referred to chapter 9 on facial sunscreens for an ingredient discussion.

SUNBURN PROTECTION FACTOR
The dermatologic community is anxiously awaiting the final version of the sunscreen monograph. Sunscreens are considered over-the-counter drugs and are therefore regulated by the monograph as to which filters may be used in which combination and in which amounts. This need to stick to the monograph allows for less variation in formulations and provides for less formulation ingenuity. One of the anticipated changes in the final sunscreen in monograph is the relabeling of SPF from sun protection factor to sunburn protection factor. This is probably a worthwhile change, since SPF only reports the UVB photoprotective properties of the sunscreen. A rating system for UVA photoprotection is anticipated, but the details have not been finalized.

> SPF has been redefined as Sunburn Protection Factor.

The SPF is currently the only comparative rating available for determining the superiority of one product over another in terms of possible sun protection. Patients are misled, however, when they purchase products on the basis of SPF alone. There is no substitute for a quality formulation from a reputable manufacturer. Further, on the only way a consumer would know that they are getting adequate UVA photoprotection is by looking for products with an SPF above 30 and finding the words "broad spectrum" on the label (Fig. 20.1). It is not possible to make a sunscreen with an SPF above 30 that does not have some UVA photoprotection. The current inflation in SPF values is an attempt by the manufacturers to report their superior UVA photoprotective qualities. While a higher SPF

Table 20.1 Natural Ultraviolet Protective Mechanisms

Cutaneous structure	Sun protective mechanism
Compact horny layer	Absorbs and scatters UV
Keratinocyte melanin	1. UV absorbing filter
	2. Free radical scavenger
	3. Dissipates UV as heat
	4. Undergoes oxidation in 300–360 nm range to produce immediate pigment darkening
Carotenoid pigments	1. Membrane stabilizers
	2. Quench oxygen radicals
Urocanic acid	Oxidized to stabilize UV-induced oxygen radicals
Superoxide dismutase	1. Oxygen radical scavenger
	2. Protects cell membrane from lipoprotein damage
Epidermal DNA excision repair	Repairs UV-induced DNA damage

Table 20.2 Category 1 Monographed Sunscreen Active Ingredients

Active sunscreen ingredient	Maximum concentration (%)
Aminobenzoic acid (p-Aminobenzoic acid, PABA)	15
Avobenzone	3
Cinoxate	3
Dioxybenzone (benzophenone-8)	3
Homosalate	15
Menthyl anthranilate	5
Octocrylene	10
Octyl methoxycinnamate	7.5
Octyl salicylate	5
Oxybenzone (benzophenone-3)	6
Padimate-O (octyl dimethyl PABA)	8
Phenylbenzimidazole sulfonic acid	4
Sulisobenzone (benzophenone-4)	10
Titanium dioxide	25
Trolamine salicylate	12
Zinc oxide	25

has little meaning in terms of UVB photoprotection, it is an important indicator of UVA photoprotection. Patients at present should be encouraged to use higher SPF formulations in the range of 40–55 for excellent body photoprotection.

Both chemical and biologic methods are used to determine the SPF; however, only the biologic evaluation will be discussed in this chapter. Most commonly, the lower back of untanned individuals is divided into small test sites and exposed to UVB light until a minimum amount of erythema develops, known as the minimal erythemal dose (MED). Lightproof barriers are placed around the test sites to prevent light contamination from one test site to another. Once the MED for the test subject has been determined, the subject is invited to return to the test site the next day for application of sunscreen. The sunscreen is placed on the test sites and allowed to dry. The skin is then exposed to UVB light at the expected SPF of the sunscreen product. The expected

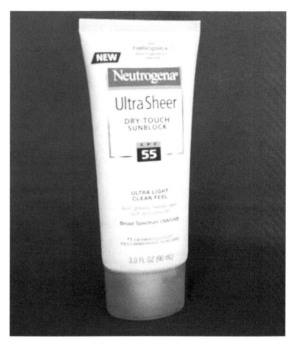

Figure 20.1 A sunscreen label containing the wording "broad spectrum" with an accompanying high SPF.

SPF is roughly determined by spectrophotometric absorption. The amount of UVB light required to obtain the same degree of erythema as the preceding day is determined and the SPF calculated.

This measurement is the optimum SPF the product can deliver under optimum conditions. The subjects have a measured amount of the product rubbed into the skin by a skilled technician. This eliminates the complicating factor of too little sunscreen applied in an erratic manner. Subjects are also evaluated indoors, eliminating the effects of wind, humidity, and perspiration due to high temperature. In my opinion, the biologic SPF determined under laboratory conditions in human test subjects should be halved to give an approximation of what can actually be expected under actual use conditions.

WATER RESISTANCE

Water-resistant qualities are very important in body photoprotection where sweating and water contact are common. Separate testing must be conducted to meet criteria required by the FDA to place the water-resistant label on a body sunscreen bottle. Water resistance is determined by applying the sunscreen with a predetermined SPF to human volunteers over a body surface area of 50 cm². The product is allowed to dry for 20 minutes and reapplied with another 20 minutes allowed for drying. The subjects are then asked to swim in an indoor pool for 20 minutes. The skin is then dried and the subjects sit outside the pool and rest for 20 minutes. The subjects then re-enter the pool for another 20 minutes. Thus, a total of 40 minutes of water contact is required to substantiate water-resistant claims (1).

Sunscreen water resistance is determined by two 20-minute water exposures.

Table 20.3 Water-Resistant Sunscreens

Chemical technology	Mechanism of efficacy
Water-in-oil emulsions	Oil is the main ingredient and resists removal by water
Silicones	Hydrophobic oily liquid that resists removal by water and forms film over skin surface
Acrylate crosspolymer	No emulsifier required which prevents water from dissolving the sunscreen, used in titanium dioxide preparations
Liquid crystal gels	Hydrophobic emulsifiers used that resist water, used in titanium dioxide preparations
Phospholipid emulsifiers	Substances engineered to mimic natural sebum (potassium cetyl phosphate) with water-resistant properties
Film forming polymers	Thin polymer film formed over the skin with inherent water resistance

Table 20.4 Methods of Sunscreen Removal by Water

1. Emulsification of the sunscreen film by water
2. Removal of the sunscreen film by rubbing
3. Separation of the UV filters from the sunscreen film

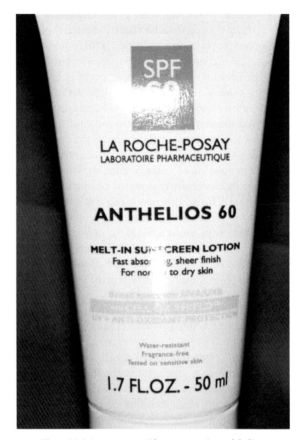

Figure 20.2 A sunscreen with a water-resistant labeling.

The SPF of the product is determined after this routine of water contact and skin drying. If the SPF following water contact is the same as the SPF prior to water contact, the product is considered to be water resistant. This testing also maximizes the water-resistant characteristics of the sunscreen. Notice that two applications of the sunscreen are performed prior to water contact. Also notice that the sunscreen is allowed to dry for 20 minutes prior to water contact. Double application ensures good coverage while the drying period maximizes the substantivity of the product for the skin. This is the advice that should be given to patients who expose themselves and their children to the sun at the beach. The patient should do everything possible to maximize the water-resistant qualities of the sunscreen since the product will not perform up to standards in real life at the beach, since the effects of wind and sand have been eliminated in the indoor pool environment used to perform the testing.

WATER-RESISTANT SUNSCREEN FORMULATIONS
There is a great deal of chemical science that goes into the development of a successful water-resistant sunscreen. The basic methods of imparting water resistance are listed in Table 20.3. All of the technologies for imparting water resistance are predicated on the fact that water-soluble and oil-soluble substances do not mix meaning that water can dissolve water-soluble substances, but not oil-soluble substances. Thus, if a sunscreen is predominantly oil with minimal water, it will not solubilize in the presence of water or perspiration. However, oil-dominant sunscreens are greasy and sticky. This has led to development of silicone liquid-based sunscreens, since silicone is an oil that is not greasy or sticky with excellent water-resistant properties.

Another method of creating water resistance is to alter or eliminate the emulsifier. Remember that the function of an emulsifier is to allow water- and oil-loving substances to mix into one continuous phase. The emulsifier in the sunscreen formulation can allow perspiration or swimming pool water to mix with the oily ingredients facilitating removal. Thus, acrylate crosspolymers and liquid crystal gels are being used where no emulsifier or hydrophobic emulsifiers can prevent solubilization of the sunscreen film by water.

The last methods used to confer water resistance are predicated on creating a film that is resistant to water removal. One technique involves the use of phospholipids, which are structurally similar to natural sebum, and create a thin oily film on the skin. The other technique involves the use of polymers that leave a thin water-resistant film on the skin surface.

WATER-RESISTANT SUNSCREEN FAILURE
Unfortunately, water-resistant sunscreens fail. All dermatologists have seen patients who have experienced severe, blistering, second-degree sunburns at the beach while wearing sunscreen. The methods by which sunscreens can be removed from the skin by water are listed in Table 20.4 (2). It is important to understand why body sunscreens fail so that better advise patients on superior sunscreen selection and use (Fig. 20.2).

Sunscreens are removed by water due to emulsification, rubbing, and separation of the sunscreen film.

There are three primary mechanisms that account for the removal of sunscreens from the skin surface. One method is water which actually dissolves the oily sunscreen film by interacting with the emulsifier in the formulation. This means that the emulsifier in water-resistant sunscreens must be of low concentration or possibly eliminated. For this reason, many of the best water-resistant and water proof sunscreens are anhydrous, meaning they contain no water. Products that are anhydrous do not require an emulsifier. This point should be emphasized to patients when selecting water-resistant sunscreens. Even though the patient may prefer a lighter feel in sunscreens, money, and application time are wasted if the product is immediately removed upon water contact.

The second manner in which water-resistant sunscreens can fail is with rubbing removal. This can be the case if the sunscreen does not stick well to the skin, a quality known as substantivity. The rubbing of water over the sunscreen film on the skin can also mechanically remove the product by lifting it off the skin surface. This quality of a sunscreen is tested in part by the evaluation of the SPF following two 20-minute swims. Dermatologists who are interested in personally testing the ability of a sunscreen to remain in place on the skin should apply the sunscreen to a glass slide and allow it to thoroughly dry. The glass slide should then be swirled in a glass of water. If the sunscreen film is even and continuous, it will remain on the slide and the water will remain clear. If a thin film is seen in the glass or the water becomes cloudy, the sunscreen has failed the test.

Lastly, the sunscreen film can physically degrade, a phenomenon most commonly seen with particulate sunscreens containing micronized titanium dioxide or microfine zinc oxide. In this case, the oily sunscreen film or polymer film adheres well to the skin, but the water-soluble titanium dioxide or zinc oxide does not remain contained within the film. Water washes away the water-soluble particulates, leaving behind a film lacking some of the ingredients required to achieve the labeled SPF. This problem can be overcome by using hydrophobic grades of titanium dioxide.

SUNSCREEN DEGRADATION AND INCOMPATIBILITIES

Sunscreen failure can also occur from degradation or interaction between the filters. This is why sunscreens are expiration dated and outdated sunscreen should not be used by the patient. Sunscreens are complex formulations without an unlimited shelf life. Some of the unwanted interactions can be suspected by the patient if the normally white sunscreen discolors to a pale yellow or brown color. These discolored products will not provide optimal sun protection and should be discarded. Discoloration may be seen in sunscreens containing octyl methoxycinnamate, which can undergo a photochemical reaction to form an intensely yellow pigment when exposed to sunlight. This can be prevented by packaging the sunscreen in an opaque container. Adding other UV absorbers, such as benzophenone-3 or zinc oxide, can stabilize the octyl methoxycinnamate while acting as active sunscreens and increasing the product SPF.

Degradation of another sort can occur with particulate sunscreens, such as micronized titanium dioxide or microfine zinc oxide. In order to be an effective sunscreen, the particles must

Table 20.5 Methods of Improving Sunscreen Compliance

1. Begin developing habits during childhood for good hygiene: brush teeth, wash face, apply sunscreen
2. Select sunscreen formulations that are appropriate for the body area of application
3. Use sunscreen-containing moisturizers instead of plain moisturizers on face, neck, upper chest, and hands
4. Select a sunscreen-containing facial foundation for a female face
5. Use a sunscreen-containing lip balm or lipstick
6. Use a gel sunscreen as an aftershave on the male face
7. Apply a quarter sized dab of sunscreen to the hand and use the entire amount on the face, neck, and ears
8. Develop a routine for sunscreen application to include face, front of neck, back of neck, ears, behind the ears, and central chest
9. Select separate products with different aesthetics for daily wear and beach wear
10. Use clothing effectively in the form of long pants, long sleeves, hats, scarves, and umbrellas as photoprotection

be dispersed evenly within the sunscreen lotion. If the particles coalesce, an even film of the active sunscreen is not achieved on the skin and the SPF of the product is that of the unprotected skin. It is important that physical sunscreens are used within their expiration period so that the suspension remains intact. The suspension should be a white color and discolored products should also be discarded. The fragrance of particulate sunscreens can also disappear with time in suboptimal formulations as it is absorbed by the titanium dioxide or zinc oxide. One of the newest developments that has improved the feel, water resistance, and SPF of physical sunscreens is the incorporation of film-forming polymers, such as acrylate copolymers or polyvinyl pyrolidone (PVP).

UV filters can also be absorbed by plastic packaging or the cap inserts. For example, polystyrene and low-density polyethylene can absorb the UV filters. For this reason, high-density polyethylene or high-density polypropylene must be chosen for packaging.

Sunscreens can interact with plastic packaging making bottle construction important in sunscreen efficacy.

SUNSCREEN COMPLIANCE

Compliance is key to sunscreen efficacy. Sunscreens do not work if they remain in the bottle. It is estimated by sunscreen manufacturers that an average U.S. adult uses less than one bottle of sunscreen per year. Clearly, this is indicative of poor compliance, since one bottle, if applied as directed on a daily basis, should last one month. The major issues in sunscreen compliance are examined next and presented in Table 20.5.

Issue 1. Sunscreens Are Sticky

One of the most common reasons patients do not like sunscreens is because they can be sticky (Fig. 20.3). Perhaps it may be helpful to obtain more insight into this issue. Most of the chemical sunscreen actives are sticky oils, such as methyl anthranilate. Usually a sunscreen formulation will combine at least two to three different actives to get

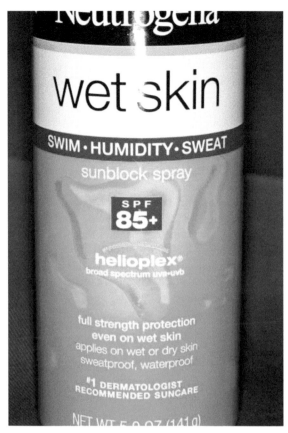

Figure 20.3 Some of the spray sunscreen formulations may offer an alternative for patients who do not like sticky creams.

broader-spectrum coverage and a higher SPF. The SPF is increased as the concentration of the active is increased. Thus, higher SPF products are usually stickier. Sunscreens with an SPF of 30 or higher are usually stickier than sunscreens with an SPF of 15 or lower. Yet, an SPF of 15 blocks about 93% of the UVB radiation while an SPF of 30 blocks out 97% of the UV radiation. This is only a 4% difference in UVB photoprotection that may make the difference between an aesthetically pleasing sunscreen and one that is undesirable. For this reason, dermatologists should reconsider advising patients to use the highest SPF product possible. Lower SPF products generally have better aesthetics and may yield better compliance. My recommendation is that patients should use an SPF 30+, which provides excellent photoprotection and optimal aesthetics.

Issue 2. Sunscreens Make you Hotter in the Sun

Another common complaint regarding sunscreen use is that patients feel hot and sweaty while they are wearing sunscreens. While some of this may be due to the fact that sunscreens are worn in the hot sun, chemical sunscreens, such as octyl methoxycinnamate, benzophenone, methyl anthranilate, and homosalate, actually function by transforming UVB radiation to heat energy. This generation of heat by the sunscreen contributes to the feeling of skin warmth. This should not be a deterrent to wearing sunscreen; however, physical sunscreen agents, such as zinc oxide or titanium dioxide, do not produce heat. Selecting the proper sunscreen can help minimize this problem which may lead to decreased compliance.

Issue 3. Sunscreens Cause Acne

Many patients have the perception that sunscreens cause acne. Usually the acne is in the form of inflammatory papules, not open or closed comedones, and presents within 48 hours after initial application. This is not true acne because sufficient time has not passed since the sunscreen application for follicular rupture to occur. The acne seen with sunscreens is more of an acneiform eruption, which I personally feel is indicative of irritant contact dermatitis. Some of the more extended wear water-resistant sunscreens are more occlusive by nature and may cause difficulty at the follicular ostia. The solution to this problem is sorting through a variety of sunscreen formulations by trial and error. Major problems can be avoided by applying the sunscreen for five consecutive nights to a small area of skin in front of the ear. The skin should be observed for the presence of inflammatory papules and pustules. Another helpful tip is the avoidance of long wearing sunscreen products. For daily use, long wearing products are not necessary and a sunscreen containing moisturizer may be a good alternative. If a beach wear product is desired, the vehicle of gel sunscreens, which may contain a polymer, should be avoided. Instead, a light-weight cream formulation should be selected and then applied frequently to obtain maximal protection.

Issue 4. Sunscreens Sting When Applied

It is true that some sunscreens sting when applied and this is more common in gel sunscreen formulations with a high concentration of a volatile vehicle, such as alcohol. Creamy sunscreens are a possible solution to this problem, as well (Fig. 20.4). Sunscreens may also sting when they enter the eye. One option is to use one of the waxy stick sunscreens in the eye area that will not melt or run when combined with sweat. These sunscreens can be stroked above the eyebrows and on the upper and lower eyelid. One of the methods for improving compliance is to pick the proper sunscreen for the proper skin site. No one sunscreen formulation will work in all body areas (Fig. 20.5).

Issue 5. Sunscreens Do Not Work

There are some who are skeptical of sunscreen efficacy from the start. This concern may be well founded, since sunscreens can fail. How does this occur? It is important to remember that sunscreens do not work unless present on the skin surface. Thus, failure to coat the entire exposed skin surface with sunscreen and sunscreen removal from rubbing or sweating are two of the most common causes of sunscreen failure. Sunscreens may also fail if the film applied to the skin is too thin. A thin film, created by failure to apply the proper amount of sunscreen, yields skin areas leaving the skin unprotected. Formulation issues are also important. Some sunscreens have better skin substantivity. Substantivity is a term used by the cosmetic chemist to explain the ability of the sunscreen to remain in place on the skin. Not all bottles of sunscreen with an identical SPF are equivalent. There is no substitute for the formulation knowledge of an experienced sunscreen manufacturer. By law, all products labeled with an SPF of 15, will provide consistent sun protection under optimal conditions. These optimal conditions include minimal perspiration, no water contact, low humidity, minimal activity, no wind, thick

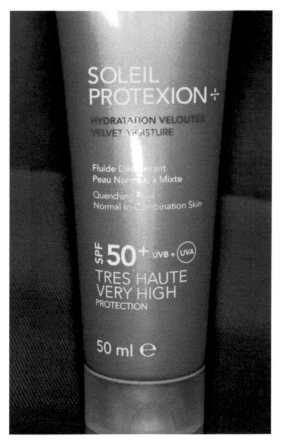

Figure 20.4 Many of moisturizing sunscreens do not sting when applied to sensitive complexion patients.

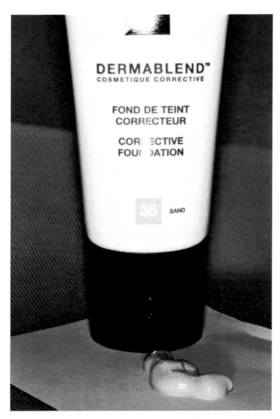

Figure 20.5 For female patients who experience problems with many sunscreen formulations, an opaque facial foundation can be used for photoprotection.

film application, etc. In reality, sunscreens are not worn under these conditions. The sunscreen in the bottle may be an SPF 15, but its performance on the skin may differ depending on formulation. I encourage my patients to avoid off brand sunscreens in favor of well-established branded products.

SUMMARY

It is evident from this discussion that tremendous science, art, chemistry, and testing must be combined to achieve a successful sunscreen product. The UV filters selected must be placed in a stable vehicle that not only creates an even water-resistant film on the skin to maintain the labeled SPF, but also is perceived by the patient as aesthetically pleasing. The best sunscreen formulations combine oil-soluble and water-soluble UV filters that are attracted to both the hydrophobic and hydrophilic areas of the skin to provide maximum coverage. The packaging is selected to maintain the integrity of the sunscreen. Dermatologist should be aware of these factors when considering sunscreen recommendations.

REFERENCES

1. Schueller R, Romanowski P. The ABCs of SPFs. Cosmet Toilet 1999; 114: 49–57.
2. Hewitt JP. Formulating water-resistant titanium dioxide sunscreens. Cosmet Toilet 1999; 114: 59–63.

SUGGESTED READING

Bissett DL, Oelrich DM, Hannon DP. Evaluation of a topical iron chelator in animals and in human beings: short-term photoprotection by 2-furil-dioxime. J Am Acad Dermatol 1994; 31: 572–8.
Cole C. Multicenter evaluation of sunscreen UVA protectiveness with the protection factor test method. J Am Acad Dermatol 1994; 30: 729–36.
Dromgoole SH, Maibach HI. Sunscreening agent intolerance: contact and photocontact sensitization and contact urticaria. J Am Acad Dermatol 1990; 22: 1068–78.
Fisher AA. Sunscreen dermatitis: para-aminobenzoic acid and its derivatives. Cutis 1992; 50: 190–2.
Fisher AA. Sunscreen dermatitis: part IV the salicylates, the anthranilates and physical agents. Cutis 1992; 50: 397–6.
Fisher AA. Sunscreen dermatitis: part II the cinnamates. Cutis 1992; 50: 253–4.
Food and Drug Administration. Sunscreen drug products for over the counter human drugs: proposed safety, effective and labeling conditions. Fed Reg 1978; 43: 38206.
Freeman S, Frederiksen P. Sunscreen allergy. Am J Contact Dermatitis 1990; 1: 240.
Geiter F, Bilek PK, Doskoczil S. History of sunscreens and the rationale for their use. In: Frost P, Horwitz SN, eds. Principles of Cosmetics for the Dermatologist. St. Louis: CV Mosby Company, 1982: 187–206.
Knobler E, Almeida L, Ruzkowski A, et al. Photoallergy to benzophenone. Arch Dermatol 1989; 125: 801–4.
Kollias N, Bager AH. The role of human melanin in providing photoprotection from solar mid-ultravioet radiation (280–320 nm). J Soc Cosm Chem 1988; 39: 347–54.
Lowe NJ. Sun protection factors: comparative techniques and selection of ultraviolet sources. In: Lowe NJ, ed. Physician's Guide to Sunscreens. New York: Marcel Dekker, Inc., 1991: 161–5.
Mathews-Roth MM, Pathak MA, Parrish JA, et al. A clinical trial of the effects of oral beta-carotene on the response of skin to solar radiation. J Invest Dermatol 1972; 59: 349–53.
Mathias CGT, Maibach HI, Epstein J. Allergic contact photodermatitis to para-aminobenzoic acid. Arch Dermatol 1978; 114: 1665–6.
Menter JM. Recent developments in UVA photoprotection. Int J Dermatol 1990; 29: 389–94.
Menz J, Muller SA, Connolly SM. Photopatch testing: a six year experience. J Am Acad Dermatol 1988; 18: 1044–7.
Murphy EG. Regulatory aspects of sunscreens in the United States. In: Lowe NJ, Shaath NA, eds. Sunscreens Development, Evaluation and Regulatory Aspects. New York: Marcel Dekker, Inc., 1990: 127–30.

Ramsay DL, Cohen HS, Baer RL. Allergic reaction to benzopenone. Arch Dermatol 1972; 105: 906–8.

Rietschel RL, Lewis CW. Contact dermatitis to homomenthyl salicylate. Arch Dermatol 1978; 114: 442–3.

Roelandts R. Which components in broad-spectrum sunscreens are most necessary for adequate UVA protection? J Am Acad Dermatol 1991; 25: 999–1004.

Shaath NA. Evolution of modern chemical sunscreens. In: Lowe NJ, Shaath NA, eds. Sunscreens Development, Evaluation and Regulatory Aspects. New York: Marcel Dekker, Inc., 1990: 3–4.

Shaath NA. The chemistry of sunscreens. In: Lowe NJ, Shaath NA, eds. Sunscreens development, evaluation and regulatory aspects. New York: Marcel Dekker, Inc., 1990: 223–5.

Shaath NA. Evolution of modern chemical sunscreens. In: Lowe NJ, Shaath NA, eds. Sunscreens development, evaluation and regulatory aspects. New York: Marcel Dekker, Inc., 1990: 9–12.

Sterling GB. Sunscreens: a review. Cutis 1992; 50: 221–4.

Thompson G, Maibach HI, Epstein J. Allergic contact dermatitis from sunscreen preparations complicating photodermatitis. Arch Dermatol 1977; 113: 1252.

Thune P. Contact and photocontact allergy to sunscreens. Photodermatology 1984; 1: 5–9.

21 Sunless tanning creams

Skin color has always been a source of preoccupation for the human race. There are reports of ancient man using burnt ashes to blacken the skin, Egyptians applying burnt ochre and beetle shells to adorn the face, and American Indians decorating their bodies with vivid pigments. This concept of self-adornment still persists in the form of recreational tanning. The desirability of a tan was popularized by Coco Chanel, who was famous for her Couture Fashions. She conceived the idea of using tanned women in advertisements designed to promote her clothing and perfume. Prior to this time, women had shunned the sun, since tanned skin indicated that a woman performed manual labor outdoors. Society women, who dwelled indoors, used their fair skin color as a sign of class status. With the industrial revolution, more and more women were leaving their jobs in the fields to live in the city and work indoors in factories. These women had little time for recreational sunning. Thus, skin tanning became popular as a sign that northerners were able to vacation in a sunny locale.

Despite the known risks of premature aging and skin cancer associated with tanning, this remains a popular practice. Tanning from natural sun exposure or from artificial tanning booth light poses a health risk that is ignored by many. Since the societal desirability of tanned skin among Caucasians has not decreased, skin care manufacturers have searched for ways of achieving tanned skin without photodamage. Products designed to simulate a tan without sun exposure are known as sunless tanning creams.

Sunless tanning creams utilize dihydroxyacetone (DHA) as the active agent (1). This chemical was originally discovered in the 1920s as a possible substitute for sweetener in diabetic diets by Procter & Gamble, Cincinnati, OH. When the DHA was chewed in concentrated form as a candy, it was noted that the saliva turned the skin brown without staining clothing or the mouth. This side effect made the substance unsuitable as a glucose substitute and DHA was not marketed until the 1950s when the first sunless tanning cream was introduced into the marketplace.

SUNLESS TANNING CREAM FORMULATION
DHA is a 3-carbon sugar that is manufactured as a white, crystalline hygroscopic powder. It interacts with amino acids, peptides, and proteins to form chromophobes known as melanoidins (2). Melanoidins structurally have some similarities to skin melanin (3). The browning reaction that occurs when DHA is exposed to keratin protein is known as the Maillard reaction (4). DHA is technically categorized as a colorant or colorless dye that glycates the protein found in the stratum corneum.

> Dihydroxyacetone (DHA) glycates proteins in the outer stratum corneum to produce a brown stain, known as melanoidins.

DHA is usually added to a creamy base in concentrations of 3–5% (5). Lower concentrations of DHA produce mild tanning while higher concentrations produce greater darkening (6). This allows sunless tanning creams to be formulated in light, medium, and dark shades. The depth of color produced by sunless tanning creams can be enhanced by increasing the protein content of the stratum corneum. This is accomplished by applying a sulfur-containing amino acid, such as methionine sulfoxide, to the skin just before applying the DHA.

As might be expected, skin areas with more protein stain a darker color. For example, keratotic growths such as seborrheic keratoses or actinic keratoses will hyperpigment. Protein-rich areas of the skin, such as the elbows, knees, palms, and soles, also stain more deeply. For this reason, it is advisable to remove all dead skin through exfoliation prior to applying the sunless tanning cream. DHA does not stain the mucous membranes, but will stain the hair and nails.

The chemical reaction is usually visible within one hour after DHA application, but maximal darkening may take 8 to 24 hours (7). Many sunless tanning preparations contain a temporary dye to allow the user to note the sites of application and to promote even application, but this immediate color should not be confused with the Maillard reaction.

Sunless tanning creams have enjoyed a renewed popularity since their original introduction in the 1950s. The original self-tanners produced a somewhat unnatural orange skin color. This problem has been corrected through the use of more purified sources of DHA that yield a more natural golden color. Yet, for persons with pink skin tones, the sunless tanning creams may still appear unnatural.

SUNLESS TANNING AND PHOTOPROTECTION
DHA is a nontoxic ingredient both for ingestion and topical application. It has a proven safety record with only a few reported cases of allergic contact dermatitis (8). Unfortunately, the browning reaction does not produce adequate photoprotection. At most, sunless tanning preparations may impart an SPF of 3 to 4 to the skin for up to one hour after application (9). The photoprotection does not last as long as the artificial tan. The brown color imparts limited photoprotection at the low end of the visible spectrum with overlap into the UVA portion of the spectrum (10). DHA used to be approved as a sun protective agent in combination with lawsone; however, the new sunscreen monograph has removed this ingredient largely due to its lack of popularity.

> Sunless tanning creams confer no photoprotection and must be used with sunscreen when going outdoors.

The staining reaction that occurs with DHA is limited strictly to the stratum corneum and can be readily removed with tape stripping and exfoliation. Thus, the product must be

Table 21.1 Tips for Sunless Tanning Cream Application

1. Bathe the areas for application to eliminate any other creams or sebum from the skin surface. Always start with clean skin
2. Use an abrasive scrub with polyethylene beads to thoroughly exfoliate the skin after bathing
3. Dry the skin thoroughly
4. Apply petroleum jelly to these areas of the body that will overstain with the sunless tanning cream: wrists, back of the neck, ankles, toes, fingers, antecubital fossae, and popliteal fossae
5. Put on disposable gloves to avoid staining the palms
6. Squeeze out of the bottle a small amount of cream and rub evenly between the palms. Rub the palms over the application area. Rub until the cream is evenly distributed to avoid streaking. Apply to one body area at a time working from the arms to the legs
7. Remain still until the cream has thoroughly dried to avoid removal and unintentional application to hair and cloth items
8. Repeat every two weeks or as necessary

reapplied daily to maintain the optimal skin darkening. There are no known side effects, except for possible irritation, from frequent application. The DHA does have a distinct odor, which is difficult to mask with fragrances.

SUNLESS TANNING CREAM APPLICATION

Sunless tanning creams can produce a natural appearing tan if artistically applied. One of the problems is that the cream will stain everything it touches, including the palms of the hands that do not tan with sun exposure. It will also stain hair and clothing. There are several tips summarized in Table 21.1, which can assist in achieving an even application. The key to a good result is aggressive exfoliation of the skin with an abrasive scrubbing cream. These creams contain particulates, such as polyethylene beads, which mechanically remove desquamating corneocytes from the surface. An accumulation of corneocytes will stain the area darker as there is more protein for the DHA to glycate. Gloves should be worn during application. The cream has to be applied in an even thin layer. Less cream should be applied to areas where the skin is hyperkeratotic, such as the wrists, back of the neck, ankles, toes, fingers, antecubital fossae, and popliteal fossae. These areas tend to stain unnaturally darker. The brown stain will last about two weeks until the stained corneocytes have sloughed.

A newer technique of applying sunless tanning cream is known as a spray tan. Spray tans are applied professionally in hair salons, nail salons, and artificial UV tanning booths. The client is placed in a booth naked surrounded by a curtain and the DHA solution is sprayed on the body for a more even application. Petroleum jelly is placed over the easily overstaining

areas mentioned above to more closely simulate a natural tan. Professional application eliminates the mess and odor of at-home application.

SUMMARY

Sunless tanning creams show a safe, cost-effective, efficient manner to obtain temporary skin darkening. They should not be used in place of a sunscreen, however. A natural simulated tan can be achieved by applying the sunless tanning cream evenly to the desired areas. Care should be taken to apply less cream to the easily staining areas, such as the ankles, knees, elbows, and toes. Since a tan remains fashionable in our modern millennium society, sunless tanning creams should be used to stain the skin rather than risking sun exposure that will ultimately result in premature skin aging and skin cancer.

REFERENCES

1. Maibach HI, Kligman AM. Dihydroxyacetone: a sun-tan-simulating agent. Arch Dermatol 1960; 82: 505–7.
2. Wittgenstein E, Berry KH. Reaction of dihydroxyacetone (DHA)jwith human skin callus and amino compounds. J Invest Dermatol 1961; 36: 283–6.
3. Meybeck A. A spectroscopic study of the reaction productsof dihydroxyacetone with aminoacids. J Soc Cosmet Chem 1977; 28: 25–35.
4. Wittgenstein E, Berry KH. Staining of skin with dihydroxyacetone. Science 1960; 132: 894–5.
5. Kurz T. Formulating effective self-tanners with DHA. Cosmet Toilet 1994; 109: 55–61.
6. Maes DH, Marenus KD. Self-tanning products. In: Baran R, Maibach HI, eds. Cosmetic Dermatology. London: Martin Dunitz, 1994.
7. Goldman L, Barkoff J, Glaney D, et al. The skin coloring agent dihydroxyacetone. GP 1960; 12: 96–8.
8. Morren M, Dooms-Goossens A, Heidbuchel M, et al. Contact allergy to dihydroxyacetone. Contact Dermatitis 1991; 25: 326–7.
9. Muizzuddin N, Marenus KD, Maes DH. UVA and UVB protective effect of melanoids formed with dihydroxyacetone and skin. San Francisco: Poster presentation, AAD meeting, 1997.
10. Johnson JA, Fusaro RM. Protecton against long ultraviolet radiation: topical browning agents and a new outlook. Dermatologica 1987; 175: 53–7.

SUGGESTED READING

Chaudhuri RK, Hwang C. Self-Tanners: formulating with Dihydroxyacetone. Cosmet Toilet Magazine 2001; 116: 87–94.
Gonzalez AD, Kalafsky RE. Sunless Tanning and Tanning Accelerators (Chapter 29). In: Shaath N, ed. Sunscreens. 3rd edn. Taylor & Francis Group, 2005: 574–99.
Herman S. Non-Enzymatic Browning: Tan Minus Sun. GCI, 2002: 22–4.
Levy S. Cosmetics that imitate a tan. Dermatol Ther 2001; 14: 1–5.
Levy S. Skin Care Products: Artificial Tanning. In: Paye M, Barel A, Maibach HI, eds. Handbook of Cosmetic Science and Technology. 3rd edn. Informa Healthcare USA, Inc., 2009.
Levy S. Tanning Preparations. Dermatol Clin 2000; 18: 591–6.
Whitmore SE, Morison WL, Potten CS, Chadwick C. Tanning salon exposure and molecular alterations. J Am Acad Dermatol 2001; 44: 775–9.

22 Cellulite

DEFINITION

Cellulite is the most common poorly understood aesthetic condition affecting women worldwide (1). This can be verified by the many names ascribed to this uneven bumpy skin texture appearing on the buttock and thighs (Fig. 22.1), including adiposis edematosa, dermopanniculosis deformans, status protrusus cutis, and gynoid lipodystrophy (2). Under ultrasound visualization, cellulite appears as low-density fat herniations into the denser dermal tissue (3). There are many theories purported to describe the pathophysiology of cellulites, none can be verified however. These theories include dietary influences, genetically determined fat deposition, vascular insufficiency, excess adipose tissue, and chronic inflammation (Table 22.1) (4). Although there are a variety of treatments for cellulite, none of which can permanently erase the unattractive dimpled skin. Yet, a sizeable number of cosmetic products can be purchased, which promise a smoother skin. This chapter is presented largely for informational purposes to assist the dermatologist in discussing cellulite with patients.

DIETARY INFLUENCES

The theory that diet contributes to the pathophysiology of cellulite has been popularized by the consumer press. Articles abound stating that a low carbohydrate, low fat, low salt, high fiber diet can minimize cellulite. A controlled medical study to verify the effect of diet on cellulite minimization has never been conducted; however, a low calorie diet, which might be low in high calorie carbohydrates and fats, may decrease adipose tissue and improve cellulite (5). Low salt, high fiber diets may indeed decrease extracellular fluid volume thus minimizing vascular effects.

When considering how diet affects the pathophysiology of cellulite, it is interesting to look at how cultural eating habits may contribute. Cellulite is more commonly seen in Caucasian women than Oriental women. It is true that visualization of skin texture irregularities is easier in fair skin, yet Oriental women seem to demonstrate less cellulite. One theory regarding the pathophysiology of cellulite is the effect of diet on circulating estrogens. The consumption of cow's milk in the Orientals is low; however, much of the milk consumed in the U.S.A. contains estrogens that enter the milk from the food fed to the cows. Another possible explanation is reduced endogenous estrogen production in Oriental women who consume large amounts of fermented soy in the form of tofu or soy nuts. Fermented soy is high in phytoestrogens, which may suppress adrenal and ovarian estrogen production, which is not the case with the estrogens ingested in cow's milk.

Thus, one explanation for cellulite is a poor diet leading to the deposition of excess fat, fluid retention, and a high circulating estrogen level (6). Another theory is that cellulite is present due to predetermined genetic influences.

GENETICALLY DETERMINED FAT DEPOSITION

Many researchers believe that the pattern of adipose deposit that leads to cellulite is genetically determined (7). Thus, women will age and deposit fat in the same areas as their mother regardless of diet or estrogen stimulation (8). This may be due to a hormone receptor allele that determines the receptor number and sensitivity to estrogen. This may determine the distribution of subcutaneous fat. Pierard espoused this theory noting that cellulite is not a result of increase body mass, but rather can be influenced by the inherited waist-to-hip ratio (9).

VASCULAR INSUFFICIENCY

One of the most widely held theories about the pathophysiology of cellulite is the effect of vascular insufficiency. Smith postulates that cellulite is a degradation process initiated by the deterioration of the dermal vasculature, particularly loss of the capillary networks (10). As a result, excess fluid is retained with the dermal and subcutaneous tissues (11). This loss of the capillary network is thought to be due to engorged fat cells clumping together and inhibiting the venous return (12).

After the capillary networks have been damaged, vascular changes begin to occur within the dermis resulting in decreased protein synthesis and an inability to repair tissue damage. Clumps of protein are deposited around the fatty deposits beneath the skin causing an "orange peel" appearance to the skin as it is pinched between the thumb and forefinger. At this stage, however, there is no visual evidence of cellulite.

The characteristic appearance of cellulite is only seen after hard nodules composed of fat surrounded by hard reticular protein form within the dermis. Ultrasound imaging of skin affected by cellulite at this stage reveals thinning of the dermis with subcutaneous fat pushing upward, which translates into the rumpled skin known as cellulite.

Thus, this theory holds that hormonally mediated fat deposition, fat lobule compression of capillary vasculature, decreased venous return, formation of clumped fat lobules, and deposition of protein substances around clumped fat lobules lead to the appearance of cellulite.

EXCESS ADIPOSE TISSUE

Some investigators have observed that cellulite is more common in overweight and obese women. This was felt to be due to the presence of copious fat lobules within the subcutaneous tissue encased in fibrous septae with dermal attachments (13) (Fig. 22.2). These fibrous attachments surrounding abundant fat lead to the rumpled appearance of the skin characteristic of cellulite (14). Thus, weight loss, which reduces the size of the fat lobules and removes the metabolic influences of excess adiposity, improves the appearance of cellulite (15). Improvement can also be achieved with exercise, since improved muscle tone creates a better foundation to support the overlying fat.

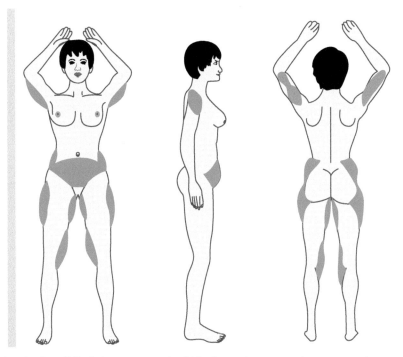

Figure 22.1 The most common location for cellulite is the upper posterior thighs. It may also occur on the upper posterior arms, buttocks, and anterior thighs.

Table 22.1 Cellulite Pathophysiology Controversy

Cellulite theory	Pros	Cons
Dietary influences	Oriental women who consume phytoestrogens in soy exhibit less cellulite	80% of women worldwide exhibit cellulite regardless of diet
Genetically determined fat deposition	Daughters of mothers with cellulite are also likely to exhibit cellulite	Cellulite can be minimized by less body fat, which is self-determined
Vascular insufficiency	Deterioration of dermal vasculature results in increased fluid retention and cellulite appearance	Ultrasound imaging of cellulite shows adipose tissue impinging on dermis, not only fluid
Excess adipose tissue	Women with more body fat tend to exhibit more cellulite	Weight loss does not eliminate cellulite
Chronic inflammation	Inflammation from collagenase breaks down dermal collagen allowing for adipose herniations	Not all menstruating women exhibit cellulite to the same degree

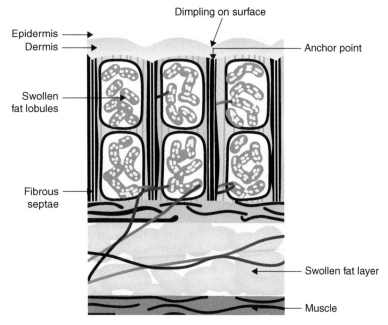

Figure 22.2 Shrinking of the fibrous septae has been argued to result in the dimpling of the skin characteristic of cellulite.

CHRONIC INFLAMMATION

The final theory espouses that cellulite is an inflammatory process resulting in the breakdown of the collagen in the dermis providing for the subcutaneous fat herniations seen on ultrasound (Fig. 22.3). The onset of cellulite with puberty and menstruation has caused some researchers to evaluate the hormonal changes necessary for sloughing of the endometrium (16). It appears that menstruation requires the secretion of metalloproteases, (MMP) such as collagenase (collagenase-1, MMP-1) and gelatinase (gelatinase A, MMP-2) (17). The endometrial glandular and stromal cells secrete these enzymes to allow menstrual bleeding to occur. Collagenases cleave the triple helical domain of fibrillar collagens at a neutral pH and are secreted just prior to menstruation. However, the collagenase may break down the fibrillar collagens present not only in the endometrium but in the dermis also.

Furthermore, gelatinase B is produced by stromal cells or mast cells during the late proliferative endometrial phase and just after ovulation. Gelatinase B is associated with an influx of polymorphonuclear leukocytes, macrophages, and eosinophils, which also contribute to inflammation (18). A marker for this inflammation is the synthesis of dermal glycosaminoglycans, which enhance water binding further worsening the appearance of the cellulite through swelling. The presence of these glycosaminoglycans has been observed on ultrasound as low-density echoes at the lower dermal/subcutaneous junction (19).

The secretion of endometrial collagenase to initiate menstruation also provides for collagen breakdown in the dermis (20). With repeated cyclic collagenase production, more and more dermal collagen is destroyed accounting for the worsening of cellulite seen with age. Eventually, enough collagen is destroyed to weaken the reticular and papillary dermis and allow subcutaneous fat to herniate between the structural fibrous septa found in female fat. Obviously, if more subcutaneous fat is present, more pronounced herniation can occur.

CELLULITE TREATMENTS

A variety of cellulite treatments are available for consumer purchase. None of them can completely resolve cellulite, but a discussion of the options is useful to better understand how to scientifically discuss cellulite with inquiring patients. Presently marketed over-the-counter (OTC) treatments include topical herbals, wraps, devices, massage, and oral supplements, which are discussed next. Surgical and laser interventions are beyond the scope of this cosmetic text.

Topical Herbals

Topical herbals are placed in creams designed to improve the appearance of cellulite in the OTC market. They can only claim to improve the appearance of cellulite or they would be classified as drugs. It is very challenging for any topical agent to reach the subcutaneous tissue as it must be both water- and fat-soluble to traverse the skin and then affect the adipocyte. Herbals such as caffeine, theophylline, and coleus forskohlii are found in moisturizing cellulite creams to stimulate the breakdown of the lipids into triglycerides. Most of these creams make claims of skin smoothness and softness based on their ability to moisturize the skin, not reduce cellulite.

> Herbals such as caffeine, theophylline, and coleus forskohlii are found in moisturizing cellulite creams.

Wraps

Wraps are used for cellulite at home, in spas, and in body slimming franchise businesses to reduce the appearance of cellulite. Cloth strips are impregnated with herbal solutions and wrapped around the legs, buttocks, or any other area exhibiting cellulite. Sometimes the wraps are warmed and sometimes the wrap environment is set to a high temperature to encourage sweating for "fat detoxification" treatment. Herbs that are used in the wraps include gotu kola, Paraguay tea, coleus forskohlii, and fennel. Again, it is doubtful that these herbs can actually reach the subcutaneous tissue. In some cases, the tight wrap may reduce the extracellular fluid in the leg to minimize cellulite, and weight loss may be seen due to sweating. It is doubtful that the wrap has any permanent effect and even spas state that weekly sessions are necessary to maintain any result.

Devices

Several OTC devices have been purported to improve the appearance of cellulite. These devices usually manipulate the skin by suction, rolling, and/or pressure. The suction devices draw up the skin and claim to "break up" the cellulite as if the lumps were due to something that could be crushed. Sometimes the suction is combined with rolling and pressure. If extracellular fluid is present due to poor venous return in the legs, removal of this fluid can improve the appearance of cellulite. Support stockings or reclining has much the same effect. Of course, the effect is temporary unless something is done to prevent fluid reaccumulation. These devices attempt to mimic the effect of massage, which is discussed next.

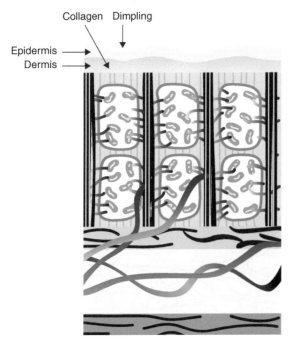

Figure 22.3 Chronic inflammation leading to degrading of collagen is another theory proposed for the development of cellulite.

Massage

One common method adopted by aestheticians for improving cellulite is massage. Deep venous massage can remove extracellular fluid and improve lymphatic drainage. Sometimes herbals that produce vasoconstriction, such as wild horse chestnut, is used in the massage cream as "circulation enhancers" and said to have "venotonic" effects. Massage can be relaxing and enjoyable, but 20 mmHg or higher compression support stockings produce the same effect.

> Massage can improve lymphatic drainage and temporarily improve the appearance of cellulite.

ORAL SUPPLEMENTS

The recent market has seen the introduction of oral supplements for cellulite, some of which have been challenged by consumer groups for false advertising claims. Cellulite claims are always very carefully worded so as not to promise too much. One category of compounds found in oral cellulite supplements are xanthines. Xanthines are found in foods containing caffeine, such as coffee, tea, and chocolate. Xanthines inhibit phosphodiesterase, which destroys cAMP and stimulates lipolysis. The lipolysis is thought to decrease cellulite. The most effective xanthine is aminophylline, but no reduction in cellulite has been noticed in persons taking this drug for respiratory disease.

Another oral supplement for cellulite contains bioflavonoids, such as proanthocyanidins, which are derived from berries and extensively studied in animals as caloric restriction mimetics and as potent antioxidants. In mice, proanthocyanidins have been shown to reduce the breakdown of collagen and elastin, possibly through modulation of collagenase and elastase. This has not been demonstrated in humans.

> Xanthines and proanthocyanidins are found in some oral cellulite supplements.

SUMMARY

The etiology of cellulite is still unknown and the efficacy of cellulite treatments is highly controversial. Perhaps if the pathophysiology were understood, more effective treatments could be developed. It is most likely that cellulite is due to a combination of all the factors discussed including hormones, genetics, adipose tissue, microcirculation, and chronic inflammation. It cannot be denied that cellulite is a widespread human condition more commonly observed in women that worsens with advancing age and may even represent part of normal human anatomy. Only prepubertal women are without cellulite. Patients frequently ask for cellulite treatments and it is unfortunate that we have little to offer in dermatology.

REFERENCES

1. Nurnberger F, Muller G. So-called cellulite: an invented disease. J Dermatol Surg Oncol 1978; 4: 221–9.
2. Dahl PR, Salla MJ, Winkelmann RK. Localized involutional lipoatrophy: a clinicopathologic study of 16 patients. J Am Acad Dermatol 1996; 35: 523–8.
3. Mirrashed F, Sharp JC, Krause V, Morgan J, Tomanek B. Pilot study of dermal and subcutaneous fat structures by MRI in individuals who differ in gender, BMI, and cellulite grading. Skin Res Technol 2004; 10: 161–8.
4. Avram MM. Cellulite: a review of its physiology and treatment. J Cosmet Laser Ther 2004; 6: 181–5.
5. Rawlings AV. Cellulite and its treatment. Int J Cosmet Sci 2006; 28: 175–90.
6. Draelos ZD, Marenus KD. Cellulite-etiology and purported treatment. Dermatol Surg 1997; 23: 1177–81.
7. Scherwitz C, Braun-Falco O. So-called cellulite. J Dermatol Surg Oncol 1978; 4: 230–4.
8. Ortonne JP, Zartarian M, Verschoore M, Queille-Roussel C, Duteil L. Cellulite and skin ageing: is there any interaction? J Eur Acad Dermatol Venereol 2008; 22: 827–34.
9. Pierard GE. Commentary on cellulite: skin mechanobiology and the waist-to-hip ration. J Cosmet Dermatitis 2005; 4: 151–2.
10. Smith WF. Cellulite treatments: snake oil or skin science. Cosmet Toilet 1995; 110: 61–70.
11. Curri SB. Cellulite and fatty tissue microcirculation. Cosmet Toilet 1993; 108: 51–8.
12. Curri SB, Bombardelli E. Local lipodystrophy and districtual microcirculation. Cosmet Toilet 1994; 109: 51–65.
13. Quatresooz P, Xhauflaire-Uhoda E, Pierard-Franchimont C, Pierard GE. Cellulite histopathology and related mechanobiology. Int. J Cosmet Sci 2006; 28: 207–10.
14. Pierard GE, Nizet JL, Pierard-Franchimont C. Cellulite: from standing fat herniation to hypodermal stretch marks. Am J Dermatolpathol 2000; 22: 34–7.
15. Terranova F, Berardesca E, Maibach H. Cellulite: nature and aetiopathogenesis. Int J Cosmet Sci 2006; 28: 157–67.
16. Marbaix E, Kokorine I, Henriet P, et al. The expresssion of interstitial collagenase in human endometrium is controlled by progesterone and by oestadiol and is related to menstruation. Biochem J 1995; 305: 1027–30.
17. Singer CF, Marbaix E, Lemoine P, Courtoy PJ, Eeckhout Y. Local cytokines induce differrential expression of matrix metalloproteinases but not their tissue inhibitors in human endometrial fibroblasts. Eur J Biochem 1999; 259: 40–5.
18. Jeziorska M, Nagasae H, Salamonsen LA, Woolley DE. Immunolocalization of the matrix metalloproteinases gelatinase B and stromelysin 1 in juman endometrium throughout the menstrual cycle. J Reprod Fertil 1996; 107: 43–51.
19. Lotti T, Ghersetich MD, Grappone C, Dini G. Proteoglycans in so-called cellulite. Int J Dermatol 1990; 29: 272–4.
20. Marbaix E, Kokorine I, Donnez J, Eeckhout Y, Courtoy PJ. Regulation and restricted expression of interstitial collagenase suggest a pivotal role in the initiation of menstruation. Hum Reprod 1996; 11 (Suppl 2): 134–43.

23 Stretch marks

Perhaps the biggest challenge for dermatologists is discussing the presence of stretch marks with a recently pubertal female. It is disappointing for both the patient and her parents to see the presence of stretch marks, medically known as striae distensae, on the breasts, abdomen, hips, and thighs (1). Stretch marks may appear due to the rapid hormonal changes and growth associated with puberty, during pregnancy, or with medical diseases, such as Cushing's syndrome. Under the microscope, they appear as dermal atrophy accompanied by loss of the rete ridges, a finding similar to scar tissue. No curative treatment has been developed; however, moisturizers, massage, microdermabrasion, and laser resurfacing may improve their appearance.

> Histologically stretch marks appear as areas of dermal atrophy accompanied by loss of the rete ridges, a finding similar to scar tissue.

CAUSES OF STRETCH MARKS
Stretch marks may occur during various phases of life, but may be related to increased cortisol secretion or increased body mass. The most common cause of stretch marks is pregnancy, when the stretch marks are medically known as striae gravidarum. It is thought that the rapid growth of the baby may play a role, but not all pregnancies produce stretch marks. A relationship between pregnancy, obesity, and increased stretch marks has been reported (2). In obesity, it is thought that the stretching of the skin with weight gain causes the scars, but stretch marks have also been observed in persons who experience a rapid increase in muscle mass with weight lifting (3). Some medications, such as internal corticosteroids, may also produce stretch marks.

> Increased stretch marks are related to pregnancy and obesity.

STRETCH MARKS: SIGNS AND SYMPTOMS
Stretch marks do not generally produce any symptoms, but have a characteristic visual appearance no matter when they appear or what causes them. They initially appear as raised, pink to purple lines longitudinally arranged over the abdomen, lateral upper thighs, inner arms, or upper breasts. With time, the purplish-pink color lightens and they appear as silvery lines on the skin, similar to a scar. The purplish-pink scars are termed striae rubra, while the silvery lines are termed striae alba. Stretch marks can also occur in dark-complected persons where they appear as dark brown lines, in which case they are termed striae nigra (4). In short, stretch marks are scars that are permanent once formed (5).

STRETCH MARKS: TREATMENTS
The treatment for stretch marks is limited (6). The most invasive therapies for stretch marks involve a physician-administered laser surgery. Improvement in stretch marks with laser therapy is accomplished by wounding the scarred skin and hoping that the newly healed skin will have a more normal cosmetically acceptable appearance (7). Medical reports of Nd:YAG laser (8), radiofrequency devices (9), and fractional photothermolysis (10,11) have shown some degree of stretch mark appearance improvement, but not resolution.

The earlier the stretch mark is treated, generally the better the result. Red immature stretch marks are more amenable to treatment than those that have matured to a silvery white. This is because the reddish stretch marks are still healing and the healing can be modified by intervention. Sometimes camouflage is the best option for treatment to hide the scars (12).

A spa treatment for stretch marks is the use of microdermabrasion. Microdermabrasion uses a spray head to bombard the skin with tiny salt, baking soda, or aluminum particles to exfoliate the skin and smooth stretch marks possibly encouraging collagen production through mild wounding. While microdermabrasion can temporarily smooth the skin surface, it cannot remove the stretch mark.

A variety of products can be purchased over-the-counter for improving the appearance of stretch marks. There are anecdotal stories of cocoa butter, emu oil, vitamin E, onion extract, and other oils aiding in the prevention and treatment of stretch marks. The most common dermatologist-recommended treatment for scars, such as stretch marks, is massage. Massaging the skin in a circular motion with oil using the fingers to reduce friction is helpful in stretching the skin collagen and elastin, making it more pliable and more normal appearing.

> Topical moisturizers for stretch marks contain ingredients such as cocoa butter, emu oil, vitamin E, and/or onion extract.

The prevention of stretch marks is challenging. It appears that stretch marks do not occur when the stretching of the skin is gradual rather than abrupt. Thus, rapid changes in body size should be avoided, if possible. Since stretch marks represent small scars, the rapid growth of the body can result in more stretch marks while slower changes in body size may allow the skin to adjust more gradually. Persons with a better skin elasticity and less rigid collagen are less likely to develop stretch marks, but it is not possible to modify these skin characteristics at present (13). The presence of stretch marks during pregnancy has been associated with pelvic relaxation resulting in prolapse of the pelvic organs with advancing age (14). Other medical associations, outside of endocrinologic disease, have not been demonstrated. In summary, stretch marks remain a treatment enigma.

REFERENCES

1. Salter SA, Kimball AB. Striae gravidarum. Clin Dermatol 2006; 24: 97–100.

2. Thomas RG, Liston WA. Clinical associations of striae gravidarum. J Obstet Gynaecol 2004; 24: 270–1.

3. García Hidalgo L. Dermatological complications of obesity. Am J Clin Dermatol 2002; 3: 497–506.

4. Piérard-Franchimont C, Hermanns JF, Hermanns-Lê T, Piérard GE. Striae distensae in darker skin types: the influence of melanocyte mechanobiology. J Cosmet Dermatol 2005; 4: 174–8.

5. Zheng P, Lavker RM, Kligman AM. Anatomy of striae. Br J Dermatol 1985; 112: 185–93.

6. Elsaie ML, Baumann LS, Elsaaiee LT. Striae distensae (stretch marks) and different modalities of therapy: an update. Dermatol Surg 2009; 35: 563–73.

7. McDaniel DH. Laser therapy of stretch marks. Dermatol Clin 2002; 20: 67–76, viii.

8. Goldman A, Rossato F, Prati C. Stretch marks: treatment using the 1,064-nm Nd:YAG laser. Dermatol Surg 2008; 34: 686–91; discussion 691–2.

9. Manuskiatti W, Boonthaweeyuwat E, Varothai S. Treatment of striae distensae with a TriPollar radiofrequency device: a pilot study. J Dermatolog Treat 2009: 1–6.

10. Bak H, Kim BJ, Lee WJ, et al. Treatment of striae distensae with fractional photothermolysis. Dermatol Surg 2009; 35: 1215–20.

11. Stotland M, Chapas AM, Brightman L, et al. The safety and efficacy of fractional photothermolysis for the correction of striae distensae. J Drugs Dermatol 2008; 7: 857–61.

12. Tedeschi A, Dall'Oglio F, Micali G, Schwartz RA, Janniger CK. Corrective camouflage in pediatric dermatology. Cutis 2007; 79: 110–12.

13. Shuster S. The cause of striae distensae. Acta Derm Venereol Suppl (Stockh) 1979; 59: 161–9.

14. Watson RE. Stretching the point: an association between the occurrence of striae and pelvic relaxation? J Invest Dermatol 2006; 126: 1688–9.

III Hair: Introduction

Hair is believed to serve no current physiological function in humans, but it is of considerable appearance and social concern. Hair washing, grooming, styling, coloring, waving, and straightening are the focus of consideration attention requiring the dedication of considerable financial resources. Both men and women desire a full head of perfectly coifed hair complying with all the current fashion ideals. Hair is a nonverbal indication of our gender, health, style, and self-obsession. A great head of shiny long hair is synonymous with health, as hair is one of the first structures lost with illness or chemotherapy administration. A face full of dirty stringy hair may be the first indication of a disturbed youth. A woman who is constantly pulling, primping, and grooming her hair in front of every mirror may be the first indication of insecurity or emotional instability. Yes, hair says a lot about who we are and what we aspire to be.

Hair is a fibrous protein structure that consists of at least three different proteins. The basic structure of the hair arises from a series of six concentric rings in the hair bulb, which arise from a single stem cell group called the matrix of the hair bulb. The three major structures of the hair relevant to hair cosmetics are the medulla, the cortex, and the cuticle (Fig. III.1). Permanent hair dyes, hair straightening, and permanent hair waving affect the medulla and the cortex while all hair grooming procedures affect the cuticle. Beautiful hair is defined as hair with an intact cuticle, making the cuticle the most important structure in hair cosmetics.

The cuticle provides strength to the hair shaft and is lost with aggressive grooming and chemical hair processing. Loss of the cuticle is inevitable over time and this process is known as weathering. When the cuticle is lost, the fragile cortex is exposed. Exposure of the weak cortex leads to splitting of the hair, especially at the ends of the hair shaft, which is commonly known as a split end. The function of the medulla in the hair is unknown and not all hairs possess a medulla. With advancing age, the medulla is lost from the hair.

Hair grows at varying rates in different regions of the body. Scalp hair grows about 0.37 mm a day making it the fastest growing hair on the body. In women, hair on the scalp grows faster than in men, but men have faster growing body hair. An individual hair grows for a period of about three years in the anagen phase before entering the catagen phase and finally falling out and entering the telogen phase (Fig. III.2). The length of time the hair remains in the growth phase determines how long a person can grow their hair. People who have hairs that remain in anagen longer than five years can grow hair below their waist, while people who have hairs that remain in anagen only two years can only grow shoulder length hair or less. About 100–150 hairs a day are shed asynchronously accounting for the replacement of shed hairs in telogen being replaced with growing hairs in anagen. Without this cyclic loss and regrowth of hair, humans would be bald every three years.

This section of the book examines all the cosmetic procedures used to modify the hair appearance according to personal

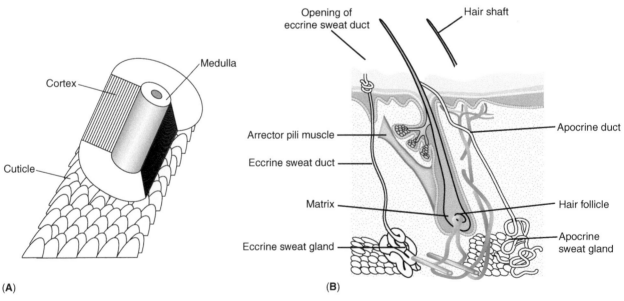

Figure III.1 (**A**) The layers of the hair shaft. (**B**) The structures of the hair unit.

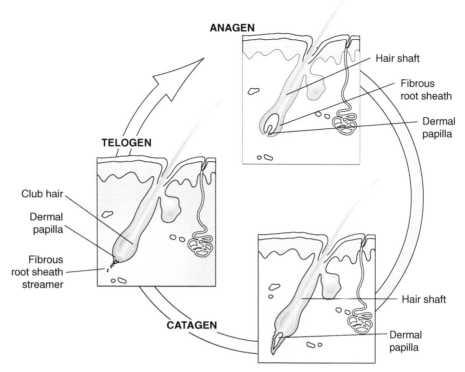

Figure III.2 The hair cycle through anagen (active growth phase), catagen (transitional phase), and telogen (resting phase).

grooming desires. It explores shampoos and conditioners to maintain scalp hygiene and beautify the hair. It examines chemical processing resulting in color and shape changes to the hair shaft. It discusses hair removal techniques and evaluates the use of hair cosmetics in common scalp diseases. Even though the hair is a useless nonliving structure, patients frequently visit the dermatologist requesting hair care advice. It is hoped that this section will provide ideas for dealing with the challenges posed by patients looking for assistance in obtaining that great looking head of hair.

24 Shampoos for hair health

Shampoo is a specialized cleanser designed to beautify the hair and to either treat or prevent scalp disease. While this sounds like a simple task, the average woman has 4 to 8 m² of hair surface area to clean (1). Shampoos are intended to remove sebum, sweat components, desquamated stratum corneum, styling products, and environmental dirt deposited on the hair and to maintain scalp health (2). It is very easy to formulate a shampoo that will remove sebum and dirt to ensure scalp health, but studies have shown that consumers do not favor a shampoo that only cleans efficiently without beautifying the hair. Hair that has been thoroughly cleaned and is devoid of sebum is dull in appearance, coarse to touch, subject to static electricity, and more difficult to style. Therefore, consumers want a shampoo that cleans the scalp, but also beautifies the hair, which is a formulation challenge. This challenge is not optimally met by any one shampoo, which has led to the tremendous variety of shampoo formulations on the market for various hair types and amounts of sebum production.

Shampoo is a relatively new concoction, as the bar soap was used to clean the hair and scalp until the middle 1930s. Bar soap was an unsatisfactory hair cleanser since hard water in combination with soap formed a nonrinsable scum that dulled the hair and irritated the scalp. Early shampoo formulations were liquid coconut oil soaps that lathered and rinsed better than bar soap, but shampoos really came of age with the development of synthetic detergents (3). This chapter examines shampoos and their appropriateness for the various therapeutic requirements of the dermatologist.

FORMULATION

Shampoos are a complex formulation containing detergents, foaming agents, conditioners, thickeners, opacifiers, softeners, sequestering agents, fragrances, preservatives, and specialty additives (4). These ingredients and their function are summarized in Table 24.1. Detergents are the primary sebum and dirt removal shampoo components; however, excessive removal of sebum leaves the hair dull, susceptible to static electricity and difficult to comb. Furthermore, consumers equate cleansing ability with foaming ability thus demanding shampoos that produce abundant, long-lasting foam. Excessive bubbles are not a technical requirement for good hair cleansing and bacteria removal, but shampoo manufacturers add increased amounts of detergents, in addition to foam boosters, to obtain the foam that consumers desire (Fig. 24.1). This increased concentration of detergent creates the need for conditioners and other additives in shampoos to improve their cosmetic acceptability.

> Shampoos are a complex formulation which contain detergents, foaming agents, conditioners, thickeners, opacifiers, softeners, sequestering agents, fragrances, preservatives, and specialty additives.

Our discussion now turns to an evaluation of each of the shampoo ingredients to better understand how shampoos can be formulated to assist in the maintenance of scalp health and the improvement of scalp disease.

Shampoo Detergents

Shampoos function by employing detergents, also known as surfactants, which are able to bind both oil-soluble dirt and water. The oil-soluble dirt binds to the detergent that is then washed down the drain with water. Cleansing occurs when the oil-soluble, or lipophilic, sebum and oily hair care products bind to the detergent while the water soluble, or hydrophilic, styling products and environmental dirt are removed during the rinse phase along with the emulsified oils. Thus, detergents are amphiphilic substances that can emulsify oils into water (5). A tremendous variety in detergents is available to the cosmetic chemist formulating a shampoo (Table 24.2), including those listed in Table 24.3 (6), which are the most common detergents in use today.

> Shampoo detergents can be chemically characterized as anionics, cationics, amphoterics, nonionics, and natural surfactants.

Shampoo detergents can be chemically characterized as anionics, cationics, amphoterics, nonionics, and natural surfactants (Table 24.4). Anionic detergents are named for their negatively charged hydrophilic polar group. The commonly used anionics are fatty alcohols that clean well, but may leave the hair harsh (7). There are several detergents contained within the anionic group:

1. Lauryl sulfates (sodium lauryl sulfate, triethanolamine lauryl sulfate, ammonium lauryl sulfate) are found in most shampoos as the main surfactant since they work well in both hard and soft water, produce rich foam, and are easy to remove. This group produces good cleansing but is hard on the hair.
2. Laureth sulfates (sodium laureth sulfate, triethanolamine laureth sulfate, ammonium laureth sulfate) produce rich foam, provide good cleansing, and leave hair in good condition. They also are a common main surfactant.
3. Sarcosines (lauryl sarcosine, sodium lauryl sarcosinate) are poor cleansers but are excellent conditioners. This group is commonly used as a secondary surfactant.
4. Sulfosuccinates (disodium oleamine sulfosuccinate, sodium dioctyl sulfosuccinate) are strong degreasers and commonly used as a secondary surfactant in oily hair shampoos.

Table 24.1 Basic Shampoo Ingredient Formulation and Function

Ingredient formulation	Function
Detergents	Remove environment dirt, styling products, sebum, and skin scale from the hair and scalp
Foaming agents	Allow the shampoo to suds, since consumers equate cleansing with foaming even though the two are unrelated
Conditioners	Leave the hair soft and smooth after sebum removal by the detergent
Thickeners	Thicken the shampoo, since consumers feel that a thick shampoo works better than a thin shampoo
Opacifiers	Make a shampoo opaque as opposed to translucent for aesthetic purposes, unrelated to cleansing
Sequestering agents	Prevent soap scum from forming on the hair and scalp in the presence of hard water. The basic difference between a liquid shampoo and a bar cleanser
Fragrances	Give the shampoo a consumer acceptable smell
Preservatives	Prevent microbial and fungal contamination of the shampoo before and after opening
Specialty additives	Treatment ingredients or marketing aids added to impart other benefits to the shampoo besides hair and scalp cleansing

Table 24.2 Shampoo Detergents by Chemical Category

1. Alkyl sulfates
2. Alkyl ether sulfates
3. Alpha-olefin sulfonates
4. Paraffin sulfonates
5. Isethionates
6. Sarcosinates
7. Taurides
8. Acyl lactylates
9. Sulfosuccinates
10. Carboxylates
11. Protein condensates
12. Betaines
13. Glycinates
14. Amine oxides

Table 24.3 The Most Common Shampoo Detergents

1. Sodium laureth sulfate
2. Sodium lauryl sulfate
3. TEA lauryl sulfate
4. Ammonium laureth sulfate
5. Ammonium lauryl sulfate
6. DEA lauryl sulfate
7. Sodium olefin sulfonate

Table 24.4 Shampoo Detergent Characteristics

Surfactant type	Chemical class	Characteristics
Anionics	Lauryl sulfates, laureth sulfates, sarcosines, sulfosuccinates	Deep cleansing, may leave hair harsh
Cationics	Long chain amino esters, ammonioesters	Poor cleansing, poor lather, impart softness and manageability
Nonionics	Polyoxyethylene fatty alcohols, polyoxyethylene sorbitol esters, alkanolamides	Mildest cleansing, impart manageability
Amphoterics	Betaines, sultaines, imidazolinium derivatives	Nonirritating to eyes, mild cleansing, impart manageability
Natural surfactants	Sarsaparilla, soapwort, soap bark, ivy, agave	Poor cleansing, excellent lather

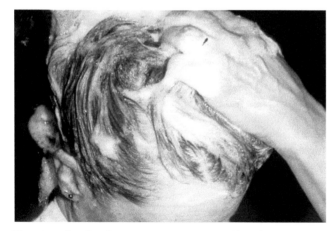

Figure 24.1 Abundant foam is not necessary for good hair cleansing, but is a consumer requirement.

The cationic detergents are named for their positively charged polar group. They are relatively poor detergents and do not lather well, but their unpopularity is largely due to their incompatibility with other anionic surfactants. Some shampoos designed for dyed or bleached hair use cationic detergents, as they are excellent at imparting softness and manageability (1).

Shampoos designed for dyed or bleached hair use cationic detergents because they impart hair softness and manageability.

The nonionic detergents are the second most popular and have no polar group. These are the mildest of all surfactants and are used in combination with ionic surfactants as a secondary cleanser (8). Examples include polyoxyethylene fatty alcohols, polyoxyethylene sorbitol esters, and alkanolamides.

The amphoteric detergents contain both an anionic and a cationic group such that they behave as cationics at lower pH values and anionics at higher pH values. The detergents that fall within this group are the betaines, sultaines. and imidazolinium derivatives. Ingredients such as cocamidopropyl betaine and sodium lauraminopropionate can be found in baby shampoos since they are nonirritating to the eyes. These surfactants foam moderately well and leave the hair manageable, making them a good choice for chemically treated and fine hair.

The last group of detergents is the natural surfactants, such as sarsaparilla, soapwort, soap bark, and ivy agave. These natural saponins have excellent lathering capabilities, but are poor cleansers, thus must be present at high concentration. Usually, they are combined with the other synthetic detergents outlined above (5).

Foaming Agents

Foaming agents in shampoos introduce gas bubbles into the water. Many consumers believe that shampoos that generate copious foam are better cleansers than poorly foaming shampoos. This is not true. As the shampoo removes sebum from the hair, the amount of foam will decrease because sebum inhibits bubble formation. This accounts for the increased foam seen on the second shampooing, when the majority of the sebum has been removed.

> As the shampoo removes sebum from the hair, the amount of foam will decrease because sebum inhibits bubble formation.

Thickeners and Opacifiers

Thickeners and opacifiers have no part in hair cleansing; they simply make the product more appealing to the consumer. Many people incorrectly believe that a thick shampoo is more concentrated than a thin shampoo; others want a shampoo that appears opaque or pearlescent.

Conditioners

Conditioners impart manageability, gloss, and antistatic properties to the hair. They are found in most shampoos for dry, damaged, or treated hair. These are usually fatty alcohols, fatty esters, vegetable oils, mineral oils, or humectants. Many conditioners are used in dry hair shampoos, including hydrolyzed animal protein, glycerin, dimethicone, simethicone, polyvinylpyrrolidone, propylene glycol, and stearalkonium chloride (9). Other protein sources, such as lanolin, beer and egg yolk, containing lecithin and cholesterol, are also used in dry hair shampoos that claim to be "natural." Of all these conditioners, hydrolyzed animal protein is probably the best for extremely dry hair since it has some substantivity for keratin and can mend split ends (trichoptilosis) (10).

Sequestering Agents

Sequestering agents make shampoos function better than bar soaps in cleansing the hair. They chelate magnesium and calcium ions so that other salts or insoluble soaps known as "scum" are not formed. Without sequestering agents, shampoos would leave a film on the hair rendering it dull. For this

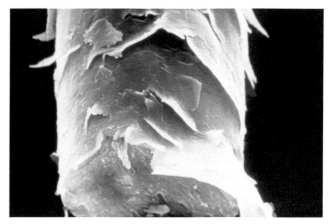

Figure 24.2 High pH results in cuticle swelling and excessive hair damage, thus most shampoos are formulated at a slightly acidic pH.

reason, patients should be encouraged to use shampoo and not bar soap when cleansing the hair. In areas of extremely hard water, the film that remains may contribute to scalp pruritus.

> Sequestering agents are the major difference between a shampoo and a bar soap, and function to prevent soap scum from adhering to the hair shafts.

pH Adjusters

Some shampoos contain ingredients designed to alter pH allowing the marketing claim of "pH balanced." Most shampoos are alkaline, which can swell the hair shaft and render it more susceptible to damage. This is not a problem for patients with healthy, nonporous hair containing an intact cuticle. Patients with damaged or chemically treated hair with a fragmented cuticle may wish to avoid hair swelling by selecting a shampoo that has an acid added to balance the pH (Fig. 24.2).

Specialty Additives

The key differences between similar purpose shampoos manufactured by various personal care product companies are the fragrance and special care additives. Additives such as wheat germ oil (containing vitamin E) and panthenol (a form of vitamin B) are added mainly for marketing reasons but are thought to leave hair more silky and manageable. Other producers add fatty substances such as plant extracts or mink oil. Proteins such as ribonucleic acid, collagen, and placenta may be added to act somewhat as conditioners. Some shampoos now include a chemical sunscreen.

TYPES OF SHAMPOO

Shampoos have been formulated in liquids, gels, creams, aerosols, and powders. Only the liquids will be discussed, as these are the most popular. A number of different types of shampoos are also available: basic shampoos (normal, dry, oily, and chemically treated hair shampoos), baby shampoos, conditioning shampoos, medicated shampoos, and professional shampoos.

Basic Shampoos

Basic shampoos may be selected from several formulations depending on the amount of scalp sebum production, hair shaft diameter, and hair shaft condition. The label usually defines the intended consumer by stating normal hair, oily hair, dry hair or damaged, colored-treated hair. Some companies alter the concentrations of detergents and conditioners to make the different formulations, so the ingredient lists may be identical for all formulations. Other product lines have different formulations for each type.

Normal hair shampoos use lauryl sulfate detergents, giving them good cleansing and minimal conditioning characteristics. These products work well for adults with moderate sebum production and coarse hair; however, they do not work well for persons with fine, unmanageable hair.

Oily hair shampoos have excellent cleansing and minimal conditioning properties. They may use lauryl sulfate or sulfosuccinate detergents and are intended for adolescents with oily hair or persons who have extremely dirty hair. They can be drying to the hair shaft if used daily. Following an oily hair shampoo with a heavy conditioner is self-defeating.

Dry hair shampoos provide mild cleansing and good conditioning. Some companies recommend the same product for dry hair and damaged hair. These products are excellent for mature persons and those who wish to shampoo daily. They reduce static electricity and increase manageability in fine hair; however, some products provide too much conditioning, which may result in limp hair. Dry hair shampoos may also cleanse so poorly that the conditioner can build up on the hair shaft. This condition has been labeled as the "greasies" in popular advertising and may account for the observation that hair sometimes has more body after using a different shampoo.

> Dry hair shampoos provide mild cleansing and good conditioning to prevent further drying of the hair.

Damaged hair shampoos are intended for hair that has been chemically treated with permanent hair colors, hair bleaching agents, permanent waving solutions, or hair straighteners. Hair can also be damaged physically by overcleansing, excessive use of heated styling devices, and vigorous brushing or combing. Longer hair is more likely to be damaged than shorter hair since it undergoes a natural process known as "weathering," whereby the cuticular scales are decreased in number from the proximal to distal hair shaft (Fig. 24.3). As mentioned previously, damaged hair shampoos may be identical to dry hair shampoos or may contain mild detergents and increased conditioners. Hydrolyzed animal protein is the superior conditioner for damaged hair since it can minimally penetrate the shaft and temporarily plugging surface defects, resulting in hair with a smoother feel and more shine. It is important that the protein is hydrolyzed: larger protein molecules cannot penetrate the hair shaft.

> Weathering is the loss of cuticular scale from the shaft due to trauma from combing, brushing, wind, etc.

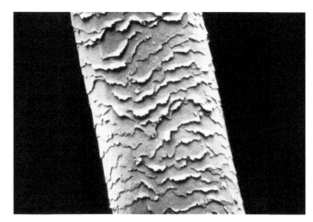

Figure 24.3 Weathering of the hair shaft as evidenced by an uplifted cuticle leads to the feel and appearance of damaged hair.

Baby Shampoos

Baby shampoos are nonirritating to the eyes and designed as mild cleansing agents since babies produce limited sebum. These shampoos use detergents from the amphoteric group (11). Baby shampoos are also appropriate for mature hair and for individuals who wish to shampoo daily.

> Baby shampoos are nonirritating to the eyes due to their anesthetic effect.

Conditioning Shampoos

Conditioning shampoos may be labeled as such or may be labeled as shampoos for dry or damaged hair. These products may actually be self-defeating since the shampoo is intended to remove sebum, the body's natural conditioner, and replace it with a synthetic conditioner, which consumers somehow interpret as cleaner. As a consequence, conditioning shampoos neither clean nor condition well (12). Detergents used in conditioning shampoos are generally amphoterics and anionics of the sulfosuccinate type. These products are sometimes known as one-step shampoos, since a conditioner need not be applied following shampooing. Patients should not use a conditioning shampoo prior to permanent dyeing or permanent waving because maximum color uptake or curling may be inhibited.

Medicated Shampoos

Medicated shampoos, also known as dandruff shampoos, contain additives such as tar derivatives, salicylic acid, sulfur, selenium disulfide, polyvinylpyrrolidone-iodine complex, chlorinated phenols, or zinc pyrithione (13). Medicated shampoos have several functions: to remove sebum efficiently, to remove scalp scale, to decrease scalp scale production, and to act as an antibacterial/antifungal. The shampoo base removes sebum while mechanical scrubbing removes scalp scale. Tar derivatives are commonly used as anti-inflammatory agents. Sulfur and zinc pyrithione are used for their antibacterial/antifungal qualities. Menthol is added to some shampoos to produce a tingling sensation some patients find aesthetically pleasing (Fig. 24.4).

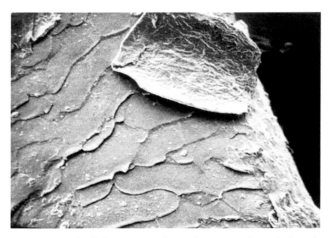

Figure 24.4 Dandruff shampoos are designed to remove skin scale from the scalp and hair.

Professional Shampoos

There are two types of professional shampoos: those intended for hair washing prior to cutting or styling and those intended to precede or follow a chemical process. Professional shampoos for hair washing are of the same formulation as the over-the-counter varieties except that they are more concentrated and must be diluted 8 to 10 times before to use. Special anionic, acidic professional shampoos are used after bleaching to neutralize residual alkalinity and prepare the hair for subsequent dyeing. Acidic, cationic shampoos are used after dyeing to act as a neutralizing rinse. A subset of these shampoos includes those designed to maintain the color of bleached or dyed hair. These shampoos are only available to licensed cosmetologists.

Our attention now turns to shampoos for scalp conditions that require both medical and cosmetic treatment. These conditions include dry postmenopausal scalp, thinning hair, seborrheic dermatitis, and scalp psoriasis.

SHAMPOOS FOR DRY POSTMENOPAUSAL SCALP

Dry postmenopausal scalp is a challenging condition for the dermatologist to treat. Postmenopausal women will note extreme itching, stinging, and burning of the scalp, but there is little to see on physical examination except a few powdery dry flakes on the scalp and perhaps a few excoriations. The thick silvery scales of scalp psoriasis and the yellow sticky scales of seborrheic dermatitis are absent. At first glance, the clinician might be tempted to wonder if the scalp symptoms are either nonexistent or a sign of depression. They are neither. Dry postmenopausal scalp, a descriptive term for the condition that will not be found as a scalp dermatosis in a dermatology textbook, really relates all about this condition. It is found in postmenopausal women who usually have accompanying body eczema. It can be best described as scalp eczema where the lack sebum production results in the powdery dry scale and the clinical symptoms of barrier disruption.

The problem in postmenopausal dry scalp is underproduction of sebum and overlying aggressive removal of sebum. The best solution is to recommend a 2-in-1 shampoo for dry hair containing dimethicone, and cool water when shampooing and rinsing to minimize further scalp dryness. The 2-in-1 shampoo will remove less sebum and leave behind a thin film

of dimethicone on the hair and scalp. Dimethicone will not leave the scalp or hair feeling greasy and also will not support the growth of bacteria or malassezia organisms. The shampoo should be followed by a dimethicone-containing instant conditioner, which is applied in the shower and rinsed again with cool water. Finally, a leave-in conditioner should be applied again with dimethicone and massaged into the scalp. The leave-in conditioner remains on the scalp as a moisturizer and is not rinsed. The next chapter provides more information on conditioners.

SHAMPOOS FOR THINNING HAIR

There are a variety of scalp conditions that can be characterized as thinning hair. They include lichen planopilaris, alopecia areata, and androgenetic alopecia. No matter what the cause of hair thinning, the shampoo recommendations are the same. Most people with thin hair like to maximize the appearance of the hair remaining by grooming it to stand away from the scalp as much as possible, since the appearance of full hair is measured by the distance the hair protrudes above the scalp. Aggressive shampooing that removes all of the sebum from the hair shafts and slightly damages the cuticle will produce the "fluffiest" hair because the hair will be more subject to static electricity and friction effects. While this is the appearance of damaged hair, it is felt to be desirable by those with thinning, which is somewhat of a contradiction. Healthy hair lays flat and smooth on the scalp while damaged hair is frizzy and unmanageable.

Shampoos for persons with hair loss should be selected from those labeled for fine hair. Fine hair shampoos do not have heavy conditioning agents that can make the hair heavy and limp. They clean away the sebum modestly, but do not deposit much conditioner on the hair. Baby shampoo is also an excellent selection in persons with thinning hair who are on a limited budget.

SHAMPOOS FOR SEBORRHEIC DERMATITIS

Seborrheic dermatitis is a shampoo challenge! The ideal shampoo will contain salicylic acid, tar, and zinc pyrithione. This will provide excellent control of the condition because the salicylic acid will remove the scalp skin scale, the tar will function as an anti-inflammatory, and the zinc pyrithione will keep the fungal organisms at bay addressing all three causative factors. This combination is not possible because dandruff shampoos are considered OTC drugs and only one active agent from the monograph can be placed in a shampoo. It is for this reason that the best control of seborrheic dermatitis is achieved by rotating shampoos. Salicylic acid is excellent at removing scalp scale, but it can also remove the hair shaft cuticle resulting in harsh feeling hair. Every third shampoo exposure to salicylic acid limits this damage. Tar is a good anti-inflammatory, but it can stain light colored hair if it has not been purified to remove the creosote. Many believe that the creosote is the key natural anti-inflammatory, but it will change white or silver hair to a yellowish-brown color that is not easily removed. Using purified tar is best and also reduces the topical carcinogen exposure. Finally, zinc pyrithione is an excellent anti-fungal, but it must be left behind on the scalp to be effective. The newer zinc pyrithione shampoos contain a smaller particle size material that can deposit on the scalp during the rinse phase of shampooing. In addition, zinc pyrithione-containing conditioners can increase the deposition. Since recolonization with malassezia occurs very rapidly in seborrheic dermatitis patients, the ability of the zinc pyrithione to prevent the release of free fatty acids by the malassezia can result in better symptom control.

SHAMPOOS FOR SCALP PSORIASIS

There is no doubt that the most challenging scalp condition to treat with shampoos is psoriasis. The thick, silvery scale resists detergent breakdown and removal. Salicylic acid is best at removing the scale, but it only works in an oily environment making it less effective in persons with thick dry scalp scale. In these patients, it is best to first soften the scale with an oily substance, such as mineral oil or peanut oil, for one hour prior to shampooing with a salicylic acid shampoo. The oil softens the scale and enhances the ability of the salicylic acid to dissolve the clumped corneocytes. Many psoriasis sufferers aggressively scrub their scalp to remove the scale, but this should be avoided as the scalp is subject to the Koebner effect and damage to the scalp can result in worsening psoriasis. Gentle rubbing with the fingertips and fingernails is best since the amount of pressure exerted is felt. Scalp brushes and other implements should be avoided.

SHAMPOOS AND CONTACT DERMATITIS

Shampoos do not represent a common cause of cutaneous irritant or allergic contact dermatitis due to their relatively brief contact with the skin prior to rinsing. Eye irritation, however, can be a problem which some shampoos overcome with the addition of imidazoline-type amphoteric surfactants, succinic ester sulfonates, silicone glycols, and fatty acid–peptide condensates (3). Ingredients in shampoos that are possible sensitizers include formalin, parabens, hexachlorophene, and miranols (14).

> Ingredients in shampoos that are possible sensitizers include formalin, parabens, hexachlorophene, and miranols.

Shampoos should be diluted to form a 1–2% aqueous solution for closed patch testing and a 5% aqueous solution for open patch testing. However, it should be recognized that false-positive reactions due to irritation may still occur. A better assessment may be obtained by patch testing individual ingredients separately (15).

REFERENCES

1. Bouillon C. Shampoos and hair conditioners. Clin Dermatol 1988; 6: 83–92.
2. Robbins CR. Interaction of shampoo and creme rinse ingredients with human hair. In: Chemical and Physical Behavior of Human Hair, 2nd edn. New York: Springer-Verlag, 1988: 122–67.
3. Markland WR. Shampoos. In: deNavarre MG, ed. The Chemistry and Manufacture of Cosmetics. Vol. 4. 2nd edn. Wheaton IL: Allured Publishing Corporation, 1988: 1283–312.
4. Fox C. An introduction to the formulation of shampoos. Cosmet Toilet 1988; 103: 25–58.
5. Zviak C, Vanlerberghe G. Scalp and hair hygiene. In: Zviak C, ed. The Science of Hair Care. New York: Marcel Dekker, 1986: 49–86.
6. Shipp JJ. Hair-care products. In: Williams DF, Schmitt WH, eds. Chemistry and Technology of the Cosmetics and Toiletries Industry. London: Blackie Academic & Professional, 1992: 32–54.
7. Tokiwa F, Hayashi S, Okumura T. Hair and surfactants. In: Kobori T, Montagna W, eds. Biology and Disease of the Hair. Baltimore: University Park Press, 1975: 631–40.
8. Powers DH. Shampoos. In: Balsam MS, Gershon SD, Rieger MM, Sagarin E, Strianse SJ, eds. Cosmetics Science and Technology. 2nd edn. New York: Wiley-Interscience, 1972: 73–116.
9. Harusawa F, Nakama Y, Tanaka M. Anionic-cationic ion-pairs as conditioning agents in shampoos. Cosmet Toilet 1991; 106: 35–9.
10. Karjala SA, Williamson JE, Karler A. Studies on the substantivity of collagen-derived peptides to human hair. J Soc Cosmet Chem 1966; 17: 513–24.
11. Wilkinson JB, Moore RJ. Harry's Cosmeticology. New York: Chemical Publishing, 1982: 457–8.
12. Hunting ALL. Can there be cleaning and conditioning in the same product? Cosmet Toilet 1988; 103: 73–8.
13. Spoor HJ. Shampoos. Cutis 1973; 12: 671–2.
14. Bergfeld WF. The side effects of hair products on the scalp and hair. In: Orfanos CE, Montagna W, Stuttgen G, eds. Hair Research. New York: Springer-Verlag, 1981: 507–11.
15. De Groot AC, Weyland JW, Nater JP. Unwanted effects of cosmetics and drugs used in dermatology. Amsterdam: Elsevier, 1994: 473–6.

SUGGESTED READING

Andrasko J, Stocklassa B. Shampoo residue profiles in human head hair. J Forensic Sci 1990; 35: 569–79.
Beauquey B. Scalp and hair hygiene: shampoos (Chapter 3). In: Bouillon C, Wilkinson J. The science of hair care. 2nd edn. Taylor & Francis Group, 2005: 83–127.
Bolduc C, Shapiro J. Hair care products: waving, straightening, conditioning, and coloring. Clin Dermatol 2001; 19: 431–6.
Bulmer AC, Bulmer GS. The antifungal action of dandruff shampoos. Mycopathologia 1999; 147: 63–5.
Draelos ZD. The biology of hair care. Dermatol Clin 2000; 18: 651–8.
Draelos ZK. Hair cosmetics. Dermatol Clin 1991; 9: 19–27.
Draelos ZD, Kenneally DC, Hodges LT, . A comparison of hair quality and cosmetic acceptance following the use of two ant-dandruff shampoos. J Investig Dermatol Symp Proc 2005; 10: 201–4.
Garlen D. Shampoos (Chapter 29). In: Rieger MM, ed. Harry's Cosmeticology. 8th edn. Chemical Publishing Co., Inc., 2000: 601–34.
Gray J. Hair care and hair care products. Clin Dermatol 2001; 19: 227–36.
Hossel P, Dieing R, Norenberg R, Pfau A, Sander R. Conditioning polymers in today's shampoo formulations-efficacy, mechanism and test methods. Int J Cosmet Sci 2000; 22: 1–10.
Nagahara Y, Nishida Y, Isoda M, . Structure and performance of cationic assembly dispersed in amphoteric surfactants solution as a shampoo for hair damaged by coloring. J Oleo Sci 2007; 56: 289–95.
Rushton H, Gummer CL, Flasch H. 2-in-1 shampoo technology: state-of-the-art shampoo and conditioner in one. Skin Pharmacol 1994; 7: 78–83.
Warner RR, Schwartz JR, Boissy Y, Dawson T. Jr. Dandruff has an altered stratum corneum ultrastructure that is improved with zinc pyrithione shampoo. J Am Acad Dermatol 2001; 45: 897–903.
Wolf R, Wolf D, Tuzun B, Tuzun Y. Soaps, shampoos, and detergents. Clin Dermatol 2001; 19: 393–7.
Wong M. Cleansing of hair (Chapter 3). In: Johnson DH, ed. Hair and hair care. Marcel Dekker, Inc., 1997: 33–64.
Wong M. Multifunctional shampoo: the two-in-one (Chapter 4). In: Schueller R, Romanowski P, eds. Multifunctional cosmetics. Marcel Dekker, Inc., 2003: 64–81.

25 Hair conditioners

The need for hair conditioners arose following the development of shampoos with extremely good detergent action (1). These new shampoos cleaned too well: they removed sebum from the hair shaft so thoroughly that the hair became unmanageable, dull, and harsh to touch. The role of a conditioner is to mimic sebum in making the hair manageable, glossy, and soft. Conditioners also attempt to recondition hair that has been damaged by chemical or mechanical trauma (2). Common sources of trauma include excessive brushing, hot blow-drying, detergent shampoos, alkaline permanent waves, bleaching, etc. Obviously, since hair is a nonliving tissue, any reconditioning that occurs is minimal and temporary until the next shampooing.

Hair conditioners were developed during the early 1930s when self-emulsifying waxes became available. These waxes were combined with protein hydrolysates, polyunsaturates, and silicones to give the hair an improved feel and texture. Early sources of the proteins included gelatin, milk, and eggs (3). The discovery of silicone and its adaptation to the hair care industry has revolutionized hair conditioners. Silicone is found in hair conditioners in several different forms including dimethicone, cyclomethicone, and amodimethicone. This chapter examines hair conditioners and their use in beautifying the hair.

CONDITIONER MECHANISM OF ACTION

Healthy, undamaged hair is soft, resilient, and easy to disentangle (4). Unfortunately, the trauma caused by shampooing, drying, combing, brushing, styling, dyeing, and permanently waving damages the hair making it harsh, brittle, and difficult to disentangle (5). Hair conditioners are designed to reverse this hair damage by improving sheen, decreasing brittleness, decreasing porosity, increasing strength, and restoring degradation in the polypeptide chain. Damage to the hair shaft can also occur through environmental factors such as exposure to sunlight, air pollution, wind, seawater, and chlorinated swimming pool water (6). This type of hair damage is technically known as "weathering" (7).

> Hair conditioners are designed to reverse hair damage by improving sheen, decreasing brittleness, decreasing porosity, and increasing strength.

Hair conditioners improve manageability by decreasing static electricity. Following combing or brushing, the hair shaft becomes negatively charged, thus repelling one another to prevent the hair from lying smoothly in a given style. Conditioners deposit positively charged ions on the hair shaft neutralizing the electrical charge. Improved manageability also derives from cuticle alterations and reduction of friction between hair

> Weathering is damage to the hair shaft that occurs over time from any external source including grooming, wind, sun, and tangling.

shafts by as much as 50% (8). This leads to enhanced disentangling of the hair, as well.

Hair gloss results from light reflected by individual hair shafts. The smoother the hair surface, the more light reflected (9). Conditioners increase hair gloss primarily by increasing the adherence of cuticular scale to the hair shaft. Gloss is also related to the hair structure. Maximum gloss is produced by large-diameter, elliptical hair shafts with a sizable medulla and intact, overlapping cuticle scales. Hair softness too results from an even overlap of cuticular scales (10).

Conditioners attempt to mend the split ends resulting from missing cortex, the structural component responsible for hair shaft strength. The resulting exposure of the soft keratin medulla results in a condition known as trichoptilosis, or split ends. Conditioners temporarily reapproximate the frayed remnants of remaining medulla and cortex.

All the problems associated with damaged hair are magnified if the hair is fine in texture. There are more fine hair fibers per weight than coarse hair fibers, so the net surface area of fine hair is greater. Proportionally, more irregular cuticle scales can develop and more of these fine hair fibers are subject to static electricity. Thus, special conditioner formulations are designed to meet the grooming needs of fine hair.

FORMULATION OF A CONDITIONER

Hair conditioners may contain as many as nine different conditioning agents from the chemical classes listed in Table 25.1 (11).

Of these, the quaternaries, protein derivatives, and alkanolamides are the most frequently used (12). Each of these categories is discussed in detail next (Table 25.2).

> The quaternaries, protein derivatives, and alkanolamides are the most frequently used compounds in modern hair conditioners.

Quaternary Conditioning Agents

The cationic detergents, also known as quaternaries or quaternary ammonium compounds or quats, are conditioning agents found in both shampoos and hair conditioners (13). They are excellent at increasing the adherence of the cuticular scales to the hair shaft, which increases the light reflective abilities of the hair, adding shine and luster. Additionally, they are able to electrically neutralize static electricity based on the

Table 25.1 Chemical Classes of Conditioners

Alkanolamides
Glycols
Lipids
Protein derivatives
Quaternaries
Surface active agents
Specialty ingredients

Table 25.2 Hair Conditioner Formulations

Type	Ingredient	Advantage	Hair type
Cationic detergent	Quaternary ammonium compounds	Smooth cuticle, decrease static	Chemically processed hair
Film former	Polymers	Fill shaft defects, decrease static, add shine	Dry hair, not fine hair
Protein-containing	Hydrolyzed proteins	Penetrate shaft	Temporarily mend split ends

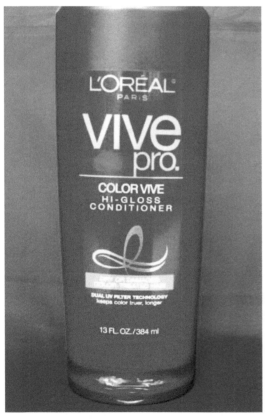

Figure 25.1 An instant conditioner for damaged dyed hair containing quaternary ammonium compounds.

negative (anionic) charge of processed or damaged hair, which attracts the positively (cationic) charged quaternary compound to adhere to the hair shaft, thus improving manageability (14). These qualities make them an excellent conditioner choice in patients with permanently dyed or permanently waved hair (Fig. 25.1).

Film-Forming Conditioning Agents

Film-forming conditioners apply a thin layer of polymer, such as polyvinylpyrrolidone (PVP), over the hair shaft (15). The polymer fills hair shaft defects creating a smooth surface to increase shine and luster while eliminating static electricity due to its cationic nature. The polymer also coats each individual hair shaft, thus "thickening" the hair shaft. Film-former conditioners should not be used on fine hair as the added weight of the polymer decreases the ability of the hair to hold a style. They are excellent, however, on normal to dry hair.

Protein Conditioning Agents

Protein-containing conditioners are the only product that can actually penetrate and alter the damaged hair shaft. These proteins, derived from animal collagen, keratin, placenta, etc., are hydrolyzed to a particle size (molecular weight 1000 to 10,000) able to enter the hair shaft (16). Hydrolyzed protein conditioners can temporarily strengthen the hair shaft and mend split ends until the subsequent shampooing when the product must be reapplied. The source of the protein is not as important as the protein particle size (17).

> Hair conditioners are available in three forms: instant conditioners and rinses, deep conditioners, and leave-in conditioners.

CONDITIONER TYPES

Hair conditioners are available in three forms: instant conditioners and rinses, deep conditioners, and leave-in conditioners (Table 25.3). Their names describe their use as instant conditioners and rinses are applied and immediately removed in the shower. Deep conditioners remain in contact with the hair for 30 minutes and leave-in conditioners remain in place until the subsequent shampooing.

Instant Conditioners

Instant conditioners are so named as they are applied following shampooing, left on the hair for five minutes and subsequently rinsed. These products provide minimal conditioning due to their short contact time with the hair and are basically useful to aid in wet combing and manageability. Their ability to repair damaged hair is somewhat limited. Nevertheless, they are the most popular type of conditioner for both home and salon use. Instant conditioners contain water, conditioning agents, lipids, and thickeners. The conditioning agents consist of combinations of cationic detergents, film formers, and proteins.

Rinses

Rinses are similar to instant conditioners in that they are applied immediately following shampooing and removed prior to drying the hair. There are two types: clear rinses and cream rinses. Clear rinses, formed from lemon juice and vinegar, were used prior to the development of pH-balanced shampoos with sequestering agents designed to prevent soap scum formation on the hair. These acidic chemicals removed calcium and magnesium soap residue and returned the hair to a neutral pH following the use of an alkaline shampoo. Residue removal restores hair shine while pH neutralization

Table 25.3 Hair Conditioner Products

Type	Use	Indication
Instant	Apply after shampoo, rinse	Minimally damaged hair, aids wet combing
Deep	Apply 20–30 min, shampoo, rinse	Chemically damaged hair
Leave-in	Apply to towel dried hair, style	Prevent hair dryer damage, aid in combing and styling
Rinse	Apply following shampoo, rinse	Aid in disentangling if creamy rinse, remove soap residue if clear rinse

restores hair manageability. Clear rinses work well in patients with oily hair, but are not recommended for patients with normal to dry hair.

Cream rinses utilize cationic quaternary ammonium compounds, such as stearalkonium chloride and benzalkonium chloride. Cream rinses are thinner than conditioners, but the differences in formulation are small. Some companies even label their products as "cream rinse/conditioners." As a general rule, cream rinses provide less conditioning than conditioners and are intended for oily to normal hair.

Deep Conditioners

Deep conditioners are creams, compared to instant conditioners, which are liquids. They contain the same conditioning agents as instant conditioners, but are more concentrated (18). They remain on the hair for 20 to 30 minutes and may include the application of heat from a hair dryer or warm towel. The extended application time allows more conditioner to coat the hair shaft, while heat causes hair shaft swelling and allows increased conditioner penetration. These products are intended for extremely dry hair. Deep conditioners used prior to some permanent coloring or permanent waving procedures are called "fillers." Fillers are designed to condition the distal hair shaft and reverse some of the effects of weathering, allowing even application of the subsequent coloring or waving procedure.

Some salons offer a deep conditioning treatment known as trichotherapy or aromatherapy. Aromatherapy involves several steps, the first of which is to condition the hair and scalp with rare oils and herbal extracts. The scalp is then vigorously brushed. A scalp and facial massage are also performed with fragrant oils to release tension and soothe the senses. The hair is then shampooed and conditioned. The value of this treatment is primarily aesthetic.

Leave-in Conditioners

Leave-in conditioners are applied following towel drying of the hair and designed to remain on the hair shaft through styling. They are removed with the next shampooing. Products designed for straight hair are known as blow drying lotions or hair thickeners. Blow drying lotions are massaged through the scalp after towel drying and prior to heat drying. Since they contain no oils, they are not rinsed from the hair. They contain the same conditioning agents previously described for instant

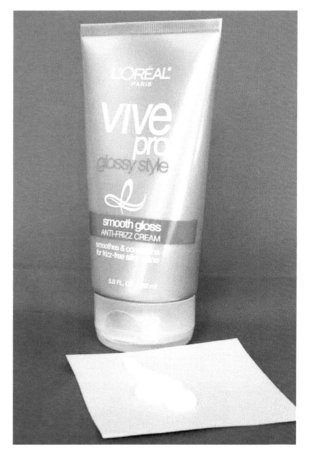

Figure 25.2 A leave-in cream conditioner that is applied to towel-dried hair.

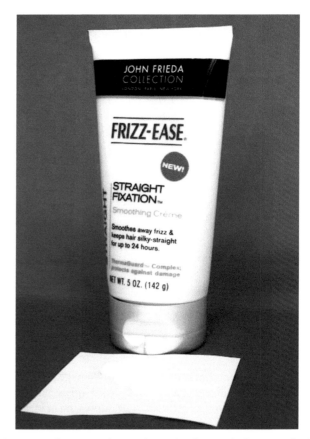

Figure 25.3 A leave-in conditioner designed to decrease the frizziness of curly hair.

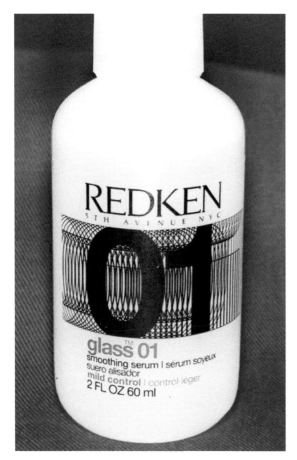

Figure 25.4 A hair thickener and hair shine formulation based on dimethicone that can be applied to wet or dry hair.

conditioners. The thin coating of conditioner on the hair only minimally prevents heat damage (Figs. 25.2 and 25.3).

Hair thickeners are another form of leave-in conditioner. They do not thicken hair by increasing the number of hair shafts, but rather provide a coating on each shaft that increases its diameter minutely. These products are protein-containing, conditioning liquids that are massaged through a towel-dried scalp before styling to increase shine, improve manageability, and impart softness. A hair thickener is thicker than a blow drying lotion and intended for persons with dry, damaged hair. Some of the newer hair thickeners are dimethicone-containing liquids (Fig. 25.4).

Special leave-in conditioners are used by Black and Asian individuals with tightly kinked hair to aid in combing, provide additional shine, improve manageability, and enhance styling options. These products are discussed more fully in the chapter on ethnic hair.

ADVERSE REACTIONS TO CONDITIONERS

Since hair conditioners are applied to the hair and eventually rinsed, they must be nonirritating to the eyes as well as the skin (19). The most popular instant conditioners only remain in contact with the skin for a brief period of time and are therefore infrequent causes of allergic and/or irritant contact dermatitis. These products can be patch tested "as is" in an open or closed manner.

The leave-in conditioners based on film-forming polymers too are infrequent causes of contact dermatitis; however, contamination with monomeric impurities, such as acrylamide, ethyleneimine, or acrylic acid, can cause problems. Acrylamide is highly toxic, ethyleneimine is carcinogenic, and acrylic acid is highly irritating to the skin. The safety and performance of polymers used in hair conditioners are related to their purity (20).

There have been some reports of reactions to proteins in some conditioners in the form of contact urticaria (21). While this is rare, it should be considered when evaluating the patient with the elusive chronic case of urticaria.

REFERENCES

1. Goldemberg RL. Hair conditioners: the rationale for modern formulations. In: Frost P, Horwitz SN, eds. Principles of Cosmetics for the Dermatologist. St. Louis: CV Mosby Company, 1982, 157–9.
2. Swift JA, Brown AC. The critical determination of fine change in the surface architecture of human hair due to cosmetic treatment. J Soc Cosmet Chem 1972; 23: 675–702.
3. deNavarre MG. Hair conditioners and rinses. In: deNavarre MG, ed. The Chemistry and Manufacture of Cosmetics. Vol. 4, 2nd edn, Wheaton, IL: Allured Publishing Corporation, 1988, 1097–109.
4. Garcia ML, Epps JA, Yare RS, Hunter LD. Normal cuticle-wear patterns in human hair. J Soc Cosmet Chem 1978; 29: 155–75.
5. Corbett JF. Hair conditioning. Cutis 1979; 23: 405–13.
6. Zviak C, Bouillon C. Hair treatment and hair care products. In: Zviak C, ed. The Science of Hair Care. New York: Marcel Dekker, Inc, 1986, 115–16.
7. Rook A. The clinical importance of "weathering" in human hair. Br J Dermatol 1976; 95: 111–12.
8. Price VH. The role of hair care products. In: Orfanos CE, Montagna W, Stuttgen G, eds. Hair Research. Berlin: Springer-Verlag, 1981, 501–6.
9. Robinson VNE. A study of damaged hair. J Soc Cosmet Chem 1976; 27: 155–61.
10. Zviak C, Bouillon C. Hair treatment and hair care products. In: Zviak C, ed. The Science of Hair Care. New York: Marcel Dekker, Inc, 1986, 134–7.
11. Rieger M. Surfactants in shampoos. Cosmet Toilet 1988; 103: 59.
12. Corbett JF. The chemistry of hair-care products. J Soc Dyers Colour 1976; 92: 285–303.
13. Allardice A, Gummo G. Hair conditioning. Cosmet Toilet 1993; 108: 107–9.
14. Idson B, Lee W. Update on hair conditioner ingredients. Cosmet Toilet 1983; 98: 41–6.
15. Finkelstein P. Hair conditioners. Cutis 1970; 6: 543–4.
16. Fox C. An introduction to the formulation of shampoos. Cosmet Toilet 1998; 103: 25–58.
17. Spoor HJ, Lindo SD. Hair processing and conditioning. Cutis 1974; 14: 689–94.
18. Bouillon C. Shampoos and hair conditioners. Clin Dermatol 1988; 6: 83–92.
19. Whittam JH. Hair care safety. In: Whittam JH, ed. Cosmetic Safety. New York: Marcel Dekker, Inc., 1987, 335–43.
20. Robbins CR. Polymers and polymer chemistry in hair products. In: Chemical and Physical Behavior of Human Hair, 2 edn. New York: Springer-Verlag, 1988, 196–224.
21. Niinimäki A, Niinimäki M, Mäkinen-Kilunen S, Hannuksela M. Contact urticaria from protein hydrolysates in hair conditioners. Allergy 1998; 53: 1078–82.

SUGGESTED READING

Bhushan B. Nanoscale characterization of human hair and hair conditioners. Prog Mater Sci 2008; 53: 585–710.
Bolduc C, Shapiro J. Hair care products: waving, straightening, conditioning, and coloring. Clin Dermatol 2001; 19: 431–6.
Erazo-Majewicz PE, Su SC. Cationic conditioning-polymer deposits on hair. J Cosmet Sci 2004; 55: 125–7.
Goddard ED. Mechanisms in combination cleaner/conditioner systems. J Cosmet Sci 2002; 53: 283–6.

Hoshowski MA. Conditioning of hair (Chapter 4). In: Johnson DH, ed. Hair and Hair Care. Marcel Dekker, Inc., 1997, 65–104.

Idson B. Polymers as conditioning agents for hair and skin (Chapter 11). In: Schueller R, Romanowski P, eds. Conditioning Agents for Hair and Skin. Marcel Dekker, Inc., 1999, 251–79.

Ruetsch SB, Kamath YK, Kintrup L, Schwark HJ. Effects of conditioners on surface hardness of hair fibers: an investigation using atomic force microscopy. J Cosmet Sci 2003; 54: 579–88.

Trüeb RM, the Swiss Trichology Study Group. The value of hair cosmetics and pharmaceuticals. Dermatology 2001; 202: 275–82.

26 Hair styling aids

Nothing beats a great looking head of hair, and styling aids are an important part of this quest for men and women. Preparations for hair adornment are some of the oldest cosmetic products known. Even the ancient Assyrians invented elaborate hair styles with layered cuts combined with oiling, perfuming, and hot iron curling. Hair styles assumed a great significance in their society as the more elaborate coifs were indicative of a high social status (1). Still today many products and devices are used to shape, mold, fix, set, and rearrange hair into a fashionable personal statement discussed in this chapter.

The key concept in hair styling is fashion. Each modern era can be characterized by a certain hair style so much so that most can identify the decade in which an old magazine was published by the hair style of the cover model. Hair styles in the 1960s were long, straight, and ungroomed, so styling aids were minimal and consisted of hair spray alone. Hair styles in the 1970s were curly and short so styling aids were destined to condition damage induced by permanent waving. Hair styles of the 1980s were gravity defying and demanded styling aids that provided the maximum hold. The 1990s were marked by hair styles with emphasis on smoothness and shine, requiring styling products that impart gloss. The millennium saw the popularity of the "bed head" look requiring hair waxes to make the hair clump and mold. And, finally, 2010 is characterized by the sleek straight look resembling 1960s hair styles and lending credence to the old fashion saying that what "goes around comes around."

HAIR STYLING PRODUCTS

Hair styling products are applied following shampooing and are completely removed with the subsequent shampooing. There are four categories of modern styling products: sprays, mousses, gels, and serums (Table 26.1).

Hair Spray

Hair sprays are used to keep the hair in a desired style (Fig. 26.1). They are a temporary water removal fixative that can hold hair in gravity-defying positions or simply smooth a few fly-away hairs, depending on their composition. Early hair sprays were aerosolized shellac, a natural resin composed of polyhydroxy acids and esters. Shellacs are no longer used since they form insoluble films that are not easily removed. In addition, chlorinated propellants have not been used since the 1979 U.S. Food and Drug Administration ban and states are now imposing limits on volatile organic compound emissions from hair sprays and other personal care products (2). Copolymers such as polyvinylpyrrolidone (PVP) are the main ingredient in hair sprays, now widely available in aerosol pumps. PVP is a resin that is soluble in water and easily removed by shampooing. However, it is also hydroscopic: the film becomes sticky upon water contact from rain, humidity, or perspiration. Once wet, the film loses its holding ability.

Vinyl acetate (VA) was added to PVP to make the product less hydroscopic, but this also made the removal difficult. Most hair sprays now combine PVP/VA and utilize anywhere from 30–70% PVP (3). Other newer polymer combinations are constantly being developed, such as copolymer resins of vinyl methyl ether and maleic acid hemiesters (PVP/MA) or copolymer resins of vinyl acetate and crotonic acid or dimethyl hydantoin-formaldehyde resins, with a few products now containing methacrylate copolymer (polyvinylpyrrolidone dimethyl aminoethyl methacrylate or PVP/DMAEMA) (4,5).

Besides polymer resins, hair sprays also contain plasticizers (mineral oil, lanolin, castor oil, and butyl palmitate), humectants (sorbitol and glycerol), solvents (SD alcohol 40, isopropyl alcohol, etc.), and conditioners (panthenol, plant proteins, hydrolyzed animal proteins, quaternium-19, and so on). More expensive hair sprays contain panthenol and quaternium-19, which are more expensive conditioners while low-priced conditioning hair sprays use hydrolyzed animal protein (6). High-priced hair sprays may also include a more costly fragrance than the low-priced brands.

Hair sprays are usually applied following hair styling, but may also function as a setting lotion, although this is not recommended. Hair sprays are available in several formulations providing varying degrees of hold. Regular hold hair sprays are designed to simply keep the hair in place. Super or extra hold hair sprays, hair styling fixes, and hair spritzes contain more copolymer than regular hold products and afford tremendous gravity-defying hold. These products also contain a less volatile vehicle than standard hair sprays, thus prolonging the drying time and allowing complex hair styling.

There was some concern in the 1960s regarding inhalation of PVP/VA aerosolized particles. These copolymers were originally developed in the medical industry for use as plasma diluents and were subsequently adopted by the cosmetics industry. Some reports indicated that thesaurosis was due to hair sprays, and inhalation of PVP solid particles could induce foreign body granuloma formation in the lung. After extensive animal testing, it was concluded that PVP resin did not provoke pulmonary lesions (7,8). Nevertheless, persons who are predisposed to lung conditions or those with allergic tendencies should use hair spray products with care (9).

> Hair sprays are applied to dry hair and designed to maintain the hair in a desired style after the hair has been groomed.

Hair sprays may produce dermatologic problems, such as nail damage (10). Patients who have their hair done weekly in a salon, especially if styled with an excessive amount of hair spray may develop hair spray buildup, resulting in hair shaft dullness. If applied as a coarse mist, the hair spray can bead on the hair shaft, resembling pediculosis capitis or trichorrhexis nodosa. The hair spray will also attract dirt, causing scalp irritation. Finally, once weekly shampooing may not be adequate to control seborrheic dermatitis in predisposed patients. There is some debate in cosmetic circles as to whether alcohol, an inexpensive evaporating solvent, also contributes to hair shaft dryness.

Hair Gel

Hair sprays are applied once the hair has been combed into a final position as the last step in hair styling (Fig. 26.2). This is in contrast to hair gels that can be applied to both wet and dry

hair. Hair gels are stronger fixatives used to hold the hair in more difficult to maintain positions. They contain the same PVP-type copolymers as hair sprays, except they are formulated

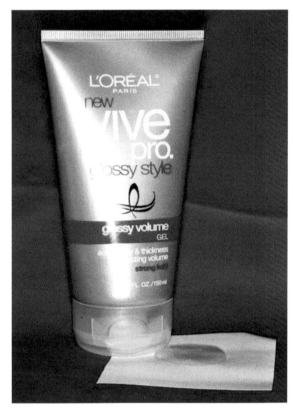

Figure 26.2 A clear hair gel contains a fixative that dries and stiffens the hair to add body and maintain a desired style.

Table 26.1 Hair Styling Aids

Styling aid	Type	Main ingredients	Purpose
Hair spray	Aerosol	Solution of film-forming resin	Hold finished hair style
Styling fix	Aerosol	Solution of film-forming resin	Add strong hold to finished hair style
Spritz	Aerosol	Solution of film-forming resin	Add strong hold to finished hair style
Styling gel	Gel	Gel of film-forming resin	Add moderate hold before styling
Sculpturing gel	Gel	Gel of film-forming resin	Add extreme hold before styling
Mousse	Foam	Aerosolized foam of film-forming resin	Add mild hold before styling

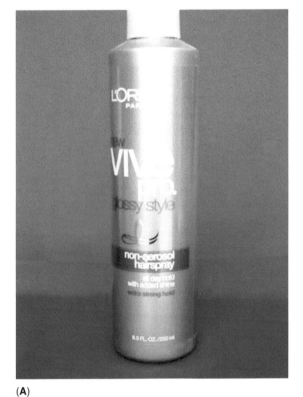

(A)

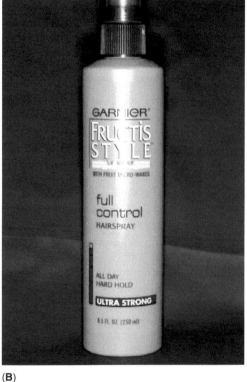

(B)

Figure 26.1 (**A**) A typical nonaerosol hair spray to maintain the hair in a desired style. (**B**) A high hold hair spray designed to maximally stiffen hair.

into a gel and packaged in soft plastic squeeze tubes. They are available in both alcohol-containing and alcohol-free forms and contain glossening agents that coat the hair shaft and restore shine. Conditioning agents, such as hydrolyzed animal proteins, panthenol, keratin polypeptides, and amino acids, are also incorporated into some hair gels for added appeal. Two formulations are available: styling gels and sculpturing gels. As the names suggest, sculpturing gels afford more hold than styling gels.

> Hair gels can be applied to dry or wet hair to create gravity defying hair styles.

Hair gels may contain synthetic color, usually in unnatural shades, such as blue, red, or purple. The colored gel coats the hair shaft, imparting tones of the color that is selected. The color molecules are too large to penetrate the undamaged hair shaft so the colored coating can be removed with one shampooing. However, persons with chemically dyed or waved hair have a porous shaft that may semi permanently absorb color molecules, requiring four to six shampooings for removal. Glitter may also be added to hair gels for effect.

Hair gels can be applied to towel-dried wet hair, damp hair, or distributed selectively on certain hair shafts depending on the desired style. If an increased hold of a hair style is desired, the gel can be combed thinly over all hair shafts prior to blow drying. If a small amount of gel is applied, the hair will have a natural look and feel. If a large amount is applied, the hair will have a wet, "spiky" look and a stiff feel. The product can also be applied to completely dry hair to get the hair to stand straight up. This is a currently popular look among teenage men.

Hair gels can be used in persons with thinning, dull hair to enhance hair fullness and restore cosmetic acceptability. The eye interprets hair thickness by the hair elevation over the crown, lateral displacement at the sides, and the extent of the visible scalp (11). Hair gels can hold the hair away from the scalp, creating the illusion of fullness (12). Glossening agents can bring shine, the visual clue to hair health based on light reflection from an intact cuticle.

These products adhere well to the hair shaft since PVP/VA has some substantivity, or increased affinity, for keratin. The films are flexible and colorless on the hair shaft, but can be removed by combing and brushing. This results in white polymer flakes in the hair that may resemble seborrheic dermatitis. The high concentration of PVP/VA also makes these products sticky with water contact. Persons who are exposed to moisture, such as athletes who perspire, should not use these styling products since the PVP/VA will fix the hair upon redrying, possibly in an undesirable position.

Hair gels can be both open and closed patch tested "as is," but they should be allowed to dry prior to occlusion. They are of low irritant potential, but may cause allergic contact dermatitis in those methacrylate-sensitive patients who choose a product containing a methacrylate-based polymer.

Hair Mousse

Hair gel is very similar in formulation to hair mousse, except hair gel is squeezed from a tube while hair mousse is a foam released under pressure from an aerosolized can. Both contain the same copolymer-containing hair styling aids to provide gloss to the hair and add an additional application of conditioner. Hair mousses can also be purchased tinted to temporarily cover gray hair. For example, persons with less than 15% gray hair can use colored mousse with brown or auburn hues to blend gray hair. Unnatural colors such as yellow, green, red, orange, purple, and blue are also available. The color is temporary and removed with one shampooing unless applied to chemically treated hair.

> Hair mousse is similar in formulation to hair gel, except that it is aerosolized foam.

Hair mousse is applied in the same manner as a hair gel to towel-dried hair. It can also be applied to dry hair to create a wet "spiky" look. Hair mousse yields a lighter copolymer application and does not provide as strong a hold as gel formulations. It also produces less flaking and less stickiness under moist conditions due to the low concentration of polymer. Many of the styling hold products for men are hair mousses, since a lighter application is desirable.

Hair styling mousses can be used to create natural-appearing fullness more easily than hair gels due to their low moisture content. A half-dollar-sized mound of mousse is placed in the palm. Small amounts are then dabbed onto the fingers and massaged into the proximal hair shaft. Drying occurs almost immediately. The mousse adds stiffness to the hair shaft, creating the illusion of fullness. This technique can be used by both men and women with thinning hair to create hair that is more attractive. A small amount of mousse applied to the palms and lightly touched to a finished style can smooth unmanageable hairs. Mature persons will probably find hair mousse more satisfactory than hair gel as a styling aid.

Hair Serums

The newest category of hair care products is hair serums. These are clear viscous liquids squirted from a nonaerosolized jar onto the palm. Hair serums are hair moisturizers based on dimethicone (Fig. 26.3). Hair becomes brittle when devoid of water, just like skin. This occurs until low humidity conditions, such as in the western U.S.A., or when the hair has been chemically processed by permanent dyeing, waving, or straightening. The disruption of the cuticle that occurs with chemical processing allows water to evaporate from the hair shaft into the environment. Remoisturization of the hair can occur with dimethicone just like remoisturization of the skin. Thus, the dimethicone functions as an occlusive agent to retard water loss (Fig. 26.4).

> Hair serums are based on dimethicone and function as a hair shaft moisturizer.

Hair serums can be useful to maintain the health of the hair shaft in persons with damaged hair. The hair serum is best applied to dry hair by rubbing the hands together and then pulling the hands through the hair to distribute an even thin

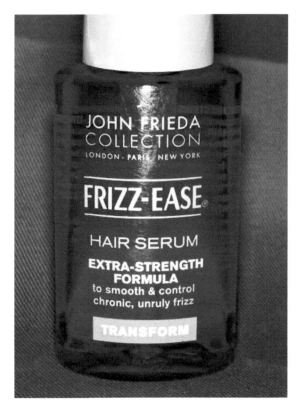

Figure 26.3 A hair serum designed to add shine and decrease hair frizz by imparting a water-resistant dimethicone layer to each hair shaft.

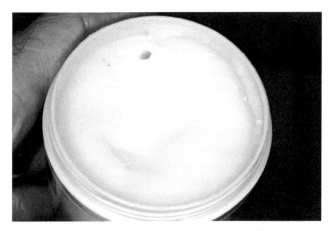

Figure 26.4 A hair cream designed to both moisturize and stiffen hair to create the popular "bed head" hair style.

film on each hair shaft. The serum can be applied daily prior to hair styling. The dimethicone smoothes down the cuticle, restoring shine and manageability, and prolongs the life of hair dye by preventing passive loss of the hair dye. It also makes the hair smooth and soft, just like on the skin. For patients who complain of "unhealthy" hair, hair serum is quickest way to restore the appearance of healthy hair.

HAIR STYLING DEVICES

Two types of modern hair styling devices are available: nonelectric and electric. Nonelectric styling devices include dry rollers, combs, brushes and a variety of hair clasps. Electric

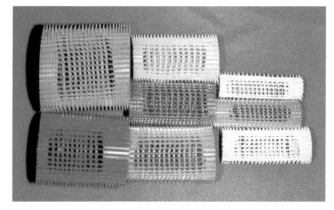

Figure 26.5 Nonelectric hair rollers come in a variety of sizes to create different curl sizes.

styling devices include hair dryers, curling irons, electric curlers, and crimping irons.

Nonelectric Hair Styling Devices

Nonelectric rollers function to impart curl and add body to create a desirable hair style. A variety of sizes and styles are available, with larger rollers forming looser curls while smaller rollers form tighter curls (Fig. 26.5). Toothed rollers are designed to hold the hair without the aid of a hair pin, but may fracture the hair shaft on removal. Hair breakage can be minimized by using toothless smooth rollers held in place with hair pins and a hair net.

Pulling and rolling wet hair onto curlers allows partial transformation of the normal alpha-keratin structure to a beta-keratin structure of the hair shaft allowing the curling of straight hair.

Wet hair is required to produce optimal curls with nonelectric rollers. Physically, wet hair is more elastic than dry hair, allowing partial transformation of the normal alpha-keratin structure to a beta-keratin structure under tension. This transformation shifts the relative position of the polypeptide chains and brings about a disruption of ionic and hydrogen bonds. During the drying process, new ionic and hydrogen bonds are formed, blocking return to the natural alpha-keratin configuration and allowing the hair to remain in its newly curled position. Wetting the hair, however, returns hair bonds immediately to the natural alpha configuration (13). Hair must be rolled under tension to provide the load required for bond breakage, but hair should not be stretched beyond the point at which more than one-third of the alpha-keratin bonds have been unfolded to beta-keratin bonds. Excessive stretching will result in permanent deformation causing the inelastic hair to fracture (Fig. 26.6).

Electric Hair Styling Devices

Electric styling devices operate on the principle that heat can temporarily reform water bonds within the hair shaft. The style can be maintained until the next water exposure when the bonds will return to the natural shape. Electric styling devices are used by professionals in the salon, as well as

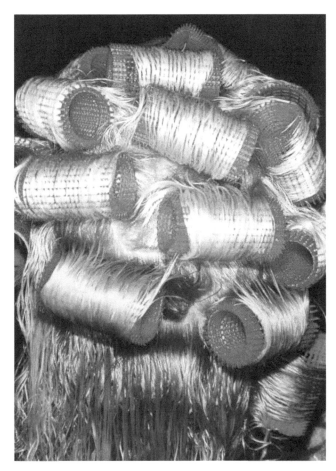

Figure 26.6 The hair is tightly wrapped around the rollers and dried to create temporary curls.

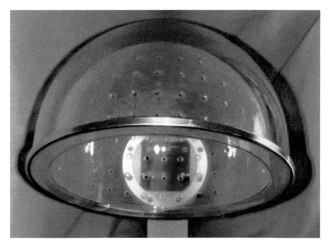

Figure 26.7 A hooded hair dryer is used in a professional salon to rapidly dry wet hair into a desired style after setting on the curlers illustrated in Figure 26.5.

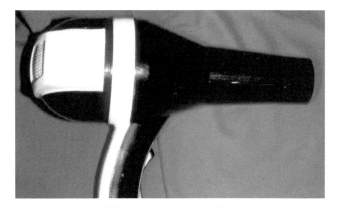

Figure 26.8 A hand-held blow dryer should be held at least 8 inches from the head to avoid burning the scalp and the hair.

consumers at home. This section highlights the use and misuse of these devices.

Hair Dryer

The most popular electric styling device is the hair dryer, which can be hooded or hand-held. Hooded hair dryers are mainly seen in professional salons and can be used for two purposes. The first is to dry the hair after it has been placed on rollers and the second is to process chemical hair treatments, such as permanent hair dyes or hair straightening. Hooded dryers are more efficient at drying the hair than blow dryers, but can cause more hair and scalp damage, especially if excess heat is present between the hood and scalp (Fig. 26.7). Second degree scalp burns have been reported when a hood hair dryer is used to process dyed hair that has been wrapped in aluminum foil to contain the hair dye only to certain hair shafts. This dyeing technique is used to dye the hair several different colors to mimic the natural variation seen in some individuals artificially. Problems can arise when the foil is heated against the scalp resulting in scarring and baldness.

Blow dryers are the most popular method of hair drying, but should be used on low heat to avoid damaging the hair protein.

Hand-held blow dryers do not dry the hair as efficiently as a hooded hair dryer, but also cannot produce scalp burns as easily (Fig. 26.8). To avoid burning the skin or the hair, the hand-held blow dryer should be positioned at least 8 inches from the scalp. High temperatures can denature hair protein resulting in permanent damage to the hair shafts perceived as easily fractured hair. A vented styling brush can be used to shape hair while blow drying to minimize overheating the hair.

Curling Iron

The second most popular hair appliance is the curling iron, which is a modern version of the oven-heated metal rods that were wrapped with hair in the pre-electric era. Modern curling irons are thermostatically controlled to prevent overheating, but temperatures capable of producing first- and second-degree burns are still attainable. Some irons come with variable temperature settings, but most patients prefer the hottest setting since the curls produced are tighter and longer lasting. It is recommended that patients remove excess heat from the curling iron prior to use by placing it in a moist towel. This lowers the rod temperature preventing burns of the hair and scalp (Fig. 26.9).

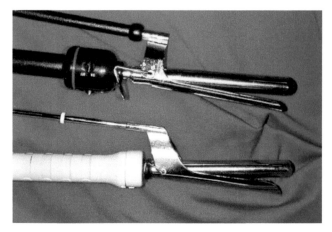

Figure 26.9 A curling iron can cause second-degree burns if not properly handled.

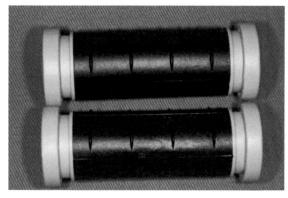

Figure 26.10 Electric curlers are less likely to cause skin burns, but to avoid hair damage only dry hair should be placed in contact with the warm curlers.

Hot curling irons can cook the water in the hair shaft causing irreversible damage in the form of bubble hair.

Removal of hair from the curling iron is another frequently encountered problem. Most curling irons have a spring loaded clip to hold the hair to the rod. Failure to release the clip completely can cause hair breakage. Newer rods are now coated with nonstick materials to facilitate hair release or made out of ceramic. However, certain styling products, such as hair spray, can melt and glue hair to the rod. Thus, patients should curl their hair first and then add hair spray or other styling products.

Electric Curlers
Electric curlers are individually heated, plastic coated rods of varying sizes (Fig. 26.10). A curler set is more expensive than a curling iron, but the chance of burning is lessened since hot metal does not come in contact with the hair or scalp. Many patients prefer curling irons since they have a shorter heating period, but fast, 60-second heating curlers are available. A variation on the firm, molded electric roller is a smaller-diameter, rubber-coated, bendable rod or disk. The shape and type of curlers available is fashion dictated.

Electric hair curlers can curl dry straight hair by affecting the water deformable bonds.

Crimping Iron
The last major type of electric hair styling appliance is a variation on the old-fashioned hair iron, known as a crimping iron or a straightening iron. This device contains two hinged metal plates that are heated with hair placed between them. If the plates are corrugated, the device is called a crimping iron and produces tight bends in the hair shaft. If the plates are smooth, the device is known as a hair straightener for those with kinky hair. This type of iron can be used to straighten mildly curly hair, but cannot be used to straighten kinky hair (Fig. 26.11). Heat straightening methods for kinky hair are covered in the chapter discussing ethnic hair.

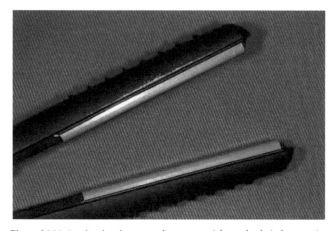

Figure 26.11 A crimping iron uses heat to straighten the hair by pressing between two warm ceramic plates.

Crimping irons are used to straighten mildly curly hair.

It is important for the physician to consider electric styling device burns in the patient with scarring alopecia, especially of the frontal and vertex areas. In these locations, it is easier for the heated device to rest on the head. Also, most women curl this area more frequently than the sides of the head, increasing the opportunity for burns.

SUMMARY
It is the artful combination of hair styling products and devices that yields a fashionable coif. From smooth and straight to curly and fluffy, all things are possible with the right sprays, gels, mousses, serums, curlers, and irons. The different hair styles that can be attained are only limited by the imagination of the artist. The many variations in hair styles can be appreciated by examining a portrait art book followed by a visit to a local mall. This chapter has educated the dermatologists on the possibilities and identified issues where possible.

REFERENCES
1. Henkin H. Hair grooming. In: The Chemistry and Manufacture of Cosmetics, 2nd edn. Wheaton, IL: Allured Publishing Corporation, 1988, 1111–24.
2. Oteri R, Tazi M, Walls E, Kosiek JC. Formulating hairsprays for new air quality regulations. Cosmet Toilet 1991; 106: 29–34.
3. Wells FV, Lubowe II. Hair grooming aids, part III. Cutis 1978; 22: 407–25.

4. Zviak, C. The Science of Hair Care. New York: Marcel Dekker, 1986, 153–65.
5. Stutsman MJ. Analysis of hair fixatives. In: Senzel AJ, ed. Newburger's Manual of Cosmetic Analysis, 2nd edn. Washington, DC: Published by the Association of Official Analytical Chemists, Inc, 1977, 72.
6. Lochhead RY, Hemker WJ, Castaneda JY. Hair care gels. Cosmet Toilet 1987; 102: 89–100.
7. Zviak, C. The Science of Hair Care. New York: Marcel Dekker, 1986, 167–8.
8. Wells FV, Lubowe II. Hair grooming aids, part IV. Cutis 1978; 22: 557–62.
9. Wilkinson JB, Moore RJ. Harry's Cosmeticology. New York: Chemical Publishing, 1982, 481–3.
10. Daniel DR, Scher RK. Nail damage secondary to a hair spray. Cutis 1991; 47: 165–6.
11. Clarke J, Robbins CR, Reich C. Influence of hair volume and texture on hair body of tresses. J Soc Cosmet Chem 1991; 42: 341–52.
12. Rushton DH, Kingsley P, Berry NL, Black S. Treating reduced hair volume in women. Cosmet Toilet 1993; 108: 59–62.
13. Robbins CR. Chemical and Physical Behavior of Human Hair, 2nd edn. New York: Springer-Verlag, 1988, 89–91.

SUGGESTED READING

Dallal JA, Rocafort CM. Hair styling/fixative products (Chapter 5). In: Johnson DH, ed. Hair and Hair Care. Marcel Dekker, 1997, 105–65.

Dallal JA. Hair setting products (Chapter 30). Rieger MM, ed. Harry's Cosmeticology, 8th edn. Chemical Publishing Co., Inc., 2000, 635–67.

Gao T, Pereira A, Zhu S. Study of hair sine and hair surface smoothness. J Cosmet Sci 2009; 60: 187–97.

Gummer CL. Hair shaft effects from cosmetics and styling. Exp Dermatol 1999; 8: 317.

Jachowicz J. Dynamic hairspray analysis. III. Theoretical considerations. J Comet Sci 2002; 53: 249–61.

Rafferty DW, Zellia J, Hasman D, Mullay J. Polymer composite principles applied to hair styling gels. J Cosmet Sci 2008; 59: 497–508.

Rafferty DW, Zellia J, Hasman D, Mullay J. The mechanics of fixatives as explained by polymer composite principles. J Cosmet Sci 2009; 60: 251–9.

Ruetsch SB, Kamath YK. Effects of thermal treatments with a curling iron on hair fiber. J Cosmet Sci 2004; 55: 13–27.

Sendelbach G, Liefke M, Schwan A, Lang G. The new method for testing removability of polymers in hair sprays and setting lotions. Int J Cosmet Sci 1993; 15: 175–80.

Trüeb RM. Dermocosmetic aspects of hair and scalp. J Investig Dermatol Symp Proc 2005; 10: 289–92.

Zhou Y, Foltis L, Moore DJ, Rigoletto R. Protection of oxidative hair color fading fram shampoo washing by hydrophobically modified cationic polymers. J Cosmet Sci 2009; 60: 217–38.

27 Hair styling with prostheses

The prior chapters have focused on methods of optimizing the appearance of the patient's natural hair through proper shampoo selection, conditioner application, and the use of styling aids and devices. Natural hair can be optimized through all of these cosmetic manipulations; however, the dermatologist may encounter patients with substantial temporary or permanent hair loss that may require the use of hair prostheses. Patients with temporary hair loss, such as chemotherapy-induced hair loss or alopecia areata, or persons with permanent scarring alopecia, such as lichen planopilaris or central centrifugal alopecia, are grateful for the advice a dermatologist can provide regarding the use of prostheses. This chapter presents knowledge on hair techniques for the patient in need of reassurance and compassion.

Hair pieces have been a part of history since the Egyptians invented them in 3000 BC, many of which still survive today. Hair pieces were popular among both ruling men and women and were fashioned from human and vegetable fibers coated with beeswax. Blond wigs were popularized by the Romans in the first century BC made of hair taken from German captives. Eventually, however, blonde wigs became the trademark of Roman prostitutes and were outlawed by the Christian Church. By 1580, wigs were again fashionable due to the influences of the English queens who developed female pattern hair loss. Even Mary, Queen of Scots, wore a wig, a fact unknown by her followers until she was beheaded. The popularity of wigs spread to France by the 18th century such that the French Court of Versailles employed 40 resident wigmakers. Today, wigs remain a part of the formal attire of some judges (1).

HAIR PIECES

The use of hair pieces can restore a positive self-image in those patients who have temporary or permanent hair loss. Both natural human hair and synthetic fiber types are available. The custom-made natural human hair products are more expensive ($100–$2000) and have a short life (2–3 yrs) due to hair breakage. Synthetic hair products are less expensive ($10–100) and have a longer life (3–5 yrs), but are limited in their styling possibilities. Synthetic fibers are designed to have a permanent curl and require less maintenance than natural fibers making them a better choice for most patients.

> Hair pieces are constructed by attaching individual fibers by hand-tying or machine-wefting to a meshwork designed to fit a specific scalp location.

A hair piece is formed by attaching individual fibers to a meshwork designed to fit a specific scalp location. Two methods of attaching hair fibers to the mesh are used: hand tied and machine wefted. Hand-tied hair pieces are more expensive because the fibers are individually knotted to the mesh.

Machine-wefted wigs are made by sewing the fibers onto strips of material and then attaching wefts to the mesh.

Synthetic and natural fiber hair pieces are cleaned in much the same manner as a head of hair. The hair piece is turned inside out, and a drop of mild shampoo is placed in the center and gently agitated under a stream of warm water. Once the shampoo is completely removed, a drop of instant conditioner is placed in the wig and again rinsed. The hair piece is allowed to air dry while inside out by attaching it with a clothespin to an indoor clothesline. Once dry, the hair piece may be styled with a specially designed wig brush.

Hair pieces come in seven basic types, depending on the scalp area to be covered. Table 27.1 and Figure 27.1 show these types.

Patients with severe alopecia areata, alopecia totalis, alopecia universalis, or chemotherapy-induced anagen effluvium require complete wigs. It is recommended that the patient select a wig prior to complete hair loss, thus allowing the patient to emotionally adjust and aid in selecting a wig that mimics the patient's natural hair color and style. If this is not possible, a picture of the patient prior to hair loss is helpful to the wig artist.

Most patients, however, only require supplementation of their natural hair by a hair piece selected to cover areas of thinning or loss. For example, female pattern alopecia can be covered with a demiwig known as a "hair thickener." This hair piece is attached to a loosely woven mesh through which the patient pulls her own hair, allowing blending of the hair fibers and also firmly securing the hair piece to the scalp. Women who note that their hair will no longer grow to a length desired may wish to consider a fall to add length or a cascade to add a bun or mass of curls.

Toupees are specifically designed for the balding men and are available in a variety of colors with the appropriate percentage of gray hair to match the patient's state of canities. Natural part line toupees, which add a small insert of sheer plastic in the part line to expose the natural color of the underlying scalp, may create a more natural appearance. Some toupees come uncut, allowing the patient to take the toupee to the barber for styling along with the patient's natural hair. Attachment of toupees to the scalp, however, remains poor relying on clips or adhesives (Fig. 27.2).

Chemotherapy patients with scalp tenderness or patients undergoing immunotherapy utilizing contact sensitization for alopecia may wish to cover their head with a soft terry cloth turban. A more natural appearance can be achieved by adding a wiglet of bangs.

HAIR ADDITIONS

Another semipermanent approach to thinning or locally absent scalp hair is the use of hair additions. Hair additions are worn continuously for approximately eight weeks, remaining in place while swimming, bathing, sleeping, and exercising.

Table 27.1 Types of Hair Pieces

1. Wigs: constructed on a flexible cap-shaped mesh designed to cover the entire head
2. Falls: long locks of hair attached to a firm contoured mesh designed to rest on the scalp vertex (Fig. 27.1A)
3. Cascades: curled locks or buns attached to a firm oblong contoured base designed to rest on the posterior scalp (Fig. 27.1B)
4. Toupees: custom fitted hair piece on a woven base to cover the top of the head (Fig. 27.1C)
5. Demiwigs: flexible cap-shaped mesh designed to cover the entire scalp except the front hairline (Fig. 27.1D)
6. Wiglets: localized hairpieces designed to create bangs or add additional hair on the top of the head (Fig. 27.1E)
7. Switches: long strands of hair in the form of braids or ponytails secured together at one end (Fig. 27.1F)

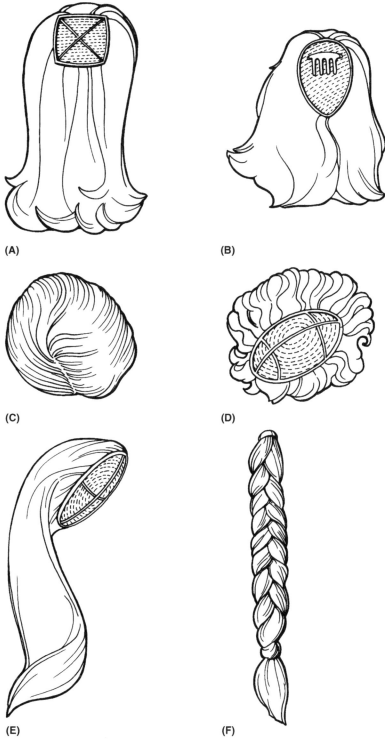

Figure 27.1 Types of artificial hair pieces. (**A**) Fall. (**B**) Cascade. (**C**) Toupee. (**D**) Demiwig. (**E**) Wiglet. (**F**) Switch.

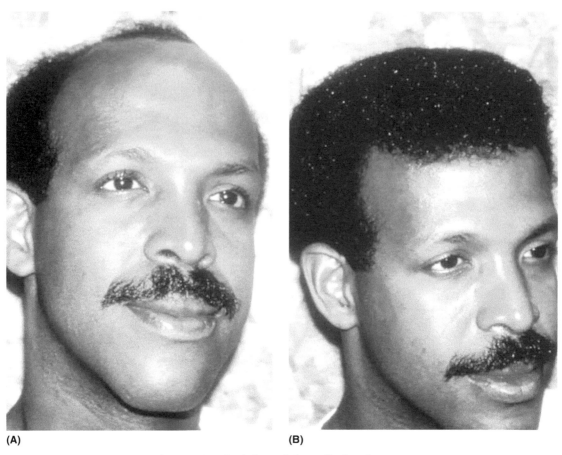

(A)   (B)

Figure 27.2 A patient before and after application of a toupee.

The technique utilizes synthetic or natural human hair fibers to supplement existing hair where needed. Hair additions can be tied, woven, or glued to the scalp or existing hair and may be obtained in full service beauty salons or at salons specializing in the technique. Augmentation of hair through additions is widely used in the entertainment industry, by Black people who wish to achieve hair length, by men who wish to camouflage androgenetic alopecia, and by women who desire special effect hair styles.

> Hair additions and wigs can be formed from synthetic modacrylic fibers or natural human hair.

There are several different types of fibers that can be used for temporary hair additions or for the construction of wigs. Synthetic fibers are man made and natural hair fibers are obtained from women who sell their hair. Most of the human hair comes from the Orient and is dyed and mixed from multiple donors to obtain a swatch that is then made into a wig. Synthetic fibers are formed from modacrylic, composed of two polymerized monomers: acrylonitrile and vinyl chloride. The polymer is drawn through a multihole metal disk, dried, and stretched. The disk design is such that fibers with an irregular cross-section and surface variations are produced to more closely mimic natural human hair. Dye may be added to the polymer either before or after extrusion to create any hair color desired. Various colored hair fibers are then combined to make a more realistic appearing wig.

The art of making a hair piece is to artistically combine fibers of varying diameters and color hues, as not all natural hair shafts are of the same thickness or color. Additionally, the fiber thickness should be varied to more accurately simulate hair shaft size in Black, Caucasian, and Oriental hair. The modacrylic can also be permanently heat formed to reproduce the appropriate amount and tightness of curl unique to the hair of different ethnic groups. Synthetic hair offers some advantages over natural human hair for use in hair additions. First, synthetic fibers are of lighter weight than natural human hair, thus exerting less pull on existing scalp hairs. Second, synthetic fibers are less expensive than human hair. Third, synthetic fibers can be melted to bond to existing scalp hair.

As mentioned previously, human hair obtained from Indian or Chinese women who grow their hair for sale is used for hair additions and wigs. Indian hair has a fine diameter and a slight natural wave whereas Chinese hair is coarser and straighter. Usually, the human hair is lightened and redyed to obtain a range of colors and may also be permanently waved to obtain the desired amount of curl. Coloring and curling of hair used in additions may be performed both before and after the added hair is attached to the scalp using standard salon products.

Human hair does not require the color and fiber diameter mixing of synthetic hair fibers as natural variations are already present. Thus, the main advantage of human hair additions is their ability to blend with existing scalp hair. Disadvantages include the weight of the natural fibers and the cost, which increases with longer lengths of hair.

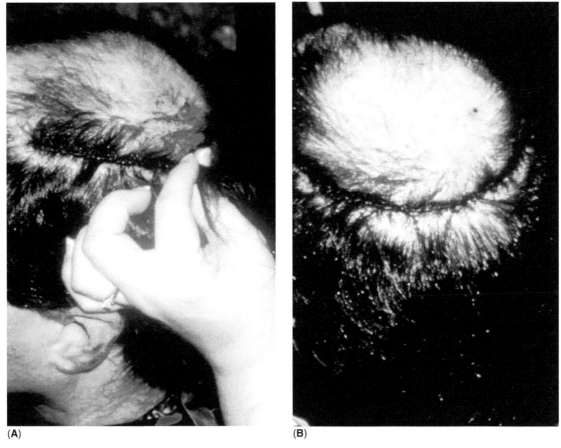

(A) (B)

Figure 27.3 Braiding on the scalp can create an attachment site for sewing a toupee to the hair braid.

METHODS OF HAIR ATTACHMENT

Hair additions use existing scalp hair to anchor the synthetic or natural human hair fibers. The added fibers may be affixed by braiding, sewing, bonding, or gluing. The attachment method selected depends on the amount of natural hair and the number or length of fibers to be added.

> Hair fibers can be attached to the scalp by braiding, sewing, bonding, or gluing.

Braiding on the Scalp

The most popular method of hair additions employs braiding on the scalp, adapted from the Black hair style known as "cornrows." Cornrows are plaited on the scalp in geometric designs with tension applied to the hair shafts exposing scalp between the braids. This is a popular hairstyle among Black individuals as it allows for organization of tightly kinked hair. Braiding on the scalp can also be used to attach a toupee (Fig. 27.3). Individual hair fibers can be woven into the braids to either thicken their appearance or, more commonly, to add length. Wefted hair, or hair fibers sewn together in a strip, can be sewn with a needle and thread to the cornrows to quickly add large amounts of hair.

Braiding off the Scalp

Braiding off the scalp employs a standard plaiting technique to which individual hair fibers are added. Fibers are attached by working them securely into the braids and leaving the loose ends for curling and styling (Fig. 27.4). This technique is

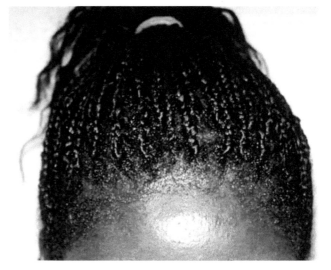

Figure 27.4 Braiding off the scalp can be used to weave in synthetic hair strands to create the illusion of long hair in African American individuals with short hair.

popular among individuals with short kinky hair, who wish to have long straight hair but long-term use can result in traction alopecia (Fig. 27.5).

Bonding

Bonding employs a hot glue gun to fuse individual synthetic hair fibers to the base of clumps of existing scalp hair. Only a few fibers can be attached at a time, due to the weight of the

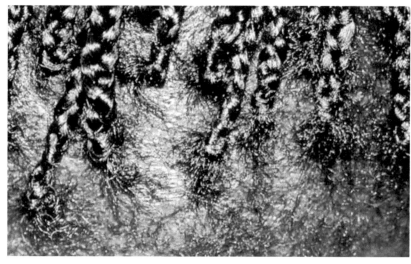

Figure 27.5 Traction alopecia is a possible permanent side effect of braiding off the scalp.

additions. This technique is used in both men and women to thicken the hair. The bonds are intended to remain in place for eight weeks; however, individuals with excessive sebum production may notice early loosening and loss of the added hair.

Gluing

This hair addition technique combines braiding on the scalp with adhesive attachment. The existing hair is initially braided into concentric arcs on the posterior scalp, known as "tracks." These tracks serve as anchors to which wefted hair is glued. The adhesive employed is a cold latex-based glue that is subject to removal by scalp sebum production (Fig. 27.6).

CARE OF HAIR ADDITIONS

Hair additions are worn continually for a period of eight weeks, or less, at which time they must be removed. Individuals with slowly growing hair may wear the hair style longer, while those with rapidly growing hair notice the added hair fibers loosen more quickly. The additions are shampooed along with the individual's existing hair using the same cleansing products and cleansing frequency. Many individuals are afraid to wash the additions as they fear loosening will occur, but good hygiene is important.

> Hair additions must be removed at 8 weeks to avoid hygiene problems and traction alopecia.

Hair additions must be removed at eight weeks to avoid hygiene problems and other complications such as traction alopecia. If the hair and scalp have been properly cleansed, hair additions begin to loosen and look ungroomed at eight weeks. Removal of braided additions simply requires undoing the braid and removing the added strands of hair which may be reused in later procedures. Bonded additions are removed by melting the hot glue with the tip of the glue gun and pulling out the individual or wefted hair fibers. Peanut oil is then rubbed through the scalp to facilitate removal of any remaining material. Latex-based glue is removed with a specially designed solvent. Lastly, sewn additions can be removed by cutting the attachment thread.

It is understandable that individuals would like to wear the additions as long as possible, since the cost may vary between $250 and $1000 depending on the complexity of the hair style, the amount and length of the added hair fibers, the salon time required and whether synthetic or human hair fibers are used. The average hair addition requires three to five hours in a salon.

Successful use of hair additions requires a hair stylist who is trained in the technique and a client who will put forth the effort to maintain the added hair. Braided and sewn hair additions pose the least problem as no adhesives are used; however, the added hair fibers put increased pull on existing scalp hair augmenting the pull already exerted by the tight braids. For these reasons, traction alopecia is a problem arising in individuals who continually wear hair additions. The traction alopecia is identical to that seen in Black patients who wear tightly pulled hair styles. Initially, only loss of the hair shaft is observed, but with continued traction, the process can result in loss of the follicular ostia and permanent alopecia. Extensive traction alopecia will eventually preclude the use of hair additions as no existing scalp hair will be available to anchor added hair.

Glued additions employ adhesives which must be patch tested prior to use. Additionally, the hair stylist must take care not to carelessly apply glue throughout the scalp which may increase hair breakage since hair combing is impeded by glue. The hot bonding gun must be kept from the scalp to avoid scalp burns which could result in permanent alopecia, if severe.

High standards of hygiene must be maintained to prevent inflammation of the scalp, in the form of seborrheic dermatitis, and infection of the scalp, in the form of bacterial folliculitis. The individual who chooses to have hair additions must realize that the new hair style requires more grooming and upkeep than natural scalp hair.

HAIR INTEGRATION SYSTEMS

Hair integration systems are a useful method of allowing the patient to supplement hair loss only where necessary. These hair pieces are custom made by fashioning a loose net to fit

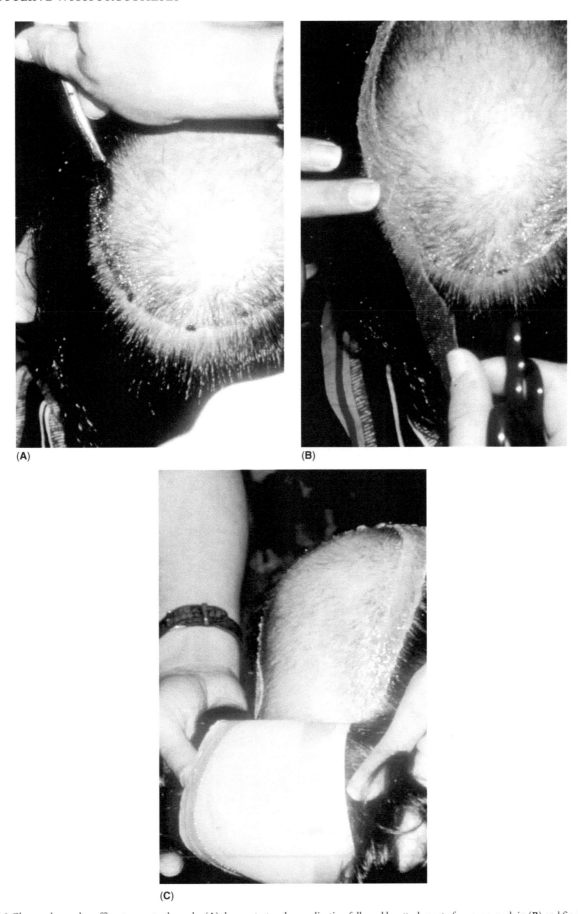

(A)

(B)

(C)

Figure 27.6 Glue can be used to affix a toupee to the scalp. (**A**) demonstrates glue application followed by attachment of a woven mesh in (**B**) and finally the toupee is glued to the woven mesh in (**C**).

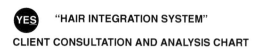

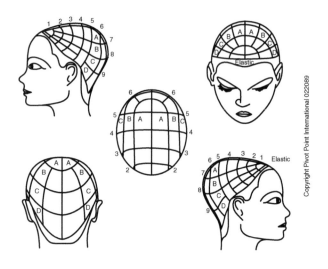

LENGTH ADDTION		TEXTURE ADDTION		COLOR ADDTION	
STRUCTURES		TEXTURE	TOOL	LEVEL	HUE
Solid					Red
Graduated					Gold
Increase					Yellow
Uniform					Blue
Combination					Violet
Textutining					Green

Figure 27.7 Hair integration systems are custom designed adding hair where needed to camouflage loss.

the scalp. Synthetic or natural human hair fibers are tied to the meshwork in the desired location, amount, length, color, and texture. Any hairstyle can be easily created (Fig. 27.7). The patient puts the integration system over their scalp and pulls their existing hair through the fenestrations in the net. This affixes the hair piece securely to the scalp and also allows a natural appearance. Integration systems can be rather costly depending upon the amount and length of hair attached. They are extremely versatile for patients with alopecia areata, androgenetic alopecia, scarring, or radiation hair loss.

> Hair integration systems are custom made by fashioning a loose net to fit the scalp to which synthetic or natural human hair fibers are tied.

CREPE HAIR TECHNIQUES
Crepe hair can be used to temporarily camouflage very small, localized areas of scalp hair loss. Its utility is in patients who have recent-onset alopecia areata with an excellent prognosis for hair regrowth who need an inexpensive, short-term camouflage. Crepe hair is made from wool and purchased as braids in a variety of colors. The wool strands are pulled from the braid and artistically glued to the scalp with adhesive.

The process must be redone with each shampooing and the adhesive removed with a specially formulated product.

> Crepe hair is composed of wool fibers that can be glued to the scalp and dusted onto the hair with a fixative.

Another more modern use of crepe hair is the fibered hair sprays or fibered powders containing the wool fibers. The fibers are charged with static electricity to allow them to adhere to the natural hair fibers and create the illusion of fuller hair. Some products also have a hair spray fixative in the formulation to increase the ability of the crepe hair to stay in place. Products are available in seven different shades to match most hair colors. These crepe hair products are popular among men to camouflage vertex balding. The product is removed with shampooing and must be reapplied as needed.

SCALP CAMOUFLAGE TECHNIQUES
Many times, it is the contrast between the pale bald scalp and the dark hair that accentuates hair loss. This contrast can be minimized by coloring the scalp to match the hair temporarily with wax crayons or vegetable dyes, or permanently with tattoo pigment. The wax crayons are stroked over the scalp artistically to mimic hair and the color is easily removed with shampoo. Tattoo pigment can also be placed in streaks to mimic hair shafts. The tattoo looks realistic when combined with hair, but if all the hair is lost in an area, the tattoo looks quite unusual. Patients should consider their natural hereditary pattern of balding prior to undergoing scalp tattooing.

> Scalp camouflaging can be performed with wax crayons, vegetable dyes, or tattoo pigment.

SUMMARY
Hair prostheses can be quite effective in camouflaging temporary or permanent alopecia. Many patients are not familiar with the options available to restore scalp hair and appreciate unbiased advice from their trusted dermatologist. This chapter has presented the basics of hair prostheses utilization. There are other cosmetic methods that can be used to optimize the appearance of thinning hair presented in the chapter on alopecia and cosmetic considerations.

REFERENCE
1. Panati C. Atop the vanity. In: Extraodinary Origins of Everyday Things. New York: Harper & Row Publishers, 1987: 234–6.

SUGGESTED READING
Beitone R, Sturla JM, Paty H, Meurice P, Samain H. Temporary restyling of the hair (Chapter 5). In: Bouillon C, Wilkinson J, eds. The Science of Hair Care. 2nd edn. Taylor & Francis Group, LLC, 2005: 187–92.

Harrison S, Sinclair R. Hair colouring, permanent styling, and hair structure. J Cosmet Dermatol 2003; 2: 180–5.

O'Hara CM, Izadi K, Albright L, Bradley JP. Case report of optic atrophy in pansynostosis: an unusual presentation of scalp edema from hair braiding. Pediatric Neurosurg 2006; 42: 100–4.

Seidel JS. The danger of scald burns during hair braiding. Ann Emerg Med 1994; 23: 1388–9.

28 Hair permanent waving

The idea of making straight hair permanently curly is appealing to both men and women who want to achieve fashionable hair styles. It always seems that those with straight want curly hair and those with curly hair want straight hair! While this seems rather silly, a whole industry is predicated on changing the conformation of hair to the likes of the individual. Hair permanent waving is a complex chemical process based on altering the 16% cystine incorporated into disulfide linkages between polypeptide chains in the hair keratin filament. These disulfide linkages are responsible for hair elasticity and can be re-formed to change the configuration of the hair shaft.

Methods of waving and curling straight hair have been practiced since ancient Egyptian times when water and mud were applied to hair wound on sticks and allowed to dry in the sun. The ancient Greeks refined the technique with hot irons, which were wrapped with hair. The use of hot irons to curl hair was rediscovered by Marcel in 1872 and is still a popular technique among Black men and women. The first hair waving solution was developed by Nessler in 1906 and consisted of borax paste, which produced longer lasting waves, but was very damaging to the hair. This method utilized external heat either in the form of electrically heated hollow iron tubes or a chemical heating pad that was attached to the curling rods with a clamp. Temperatures reached about 115°C and heating continued for 10 to 15 minutes (1).

In the 1930s, the first cold wave was introduced which virtually replaced heat methods of curling. The solution was based on ammonium thioglycolate containing free ammonia and a controlled pH. The original U.S. patent was granted to E. McDonough on June 16, 1941. Interestingly enough, this cold wave solution, with slight variations, is still popular today for both salon and home use. It is estimated that more than 65 million permanent waves are sold in salons and 45 million home waves are performed on an annual basis in the U.S.A. (2).

> Hair permanent waving is a complex chemical process based on altering the 16% cystine incorporated into disulfide linkages between polypeptide chains in the hair keratin filament.

CHEMISTRY

Permanent waving is a complex chemical process with three distinct steps: chemical softening, rearranging, and fixing (3). The basic chemistry involves the reduction of the disulfide hair shaft bonds with mercaptans (4). The process can be chemically characterized as listed in Table 28.1 (5).

> Permanent waving is a complex chemical process with three distinct steps: chemical softening, rearranging, and fixing.

APPLICATION TECHNIQUE

Cold permanent waves can be administered at home or in a salon, but involve the same application technique (6). It usually takes about 90 minutes to complete the entire process, depending on the length of the hair.

The standard procedure involves initial shampooing of the hair to remove dirt and sebum. This wetting process is the first step in preparing the hair for chemical treatment since the water enters the hair's hydrogen bonds and allows increased flexibility. The hair is then sectioned into 30 to 50 areas, depending on the length and thickness of the hair, and wound on mandrels or rods. The size of the rod determines the diameter of the curl with smaller rods producing tighter curls (Fig. 28.1). A sufficient amount of tension must be applied to the hair as it is wound around the rod to provide the stress required to encourage bond breaking. If too much tension is applied, the hair can be stretched beyond its elastic range, transforming it into a brittle substance that will easily fracture. Tissue paper squares about 5 × 5 cm, known as "end papers," are applied to the distal hair shafts to prevent irregular wrapping of the ends around the rod. Failure to use end papers can result in a frizzy appearance of the distal hair shaft (Fig. 28.2).

Next, the waving lotion is applied and left in contact with the hair for 5 to 20 minutes, depending on the condition of the hair (Fig. 28.3). The reducing action of the waving lotion is said to "soften" the hair and contains a disulfide bond-breaking agent, such as ammonium or calcium thioglycolate, and an antioxidant, such as sodium hydrosulfite, to prevent the lotion from reacting with air before it reaches the hair. Sequestering agents, such as tetrasodium EDTA, are added to prevent trace metals such as iron in tap water from reacting with the thioglycolate lotion. Other ingredients include pH adjusters, conditioners, and surfactants to remove the remaining sebum from the hair (Fig. 28.4). Coarse hair requires a longer processing time than fine hair and undyed hair requires a longer processing time than permanently dyed or bleached hair. A "test curl" is then checked to determine if the desired amount of curl has been obtained and overprocessing avoided (Fig. 28.5).

The hair disulfide bonds are subsequently reformed with the hair in the new curled conformation around the perming rods. This process is known as neutralization, fixation, or "hardening" (Fig. 28.6). The neutralization procedure, chemically characterized as an oxidation step, should involve two steps. First, two-thirds of the neutralizer should thoroughly saturate the hair with the rods in place and allowed to set for five minutes. The rods are then removed and the remaining one-third of the neutralizer applied for an additional five minutes. The hair is then carefully rinsed. Patients who complain of an undesirable odor following permanent waving, especially after shampooing, have undergone incomplete neutralization.

Repeating the neutralization process as outlined above will reduce the excessive odor (7).

The newly curled hair is now ready for drying and styling. Most companies recommend avoiding shampooing or manipulating the hair for one to two days following the cold wave procedure to ensure long lasting curls.

Table 28.1 Permanent Waving Process

1. Penetration of the thiol compound into the hair shaft.
2. Cleavage of the hair keratin disulfide bond (kSSk) to produce a cysteine residue (kSH) and the mixed disulfide of the thiol compound with the hair keratin (kSSR).

$$kSSk + RSH \rightarrow kSH + kSSR$$

3. Reaction with another thiol molecule to produce a second cysteine residue and the symmetrical disulfide of the thiol waving agent (RSSR).

$$kSSR + RSH \rightarrow kSH + RSSR$$

4. Rearrangement of the hair protein structure to relieve internal stress, which is determined by curler size and hair wrapping tension.
5. Application of an oxidizing agent to reform the disulfide cross-links.

$$kSH + HSk \xrightarrow{\text{oxidizing agent}} kSSk + water$$

A permanent wave is designed to last three to four months. Curl relaxation occurs with time as the hair returns to its original conformation. Hairdressers generally will therefore select a curl tighter than the patient desires with this fact in mind. Most of the curl relaxation occurs within the first two weeks after processing, a fact that is reassuring to the patient who has had an undesirable result. Curl relaxation can be increased slightly by frequent shampooing beginning immediately following the permanent waving procedure. Some strong detergent shampoos, such as those recommended for seborrheic dermatitis, will cause curl relaxation more rapidly than conditioning shampoos. New hair growth also decreases the curled appearance of the hair. Patients with rapidly growing hair need to repeat the permanent waving procedure more frequently. Increased hair growth during pregnancy could account for the fact that some hairdressers note permanent waves do not "take" in pregnant women. Hair at the nape of the neck also has a decreased "take."

FACTORS INFLUENCING PERMANENT WAVING

There are several factors that determine the success or failure of a cold waving procedure. Most of the suboptimal results that cause patients to seek dermatologic help result from failure to consider the key points listed in Table 28.2 while performing the procedure (8).

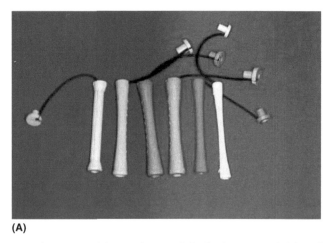

(A)

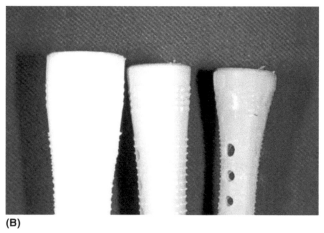

(B)

Figure 28.1 Hair is wound on mandrels of various sizes with (**A**) smaller rods producing tighter curls and (**B**) larger rods producing looser curls.

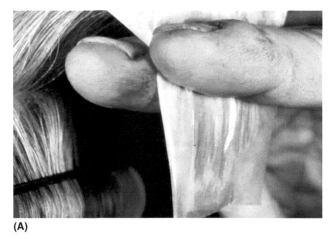

(A)

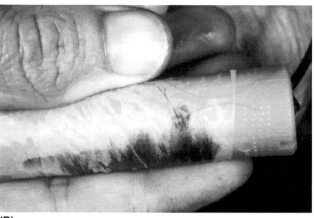

(B)

Figure 28.2 The ends of the hair are wrapped in end papers to make sure that all hairs are wound around the mandrel to prevent hair frizziness.

ASSESSING THE PERMANENT WAVE EFFECTIVENESS

Several methods are used by manufacturers of cold waving products to determine wave efficiency and degree of hair shaft damage. These are known as the deficiency in tightness (DIT) value, the curl length, and the 20% index (8).

The DIT value is determined as follows:

$$DIT = \frac{diameter\ of\ curl\ (mm) - diameter\ of\ rod\ (mm)}{diameter\ of\ rod\ (mm)} \times 100$$

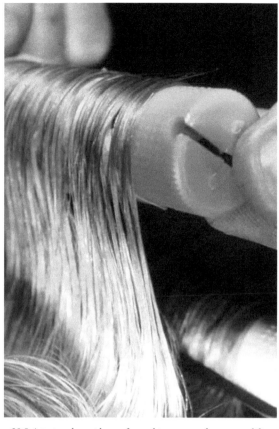

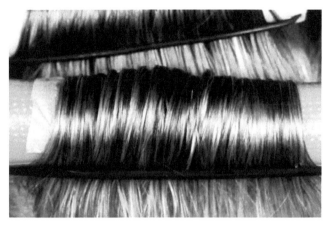

Figure 28.3 The hair is wrapped around the mandrel ready for waving lotion application.

Figure 28.5 A test curl must be performed to ensure adequate curl formation and avoid overprocessing of the hair shafts.

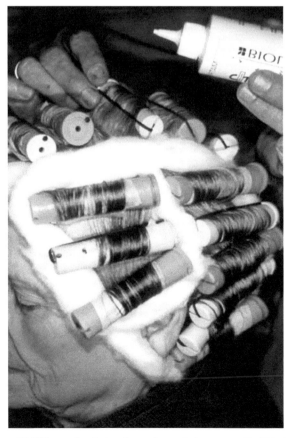

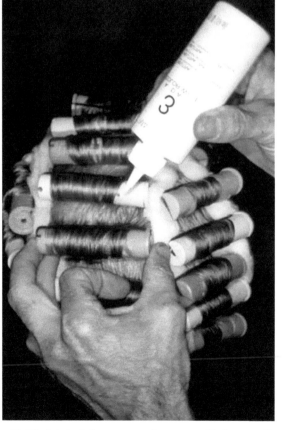

Figure 28.4 The waving lotion is evenly applied to cause disulfide bond breaking in each hair shaft for an even curl.

Figure 28.6 Each hair shaft must come in contact with the neutralizer to reform the disulfide bonds in the new curled shape and restore hair strength.

Table 28.2 Permanent Waving Guidelines

1. The hair must not be wound with excessive tension around the rods, or an increased breakage may occur (9).
2. Smaller rods will produce smaller curls, which are more damaging to the hair shaft.
3. The hair must fit around the rod at least once for complete curl formation in patients with short hair.
4. A stronger waving lotion will not produce a tighter curl. The curl diameter is determined by the rod diameter.
5. Weak waving lotions with shorter processing times should be used for damaged hair.
6. It may be necessary to use different strengths of waving lotions on new proximal growth and previously waved distal growth, especially in patients with bleached hair.
7. A test curl should be performed to avoid over-processing the hair. Long processing times can excessively damage hair, increasing the breakage.
8. Discoloration of the hair may occur in patients who have used para-phenylenediamine-based permanent dyes that have been incompletely oxidized.

The higher the DIT value, the greater the effectiveness of the curling solution. In other words, weak cold wave solutions have low DIT values.

The curl length is evaluated by suspending a fresh curl and observing the spring of the formed coil. The degree of laxity is indicative of the efficiency of the wave and also of the degree of hair shaft damage. Thus, longer curls are indicative of greater hair shaft damage.

The 20% index is determined by stretching freshly permed hair with a uniformly increasing load. The ratio of the load required after perming to the load required prior to perming to stretch a wet strand of 12 hairs to 20% of their original length is known as the 20% index. The higher the index, the lower the reduction in hair strength due to the cold wave procedure.

Cold wave chemists use these three criteria to determine not only the success of the permanent wave procedure, but also the degree of hair shaft damage. Factors affecting the efficacy of a permanent waving product are processing time, processing temperature, concentration of reducing agent, ration of lotion to hair quantities, penetration of the lotion, pH and the nature and condition of the untreated hair (10). A marketable permanent wave solution must produce the best curl with the least amount of hair damage (11).

Factors affecting the efficacy of a permanent waving product are processing time, processing temperature, concentration of reducing agent, ration of lotion to hair quantities, penetration of the lotion, pH and the nature and condition of the untreated hair.

HAIR ALTERATIONS FOLLOWING PERMANENT WAVING

Following the permanent waving process, the hair has been irreversibly altered. These changes contribute to some of the dermatologic problems noted in chemically waved hair. First, the dry waved hair shaft is shorter than the original hair shaft (12). This may account for the perception by many patients that their hair was cut too short following a perming procedure. Second, the chemically treated hair shaft is 17% weaker and thus less able to withstand the trauma of combing and brushing (13). Patients comment that their hair is falling following permanent waving when in actuality the hair shaft is fracturing more readily. Third, the hair demonstrates more frictional resistance following permanent waving (14). This means it is more difficult to comb. Lastly, the hair demonstrates increased swelling capacity, which is evidence of cortical damage (15). This swelling accounts for the increased penetration of other chemicals applied to the hair, such as dyes, yielding unexpected results (Fig. 28.7).

TYPES OF PERMANENT WAVES

Waving lotions consist primarily of a reducing agent in an aqueous solution with an adjusted pH (16). Table 28.3 summarizes waving lotion ingredients and their function (1). The most popular reducing agents are the thioglycolates, glycerol thioglycolates, and sulfites. On the basis of waving lotion type, permanent waves can be classified into the following groups (4,17):

1. Alkaline permanents
2. Buffered alkaline permanents
3. Exothermic permanents
4. Self-regulated permanents
5. Acid permanents
6. Sulfite permanents

Table 28.4 summarizes differences between each of the permanent wave types.

Alkaline Permanents

Alkaline permanents utilize ammonium thioglycolate or ethanolamine thioglycolate as the reducing agent in the waving lotion. The pH is adjusted to between 9 and 10 since the thioglycolates are not as effective at lower pH. These products process extremely rapidly and produce a tight, long-lasting curl; however they are harsh on the hair. The alkalinity allows hair shaft swelling which can cause problems in individuals with color-treated hair, especially bleached hair. For this reason, the concentration of the thioglycolate waving lotion is adjusted from the 7% used on natural hair to1% used on heavily bleached hair.

Buffered Alkaline Permanents

In order to decrease hair swelling encountered due to the high pH of alkaline permanent waves, a buffering agent such as ammonium bicarbonate is employed. These products are known as buffered alkaline permanents and result in a tight curl at a pH of 7 to 8.5. Their advantage is the production of a tight, long-lasting curl with less hair damage.

Exothermic Permanents

Exothermic permanent waves produce heat as a by-product to increase client comfort as some individuals may feel chilled during the permanent waving process. The heat is produced when an oxidizing agent, such as hydrogen peroxide, is mixed with the thioglycolate-based waving lotion immediately prior to scalp application. The reaction of the thioglycolate with the peroxide produces dithiodiglycolate (the disulfide of thioglycolate) which

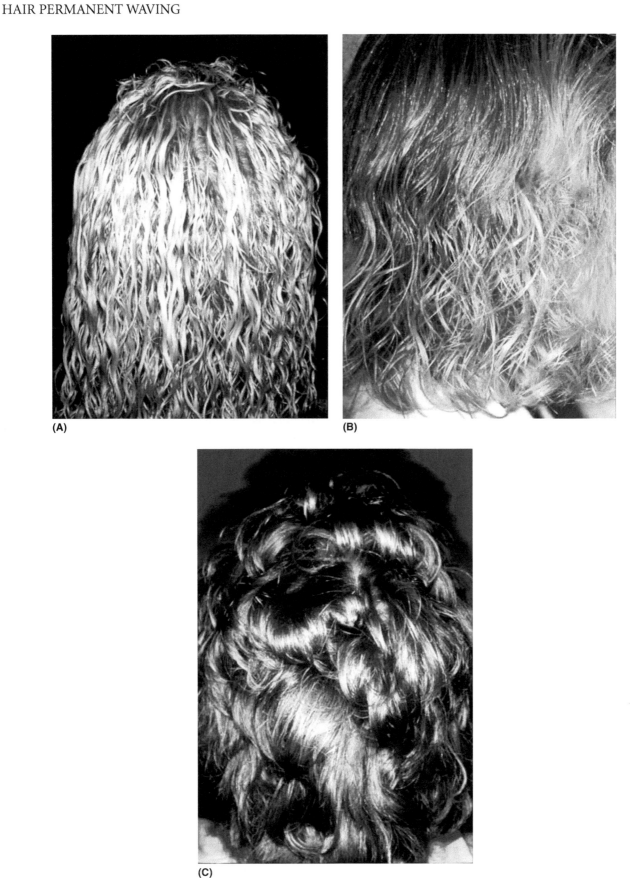

Figure 28.7 (**A**) A tight permanent wave as evidenced by tightly curled hair. (**B**) A medium permanent wave showing relaxed ringlets. (**C**) A loose permanent wave, also known as body wave, demonstrating loose curls.

Table 28.3 Permanent Waving Lotion Ingredients

Ingredient	Chemical examples	Function
Reducing agent	Thioglycolates sulfites	Break disulfide bonds
Alkaline agent	Ammonium hydroxide, triethanol-amine	Adjust pH
Chelating agent	Tetrasodium EDTA	Remove trace metals
Wetting agent	Fatty alcohols	Improve hair saturation with waving lotion
Conditioner	Proteins, humectants, quaternium compounds	Protect hair during waving process
Opacifier	Polyacrylates, polystyrene latex	Opacify waving lotion

Source: Adapted from Ref. 1.

Table 28.4 Function of Neutralizer Ingredients

Ingredient	Chemical example	Function
Oxidizing agent	Hydrogen peroxide, sodium bromated	Reform broken disulfide bonds
Acid buffer	Citric acid, acetic acid, lactic acid	Maintain acidic pH
Stabilizer	Sodium stannate	Prevent hydrogen peroxide breakdown
Wetting agent	Fatty alcohols	Improve hair saturation with neutralizer
Conditioner	Proteins, humectants, quaternium compounds	Improve hair feel
Opacifier	Polyacrylates, polystyrene latex	Make neutralizer opaque

Source: Adapted from Ref. 1.

limits the extent to which the permanent wave can process. Irreversible hair damage will result if the waving lotion is not mixed with the oxidizing agent prior to application. For this reason, exothermic permanent waves are mainly available for professional use only.

Self-Regulated Permanents

Self-regulated permanent waves are designed to limit the amount of hair disulfide bond breakage so that irreversible hair damage is prevented. Overprocessing, due to leaving the permanent wave solution on the hair longer than recommended, causes extensive hair breakage acting like a depilatory. It is not unusual for a busy beautician to have three to four permanent waves processing at the same time. Self-regulated permanent waves are designed to form a chemical equilibrium such that the disulfide bond breakage is stopped. This is accomplished by adding dithioglycolic acid to the thioglycolate-based waving lotion. This is the same chemical reaction discussed for exothermic permanent waves.

Acid Permanents

Acid permanent waves occur in an acidic environment with a pH of 6.5 to 7. They are based on thioglycolate esters such as

glycerol monothioglycolate. The lower pH is an advantage since less hair shaft swelling occurs than at higher pH levels, thus hair damage is minimized. These products result in a looser, shorter-lasting curl, but leave the hair soft. They are ideal for bleached or color-treated hair. It is possible to achieve a tighter curl if the permanent wave is processed with added heat under a hair dryer, but more hair shaft damage results.

The glycerol monothioglycolate in this type of permanent wave is responsible for allergic contact dermatitis in both beauticians and clients (18). Interestingly enough, the hair may continue to be allergenic even after all products have been thoroughly rinsed from the hair.

> Glycerol monothioglycolate found in acid permanent waves is responsible for allergic contact dermatitis in both beauticians and clients.

Sulfite Permanents

Sulfite permanent waves are mainly marketed for home use and have not found popularity among salons in the U.S.A. These products differ in that the reducing agent is a sulfite or bisulfite, instead of a mercaptan. This accounts for the reduced odor which is their primary advantage. They require a long processing time at a pH of 6 to 8 and result in loose curls. A conditioning agent must be added to the formulation as the sulfite permanent waves can leave the hair feeling harsh.

Home Permanents

Home permanents are designed for the nonprofessionals and are of two types: ammonium thioglycolate permanents and sulfite permanents. The ammonium thioglycolate permanents have the same characteristics as the salon solutions except they are one-third strength. This is to prevent excessive hair damage by the novice. Thus, home thioglycolate permanents produce looser curls that are not as long lasting as salon permanents.

As mentioned previously, sulfite permanents are manufactured only for home use and have no professional counterpart. The major advantage of this type of permanent wave is decreased odor. The head is covered with a plastic cap to use body heat for processing and an alkaline rinse is applied as a neutralizer. The mild curls produced are not long lasting.

Neutralizers

Neutralizers function to reform the broken disulfide bonds and restore the hair to its original condition. Two methods are available: self-neutralization and chemical neutralization. Both methods rely on oxidation. Self- neutralization allows air to oxidize the permanent wave, but this requires 6 to 24 hours. During this time, the hair must be left on the permanent wave rods. This method is rarely used. Chemical neutralization is more popular, due to its speed, and relies upon the use of an oxidizing agent. The oxidizing agent is usually 2% hydrogen peroxide adjusted to an acidic pH. Bromates may also be used, but are more expensive. The ingredients found in a chemical neutralizer and their functions are summarized in Table 28.4 (1).

ADVERSE REACTIONS

The use of permanent wave solutions is considered safe; however, incidence of both irritant and allergic contact dermatitis has been reported to thioglycolate-containing waving lotions (19).

Irritant contact dermatitis is more common and can be avoided by minimizing skin contact with the solution (20). This is especially important in patients using topical tretinoin, who seem to experience skin irritation more readily with permanent waving. Prior to application of the waving lotion, a layer of petroleum jelly should be applied to the margins of the scalp and covered with a band of absorbent cotton. This provides a protective covering for the non-hair bearing skin that might contact any waving lotion running over the scalp. Patients with a sensitive scalp can even apply petroleum jelly to the scalp as protection. The petroleum jelly contacts the proximal hair shaft, however, preventing curling in this region.

Allergic contact dermatitis can occur immediately after permanent waving or persist due to an allergen in the hair of patients who undergo permanent waving procedures involving glyceryl monothioglycolate (18,21). The North American Contact Dermatitis Group found this chemical to be the fifth most common cause of dermatitis (22). The substance should be patch tested at a 1% concentration in petrolatum (23).

SUMMARY

Permanent waving is a popular hair styling technique for both men and women. The increased curl makes straight hair appear fuller and provides for fashionable styles. Unfortunately, there is no such thing as a body building permanent wave or a hair restorative permanent wave. All permanent wave processes damage and weaken the hair fiber. This chapter has evaluated the chemistry of the various permanent waves on the market for their effect of the hair shaft presenting information to help the dermatologist understand the procedure and advise patients in a meaningful way when they present with problems from permanent waving.

REFERENCES

1. Lee AE, Bozza JB, Huff S, de la Mettrie R. Permanent waves: an overview. Cosmet Toilet 1988; 103: 37–56.
2. Wickett RR. Disulfide bond reduction in permanent waving. Cosmet Toilet 1991; 106: 37–47.
3. Wickett RR. Permanent waving and straightening of hair. Cutis 1987; 39: 496–7.
4. Zviak C. Permanent waving and hair straightening. In: Zviak C, ed. The Science of Hair Care. New York: Marcel Dekker, 1986, 183–209.
5. Cannell DW. Permanent waving and hair straightening. Clin Dermatol 1988; 6: 71–82.
6. Draelos ZK. Hair cosmetics. Dermatol Clin 1991; 9: 19–27.
7. Brunner MJ. Medical aspects of home cold waving. Arch Dermatol 1952; 65: 316–26.
8. Heilingotter R. Permanent waving of hair. In: de Navarre MG, ed. The Chemistry and Manufacture of Cosmetics. Illinois: Allured Publishing Co, 1988, 1167–227.
9. Wortman FJ, Souren I. Extensional properties of human hair and permanent waving. J Soc Cosmet Chem 1987; 38: 125–40.
10. Shipp JJ. Hair-care products. In: Chemistry and Technology of the Cosmetics and Toiletries Industry, London: Blackie Academic & Professional, 1992, 80–6.
11. Szadurski JS, Erlemann G. The hair loop test—a new method of evaluating perm lotions. Cosmet Toilet 1984; 99: 41–6.
12. Garcia ML, Nadgorny EM, Wolfram LJ. Letter to the editor. J Soc Cosm Chem 1990; 41: 149–54.
13. Feughelman M. A note on the permanent setting of human hair. J Soc Cosmet Chem 1990; 41: 209–12.
14. Robbins CR. Chemical and Physical Behavior of Human Hair. New York: Springler-Verlag, 1988, 94–8.
15. Shansky A. The osmotic behavior of hair during the permanent waving process as explained by swelling measurements. J Soc Cosm Chem 1963; 14: 427–32.
16. Ishihara M. The composition of hair preparations and their skin hazards. In: Koboir T, Montagna W, eds. Biology and Disease of the Hair. Baltimore: University Park Press, 1975, 603–29.
17. Gershon SD, Goldberg MA, Rieger MM. Permanent waving. In: Balsam MS, Sagarin E, eds, Cosmetics Science and Technology, 2nd edn, Vol. 2, New York: Wiley-Interscience, John Wiley & Sons, 1972, 167–250.
18. Morrison LH, Storrs FJ. Persistence of an allergen in hair after glyceryl monothioglycolate-containing permanent wave solutions. J Am Acad Dermatol 1988; 19: 52–9.
19. Lehman AJ. Health aspects of common chemicals used in hair-waving preparations. JAMA 1949; 141: 842–5.
20. Fisher AA. Management of hairdressers sensitized to hair dyes or permanent wave solutions. Cutis 1989; 43: 316–18.
21. Storrs FJ. Permanent wave contact dermatitis: contact allergy to glyceryl monothioglycolate. J Am Acad Dermatol 1984; 11: 74–85.
22. Adams RM, Maibach HI. A five-year study of cosmetic reactions. J Am Acad Dermatol 1985; 13: 1062–9.
23. White IR, Rycroft RJG, Anderson KE, et al. The patch test dilution of slyceryl thioglycolate. Contact Dermatitis 1990; 23: 198–9.

SUGGESTED READING

Bolduc C, Shapiro J. Hair care products: waving, straightening, conditioning, and coloring. Clin Dermatol 2001; 19: 431–6.
Borish ET. Hair waving (Chapter 6). In: Johnson DH, ed. Hair and Hair Care. Marcel Dekker, 1997, 167–90.
DeGeorge, MS. Permanent waving, hair straightening, and depilatories (Chapter 32). Harry's Cosmeticology, 8th edn. Chemical Publishing Co., Inc., 2000, 695–723.
Han MO, Chun JA, Lee JW, Chung CH. Effects of permanent waving on changes of protein and physicomorphological properties in human head hair. J Cosmet Sci 2008; 59: 203–15.
Hishikawa N, Tanizawa Y, Tanaka S, Honiguchi Y, Asakura T. Structural change of keratin protein in human hair by permanent waving treatment. Polymer 1998; 39: 3835–40.
Kuzuhara A. Analysis of structural changes in permanent waved human hair using Raman spectroscopy. Biopolymers 2007; 85: 274–83.
Syed AN, Ayoub H. Correlating porosity and tensile strength of chemically modified hair. Cosmet Toilet 2002; 117: 1245–30.
Wickett RR. Permanent waving and straightening of hair. Cutis 1987; 39: 496–7.
Zviak C, Sabbagh A. Permanent waving and hair straightening (Chapter 6). In: Bouillon C, Wilkinson J, eds. The Science of Hair Care, 2nd edn. Taylor & Francis Group, LLC, 2005, 201–27.

Hair straightening is truly an art. It is a commonly practiced procedure among persons with wavy and curly hair to allow versatility in hair styling that otherwise could not be achieved (1). Hair straightening requires skill, dexterity, and knowledge to obtain an optimal result. Skill is required to apply the straightening cream evenly to the entire hair shaft in an organized methodical fashion. Dexterity is required to apply the straightening cream, comb the hair straight, and remove the cream within a 20-minute time period. Lastly, knowledge is required to select the hair straightening chemical that will break enough disulfide bonds in the hair shaft to allow straightening to occur without weakening the hair shaft to the point of fracture. There is no substitute for the skill of a well-trained beautician when it comes to straightening hair. It is infinitely more difficult than permanent waving or dyeing hair.

> Permanent hair straightening is a procedure technically known as lanthionization.

Hair can be straightened with heat or chemical techniques (2). Heat straightening techniques are temporary and have already been covered. This chapter shall discuss the permanent method of hair straightening, also known as lanthionization. Hair straightening is undertaken for many reasons including those listed in Table 29.1 (3).

The first permanent hair straighteners, also known as hair relaxers or perms, were developed around 1940 and consisted of sodium hydroxide or potassium hydroxide mixed into potato starch. Once the disulfide bonds were broken, the hair was pulled straight and the disulfide bonds reformed in their new configuration. This section examines the physical and chemical differences between African American hair and Caucasian hair, discusses the chemistry of hair straightening, reviews the unique aspects of the hair straightening techniques, and presents the relevant dermatologic considerations.

HAIR STRAIGHTENING CHARACTERISTICS

There are some unique differences between Caucasian hair and African American hair. Table 29.2 summarizes some of the key differences (4). It is interesting to note that African American hair has a greater thickness but requires less strength to break than Caucasian hair. Notice that Asian hair grows the longest and is the most resistant to breakage. This may account for the fact that most human hair wigs for African Americans are woven from treated Asian hair. There are also subtle differences in the chemical substances such as amino acid, sulfur, and ammonia between African American and Caucasian hair (Table 29.3).

> African American hair has a greater thickness than Caucasian hair, but requires less force to break.

In summary, it can be said that African American hair has fewer cuticle layers than Caucasian hair, 7 as compared to 12. The hair shafts have a larger diameter, but tend to break where the hair begins to kink at pinch points (5). Lastly, African American hair has a lower moisture content than Caucasian hair, which reduces the hair shaft elasticity and encourages breakage.

> African American hair has a lower moisture content than Caucasian hair, reducing the hair shaft elasticity and encouraging breakage.

HAIR STRAIGHTENING CHEMISTRY

Hair relaxing, also known as lanthionization, is a chemical process whereby extremely curly hair is straightened through the use of metal hydroxides, such as sodium, lithium, potassium, or guanidine hydroxide, to change about 35% of the cysteine contents of the hair to lanthionine along with minor hydrolysis of the peptide bonds. Chemical relaxing can be accomplished with lye-based, lye-free, ammonium thioglycolate, or bisulfite creams (6).

Lye-based, or sodium hydroxide straighteners are alkaline creams with a pH of 13. Sodium hydroxide is a caustic substance that can damage hair, produce scalp burns, and cause blindness if exposed to the eye. These products are generally restricted to professional or salon use and may contain up to 3.5% sodium hydroxide. The basic chemistry of hair relaxing with lye products is depicted in Table 29.4 while the hair rearrangement schematic is presented in Table 29.5 (7).

> Lye-based hair straighteners are the most popular straighteners and are alkaline creams with a pH of 13.

Lye relaxers are available in "base" and "no-base" forms (Table 29.6). The "base" is usually petrolatum that is applied to the scalp and hair line prior to application of the sodium hydroxide. This prevents scalp irritation and burns. The "base" relaxers contain between 1.5% and 3.5% sodium hydroxide and therefore require that the scalp and hairline be coated with a petrolatum base prior to application. These high-concentration lye products are necessary for hard-to-straighten hair. "No-base" relaxers, on the other hand, contain 1.5% to 2.5% sodium hydroxide and only require base application to the hairline (8). They are more popular since it is time consuming for the beautician to apply the base to the scalp and most individuals are re-straightening hair that has already been chemically weakened.

Other strong alkali chemicals sometimes used in place of sodium hydroxide are guanidine hydroxide and lithium hydroxide, which are known as "no-lye" chemical hair straighteners

Table 29.1 Rationale for Permanent Hair Straightening

1. Hair manageability is improved
2. The hair can be more easily combed and styled
3. Hair breakage may be decreased due to less combing friction
4. Hair shine is improved with a straighter hair shaft
5. Fashion may dictate the need for straight hair
6. Versatility in straightening techniques allows multiple styling options: completely straightened, minimally straightened, texturized, or straightened and recurled

Table 29.2 Comparative Physical Characteristics of African American Hair

Property evaluated	African American	Caucasian	Asian
Maximum length (mm)	15–30	60–100	100–150
Thickness	High	Medium	Low
Shape	Kidney	Oval	Round
Force (g)	33	43	63
Breaking strength dry (N/m^2)	0.153	0.189	
Breaking strength wet (N/m^2)	0.089	0.165	
Elongation at breaking point wet (%)	42	62	
Elongation at breaking point dry (%)	39	50	

Source: Adapted from Vermeulen S, Banham A, Brooks G. Ethnic hair care. Cosmet Toilet 2002; 117: 69–78.

Table 29.3 Comparative Chemical Amino Acid Characteristics of African American Hair

Amino acids and other hair components	African American hair content	Caucasian hair content
Glycine	541	539
Alanine	509	471
Valine	568	538
Leucine	570	554
Isoleucine	277	250
Serine	672	870
Threonine	615	653
Tyrosine	202	132
Phenylalanine	179	130
Aspartic acid	436	455
Glutamic acid	915	871
Lysine	23	213
Arginine	482	512
Histidine	84	63
Sulfur	1380	1440
Half cystine	1370	1380
Cysteic acid	10	55
Proline	662	672
Ammonia	935	780

Source: Adapted from Vermeulen S, Banham A, Brooks G. Ethnic hair care. Cosmet Toilet 2002; 117: 69–78.

(Table 29.7). These relaxing kits contain 4–7% cream calcium hydroxide and liquid guanidine carbonate. The guanidine carbonate activator is then mixed into the calcium hydroxide cream to produce calcium carbonate and guanidine hydroxide, the

Table 29.4 Chemistry of Hair Relaxing

Strong alkali chemical relaxing

$$NaOH + K\text{-}S\text{-}S\text{-}K \xrightarrow{OH^-} K\text{-}S\text{-}K + Na_2S + H_2O$$

(Alkali can be Na+, K+, or Li+)

Source: Adapted from Obukowho P, Birman M. Hair curl relaxers: a discussion of their function, chemistry, and manufacture. Cosmet Toilet 1995; 110: 65–9.

Table 29.5 Two-Part Guanidine Carbonate Relaxing

Part One

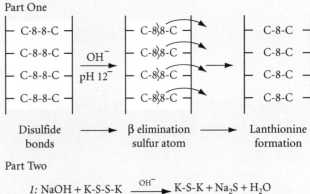

Part Two

$$1\text{: } NaOH + K\text{-}S\text{-}S\text{-}K \xrightarrow{OH^-} K\text{-}S\text{-}K + Na_2S + H_2O$$

(Alkali can be Na^+, K^+, Li^+)

$$2a\text{: } \overset{+NH_2\text{-}CO_3^-}{\underset{\parallel}{NH_2\text{-}C\text{-}NH_2}} + Ca(OH)_2 \xrightarrow{OH^-} \overset{+NH_2\text{-}OH^-}{\underset{\parallel}{NH_2\text{-}C\text{-}NH_2}} + CaCO_3$$

$$2b\text{: } \overset{+NH_2\text{-}OH^-}{\underset{\parallel}{NH_2\text{-}C\text{-}NH_2}} + K\text{-}S\text{-}S\text{-}K \xrightarrow{OH^-} K\text{-}S\text{-}K + (NH_4)_2\text{-}S + H_2O \text{ etc.}$$

Source: Adapted from Obukowho P, Birman M. Hair curl relaxers: a discussion of their function, chemistry, and manufacture. Cosmet Toilet 1995; 110: 65–9.

Table 29.6 Ingredients in a Lye No-Base Relaxer

Petrolatum
Mineral oil
Fatty alcohol
Emulsifying wax
Simethicone
Water
Propylene glycol
Sodium lauryl sulfate
Sodium hydroxide (lye)

active agent. These products do not require basing of either the scalp or the hairline. The chemical reaction that occurs with a guanidine hydroxide product is illustrated in Table 29.5.

No lye relaxers are based on guanidine hydroxide and lithium hydroxide, which may be more damaging to the hair shaft than lye relaxers, if not properly applied.

Table 29.8 compares the lye and no-lye relaxers in terms of their effect on the hair shaft.

Table 29.7 Ingredients in a No-Lye Cream Relaxer

Cream Relaxer Components
    Petrolatum
    Mineral oil
    Fatty alcohol
    Emulsifying wax
    Simethicone
    Water
    Propylene glycol
    Calcium hydroxide
Liquid Activator Components
    Water
    Propylene glycol
    Xanthan gum
    Guanidine carbonate

Table 29.8 Comparison of Lye and No-Lye Chemical Relaxers

Hair quality	Lye chemical relaxer	No-Lye chemical relaxer
Relative strength on a scale of 1–3 (higher no. is stronger)	3	1
Alkaline relaxing agent	NaOH or KOH	Guanidine hydroxide
Chemical agent	OH	OH
PH	12.5–14	12.5–13.5
Hair shaft penetration	Faster	Slower
Processing time	Shorter	Longer
Irritation	High	Low
Hair drying potential	Less drying to hair and scalp	More drying to hair and scalp

Source: Adapted from Obukowho P, Birman M. Hair curl relaxers: a discussion of their function, chemistry, and manufacture. Cosmet Toilet 1995; 110: 65–9.

Thioglycolate can also be used as an active agent in hair straightening (9). These are the same thioglycolate chemicals that were described as permanent wave solutions, except that they are formulated as thick creams, rather than lotions. The cream adds weight to hair and helps to pull it straight. Also, instead of the hair being wound on mandrels, it is combed straight while the thioglycolate cream is in contact with the hair shaft. Thioglycolate hair straighteners are extremely harsh on the hair and are the least popular of all the relaxing chemicals for this reason. The thioglycolate cream has a pH of 9.0 to 9.5, which removes the protective sebum and facilitates hair shaft penetration. Chemical burns can also occur with this variety of chemical hair straightener (10).

The least damaging of all hair straightening chemicals are the ammonium bisulfite creams. These products contain a mixture of bisulfite and sulfite in varying ratios depending on the pH of the lotion. Many of the home chemical straightening products are of this type, but can only produce short lived straightening. These are very similar to the home sulfite permanent waves, except here again the hair is combed straight instead of being wound on curling rods.

Table 29.9 Considerations for Selecting a Hair Relaxer

1. Relaxer must effectively straighten hair
2. Relaxer must contain adequate petrolatum and other oils to protect against scalp and hairline irritation
3. Relaxer must be stable at room temperature
4. Relaxer must be an easy-to-apply cream that spreads over hair with sufficient weight to pull hair straight
5. Relaxer must rinse easily with warm water
6. Relaxer must not damage hair beyond acceptable limits

Table 29.10 Hair Relaxing Steps

1. Do not shampoo
2. Apply petrolatum base to scalp and hairline
3. Section hair
4. Apply cream relaxer from hair root to end beginning at nape of neck
5. Gently comb hair straight for 10 to 30 min until the degree of relaxation is achieved
6. Rinse thoroughly with water
7. Apply neutralizer
8. Shampoo
9. Apply conditioner
10. Style
11. Apply styling conditioner

Chemical hair straightening chemicals that produce the longest-lasting hair straightening are also the most damaging to the hair shaft.

As a general rule, the chemicals that produce the greatest, longest-lasting hair straightening are also the most damaging to the hair shaft. Table 29.9 presents the important considerations when selecting a relaxer product.

APPLICATION TECHNIQUE
This section has presented the basic chemistry involved in hair relaxing and now presents the application technique. Whether the patient chooses to utilize lye-based, no-lye, thioglycolate, or sulfite chemicals to induce the straightening, the application technique is similar (Table 29.10) (11). The relaxing process is illustrated in Figure 29.1. Shampooing is the first step in the permanent waving technique for straight hair, but the hair is not shampooed when straightening is undertaken. This is because hair straightening chemicals are far more irritating and shampooing would remove the protective sebum from the scalp. As a matter of fact, the protective sebum is supplemented with a petrolatum base applied to the scalp and hairline to prevent skin burns. Following application of the base, the hair is divided into quadrants allowing the hair stylist to work systematically. For previously untreated hair, the chemical straightener is applied from hair root to distal end beginning at the nape of the neck and moving forward to the anterior hairline. The hair at the nape of the neck receives the chemical first, since it is subject to less weathering, resulting in the presence of more cuticular scale. This means it will be more resistant to the lanthionization process. The chemicals are left in contact with the hair only 20 to 30 minutes during which time the hair stylist is

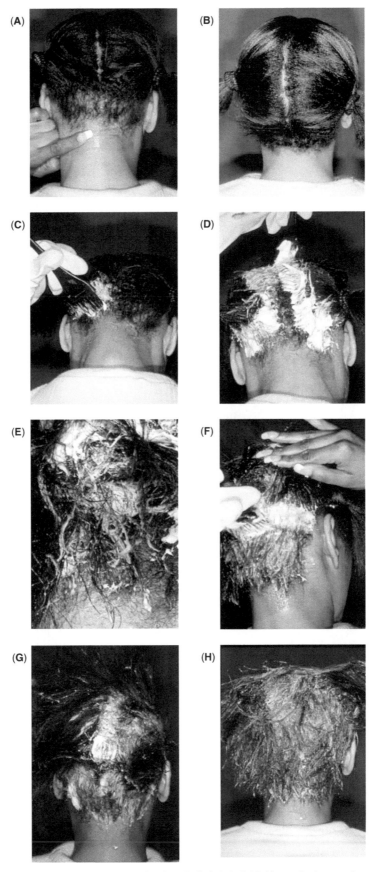

Figure 29.1 (**A**) A petrolatum base is applied to the entire hairline and scalp. (**B**) The hair is divided by parting into quadrants. (**C**) The cream is scooped from its jar and applied to the scalp with a stiff brush. (**D**) Application of the straightener to the hair close to the scalp at the nape of the neck. (**E**) The straightener is applied to the hair next to the scalp over the entire head. (**F**) A protective rubber glove is worn to prevent the strong alkali from producing cutaneous burns. (**G**) The relaxer has been applied to the entire scalp within 10 minutes. (**H**) The hair is combed and pulled straight.

combing the hair straight. The hair stylist must work quickly to get the straightening cream worked through all areas of the scalp quickly. Longer contact of the chemicals with the hair shafts will result in irreversible damage.

The hair stylist must work quickly to get the hair straightening chemicals in and out of the hair as quickly as possible to avoid overprocessing, which irreversibly weakens the hair shafts.

For previously treated hair, the chemical straightener is applied to the new growth only taking care to minimize scalp contact. Usually, the straightening cream is applied to the hair closest to the scalp first and then combed through the previously relaxed distal ends for the last 10 minutes of the process. The hair is combed to pull it straight concurrently with the straightening cream application. The hair stylist should completely remove all of the straightening chemicals within 20 minutes. This requires skill and organization. It is for this reason that hair straightening should not be attempted by someone without education and experience.

(A)
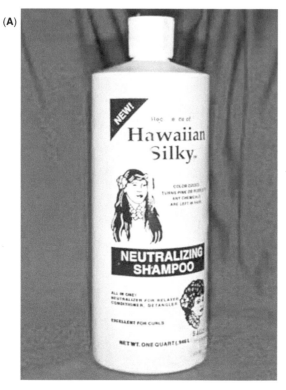

(B)
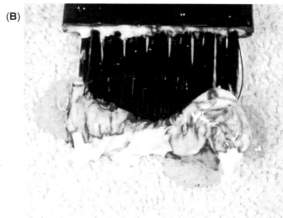

(C)
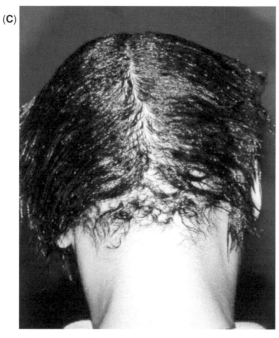

(D)
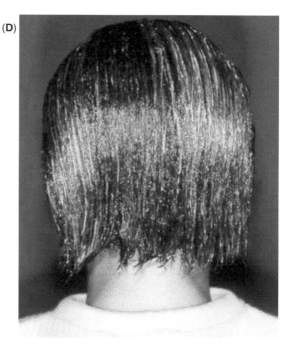

Figure 29.2 (**A**) The neutralizer lotion. (**B**) The neutralizer has a pH indicator and turns pink when applied to any hair that still contains the alkaline lye. (**C**) The hair has been shampooed and conditioned. (**D**) The appearance of the newly straightened hair.

When the hair has relaxed to desired degree of straightening, the cream must be thoroughly removed with water rinsing (Fig. 29.2). A neutralizer is then smoothed on the hair taking care to keep it straight and untangled, since the hair shafts can very easily fracture until the neutralization process is complete. Once the hair has been thoroughly neutralized, it is shampooed with a nonalkaline shampoo to minimize hair shaft swelling. A conditioner must be applied immediately following shampooing to decrease water loss from the hair shaft. The hair straightening chemicals produce holes in the hair shaft cuticle through which the hair shaft water evaporates leaving the hair shaft dry and inelastic. The remoisturizing poststraightening conditioner minimizes hair shaft brittleness and breakage. The formulation presented in Table 29.11 contains panthenol as a humectant, stearaylkonium chloride and dicetyldimonium chloride as conditioners, cetearyl alcohol and mineral oil as emollients, and octyl dimethyl PABA as a UV protectant. The hair is then dried and styled. Following styling, a second conditioner is applied to further condition the hair shafts. The formulation presented in Table 29.12 contains petrolatum, mineral oil, and beeswax to prevent water loss and add hair shaft shine.

If the hair is not properly neutralized, it will easily break after the relaxing procedure because the disulfide bonds have not been restored.

There are two other styling variations of hair relaxers known as blow-out relaxers and texturizing relaxers. The chemicals employed and the lanthionization process are identical to that

Table 29.11 Remoisturizing Post-Straightening Conditioner

Water
Methyl paraben
Imidazolidinyl urea
Panthenol
Sodium PCA
Cetearyl alcohol
Dicetyldimonium chloride
Mineral oil
Polysorbate-20
Propyl paraben
Octyl dimethyl PABA
Fragrance

Table 29.12 Ingredients in Oil Moisturizing Lotion Styling Conditioner

Petrolatum
Mineral oil
Propyl paraben
Beeswax
Stearic hydrazide
Sorbitan sesquioleate
Polysorbate-80
Water
Methylparaben
Imidazolidinyl urea
Sodium borate
Fragrance

previously discussed. The blow-out relaxers minimally straighten the hair shaft leaving it more manageable, but preserving some of the curl. Texturizing relaxers leave the hair wavy and not completely straight. Both of these relaxer varieties are most popular among men with short hair.

The key to successful hair relaxing is an experienced beautician who can quickly apply and remove the chemicals and determine when the desired degree of disulfide bond breaking has occurred. It is estimated that virgin hair loses about 30% of its tensile strength following a properly performed chemical straightening procedure. It also becomes more porous allowing future relaxing procedures to process more quickly (12). Hair relaxing is a careful balance between achieving the straightening of kinky hair and minimizing irreversible hair shaft damage.

It is estimated that virgin hair loses about 20% of its tensile strength following a properly performed chemical straightening procedure.

HAIR PERMING APPLICATION TECHNIQUE
Another technique for relaxing kinky hair is known as hair perming. The products used are similar to Caucasian permanent waves, in that they are based on ammonium thioglycolate, which is neutralized with ammonium hydroxide. The main differences between a straight hair perm and a kinky hair perm are the level of the active ingredients and the application technique. Perming is performed in four stages consisting of rearranging, boosting, neutralizing, and conditioning (Table 29.13).

Permanent waving of kinky hair begins by shampooing and sectioning the hair as described for hair straightening. A cream is then applied containing high levels of ammonium thioglycolate in the range of 7–7.5%. This cream is known as the reducing cream or rearranger. It is applied from the hair root to distal end on virgin hair starting at the nape of the neck proceeding to the anterior hair line. In previously chemically treated hair, the rearranger is only applied to new growth. Its purpose is to straighten the hair in preparation for the curling

Table 29.13 Kinky Hair Permanent Waving Technique

1. Shampoo hair
2. Section hair into quadrants
3. Apply rearranger from hair root to distal hair shaft starting with hair at the nape of the neck and moving forward
4. Rinse rearranger with water
5. Apply booster from hair root to distal hair shaft starting with the hair at the nape of the neck and moving forward
6. Section hair
7. Wrap hair around rods
8. Place patient under hooded hair dryer for 15–20 min
9. Perform test curl
10. Rinse hair thoroughly
11. Apply neutralizer to each rod for 15–20 min
12. Remove curling rods
13. Rinse hair thoroughly
14. Apply conditioner for 10–20 min
15. Dry hair
16. Apply glycerin curl activator
17. Style hair

procedure. The rearranger is then rinsed and a reducing lotion or curl booster is applied from the hair root to the distal end. The hair is then sectioned and wrapped around perming rods. The patient is placed under a hooded hair dryer to increase the rate of the chemical reaction with heat. After 15–20 minutes, a test curl is performed to determine whether the desired amount of curl has been obtained. This is assessed by unwrapping several rods and observing whether the hair makes a complete "s", meaning that the desired amount of curl has been achieved. This is identical to the reducing step in a permanent wave on straight hair. The hair is then thoroughly rinsed.

Next the hair is ready for neutralization with an oxidizing solution containing 10–13% sodium bromate for 15 to 20 minutes. This sets the curls and the rods are removed. The hair is then thoroughly rinsed. A variety of conditioners and glycerin curl activators are now applied to prevent excessive hair shaft water loss and hair brittleness. The hair is then dried and styled as desired.

These kinky hair perm products, known as the "Jheri" curl after the company that pioneered the technology, were introduced in the late 1970s. They have recently lost some of their original appeal since the curling procedure is extremely damaging to African American hair leaving it frizzy, dry, and brittle. Daily use of propylene glycol and glycerin curl activators is required prior to styling to maintain the hair style and decrease breakage. Unfortunately, the glycerin styling products leave the hair sticky and tend to stain clothing and pillow cases. It is also necessary to repeat the procedure every 12 weeks, further weakening the hair shafts and predisposing to hair loss through breakage.

ADDRESSING PATIENT PROBLEMS

The dermatologist may frequently encounter patients who are experiencing problems related to the use of hair straighteners. Most patients will complain of hair loss immediately following a relaxing procedure. It is important to verify that the relaxer is indeed the cause. Hair that has been relaxed has undergone a significant insult to the disulfide backbone of hair strength. As previously mentioned, the disulfide bonds must be broken to straighten the hair and not all of them can be reconnected resulting in weaker hair. The dermatologist can verify whether the hair has been damaged by grasping the end of the hair and pulling. If the hair breaks, it has been over-relaxed and chemically damaged. The hair should also be pulled where it exits the scalp. If breakage occurs, the damaged induced by chemical relaxing can be confirmed.

Once it has been confirmed that the hair loss is due to chemical straightening, the dermatologist should offer some helpful suggestions. Of course, the damaged hair cannot repair itself. The brittle hair must be trimmed, and overprocessing of the new growth should be avoided. Overprocessing can be avoided by decreasing the strength of the solution and, more importantly, leaving the chemicals on the hair for a shorter period of time. The beautician must get the chemicals applied quickly and removed quickly for best results and minimum hair weakening. Hair around the face experiences more trauma, a phenomenon known as weathering, than hair in other locations. For this reason, the relaxer should be applied first at the nape of the neck and moved forward. This minimizes the time the relaxer remains on this damaged hair, since it is applied last and removed first. In addition, worsening hair damage can be avoided by allowing as long as possible between hair straightening procedures.

> Hair breakage can be minimized by combing or styling the hair as little as possible, applying moisturizing conditioning agents, and avoiding any further chemical treatments such as permanent hair dyeing or bleaching.

Hair breakage can be minimized by combing or styling the hair as little as possible, applying moisturizing conditioning agents, and avoiding any further chemical treatments such as permanent hair dyeing or bleaching (13). Protein-containing deep conditioners may be helpful to temporarily strengthen the damaged hair by 5–10%. The holes that are created in the cuticle by the straightening chemicals never completely seal and can be used to passively diffuse small-molecular-weight proteins into the hair shaft. Protein-containing deep conditioners are thick creams applied to the hair and left in contact for 20–30 minutes sometimes under a hair dryer set at low. The prolonged contact and heat encourage the proteins to enter the hair shaft. Weekly protein pack leave-in conditioners may minimize hair breakage.

Hair that has been over-relaxed may also break due to decreased water content. When holes are created in the hair shaft by the relaxer to break the disulfide bonds in the cortex, water is released from the hair. Water allows the hair to behave as an elastic material. While the water cannot be replaced, moisturizing the hair shaft to restore protein flexibility may decrease breakage. Heavy occlusive hair conditioners that contain petrolatum, glycerin, and dimethicone can minimize water loss, decrease combing friction, and add shine to relaxed hair. These products were originally known as pomades, but are now called hair conditioners. It is impossible to overcondition relaxed hair. Since sebum is the best conditioning agent, once weekly or every other week shampooing also minimizes hair damage, but can compromise hair hygiene.

Dermatologists should also recognize that hair straightening chemicals are all well-known cutaneous irritants. It is for this reason that a petrolatum cream is applied as a base to the scalp and hairline. This process, known as "basing," is important not to damage the scalp skin. Hair straightening solutions are not suitable for patch testing and chemical burns are possible if a novice is performing the straightening procedure. Patients should select only experienced, salon trained professionals to perform hair straightening to avoid adverse reactions.

REFERENCES

1. Bernard B. Hair shape of curly hair. Supp J Am Acad Dermatol 2003; 48: S120–6.
2. McDonald CJ. Special requirements in cosmetics for people with black skin. In: Frost P, Horwitz SN, eds. Principles of Cosmetics for the Dermatologist. St. Louis: CV Mosby, 1982: 302–4.
3. Syed A, Kuhajda A, Ayoub H, Ahmad K. African-American hair. Cosmet Toilet 1995; 110: 39–48.
4. Franbourg A, Hallegot P, Baltenneck F, Toutain C, Leroy F. Current research on ethnic hair. Supp J Am Acad Dermatol 2003; 48: S115–19.
5. McMichael A. Ethnic hair update: past and present. Supp J Am Acad Dermatol 2003; 48: S127–33.

6. Cannell DW. Permanent waving and hair straightening. Clin Dermatol 1988; 6: 71–82.

7. Syed A. Ethnic hair care: history, trends, and formulation. Cosmet Toilet 1993; 108: 99–108.

8. Khalil EN. Cosmetic and hair treatments for the black consumer. Cosmet Toilet 1986; 101: 51–8.

9. Ogawa S, Fufii K, Kaneyama K, Arai K, Joko K. A curing method for permanent hair straightening using thioglycolic and dithiodiglycolic acids. J Cosmet Sci 2000; 51: 379–99.

10. Bulengo-Ransby SM, Bergfeld WF. Chemical and traumatic alopecia from thioglycolate in a black woman. Cutis 1992; 49: 99–103.

11. Brooks G. Treatment regimes for styled black hair. Cosmet Toilet 1983: 59–68.

12. Syed A, Ayoub H. Correlating porosity and tensile strength of chemically modified hair. Cosmet Toilet 2002; 117: 57–62.

13. Burmeister F, Bollatti D, Brooks G. Ethnic hair: moisturizing after relaxer use. Cosmet Toilet 1991; 106: 49–51.

SUGGESTED READING

De Sa Dias TC, Baby AR, Kaneko TM, Robles Velasco MV. Relaxing/straightening of afro-ethnic hair: historical overview. J Cosmet Dermatol 2007; 6: 2–5.

Draelos ZD. Understanding African-American hair. Dermatol Nurs 1997; 9: 227–31.

Etemesi BA. Impact of hair relaxers in women in Nakuru, Kenya. Int J Dermatol 2007; 46(Suppl 1): 23–5.

Grimes PE. Skin and hair cosmetic issues in women of color. Dermatol Clin 2000; 18: 659–65.

Grimes PE, Davis LT. Cosmetics in blacks. Dermatol Clin 1991; 9: 53–68.

Halder RM. Hair and scalp disorders in blacks. Cutis 1983; 32: 378–80.

Holloway VL. Ethnic cosmetic products. Dermatol Clin 2003; 21: 743–9.

Kahre J. Ethnic differences in haircare products (Chapter 52). In: Barel A, Paye M, Maibach H, eds. Handbook of Cosmetic Science and Technology. Marcel Dekker, Inc., 2001: 605–18.

Khumalo NP, Jessop S, Gumedze F, Ehrlich R. Determinants of marginal traction alopecia in African girls and women. J Am Acad Dermatol 2008; 59: 432–8.

McMichael AJ. Ethnic hair update: past and present. J Am Acad Dermatol 2003; 489(Suppl): S127–33.

Quinn CR, Quinn TM, Kelly AP. Hair care practices in African American women. Cutis 2003; 72: 280–2, 285–9.

Quinn CR, Quinn TM, Kelly AP. Hair care practices in African American women. Drug Ther Topics 2003; 72: 280–9.

Roseborough IE, McMichael AJ. Hair care practices in African-American patients. Semin Cutan Med Surg 2009; 28: 103–8.

Smith W, Burns C. Managing the hair and skin of African American pediatric patients. J Pediatr Health Care 1999; 13: 72–8.

Syed AN. Ethnic hair care products (Chapter 9). In: Johnson DH, ed. Hair and hair care. Marcel Dekker, Inc., 1997: 235–59.

30 Hair dyeing

Hair dyes represent a major hair cosmetic used by both men and women. It is estimated that 40% of women regularly use hair dyes to blend gray tones, cover gray hair, add colored highlights, produce unnatural temporary colors, and either lighten or darken the original hair color. Hair dyeing is used to cover gray and achieve a more youthful appearance, but it is also used to change the natural hair color based on personal preference. A number of different hair dye cosmetics have been developed to fulfill all of these needs: gradual, temporary, semipermanent, and permanent. Approximately 65% of the hair dye market is for permanent hair colorings, 20% for semipermanent colorings, and 15% for the remaining types.

Hair coloring is an ancient tradition that was common among the ancient Persians, Hebrews, Greeks, and Romans. The use of henna, a naturally occurring plant dye, dates to the third dynasty of Egypt 4000 years ago. The Egyptians mixed the Lawsonia plant from which henna is derived with hot water and placed the material on the head to produce an orange-red hair color. Metallic dyes containing lead acetate, obtained by dipping lead combs in sour wine, were used by Roman men to cover gray hair (1). Roman women, on the other hand, attempted to lighten their hair by applying lye followed by sun exposure.

The modern concept of permanent hair dyeing dates back to 1883 when Monnet patented a process for coloring fur using p-phenylenediamine and hydrogen peroxide. Feathers and hair were later dyed in 1888 and the first human application was in Paris in 1890 and in St. Louis, Missouri, U.S.A. in 1892 (2). Temporary and semipermanent dyes were not developed until the 1950s when they were incorporated from the textile industry into the cosmetic industry. Bleaching of the hair with hydrogen peroxide was first demonstrated at the Paris Exposition of 1867 by Thillary and Hugo (3). All of these products form the basis for modern hair coloring, which can produce a myriad of hair colors (Fig. 30.1).

HAIR COLOR PHYSIOLOGY
Pigment comprises less than 3% of the fiber mass of hair, yet is one of the most important hair cosmetic aspects (4). Three pigment types produce the tremendous variety of colors seen in human hair: eumelanins, pheomelanins, and oxymelanins. Eumelanins are insoluble polymers accounting for the brown and black hues consisting mainly of 5,6-dihydroxyindole with lesser amounts of 5,6-dihydroxyindole-2-carboxylic acid. Pheomelanins are soluble polymers accounting for the yellow to red hues containing 10–12% sulfur and 1,4-benzothiazinylalanine. Eumelanin contains less sulfur than pheomelanin (5). A lesser pigment, known as oxymelanin, is yellow or reddish in color and probably represents bleached eumelanin pigment arising from partial oxidative cleavage of 5,6-dihydroxyindole units. Oxymelanin is distinct in that it contains no sulfur (6). Hair dyes attempt to mimic these pigments in reproducing a natural appearing hair color.

The tremendous variety observed in natural human hair color is due to three pigments: eumelanin, pheomelanin, and oxymelanin.

The principal aim of hair dyeing is to cover gray hair. The mechanism of graying is not totally understood, however. It is thought that the death of some melanocytes within the hair melanocyte unit triggers a chain reaction resulting in the death of the rest of the unit melanocytes in a relatively short period (7). A possible mechanism of death is the accumulation of a toxic intermediate metabolite, such as dopaquinone (8).

Hair dyes can be divided into several types based on their formulation and permanency: gradual, temporary, semipermanent, and permanent.

TYPES OF HAIR DYES
Hair dyes can be divided into several types based on their formulation and permanency: gradual, temporary, semipermanent, and permanent (Table 30.1).

Gradual
Gradual hair dyes, also known as metallic or progressive hair dyes, require repeated application to result in gradual darkening of the hair shaft. This product will change the hair color from gray to yellow-brown to black over a period of weeks (Fig. 30.2) (9). There is no control over the final color of the hair, only the depth of color and lightening is not possible. They employ water-soluble metal salts which are deposited on the hair shaft in the form of oxides, suboxides, and sulfides. The most common metal used is lead, but silver, copper, bismuth, nickel, iron, manganese, and cobalt have also been used. In the U.S.A., 2–3% solutions of lead acetate or nitrate are used to dye the hair while 1–2% solutions of silver nitrate are used to dye eyelashes and eyebrows (10).

Gradual hair dyes employ water-soluble metal salts which are deposited on the hair shaft in the form of oxides, suboxides, and sulfides.

Metallic hair dyes are inexpensive and do not require a professional operator for application. Their disadvantages include poor color quality and stiff, brittle, or dull hair that may not withstand further chemical processing. In addition, the trace metals left on the hair will cause permanent dyes or permanent waving solutions to perform poorly. The metal can cause breakdown of the hydrogen peroxide in bleaching or permanent waving products, resulting in the rupture of the hair shaft. The hair that has been treated with the gradual hair colorant must, therefore, grow out before other dyeing or waving procedures are used, to guarantee an optimal result (11).

The gradual color change induced by metallic dyes requires continued use if the color is to be maintained; however, the hair shaft damage induced by the product is permanent. Therefore, metallic dyes are not appropriate for female patients who desire more color darkening than the product can provide and who are likely to undergo permanent waving. These products are most appropriate for male patients who cut their hair frequently, only need minimal darkening, and are unlikely to process their hair further (12).

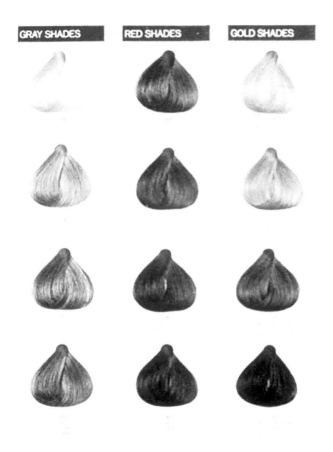

Figure 30.1 Hair coloring technology can produce a myriad of hair colors.

Temporary

Temporary hair coloring agents are designed to be removed in one shampoo washing (13). They are used to add a slight tint, brighten a natural shade, or improve an existing dyed shade. Their particle size is too large to penetrate through the cuticle, accounting for their temporary nature (1). Temporary dyes can be easily rubbed off the hair shaft, however, and will run onto clothing if the hair gets wet from rain or perspiration. They can be formulated as a liquid, mousse, gel, or spray (Fig. 30.3).

> Temporary hair dyes are designed to be removed in one shampooing to tint or brighten or improve hair color.

Liquid temporary hair colorants are also referred to as "hair rinses" since they are frequently applied in the shower following shampooing, with the excess dyestuff removed by rinsing. They contain acid dyes of the same type used to dye wool fabrics and belong to the following chemical classes: azo, anthraquinone, triphenylmethane, phenzainic, xanthenic, or benzoquinoneimine (14). These dyes are known as FDC and DC blues, greens, reds, oranges, yellows, and violets. No damage is imparted to the hair shaft by these dyes because they are composed of large molecules that are deposited on the surface of the hair, and are unable to penetrate due to size.

The liquid rinse formulation is most popular, especially among mature patients with gray hair who wish to remove undesirable yellow tones and achieve a purer platinum color. A sample product for this purpose may contain a 0.001% concentration of methylene blue, acid violet 6B, and water-soluble nigrosin in an aqueous preparation (Fig. 30.4). Temporary hair colorants are recommended for mature patients since the hair shaft is not damaged and many patients only require weekly shampooing. The liquid rinse can also be used by patients who have achieved an undesirable permanent dye color and wish to tone the bad result until the poorly colored hair grows out and is cut.

Mousse formulations of temporary hair colorants are available in both natural and party colors. They are applied soon after shampooing to towel-dried hair and are not removed. Because the coloring agent is dispersed in a styling polymer, such as polyvinylpyrrolidone/vinyl acetate, the mousse serves

Table 30.1 Hair Coloring

Type	Main ingredient	Duration of effect	Effect on hair	Advantages/disadvantages
Gradual	Aqueous solution of lead or silver oxides, suboxides, and sulfides	Color persists with continued use	Darkens gradually by "plating" hair shaft	Cannot be combined with permanent dye or permanent wave
Temporary	High-molecular-weight, textile dyes	Removal with one shampooing	Large color molecules deposited in hair shaft	Can blend or tone undesirable hair color
Semipermanent	Low-molecular-weight, natural or synthetic textile-type dye	Removal with four or six shampooings	Small color molecules penetrate hair cortex	Tone-on-tone coloring. Will cover less than 30% gray. May be allergenic
Permanent	Oxidation coloring employing primary intermediates, couplers, and an oxidant	Permanent	New color molecules formed within hair shaft	Lighten (two-step processing) or darken (one-step processing). Will cover gray 100%. Need to cover new growth with monthly dyeing. May be allergenic

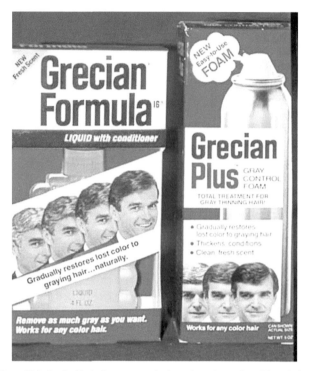

Figure 30.2 Gradual hair dyes are popular in male patients who wish to darken hair color slowly over time.

both as a styling agent and temporary colorant. This product may be used to add highlights or blend gray hair in brunette patients with less than 15% gray hair. Mousse temporary coloring agents are ideal for the female patient with minimal bitemporal graying. These products are also available in party colors such as yellow, orange, blue, green, purple, and red, which can be used to create special multicolored effects.

Gel formulations of temporary hair colorants are identical to mousse formulations, except that they are packaged as a gel in a tube rather than as foam released from an aerosol can. Gel temporary hair colorants also combine a styling aid with coloring; however, the hold provided by the gel is generally superior to that provided by the mousse. These products are only available in party colors, with some lines including a hair glitter. Gel temporary hair colorants are only appropriate for creating unusual hair styles.

Spray formulations of temporary hair colorants are also available to professional cosmetologists. A pressurized aerosol spray is used to apply the temporary liquid dyestuff to the hair (15).

Temporary, hair coloring agents should be used with care in patients with damaged or chemically treated hair because the hair shaft has increased porosity due to loss of the cuticular scale. The porous hair shafts allow entrance of the color molecules into the hair shaft, rendering them more permanent.

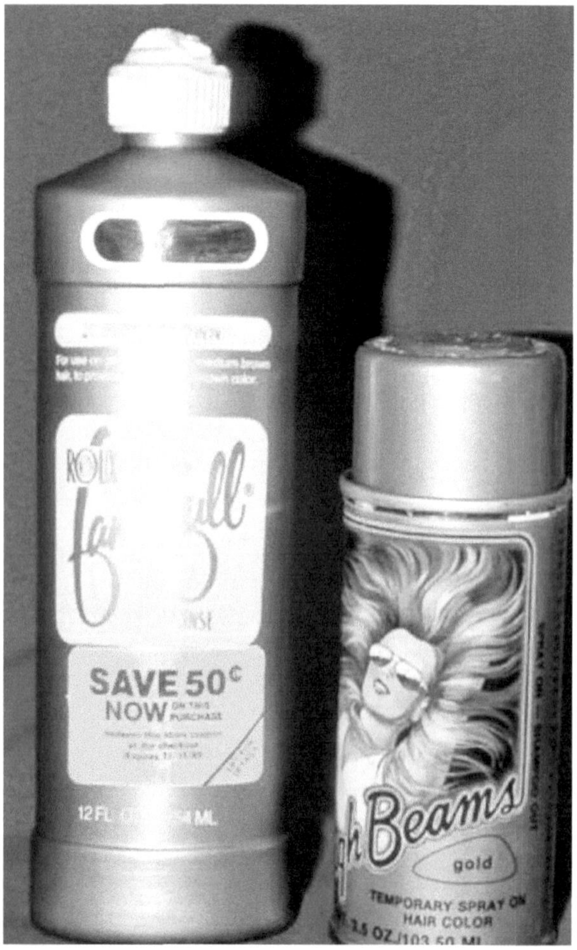

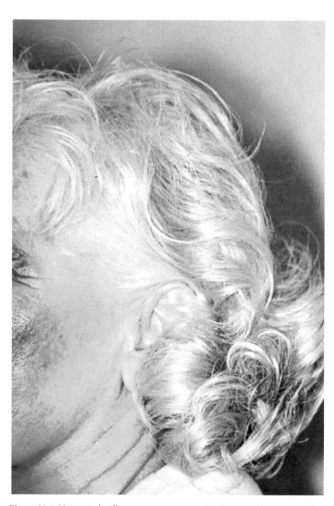

Figure 30.3 Spray temporary coloring agents are popular among teens wanting a pink, blue, or green lock of hair for fashion purposes.

Figure 30.4 Unwanted yellow overtones in graying hair can be minimized by using a purple rinse, but in some cases the rinse can inadvertently dye the hair purple as demonstrated in this image.

Under these conditions, it may take more than one shampooing to remove the color.

Semipermanent

Textile Dyes

Semipermanent hair coloring is popular with both men and women. Formulated for use on natural, unbleached hair, it can cover gray, add highlight, or rid hair of unwanted tones (Fig. 30.5). Semipermanent hair dyes are removed in four to six shampooings due to their intermediate sized particles that can both enter and exit the hair shaft (16). Recently, longer lasting products within this category incorporating hydrogen peroxide have become available. The dyes are retained in the hair shaft by weak polar and van der Waals attractive forces, thus dyestuffs with increased molecular size will remain longer. The formulation of a typical semipermanent hair dye comprises these: dyes (nitroanilines, nitrophenylenediamines, nitroaminophenols, azos, and anthraquinones), alkalizing agent, solvent, surfactant, thickener, fragrance, and water (17). Usually, 10 to 12 dyes are mixed to obtain the desired shade (18).

> Semipermanent hair dyes are removed in 4 to 6 shampooings and can cover gray, add highlights, or get rid hair of unwanted tones.

Semipermanent dyes are available as lotions, shampoos, and mousses. The shampoo-in process is most popular for home use. The dyestuff is combined with an alkaline detergent shampoo to promote hair shaft swelling so that the dye can penetrate, a thickener so that the product will remain on the scalp, and a foam stabilizer so that the product will not run and stain facial skin. The mousse formula incorporates the dyestuff in aerosolized foam. Both products are applied to wet, freshly shampooed hair and are rinsed in 20 to 40 minutes. Semipermanent dyes can become more permanent if applied to porous, chemically treated hair.

Semipermanent dyes produce tone-on-tone coloring rather than effecting drastic color changes, so their role is actually in toning rather than dyeing the hair. The less color change required by the patient, the more satisfied he or she will be with the semipermanent dye result. Semipermanent dyes are best suited for patients with less than 30% gray hair who want to restore their natural color (19). This is done by selecting a dye color that is lighter than the natural hair color since the dye will penetrate both the gray and the nongray hairs, resulting in an increased darkening of the nongray hairs. It is not possible to lighten hair with semipermanent dyes, since they do not contain hydrogen peroxide, nor is it possible to darken hair more than three shades beyond the patient's natural hair color. Thus, in the cosmetic industry, semipermanent dyes are known as suitable only for staying "on shade."

Stains

A newer type of semipermanent hair coloring is hair stain. Hair stain is a synthetic polymer, usually in unnatural shades such as reds, blues, purples, or yellows, that imparts a hue or highlight to the hair. For example, brunette hair with a red stain will have a reddish glow or blond hair with a yellow stain will have a yellow glow. The stain appears transparent so that it blends with the underlying hair color. The stain does not cover, but only tones. If heat is added to the staining process, the stain is more resistant to shampoo removal and if both heat and hydrogen peroxide are added to the staining process, the stain can penetrate the hair shaft deeply and become permanent.

> Semipermanent hair stains are synthetic polymers designed to add hues and highlights to the hair.

Rarely, individuals with multiple dye sensitivities may wish to stain hair with natural agents, such as walnut stain (Herbasol, extract of walnut leaves; Cosmetochem USA, Clifton, NJ). This extract of black walnut leaves produces a deep brownish-black color when applied to the hair.

Vegetable Dyes

Vegetable dyes, the first form of hair coloring developed, fall under the semipermanent category because they minimally penetrate the cuticle, although four to six shampooings are required for removal (Fig. 30.6). The only vegetable dye remaining today is henna, derived from the *Lawsonia alba* plant. As originally used, the dried plant leaves were ground to form a powder that was activated with water to form an acidic naphthoquinone dye that was then applied as a paste to the hair for 40 to 60 minutes. The henna imparted a reddish hue to the hair. Metallic salts were combined with henna to produce what was termed a "compound henna", to provide a wider

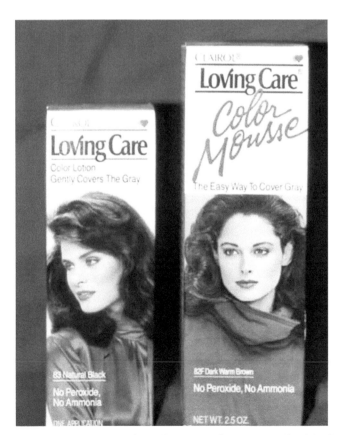

Figure 30.5 Semipermanent hair coloring is used in persons with minimal gray hair to add red or blonde highlights.

range of colors. Today, natural henna dyes have been replaced by synthetic henna-type products with dye shades ranging from auburn to blonde to gray. These synthetic henna products combine a conditioning agent with the dye, but they are still powders mixed with water to form a paste that remains in contact with the hair for 40 minutes. Hennas can be used for darkening, but not lightening, of the original hair color. Natural hennas are inferior to synthetic hennas because they leave the hair stiff and brittle after repeated applications. Henna has not been reported to cause allergic contact dermatitis when used as a hair dye.

Semipermanent vegetable dyes from henna are used to create red hair tones, but most modern hennas contain synthetic coloring ingredients.

Permanent
Permanent hair coloring accounts for $3 of every $4 dollars spent on hair dyeing in the U.S.A. It is more popular with women than men since women are more likely to effect a complete hair color change than men. Permanent hair coloring is so named because the dyestuff penetrates the hair shaft to the cortex and forms large color molecules that cannot be removed by shampooing (Fig. 30.7) (20). It can be used to both cover gray and produce a completely new hair color. Redyeing is necessary every four to six weeks, as new growth, known in the cosmetic industry as "roots," appears at the scalp.

Permanent hair dyes contain colorless dye precursors that chemically react with hydrogen peroxide inside the hair shaft to produce colored molecules.

This type of hair coloring does not contain dyes, but rather colorless dye precursors that chemically react with hydrogen peroxide inside the hair shaft to produce colored molecules (21). The process entails the use of primary intermediates (p-phenylenediamine, p-toluenediamine, and p-aminophenols) which undergo oxidation with hydrogen peroxide. These reactive intermediates are then exposed to couplers (resorcinol, 1-naphthol, m-aminophenol, etc.) to result in a

wide variety of indo dyes. These indo dyes can produce shades from blonde to brown to black with highlights of gold to red to orange. Variations in the concentration of hydrogen peroxide and the chemicals selected for the primary intermediates and couplers produce this color selection (22). Red is produced by using nitro para phenylenediamine alone or in combination with mixtures of para-aminophenol with meta phenylenediamine, alpha naphthol, or 1,5-dihydroxynaphthalene. Yellow is produced by mixtures of ortho aminophenol, ortho phenylenediamine, and nitro-ortho phenylenediamine. Blue has no single oxidation dye intermediate and is produced by combinations of para phenylenediamine, phenylenediamine, methyl toluylenediamine, or 2,4 diaminoanisol (23).

Permanent dyeing allows shades to be obtained both lighter and darker than the patient's original hair color. Higher concentrations of hydrogen peroxide can bleach melanin thus the oxidizing step functions both in color production and bleaching. Due to the use of hydrogen peroxide in the formation of the new color molecules, hair dyes must be adjusted so that hair lightening is not produced with routine dyeing (24). However, hydrogen peroxide cannot remove sufficient melanin alone to lighten dark brown or black hair to blonde hair. Boosters, such as ammonium persulfate or potassium sulfate, must be added to achieve great degrees of color lightening. The boosters must be left in contact with the hair for one to two hours for an optimal result. Nevertheless, individuals with dark hair who choose to dye their hair a light blonde color will notice the appearance of reddish hues with time. This is due to the inability of the peroxide/booster system to completely remove reddish pheomelanin pigments, which are more resistant to removal than brownish eumelanin pigments.

Permanent hair dyes are sold as two bottles containing colorless liquid within a kit. One bottle contains the dye precursors in an alkaline soap or synthetic detergent base and the other contains a stabilized solution of hydrogen peroxide. The two bottles are mixed immediately prior to use and applied to the hair. The dye precursors and hydrogen peroxide diffuse into the hair where the new color is created.

Permanent hair dyes are the most damaging to the hair. This type of hair dye alters the internal hair shaft structure and

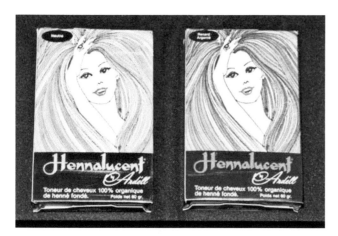

Figure 30.6 Henna has recently seen an increase in popularity as a hair dye because it is a natural dye of plant origin.

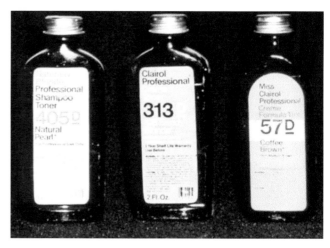

Figure 30.7 Professional salon permanent hair dyes can produce more dramatic color changes than those designed for at home use.

thereby decreases its strength. Several key points should be remembered to minimize hair shaft damage:

1. If both permanent waving and permanent dyeing are to be performed, the hair should be permanently waved first and permanently dyed second. Ten days should be allowed between the procedures.
2. Lightening, or bleaching, the hair is more damaging than dyeing the hair to a darker color.
3. Each redyeing procedure further damages the hair shaft, thus the period between redyeing should be as long as possible and the dye should be concentrated

on the new proximal hair growth, not the previously dyed distal hair shaft.

Permanent hair coloring agents are available for both home and professional salon use. The chemistry is identical for both home and salon products, except that more drastic color changes require a salon product (Fig. 30.8). Permanent hair coloring agents for home use are available in several different formulations: liquid, cream, and gel. The liquid shampoo-in formulas are most popular. All formulations come with a hair color tint and developer that must be mixed immediately before application on dry hair. The product must saturate the

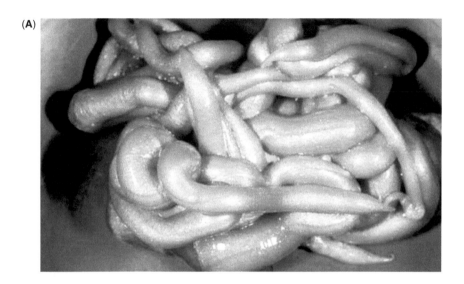

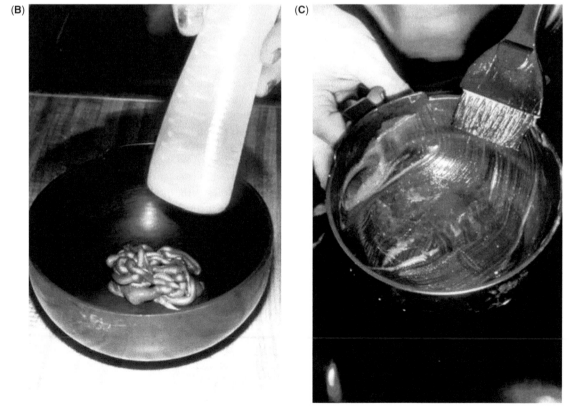

Figure 30.8 (**A**) The appearance of a cream professional permanent hair dye. (**B**) The permanent hair dye is mixed with hydrogen peroxide. (**C**) The hair dye and hydrogen peroxide are mixed to begin the chemical reaction and are now ready for hair application.

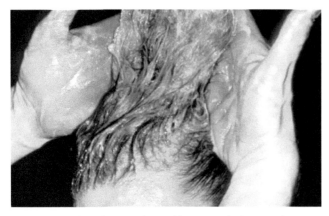

Figure 30.9 The hair dye must thoroughly saturate the hair to achieve even color.

hair, with thicker cream formulations requiring parting and sectioning of the hair to ensure an even application (Fig. 30.9). The excess dye is then rinsed and frequently a conditioner is applied. Home permanent dye products can be purchased to lighten or darken the hair by three shades. Products that lighten the hair contain ammonia and more hydrogen peroxide, thus bleaching as well as dyeing the hair. Most home products are designed to achieve a 35% coverage of gray hair. More dramatic color changes require professional products.

Even though oxidation dyes are said to be permanent, some color drift or "off-shade fading" does occur. This is due to slow chemical changes in the indo dyes, which produce a reddish to yellowish cast. Thus, permanent hair colors may become "brassy" with age. Semipermanent hair colorings may be used to cover the brassy tones until redyeing occurs. Sometimes, undesirable reddish and yellowish tones develop immediately following dyeing. In this case "drabbers" are used to remove the harshness from a color. Examples of drabbers are resorcinol to yield dark green to brown colors, pyrocatechol to yield deep gray, pyrogallol to yield gold, alpha naphthol to yield bright violet, beta naphthol to yield red brown, and hydroquinone to yield yellow brown (23).

ONE- AND TWO-STEP PROCESSING
Professional permanent hair dyeing techniques can be classified into one- and two-step processing. One-step processing permanently darkens the hair color, whereas two-step processing permanently lightens the hair color. In one-step processing, a cream tint is used in a shampoo formulation. Often a conditioner or filler must be used prior to processing to ensure even uptake of the dye by the entire hair shaft. Damaged distal hair shafts or previously treated hair will absorb or "grab" color more quickly. The filler prevents the distal hair shaft from dyeing darker than the proximal hair shaft. However, in extremely damaged hair, a filler cannot ensure an even dye uptake. In these cases the dyestuff is applied to the scalp first and the ends last so that the distal hair shafts have a shorter dyeing time. The cream tint is then rinsed and a postdyeing conditioner may be applied. Sometimes the hydrogen peroxide used in the oxidation dyeing process can lighten the existing hair color, a phenomenon known as "lift." Hair cosmetic companies formulate one-step permanent oxidation dyes to avoid lift.

HAIR BLEACHING
Two-step hair processing involves bleaching or lifting the natural hair color, with subsequent redyeing to the desired lighter shade. This technique is used when patients wish to dye their hair much lighter than their natural color. The bleaching is achieved with an alkaline mixture of hydrogen peroxide and ammonia, which causes swelling of the hair shaft to allow easier penetration of the dye, known as a toner (27). A toner must be used as the hair, when completely stripped of its color, has an undesirable appearance. The toner can be either a permanent or semipermanent dye.

> Hair bleaching to lightening hair color is achieved with an alkaline mixture of hydrogen peroxide and ammonia, which causes swelling of the hair shaft to allow easier penetration of the dye, known as a toner.

The hair must be lightened to the desired color group and then dyed to the desired shade. There are seven levels of lightening:

1. Black
2. Brown
3. Red
4. Red gold
5. Gold
6. Yellow
7. Pale yellow

A patient with a black natural hair color would have to go through all seven stages of lightening to become a pale yellow blonde, whereas a patient with a natural gold hair color would have to go through three stages of lightening to become a pale yellow blonde. The more are the stages of lightening required to achieve the end result, the stronger the bleaching agent used and the more damaging the process is to the hair (26). A "booster" such as ammonium persulfate or potassium persulfate may be added to the hydrogen peroxide and ammonia solution for patients who desire an extreme lightening of hair color (27). Allergic reactions to ammonium persulfate have been reported (28). The eumelanin pigments in the hair are easily bleached by hydrogen peroxide, but the pheomelanins are somewhat resistant. This accounts for the increased difficulty in bleaching the hair of persons with reddish hair. It is difficult to formulate a solution strong enough to degrade hair pigment without damaging the hair keratin structure.

Some patients do not wish to lighten the hair on the entire scalp. For example, if only selected hairs are lightened in color, a technique known as "highlighting," a cap with holes is applied to the scalp and only certain hairs are pulled through and exposed to the bleaching and dyeing process. If only the tips of the selected locks of hair are treated, the process is known as "tipping" whereas "streaking" involves treating the entire hair shaft of certain locks of hair. "Frosting" the hair entails bleaching a larger proportion of entire hair shafts than streaking. Fashion trends dictate the proportion of bleached to unbleached hairs in the scalp. One popular method of lightening the hair and dyeing to different shades is known as hair "foiling" (Fig. 30.10).

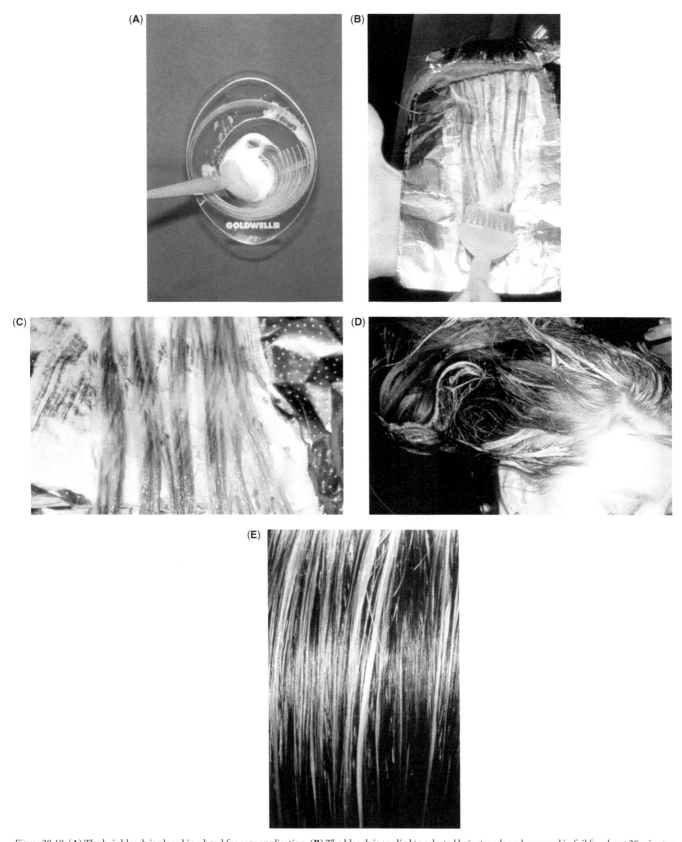

Figure 30.10 (**A**) The hair bleach is placed in a bowl for easy application. (**B**) The bleach is applied to selected hair strands and wrapped in foil for about 20 minutes. (**C**) The foil is unwrapped to expose the newly bleached hair. (**D**) The hair is rinsed to remove excess bleach and the appearance of the lightened hair is immediately apparent. (**E**) The dried hair demonstrates selectively bleached blonde strands among brunette strands, which is a popular hair fashion.

There is no doubt that the two-step processing is the most damaging form of hair coloring. Hair that has been bleached is extremely porous and as a result is brittle, hard to untangle, and lacking in luster. Conditioners can do very little to improve the appearance of hair that has sustained damage this severe. Most patients with double-processed hair who are dissatisfied with the appearance and texture of their hair are best advised to cut the damaged portion of the hair shafts and await new growth. Unfortunately, once the hair has been bleached many shades lighter than the natural hair color, the proximal dark regrowth is cosmetically unattractive. This further encourages the patient to reprocess the hair. Perhaps patients can be encouraged to change to a shorter hair style or wear a wig during the regrowth period. Another alternative is to use a semi-permanent dye to blend the bleached and naturally colored areas of the hair shaft, but if a color difference of more than three shades is present, the result will be suboptimal. Two-step processing should be minimized. It is recommended that patients stay within their own color group to maintain a natural appearance and prevent extensive hair shaft damage. Generally, a patient's natural hair color group will complement the eye color and skin tone for an overall attractive blend. Patients who distort this balance create many cosmetic problems.

Two-step processing, however, can be successful and attractive in the mature patient who had dark brown hair and now has more than 60% gray hair. If the patient does not like the appearance of this hair coloring, some dyeing procedure is required. The patient is faced with the dilemma of whether to restore the original dark brown color or to lighten the remaining dark brown hairs and redye the hair blonde. This is a personal decision, since both hair color changes require permanent dyeing. Restoring the entire scalp to a dark brown might increases the contrast between the lighter scalp and darker hair in a mature women with female pattern alopecia. In addition, the problem of new hair growth will be magnified due to the color difference between the natural gray color and dark brown dyed color. Lightening the hair by two shades followed by a toner could give the patient dark blonde hair with excellent coverage of the gray hair, a minimal scalp contrast, and a decreased color difference between dyed hair and new growth.

Melanin pigment is very resistant to reducing agents but is easily degraded by oxidizing agents. Therefore, hair bleaching can be considered an oxidative alkaline treatment. Hydrogen peroxide is the major oxidizer in the process, causing oxygen to be released from the hair keratin. The amount of hair lightening obtained is related to the amount of oxygen released, a quantity expressed as volumes by the cosmetic industry. The volume of a hydrogen peroxide solution is the number of liters of oxygen released by a liter of the bleaching solution. For example, a 20-volume solution contains 6% hydrogen peroxide and a 30-volume solution contains 9% hydrogen peroxide (29). Home bleaching products generally contain 6% hydrogen peroxide and professional bleaching products may contain up to 9% hydrogen peroxide. The hydrogen peroxide solution is mixed with an alkaline ammonia solution immediately prior to application to speed the reaction. The pH of the final solution is between 9 and 11. The amount of alkaline material added must be limited, however, because excess keratin damage and scalp irritation may result.

The hair should not be washed prior to bleaching because scalp sebum provides protection from the harsh chemicals. The hair should be shampooed following the bleaching process to remove excess solution. This is best accomplished with an acid pH shampoo with minimal detergent action. The shampooing should be done gently to avoid scalp irritation.

The ease with which pigment bleaching occurs differs throughout the length of the hair shaft, with the hair near the scalp bleaching more easily than the distal shaft. This is thought to be due to the acceleration of the bleaching process by body heat radiating from the scalp. Proper bleaching requires that the solution be applied at the ends first and then the roots to ensure an even color throughout the hair shaft.

As mentioned previously, bleaching is extremely damaging to the hair shaft. This damage results in a 2–3% weight loss from the individual shaft, which causes weakening and promotes an increased hair breakage. Small amounts of the amino acids tyrosine, threonine, and methionine are degraded. It is estimated that 15–25% of the hair's disulfide bonds are degraded during moderate bleaching with up to 45% of the cystine bonds broken during severe bleaching (30). This weakening of the hair shaft is more pronounced in wet hair, thus the hair should be handled minimally until dry (31). Bleached hair is also more porous and tends to absorb increased water, making it more susceptible to humidity changes and prolonging the drying time. Decreased overlapping of the cuticular scales also leads to increased hair friction, which allows the hair to tangle more readily. Finally, an increased porosity allows a better penetration of permanent dyeing and waving preparations, so bleached hair will dye to a darker shade than natural hair and will curl more readily than untreated hair. All further chemical processing requires weaker solutions to obtain desirable results.

HAIR DYE REMOVAL

Removal of hair dye depends upon the type of coloring process used. As discussed previously, temporary hair dyes are removed with one shampooing while semipermanent hair dyes are removed in four to six shampooings. The amount of time for a dye to wash out is equal to the time required for the dye to color the hair shaft. For example, if it takes 20 minutes for a semipermanent dye to penetrate from the cuticle to the cortex, then it will also take 20 minutes for the dye to exit the hair shaft. Thus, if the hair is shampooed for five minutes, the dye will be removed in four shampooings for a total elapsed time of 20 minutes.

> The amount of time for a hair dye to remove from the hair shaft is equal to the time required for the dye to color the hair shaft.

Permanent hair dye removal is a much different matter, however. It is actually easier to bleach hair than to remove these unnatural pigments. Permanent dyes can be removed with reducing agents or oxidants, such as high-strength peroxide. Reducing agents, such as sodium hydrosulfite or sodium formaldehyde sulfoxylate, are dissolved in water to form a 2–5% solution followed by an alkaline rinse (26). Special salon removal products are available (Clairol, Metalux). This procedure is extremely damaging to the hair, leaving it largely cosmetically unacceptable. If at all possible, the hair should be appropriately trimmed and possibly toned with other dyestuffs.

Metallic dyes should not be removed with peroxide as the hair can become darkened or discolored. Sulfonated castor oil with the addition of salicylic acid or chelating agents may be effective (32).

ADVERSE REACTIONS

Hair coloring is generally regarded as a safe product with low risk of mutagenicity and oncogenicity (33–35). A prospective study of permanent hair dye use found no increase in hematopoietic cancers (36). Furthermore, the skin penetration is minimal and limited to 0.02–0.2% of the quantity of dye applied to the head (37). Gradual and temporary hair dyes represent minimal risk for irritant and allergic contact dermatitis. However, semipermanent dyes can cause contact allergic contact dermatitis since they may contain "para" dyes (diamines, aminophenols, and phenols) or dyes that cross-react with the "para" dyes. Paraphenylenediamine (PPD) is the sensitizer in permanent hair dyeing (38), with an estimated incidence of allergic contact dermatitis of 1 in every 50,000 applications (Fig. 30.11) (39). However, patch testing may overestimate the incidence of reactions to PPD-containing hair dyes. This is due to the limited contact time during dyeing and the less than 3% concentration of PPD. Furthermore, PPD combines with oxidizing agents in hair dyes, which quickly react to create a new chemical moiety (40).

> Para phenylenediamine (PPD) is the sensitizer in permanent hair dyeing, with an estimated incidence of allergic contact dermatitis of 1 in every 50,000 applications.

Permanent and semipermanent hair dyes must be tested on the patient prior to use, preferably using a small swatch of hair and skin hidden on the posterior neck. The testing is necessary to avoid the possibility of an overwhelming allergic contact dermatitis to the dye stuff. The hair dye should be tested in addition to the following substances (41):

> para-phenylenediamine, 1% in petrolatum
> para-toluylenediamine, 1% in petrolatum
> ortho-nitro-para phenylenediamine, 1% in petrolatum

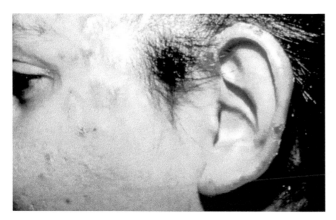

Figure 30.11 Allergic contact dermatitis due to hair dye occurs 1 in every 50,000 hair dye applications.

> meta-toluylenediamine, 1% in petrolatum
> resorcinol, 2% in petrolatum
> meta-aminophenol, 2% in petrolatum
> hydroquinone, 1% in petrolatum

In addition, the dye should be tested on the hair to prevent undesirable color results. Virgin, untreated hair does not accept the dyestuff as readily as previously treated hair. Untreated hair with an intact cuticle may even be so resistant to coloring as to require an alkaline agent to loosen the cuticle or increase porosity prior to dyeing. This type of hair is termed "dye resistant." Previously treated hair will absorb or "grab" the color readily, which can result in overdyeing if the beauty operator is careless. Hair previously treated with metallic dyes or conditioners may not respond as expected. A color test area, known as a "strand test," allows the beautician to determine if the appropriate color has been applied to the hair for the appropriate amount of time.

Once the hair has been semipermanently or permanently dyed, it is no longer allergenic (42). However, all excess dye must be removed with a final acidic shampoo, known as a neutralizing rinse. Sometimes patients with a tremendous paraphenylenediamine allergy, who have previously used home dyeing preparations, develop swelling and bullae formation immediately upon application of the dye product. In their haste to come to the dermatologist's office, they may neglect to remove all of the excess dye. Schueller recommends a chloride peroxide rinse to neutralize the excess dye, which is formulated as follows (43):

> Sodium chloride, 150 g
> Hydrogen peroxide (20 volume), 50 ml
> Water q.s. 1000 ml

This preparation can be mixed by the pharmacist and applied to the patient's hair to remove any remaining allergen. It is not necessary for the patient to cut his or her hair, but further hair dyeing should be avoided.

Hair bleaching has been reported to cause hair breakage, skin irritation, allergic sensitization, and scarring alopecia (44). Cutaneous and respiratory allergic reactions have been reported to ammonium persulfate, mentioned previously as a booster in the hair bleaching process. Reported reactions include allergic contact dermatitis, irritant contact dermatitis, localized edema, generalized urticaria, rhinitis, asthma, and syncope (45,46). Some of the reactions are thought to be truly allergic while others appear to be due to nonimmunologic histamine release (47). Patch testing may be performed with a 2–5% aqueous solution of ammonium persulfate (48).

> The cancer risk of hair dyeing is likened to the cancer risk of smoking one cigarette.

There has been some concern over the carcinogenicity of hair dyes and their appropriateness for use during pregnancy (49). There has been no link between hair dye and cancer in humans, but the cancer risk has been likened to smoking one cigarette each time the hair is dyed. Thus, the desire of the patient to dye their hair must be balanced with the chemical exposure (50).

Pregnant women frequently ask if hair dyeing is safe during pregnancy. There are no restrictions placed on hair dyes during pregnancy, but again the risks should be weighed.

REFERENCES

1. Corbett JF. Hair coloring. Clin Dermatol 1988; 6: 93–101.
2. Spoor HJ. Permanent hair colorants: oxidation dyes 1. Chemical technology. Cutis 1977; 19: 424–30.
3. Corbett JF. Changing the color of hair. In: Frost P, Horwitz SN, eds. Principles of Cosmetics for the Dermatologist. St. Louis: CV Mosby Company, 1982: 160–3.
4. Menkart J, Wolfram LJ, Mao I. Caucasian hair, negro hair, and wool; similarities and differences. J Soc Cosmet Chem 1966; 17: 769–89.
5. Arakindakshan MI, Persad S, Haberman HF, Kurian CJ. A comparative study of the physical and chemical properties of melanins isolated from human black and red hair. J Invest Dermatol 1983; 80: 202–6.
6. Brown KC, Prota G. Melanins: hair dyes for the future. Cosmet Toilet 1994; 109: 59–64.
7. Cesarini JP. Hair melanin and hair colour. In: Orfanos CE, Happle R, eds. Hair and Hair Diseases. Berlin: Springer-Verlag, 1990: 166–97.
8. Vardy DA, Marcus B, Gilead L, et al. A look at gray hair. J Geriatric Dermatol 1993; 1: 22–7.
9. Pohl S. The chemistry of hair dyes. Cosmet Toilet 1988; 103: 57–66.
10. Spoor HJ. Part II: metals. Cutis 1977; 19: 37–40.
11. O'Donoghue MN. Hair cosmetics. Dermatol Clin 1987; 5: 619–25.
12. Casperson S. Men's hair coloring. Comet Toilet 1994; 109: 83–7.
13. Spoor HJ. Hair dyes: temporary colorings. Cutis 1976; 18: 341–4.
14. Wilkinson JB, Moore RJ. Harry's Cosmeticology, 7th edn. New York: Chemical Publishing, 1982: 526–8.
15. Corbett JF. Hair dyes. In: The Chemistry of Synthetic Dyes, Vol. 5, New York: Academic Press, Inc, 1971: 475–534.
16. Spoor HJ. Semi-permanent hair color. Cutis 1976; 18: 506–8.
17. Corbett JF. Hair coloring processes. Cosmet Toilet 1991; 106: 53.
18. Robbin CR. Chemical and Physical Behavior of Human Hair, 2nd edn. New York: Springer-Verlag, 1988: 185–8.
19. Zviak C. Hair coloring, nonoxidation coloring. In: Zviak C, ed. The Science of Hair Care. New York: Marcel Dekker, Inc, 1986: 235–61.
20. Tucker HH. Formulation of oxidation hair dyes. Am J Perfum Cosmet 1968; 83: 69.
21. Corbett JF, Menkart J. Hair coloring. Cutis 1973; 12: 190.
22. Zviak C. Oxidation coloring. In: Zviak C, ed. The Science of Hair Care. New York: Marcel Dekker, Inc, 1986: 263–86.
23. Spoor HJ. Permanent hair colorants: oxidation dyes. Part II Colorist's art. Cutis 1977; 19: 578–88.
24. Corbett JF. Chemistry of hair colorant processes – science as an aid to formulation and development. J Soc Cosmet Chem 1984; 35: 297–310.
25. Spoor HJ: Hair coloring – a resume. Cutis 1977; 20: 311–13.
26. Zviak C. Hair bleaching. In: Zviak C, ed. The Science of Hair Care. New York: Marcel Dekker, Inc, 1986: 213–33.
27. Corbett JF. Hair coloring processes. Cosmet Toilet 1991; 106: 53–7.
28. Fisher AA, Dooms-Goossens A. Persulfate hair bleach reactions. Arch Dermatol 1976; 112: 1407.
29. Kass GS. Hair coloring products. In: deNavarre MG, ed. The Chemistry and Manufacture of Cosmetics, Vol. 4, 2nd edn. Allured Publishing Corporation, 1988: 841–920.
30. Robbins C, Kelly. Amino acid analysis of cosmetically altered hair. J Soc Cosmet Chem 1969; 20: 555–64.
31. Robbins CR. Physicial properties and cosmetic behavior of hair. In: Chemical and Physical Behavior of Human Hair, 2nd edn. New York: Springer-Verlag, 1988: 225–8.
32. Wall, FE. Bleaches, hair colorings, and dye removers. In: Balsam MS, Gershon SD, Rieger MM, Sagarin E, Strianse SJ, eds. Cosmet Sci Technol, Vol. 2, 2nd edn. New York: Wiley-Interscience, 1972: 279–343.
33. Marcoux D, Riboulet-Delmas G. Efficacy and safety of hair-coloring agents. Am J Contact Dermatitis 1994; 5: 123–9.
34. Morikawa F, Fujii S, Tejima M, Sugiyama H, Uzuak M. Safety evaluation of hair cosmetics. In: Kobori T, Montagna W, eds. Biology and Disease of the Hair. Baltimore: University Park Press, 1975: 641–57.
35. Corbett JF. Hair dye toxicity. In: Orfanos CE, Montagna W, Stuttgen G, eds. Hair Research, New York: Springer-Verlag, 1981: 529–35.
36. Grodstein F, Hennekens CH, Colditz GA, Hunter DJ, Stampfer MJ. A prospective study of permanent hair dye use and hematopoietic cancer. J Natl Cancer Inst 1994; 86: 1466–70.
37. Kalopissis G. Toxicology and hair dyes. In: Zviak C, ed. The Science of Hair Care. New York: Marcel Dekker, Inc, 1986: 287–308.
38. Goldberg BJ, Herman FF, Hirata I. Systemic anaphylaxis due to an oxidation product of p-phenylenediamine in a hair dye. Ann Allergy 1987; 58: 205–8.
39. Rostenberg A, Kass GS. Hair Coloring, AMA Committee of Cutaneous Health and Cosmetics, 1969
40. Corbett JF. p-benzoquinonediimine – a vital intermediate in oxidative hair dyeing. J Soc Cosmetic Chemists 1969; 20: 253.
41. DeGroot AC, Weyland JW, Nater JP. Unwanted Effects of Cosmetics and Drugs Used in Dermatology. Amsterdam: Elsevier, 1994: 481–2.
42. Reiss F, Fisher AA. Is hair dyed with para-phenylenediamine allergenic? Arch Dermatol 1974; 109: 221–2.
43. Calnan C. Adverse reactions to hair products. In: Zviak C, ed. The Science of Hair Care. New York: Marcel Dekker, Inc, 1986: 409–23.
44. Bergfeld WF. Hair research. In: Orfanos CE, Montagna E, Stuttgen G, eds. Berlin: Springer-Verlag, 1981: 534–47.
45. Brubaker MM: Urticarial reaction to ammonium persulfate. Arch Dermatol 1972; 106: 413–14.
46. Blainey AD, Ollier S, Cundell D, Smith RE, Davies RJ. Occupational asthma in a hairdressing salon. Thorax 1986; 41: 42–50.
47. Calnan CD, Shuster S. Reactions to ammonium persulfate. Arch Dermatol 1963; 88: 812–15.
48. Fisher AA, Dooms-Goossens A. Persulfate hair bleach reactions. Arch Dermatol 1976; 112: 1407–9.
49. Czene K, Tiikkaja S, Hemminki K, Cancer Risks in Hairdressers. Assessment of carcinogenicity of hair dyes and gels. Int J Cancer 2003; 105: 108–12.
50. Bolt HA, Golka K, The debate on carcinogenicity of permanent hair dyes. New insights. Crit Rev Toxicol 2007; 37: 521–36.

SUGGESTED READING

Anderson JS. Hair colorants (Chapter 31). In: Rieger MM, ed. Harry's Cosmeticology, 8th edn. Chemcial Publishing Co., Inc., 2000, 669–94.

Brown KC. Hair coloring (Chapter 7). In: Johnson DH, ed. Hair and Hair Care. Marcel Dekker, Inc., 191–215.

Corbett JF. An historical review of the use of dye precursors in the formulation of commercial oxidation hair dyes. Dyes Pigments 1999; 41: 127–36.

Harrison S, Sinclair R. Hair colouring, permanent styling, and hir structure. J Cosmet Dermatol 2003; 2: 180–5.

Krasteva M, Bons B, Ryan C, Gerberick GF, Consumer Allergy to Oxidative Hair Coloring Prouducts. Epidemiologic data in the literature. Dermatitis 2009; 20: 123–41.

Sosted H, Agner T, Andersen KE, Menne T. 55 cases of allergic reactions to hair dye: a descriptive, consumer complaint-based study. Contact Dermatitis 2002; 47: 299–303.

Takkouche B, Etminan M, Montes-Martinez A. Personal use of hair dyes and risk of cancer. JAMA 2005; 293: 2516–25.

Zviak C, Millequant J. Hair bleaching (Chapter 7). In: Bouillon C, Wilkinson J, eds. The Science of Hair Care, 2nd edn. Taylor & Francis Group, LLC, 2005: 229–301.

Zviak C, Millequant J. Hair coloring: non-oxidation coloring (Chapter 8). In: Bouillon C, Wilkinson J, eds. The Science of Hair Care, 2nd edn. Taylor & Francis Group, LLC, 2005: 251–75.

Zviak C, Millequant J. Oxidation coloring (Chapter 9). In: Bouillon C, Wilkinson J, eds. The Science of Hair Care, 2nd edn. Taylor & Francis Group, LLC, 2005: 277–312.

31 Folliculitis and shaving

Shaving is an important grooming procedure with tremendous dermatologic ramifications. Shaving removes not only hair, but also more or less of the stratum corneum depending on the quality of the shave. A successful shave requires an excellent implement, good skin conditioning, and superb hair removal. The idea of shaving was popularized by Alexander the Great who required his Greek soldiers to shave to prevent the beard from being used as an aid for throat slashing or decapitation. Shaving products necessarily developed as the practice of shaving became more common. From the 14th century to World War I, shaving soaps were the main preparation available. Lathering shaving creams were introduced in 1936 and continue in popularity (1).

Many dermatologic conditions are related to problems with unwanted hair growth necessitating some form of hair removal. While shaving can exacerbate eczema, pseudofolliculitis barbae, folliculitis, impetigo, verruca planae, and sensitive skin, most dermatologists know relatively little about this grooming activity. This chapter investigates common shaving practices and offers practical tips to optimize hair removal while minimizing dermatologic complications. The topics for consideration are razor selection, razor design, razor care, shaving cream selection, shaving technique, spread of infection, and shaving of special skin areas.

RAZOR SELECTION

Razor selection is perhaps one of the most important considerations for achieving an excellent hair removal result. Without good tools, a good result cannot be obtained. Many people with dermatologic problems complain that shaving causes pain, discomfort, and razor burn, which could be minimized through proper razor selection.

Razors can be purchased with a disposable blade and handle or only with a disposable blade. The completely disposable razors should not be selected for the dermatologic patient with folliculitis. First, the disposable razors are made out of a thin plastic shell and are not heavy. A good razor with replaceable cartridge blades will have good weight in the handle to ensure that the blades strike the skin at the proper angle. When the razor is held in the hand, the head angles the blade to meet the skin for optimal hair removal while minimizing skin removal (Fig. 31.1). Second, disposable razors generally do not have high quality laser cut, spring mounted blades.

As of late, there has been inflation in the number of blades found on the razor. The first razors to enter the market were single edged. These old fashioned blades are used by some dermatologists to remove seborrheic keratoses and nevi when longitudinally broken. While these blades may function well as a scalpel, they are not a good choice for hair removal. The double-edged razor replaced the single blade razor when it was recognized that the first blade lifts the hair from the skin surface for cutting by the second blade. This lifting of the hair increases the chances for a close shave while minimizing the

unnecessary removal of skin, a condition commonly known as razor burn.

The next development in razor design was the addition of glide strip. This strip placed on the leading edge of the blade was intended to reduce friction when the razor was dragged across the skin leading to fewer problems when shaving over curved surfaces. The strip was later loaded with skin conditioning agents, such as aloe, to provide additional skin benefits. The loaded glide strip was problematic in some of the early razor designs as the moisturizer became stringy and clogged the blades. This problem has now been overcome by the use of a thinner more flexible glide strip (Fig. 31.2).

The most significant development in razor design has been the development of five multiblade razors (Fig. 31.3). The hair is lifted and successively cut by each of the blades to produce a very close shave without using undue razor pressure on the skin. Blade pressure on the skin leads to razor burn. The multiblade razor produces a close shave without the requirement of pressure causing less razor burn, less skin irritation, and fewer skin cuts. Further shaving pressure reduction can be created by vibrating the razor and manually dragging it over the skin surface. This is the rationale behind the new battery-operated razors.

> The multiblade razor produces a close shave without the requirement of pressure causing less razor burn, less skin irritation, and fewer skin cuts.

The most expensive razor blades also have laser cut blades with spring mounts, in addition to multiple blades. The laser cut blades have a more accurate edge with fewer defects, providing for less razor burn and a closer shave. The springs help to allow the blades to rotate over the skin surface reducing cuts and providing a close shave over curved surfaces, such as the chin or the knees. While the high cost of the blades may deter some patients, the extra expense is well justified. There is no substitute for a blade that is designed for optimal performance. A blade with an angle of 28 to 32° between the blade and the skin produces the closest shave with the least amount of irritation (2).

RAZOR CARE

An expensive blade requires excellent care to deliver a superior shave over the blade lifetime. It is important to counsel patients on good blade care to prevent blade damage that compromises the shave quality. Razor blades should not be stored in the wet environment of the shower. They should be allowed to dry between shaves and kept in a dry location, such as the counter top or the drawer. Prior to drying, the blades should be thoroughly rinsed of hair and skin debris to prevent the material from sticking to the blade and compromising the sharp edge.

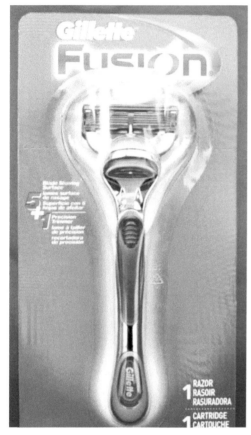

Figure 31.1 A razor blade handle with a good weight is important to allow the razor to touch the skin at the proper angle to cut the hair optimally without cutting the skin.

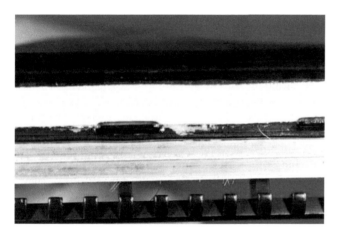

Figure 31.2 The green glide strip shown on this razor blade decreases friction between the razor blade cartridge and the skin to decrease razor burn.

It is also important not to drop the blade or bang it into other objects. Dropping the razor on the blade creates a dull spot on the edge. There is a saying in razor blade technology that "the patient always shaves with the dullest portion of the blade." This means that razor burn results from the damaged blade areas, not the sharp blade areas. If the blade is only 5% damaged and 95% undamaged, razor burn will still occur even though the majority of the blade is still in optimal condition. Most razor blades are designed to be used for five to seven shaves, meaning that the blade should be replaced at least on a weekly basis.

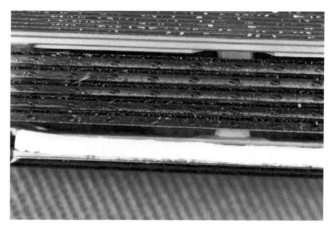

Figure 31.3 This five multiblade razor produces a close shave by allowing each successive blade to cut the hair closer and closer to the skin.

> Most razor blades are designed to be used five to seven shaves, meaning that the blade should be replaced at least on a weekly basis.

SHAVING PRODUCT SELECTION

Shaving preparations are intended to decrease the amount of trauma that results from using a sharp metal blade to remove hair from the body. Proper shaving product selection is necessary to achieve the optimal shave and the currently available products include preshave products, shaving products, and aftershave products, discussed next.

Preshave Products

Preshave products, popular among men who use an electric razor, are designed to reduce friction between the shaver and the beard, thus allowing a greater pressure to be applied on the shaver. This allows a closer shave, but with reduced irritation. These are mainly fragranced alcoholic solutions which reduce surface friction by reducing surface moisture and dry the hair allowing it to stand more upright. Some products also contain volatile silicones to function as lubricants (3).

Shaving Products

Shaving products may be formulated as soaps, sticks, powders, and creams. However, aerosol shaving creams have virtually replaced the other forms (4). Shaving creams are essentially a modern version of fatty acid shaving soaps, but with an increased amount of water and additives to ensure stability. The goal of a shaving cream is to allow a close shave without removing excess stratum corneum or promoting corrosion of the razor blade. This can only be accomplished if the hair is softened through adequate hydration and the skin lubricated. The force required to cut water-saturated beard hair is about 65% less than that for dry hair (5,6). Thus, an effective shaving cream should possess low solution viscosity, high foam density, small molecular diameter, low solute concentration, good detergent action, low film strength, and high diffusivity (7).

> The force required to cut water-saturated beard hair is about 65% less than that for dry hair.

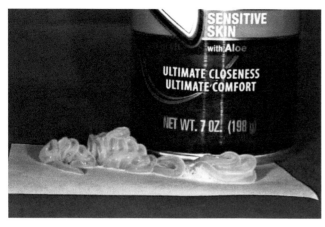

Figure 31.4 An example of a postfoaming shave gel designed for men. It dispenses as a gel and then turns into foam when rubbed into the skin.

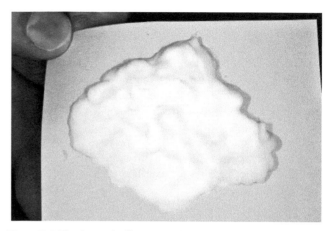

Figure 31.5 The shave gel will turn into foam when rubbed on the skin and should be left in place for three to four minutes before beginning to shave to soften the hair.

Shaving creams are formulated as foaming shaving creams and postfoaming shave gels. There is some evidence that postfoaming shave gels are superior lubricants over shave foams (Fig. 31.4). The reason for this is not clear, but may be related to the orientation of the fatty acids into the lamellar layers necessary to form a gel (8).

Shaving creams contain either sodium or potassium hydroxide, a superfatting agent (stearic acid, vegetable oils, mineral oil, or lanolin) and glycerol or propylene glycol to allow the cream to remain soft and improve lather by aiding moisture retention. Menthol is added to some preparations to provide both fragrance and a cooling effect on the skin. Beard softeners are wetting agents such as sulfuric acid esters of lauryl alcohol or fatty acid amides.

Aftershave Products

Aftershave products function to relieve the discomfort induced by shaving. They are designed to soothe and cool the skin while imparting a feeling of well being. The fragranced alcoholic lotions are the most popular. Other additives may include menthol for its cooling effect, an antibacterial to prevent infection, and glycerol or propylene glycol to act as an emollient and humectant (9). These products have enjoyed a renewed popularity as they are now formulated to cross over into the fragrance market for men.

APPLICATION OF SHAVING PRODUCTS

Proper shaving cream application is important in patients who are prone to develop irritant contact dermatitis. These patients generally do not allow the skin and hair shaft to absorb sufficient moisture prior to shaving. A shaving cream left in contact with the skin for at least four minutes will decrease razor trauma in most patients. Some patients will require additional lubrication and softening, which can be provided by applying a lipid-free cleanser to the area for an additional 15 minutes followed by shaving cream application.

A good well-maintained blade is part of the equation for a superior shave, but the shaving cream is equally important. The shaving cream creates the interface between the blade and the skin. A good interface sets the stage for a good shave and a poor interface sets the stage for a poor shave. Many patients feel that a shaving cream is extraneous and use nothing, or

other items handy in the bath such as bar soap, shampoo, or hair conditioner. It is important to remember that all personal care products are carefully designed for their intended purpose and are not well suited for any other use. Bar soaps, shampoo, and hair conditioner leave a film on the blade hastening blade dulling and do not optimally alleviate friction between the blade and the skin. Shaving cream is specially designed for this purpose.

There are many shaving products on the market. Some of them are old fashioned soaps applied with a brush, some are dispensed and warm when rubbed on the face, others are foams squirted from a can, and the best are gels dispensed from an aerosol can that foam when rubbed on the face. The latter are known as postfoaming shave gels. The postfoaming shave gel is the best choice for persons with shaving challenges because they entrain water better than any other type of shave product. Entraining water is the event that occurs when the hair shaft becomes hydrated. Hydration is the first step in preparing the hair for cutting because the keratin softens and can be cut with less force. A dry hair likened to a similar diameter copper wire while a wet hair is likened to an aluminum wire. Aluminum is much easier to cut than copper. These metals are used to model the physical dynamics of shaving.

The proper way to prepare the skin for shaving is by washing the face and then thoroughly wetting the face with lukewarm water. This wetting step places a thin layer of water over the hair and skin. Next, the shaving gel should be dispensed from the can and placed in the palm. The palms should be rubbed together to generate a rich foam, which is generously applied to the premoistened face. The shaving gel should remain on the face for three to four minutes before commencing shaving (Fig. 31.5). This allows time for more water to enter the hair shaft. At this point, the hair and skin are ready for shaving.

> The shaving gel should remain on the face for three to four minutes before commencing shaving.

OPTIMAL SHAVING TECHNIQUE

Once the skin has been properly prepared, it is necessary to execute the proper shaving technique. The blade should gently glide over the skin surface with minimal pressure. The quality of a shave is measured as the ratio of the amount of hair removed to the amount of skin removed. If the ratio is high, the shave is good. Conversely, if the ratio is low, the shave is poor. The blade should be dragged over each area for shaving only once. If the blade is rubbed multiple times over the same area, the chance for razor burn increases. Any areas that are not shaved as closely as desired should be left for shaving on the following day.

Shaving should occur in parallel strokes, even though the hair may grow in many different directions. The newer multiple blade razors provide for excellent shaving of hairs that demonstrate different skin exit angles. It is also important to rinse the blade after each stroke, to remove hair, skin, and shaving gel debris.

INFECTION PREVENTION

A common dermatologic problem related to shaving is the spread of disease. Bacterial diseases, such as impetigo and methicillin-resistant *Staphylococcus aureus* infection, can be spread on a razor blade in addition to viral diseases, such as verruca and molluscum contagiosum. A good razor and shaving cream can help in minimizing skin trauma and the opportunity for infection, but it may be necessary for shaving to be discontinued in infection areas until treatment is complete.

Razor blades can pass bacterial and viral infection to various sites on an individual patient or between family members who all use the same razor. It is best not to share razors for hygiene reasons, but also for optimal blade performance. Blades that are used to shave a male face experience a razor wear in a different manner than blades used to shave female legs. Different patterns of blade wear can lead to increased razor burn.

Allowing the razor to dry between uses can minimize the spread of infection. Soaking the razor head and blade in rubbing alcohol for a minute can also decrease spread, but can decrease razor blade life. Patients can put 2 inches of isopropyl alcohol in a jar and let the razor sit in the jar for 60 seconds, remove, and allow to dry, if recurrent infection is a problem.

Patients can put 2 inches of isopropyl alcohol in a jar and let the razor sit in the jar for 60 seconds, remove, and allow to dry, if recurrent infection is a problem.

SHAVING OF SPECIAL SKIN AREAS

Special skin areas, such as the female underarms and bikini area, deserve special mention. The underarms are unique in that they are concave, instead of convex, like most other shaved body areas. Likewise, the bikini area requires shaving areas that may be difficult to visualize again with tight concave areas that the razor must reach. There are razors designed for male and female use. Male razors are designed to shave the small curved areas of the face. Female razors are designed to shave the straight long surfaces of the legs and not necessarily the

Table 31.1 10 Tips for a Successful Shave

1. Select a multiblade razor with replaceable blades and a glide strip
2. Purchase a postfoaming shave gel
3. Change the razor blade weekly
4. Always clean the face prior to shaving
5. Wet the face with lukewarm water prior to shaving
6. Leave the shave gel on the face for three to four minutes before shaving
7. Shave with minimal pressure
8. Never shave with a damaged blade
9. Shave daily
10. Store the razor out of the bath in a dry location

armpits and the groin. It is important to pick a razor that fits nicely in the hand of the user. For patients with shaving challenges, it is well worth the money to buy several different handles with a few blades to see which one provides the best shave. Just like many people have a favorite pen, it is also necessary to find that one favorite razor.

SUMMARY

This chapter has discussed the finer points of shaving from blade design to shaving gel selection to shaving technique to minimize the presence of folliculitis. These points are summarized in Table 31.1. Shaving is a daily event for both male and female patients. Understanding the physics behind blade and razor design accompanied by the physiology of hair and skin is necessary to achieve the optimal shave.

REFERENCES

1. Saute RE. Shaving preparations. In: deNavarre MG, ed. The Chemistry and Manufacture of Cosmetics. Wheaton, IL: Allured Publishing Corporation, 1975: 1313–14.
2. Hollander J, Casselman EJ. Factors involved in satisfactory shaving. JAMA 1937; 109: 95.
3. Brooks GJ, Burmeister F. Preshave and aftershave products. Cosmet Toilet 1990; 15: 67–9.
4. Flaherty FE. Updating the art of shaving. Cosmet Toilet 1976; 91: 23–8.
5. Deem DE, Rieger MM. Observations on the cutting of beard hair. J Soc Cosmet Chem 1976; 27: 579–92.
6. Breuer MM, Sneath RL, Ackerman CS, Pozzi SJ. Perceptual evaluation of shaving closeness. J Soc Cosmet Chem 1989; 40: 141–50.
7. Saute RE. Shaving preparations. In: deNavarre MG, ed. The Chemistry and Manufacture of Cosmetics. Wheaton, IL: Allured Publishing Corporation, 1975: 1317–19.
8. Wickett RR. The effect of gels and foams on shaving comfort and efficacy. Skin Care J 1993; 2: 1–2.
9. Bell SA. Preshave and aftershave preparations. In: Balsam MD, Safarin E, eds. Cosmetics, Science and Technology. Vol. 2. 2nd edn. New York, NY: Wiley-Interscience, 1972: 13–37.

SUGGESTED READING

Foltis P. Shaving preparations (Chapter 25). Harry's Cosmeticology. 8th edn. Chemical Publishing Co., Inc., 2000: 501–21.
Olsen EA. Methods of hair removal. J Am Acad Dermatol 1999; 40(2 Pt 1): 143–55; quiz 156–7.

32 Hair removal

Hair removal is an important hygiene undertaking with both social and religious underpinnings. For example, Roman soldiers shaved all body hair prior to entering a battle as part of their worthiness for combat. Women shave their legs and underarms in western culture as it is felt that women should be devoid of terminal body hair for physical attractiveness. Men, on the other hand, sport chest hair in Mediterranean culture as a sign of virility while the present trend among young men in the U.S.A. is for shaving of chest and pubic hair. No single method of hair removal is appropriate for all body locations and all circumstances, thus there are several methods of hair removal that are presently available. Chapter 33 presented a discussion of wet shaving with a razor and this chapter discusses the remaining hair removal techniques that can be used for basic grooming and also for the cosmetic treatment of hirsutism. The various methods of hair removal are summarized in Table 32.1. Methods discussed include dry shaving, plucking, epilating, waxing, hair-removing gloves, abrasives, threading, chemical depilatories, electrolysis, and laser hair removal.

DRY SHAVING

Shaving is the most widespread method of hair removal due to its rapid speed, effectiveness, and low expense. Shaving is the preferred removal technique for facial hair in men and underarm or leg hair in women. A major limitation of this technique is rapid, bristly regrowth due to a hair shaft now devoid of a naturally tapered tip (1,2). Shaving can be accomplished with a razor blade combined with a shaving cream, a hair removal technique known as wet shaving, or with an electric shaver without moisture or shaving cream, a technique known as dry shaving. The electric shaver contains multiple blades, which rotate or vibrate thereby cutting the hair shaft. In general, an electric shaver cannot cut the hairs close to the skin surface as nearly as a razor, but skin abrasion is not as great a problem. Skin irritation and the spread of cutaneous infections may still occur (3).

Many factors influence the closeness of a dry shave, mainly achieved by the optimum interaction between the moving blades and the skin. Skin factors that contribute to dry shave closeness, which are identical to wet shave closeness, include abundant facial subcutaneous fat (resulting in improved resiliency), the absence of deep pits around hair ostia, and ostia containing only one hair (4). Factors that lead to increased dry shaving irritation are old razor blades, a large shaving angle, thin lathers, high skin tension, shave against the direction of hair growth, repeat shave over a given facial area, and increased shaving pressure (5).

Advantages of dry shaving include the rapidity and the ease with which the hair can be removed. Large surface areas can be shaved with minimal effort, as long as the hair shafts are short. Clippers, a variant of the electric razor, can be used

to easily shave longer hairs. It is difficult to injure the skin with dry shaving, which can be an advantage for persons with poor vision and/or poor manual dexterity. However, in areas where rapid hair regrowth or bristly hair is a problem, such as the face of women, dry shaving should not be used. Furthermore, the sharp regrowing hair shafts may cause irritation in intertriginous areas such as the underarms or inguinal folds (Fig. 32.1). Dry shaving may also cause irritation of the follicular ostia resulting in perifollicular pustules, a problem seen especially in the female pubic area, and the regrown hair shafts have a sharp tip, which may re-enter the skin, resulting in pseudofolliculitis barbae, commonly seen in the neck area of Black patients (6,7).

> The biggest problem with dry shaving is failure of the patient to use sharp blades.

The biggest problem with dry shaving is the failure of the patient to use sharp blades. Since the shaver blades cannot be replaced, it is important that the patient sharpen the blades as needed. Shaver blades are not designed to stay sharp for the lifetime of the electrical device. Also, the blades can be difficult to clean and the hair debris can clog the proper contact of the blade with the skin. Finally, it is possible to transmit an infectious disease from the moist skin and hair debris that remains under the protective screens in the shaver head. Proper shaver care is the secret to successful dry shaving.

PLUCKING

Plucking of the hair is a method of removing the entire hair shaft, including the bulb, with a pair of tweezers (8) (Fig. 32.2). It is an easy, inexpensive method of hair removal requiring minimal equipment, but is tedious and mildly uncomfortable. Plucking does not encourage rapid regrowth. Removal of hair from large areas is not feasible, but plucking is effective for removal of stray eyebrow hairs or isolated coarse hairs on the chin of postmenopausal women. Only terminal hairs can be efficiently plucked, as vellus hairs usually break close to the skin surface.

Plucking produces little skin damage and provides a longer regrowth period due to complete hair shaft removal. It should be remembered, however, that repeated plucking of a given hair may result in ingrown hairs or failure of the hair to regrow, due to follicular damage (9). For this reason, overplucking of the eyebrow area should be avoided (Fig. 32.3).

> Only terminal hairs can be efficiently plucked, as vellus hairs usually break close to the skin surface.

Table 32.1 Methods of Hair Removal

Technique	Equipment	Cost	Regrowth period	Body sites for use	Advantages	Disadvantages
Shaving	Razor or shaver	+	Days	Face, arms, legs, axilla	Fast, easy	Irritating, rapid regrowth
Plucking	Tweezers	+	Weeks	Eyebrows, facial hair	Longer regrowth period	Painful, slow
Epilating	Epilator	+	Weeks	Arms, legs	Longer regrowth period, fast	Painful, irritating
Waxing	Wax and melting pot	++	Weeks	Face, eyebrows, groin	Longer regrowth period	Painful, slow
Hair-removing gloves	Sand-paper gloves	++	Days	Legs, male face	None	Irritating, slow
Abrasives	Pumice stone	++	Days	Legs, male face	None	Irritating, slow
Threading	Thread	+	Days	Legs, arms	None	Painful, slow
Depilatories	Depilatory	++	Days	Legs, groin	Quick	Irritating
Electrolysis	Trained professional	++++	May be permanent	All	May be permanent	Painful, time consuming, expensive
Bleaching	Peroxide bleach	++	Does not remove hair	Female facial and arm hair	Quick	Irritating
Laser	Selective photothermolysis with laser	++++	Permanent	All body areas, does not work on unpigmented hair	Long lasting	Expensive

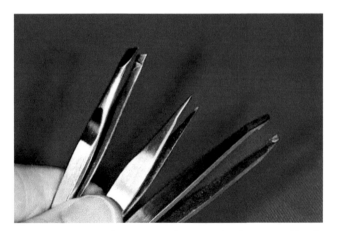

Figure 32.1 The rough cut end of a male beard hair accounting for the harsh feel of hair cut by a mechanized shaver.

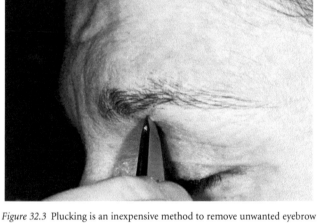

Figure 32.3 Plucking is an inexpensive method to remove unwanted eyebrow hairs, but overplucking should be avoided to minimize permanent hair loss.

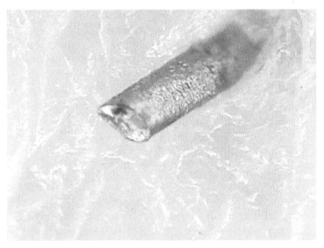

Figure 32.2 A variety of tweezers are shown. A pair of tweezers with a flat smooth tip is recommended over that with a pointed tip, shown in the middle, which can break the hair prior to complete removal.

EPILATING

Epilating has now come to refer to a mechanized method of plucking hair (10). Most electric hand-held epilating devices are stroked over the skin much like an electric shaver. They consist of a rotating, tightly coiled spring that traps the hair and pulls it out at the level of the hair bulb. Retail cost for the device is $30 to $50. This efficient plucking of the hair provides a long regrowth period, but is somewhat painful. Additionally, the device functions poorly on curved surfaces, such as the underarms, and can do considerable damage to body areas with thin skin, such as the face.

Epilating is best used on large flat surfaces such as the arms and legs, but the hair must be of sufficient length for entrapment in the coiled spring. Follicular disruption is a problem that can result in ingrown or coiled hairs beneath the skin surface (11,12). Infection may also be a problem, so use of an antibacterial agent prior to and following hair removal is

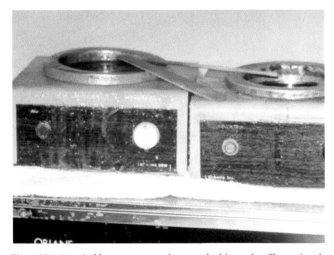

Figure 32.4 A typical hot wax pot as photographed in a salon illustrating the poor hygiene standards that may be present.

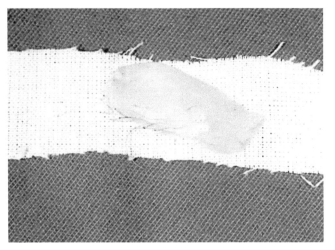

Figure 32.5 The eyebrow hairs are shown attached to the adhesive, which is affixed to the cloth. Cold waxing is an efficient method of plucking multiple hairs simultaneously.

recommended. If the epilator is pressed too firmly against the skin, purpura may result.

> Follicular disruption is a problem that can result in ingrown or coiled hairs beneath the skin surface following traumatic epilation.

WAXING

Waxing is another variation on plucking of the hair. Two waxing techniques are available: hot waxing and cold waxing. Hot wax is composed of rosin, beeswax, paraffin wax, petrolatum and mineral or vegetable oil. Some products are mentholated. The wax is melted in a double boiler or professional wax pot and applied to the hairs with a wooden spatula (Fig. 32.4). Hair becomes embedded within the wax, which is allowed to cool and harden. The hair is then pulled out at the level of the hair bulb as the wax is ripped from the skin. Care must be taken not to burn the skin.

Cold waxing, a newer method, employs a wax-like substance that is squeezed as a liquid from a pouch, thus eliminating the need for melting. Sometimes cold waxing uses a cloth piece which is initially placed on the hair removal area followed by liquid application. The cloth is then ripped from the skin with the hair and the wax (Fig. 32.5). The advantage of the cloth is that it provides strength so the wax can theoretically be removed in one piece rather than numerous smaller pieces.

Waxing has the advantage of adequate removal of both terminal and vellus hairs. This works significantly well on the upper lip, chin, eyebrows, cheeks and groin of women where removal of all hair is desirable. Men generally do not find waxing of facial hair acceptable as the hair has to grow to at least one-sixteenth of an inch before it can be reliably removed by waxing. Excess hair present in Becker's nevi, congenital hairy nevi, and benign hairy nevi can be removed in both men and women with this technique.

The major disadvantages of waxing are discomfort and poor removal of hairs shorter than one-sixteenth of an inch. Patients may also need to tweeze a few hairs that still remain and a thick hair growth may require two treatments for complete removal.

The results of waxing are identical to hair plucking. The two-week regrowth period is longer than that for shaving since the hair is removed by the root. When regrowth occurs, the hair has a tapered tip rather than the sharp, blunt tip produced by shaving. No damage to the surrounding skin occurs, but patients must test the heated wax prior to application to avoid a burn. Waxing can be done professionally in a salon or at home. Professional fees vary depending on the size of the removal area. For example, it costs about $20 to have the eyebrows professionally waxed. Home waxing is much less expensive: $4 will purchase sufficient wax to remove excess eyebrow hair for 30 treatments.

> Waxing has the advantage of adequate removal of both terminal and vellus hairs on the face.

HAIR-REMOVING GLOVES

Hair-removing gloves consist of a mitten of fine sandpaper that is rubbed over the hair-bearing skin in a circular fashion (13). This mechanically fractures the hair shaft, but is also irritating to the skin. This is a method used to remove female leg hair and male facial hair in some countries, but is not popular in the U.S.A. The most important use of hair-removing gloves is in a female patient with excessive white vellus hair on the face. It is easy to break off the vellus hairs without the irritation from depilatories or shaving.

ABRASIVES

A variation on hair-removing gloves is the use of abrasive substances to break and remove the hair. Pumice stone or other abrasives can be rubbed over the skin to remove hair through mechanical friction (13). Again, this is very irritating to skin and not a popular hair removal technique in the U.S.A. This hair removal method is more commonly found in third world nations.

THREADING

Threading is a hair removal technique popular in India that has found a following in the U.S.A., especially for the removal of eyebrow hair and unwanted vellus facial hair that is hard to pluck. Threading is performed by looping a cotton thread around the neck of the operator and twisting the other end into a loop held in one hand. Then the ends are twisted and the loop is pulled across the skin. The thread catches the hair and removes some at the level of the follicle while some hairs break above the skin surface (8). Threading is an efficient way of plucking the hair that involves minimal trauma, if properly done. The success of the hair removal result is highly operator dependent, but the supplies to perform threading are simple and inexpensive.

> Threading is performed by looping a cotton thread around the neck of the operator and twisting the other end into a loop held in one hand.

DEPILATORIES

From the mechanical methods of hair removal, the discussion now turns to chemical hair removal with products known as depilatories. Chemical depilatories function by sufficiently softening the hair shaft above the skin surface so it can be gently wiped away with a soft cloth (Fig. 32.6). Presently marketed chemical depilatories are available in pastes, powders, creams, and lotions with formulations specially adapted for use on the legs, groin area, and face. All formulations function by softening the cysteine-rich hair disulfide bonds to the point of dissolution. This is accomplished by combining five different classes of ingredients.

The agents combined to produce a chemical depilatory are detergents, hair shaft swelling agents, adhesives, pH adjusters, and bond-breaking agents (14). Together they function to prepare the hair for and facilitate removal. Detergents such as sodium lauryl sulfate, laureth-23, or laureth-4 remove protective hair sebum and allow penetration of the bond-breaking agent. Further penetration is accomplished with swelling agents such as urea or thiourea. Adhesives such as paraffin allow the mixture to adhere to the hairs while adjustment of pH, to between 9.0 and 12.5, is important to minimize cutaneous irritation. Lastly, the bond-breaking agent is able to successfully destroy the hair shaft.

Several bond-breaking agents are available: thioglycolic acid, calcium thioglycolate, strontium sulfide, calcium sulfide, sodium hydroxide, and potassium hydroxide. The most popular commercial bond-breaking agents are the thioglycolates as they minimize cutaneous irritation while effectively breaking disulfide bonds; however, they are less effective at dissolving coarse hair such as the male beard. Sulfide bond-breaking agents are faster acting, but are more irritating and sometimes produce an undesirable sulfur odor. Sodium hydroxide, also known as lye, is the best bond-breaking agent, but extremely damaging to the skin.

Chemical depilatories are designed to remain in contact with the skin for five to ten minutes, shorter for fine hair and longer for coarse hair. The products are somewhat selective for hair shaft damage since the hair shafts contain more cysteine than the surrounding skin, but are still irritating to skin, especially if the contact is prolonged. The hairs are wiped away once they assume a corkscrew appearance. Under no circumstances should chemical depilatories be applied to abraded or dermatitic skin.

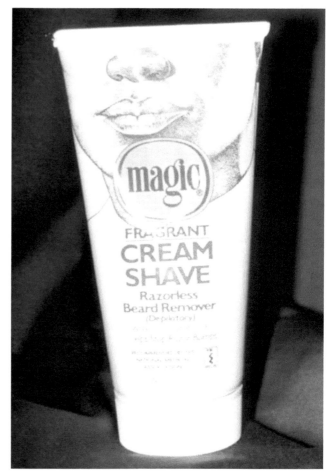

Figure 32.6 Male facial hair depilatories are popular among African American men who avoid the disfigurement of pseudofolliculitis barbae from shaving by dissolving the hair shaft at the follicular ostia.

The main advantage of chemical depilatory hair removal is slower regrowth than with shaving and, if used properly, the technique is painless and free of scarring. The major disadvantage is the skin irritancy (8).

> The main advantage of chemical depilatory hair removal is slower regrowth than with shaving.

Chemical depilatories are best used for removal of hair on the legs to include the upper thigh. Darkly pigmented hair seems somewhat more resistant to removal than lighter hair and coarse hair is more resistant than fine hair. This explains why these products are difficult to use on the male beard. However, a variety of powder depilatories, containing barium sulfide, are available for the Black male who has difficulty with pseudofolliculitis barbae (15,16). These powdered products are mixed with water to form a paste and applied to the beard with a wooden applicator for three to seven minutes. The hair and depilatory are then removed with the same applicator and the skin is rinsed with cool water. This procedure should be performed no more frequently than every other day.

Both allergic and irritant contact dermatitis can occur with the use of chemical depilatories. Allergic contact dermatitis is less common but may be seen due to fragrances, lanolin derivatives, or other cosmetic additives. Irritant contact dermatitis is common, especially in individuals who use the product more than once weekly or apply it close to mucous membranes. Generally, the product is not appropriate for any patient with dermatologic problems. Most cutaneous problems can be remedied by discontinuing use and applying a topical corticosteroid. Depilatories also can damage fabrics and furniture.

ELECTROLYSIS

Electrolysis is a permanent method of hair removal. It is not so commonly performed now that laser hair removal has become mainstream method; yet it is worth discussing. Dermatologists are well aware of the complications of electrolysis, which include scarring, failure to destroy the germinative follicular cells, and the transmission of viral and bacterial diseases. Yet, electrolysis remains a tremendously popular hair removal technique among women for unwanted hairs on the face, chin, neck, and bikini areas (17). There are three electrolysis techniques: galvanic electrolysis, thermolysis, and the blend.

The first individual to use electrolysis for hair removal was a Missouri ophthalmologist, named Dr. Charles E. Michel, who in1875 used the technique in the treatment of trichiasis. The technique became well known during the later part of the 19th century. In 1924, the technique of thermolysis was developed by Dr. Henri Bordier of Lyon, France. The combination of electrolysis and thermolysis, known as the blend, was developed by Arthur Hinkel and Henri St. Pierre in 1945 and a patent was granted for the technique in 1948 (18).

All electrolysis techniques involve the insertion of a needle into the follicular ostia down to the follicular germinative cells. The dermal papillae must be destroyed to permanently prevent hair growth. There are several important considerations in determining the effectiveness of electrolysis techniques.

Telogen vs. Anagen

Only hairs that are visible can be removed by electrolysis, and only anagen hairs can be adequately treated. On the other hand, follicles in the telogen phase, without a visible hair shaft, cannot be treated. If there is a high telogen to anagen ratio, a substantial amount of hair growth will be seen in the treated area. This ratio varies depending on the body area (19).

Many electrologists advise that their clients shave the hair in the area to be treated several days prior and refrain from other temporary hair removal techniques. This ensures that only anagen hair follicles are treated. Prior waxing or plucking of the hairs may delay regrowth thus decreasing the thoroughness of electrolysis.

Moisture Content

Moisture content of the hair follicle is also important in determining the success of electrolysis. The lower part of the hair follicle is better hydrated than the more superficial follicle. Water is necessary for transmitting electrical energy between the needle and dermal papillae. For this reason, the electrolysis needle must be inserted to the depth of the hair follicle.

Depth

The depth of needle insertion is determined by the hair shaft diameter. As is readily demonstrated in Table 32.2, larger-diameter hairs require deeper needle insertion for adequate

Table 32.2 Hair Shaft Diameter and Hair Follicle Depth

Hair shaft diameter (inches)	Description of hair	Hair follicle depth (mm)
<0.001	Very fine	<1
0.001–0.002	Fine	1–2
0.002–0.003	Medium	2–3
0.003–0.004	Coarse	3–4
0.004–0.005	Very coarse	4–5
0.005–0.006	Extra coarse	5
>0.006	Super coarse	5

Source: Adapted from Ref. 21.

destruction. Knowledge of follicular depth is necessary to ensure adequate follicular destruction without scarring.

Intensity and Duration

Dermal papillae damage depends both on the intensity and duration of the current administered. High-intensity energy may be used for a short duration or lower-intensity energy may be used for a longer duration. The decision of how much energy to use depends upon both the technique used by the electrologist and the pain tolerance of the client. As might be expected, pain increases with high-intensity energy. Low intensity energy, however, is unable to destroy some hairs. In general, coarse hairs require a longer-duration treatment than fine hairs (20).

Follicular Shape

Electrolysis is much more difficult to perform on individuals with curly, wavy, or kinky hair. This is due to difficulty in placing the needle accurately into the hair follicle.

Only visible hairs can be removed by electrolysis, thus only anagen hairs can be adequately treated.

HAIR REMOVAL TECHNIQUE

Electrolysis, thermolysis, and the blend represent the three techniques that can be used to permanently remove unwanted hair (21). Other advertised methods, such as electronic tweezers, do not work.

Electrolysis

This technique is properly known as "galvanic electrolysis" and utilizes direct current (DC) which is passed through a stainless steel needle into sodium chloride and water in the tissue surrounding the hair follicle. The DC current causes ionization of the salt (NaCl) and water (H_2O) into free sodium (Na^+), chloride (Cl^-), hydrogen (H^+) and hydroxide (OH^-) ions. These free ions then recombine into sodium hydroxide (NaOH), known as lye, and hydrogen gas (H_2). The caustic sodium hydroxide destroys the hair follicle while the hydrogen gas escapes into the atmosphere. The amount of sodium hydroxide produced is greater at the base of the hair follicle due to increased moisture content and minimal at the skin surface. Less lye production near the skin surface accompanied by the protective effect of sebum decreases the skin irritancy potential of this technique. The amount of follicular destruction induced is measured in units of lye, defined by Arthur Hinkel as: the amount of lye produced when 0.1 mA of current flows for one second (22).

Galvanic electrolysis is the most effective method of producing permanent hair removal, but is tedious and slow. This has led to the development of multiple needle techniques.

Thermolysis

Thermolysis, also known as short-wave radio frequency diathermy, differs from galvanic electrolysis in that alternating high frequency (AC) current is passed down the needle. This current causes vibration of the water molecules around the hair follicle and produces heat. Thus, heating occurs in the same manner as in a microwave oven (23).

The needle begins to heat at the tip first and spreads toward the skin surface. This means that the heat remains longer around the hair follicle than at the skin surface, minimizing discomfort and cutaneous damage. If too much AC current is administered, steam is produced which exits through the follicular ostia resulting in a burn and possible scarring.

Thermolysis is much faster than galvanic electrolysis, but does not destroy the hair follicle as reliably. Additionally, thermolysis does not work well on distorted or curved hair follicles. An extremely rapid method of thermolysis, known as the flash method, was introduced several years ago, but unfortunately was plagued by high hair regrowth rates.

Blend

The blend is a combination of both galvanic electrolysis and thermolysis (24). Both direct and high-frequency alternating current are passed down the needle at the same time to produce sodium hydroxide and heat. The hot lye is extremely effective in destroying the dermal papillae, allowing superior results with less regrowth. Furthermore, the tissue damage induced by the thermolysis allows the lye to spread through the hair follicle more rapidly. The blend requires only one-fourth the time of galvanic electrolysis alone.

NEEDLE SELECTION

Needle selection is important to the success of electrolysis. Needles are available in a variety of shapes: straight, tapered, bulbous, and insulated (25) (Fig. 32.7). Most electrologists prefer to use a straight needle with a gently rounded tip. Tapered needles (narrower at the tip than the base) are sometimes selected for the removal of deep terminal hairs. Electrolysis of these hairs requires more energy, which can be delivered at the tip without exposing the more superficial tissues to excessive damage.

A variety of sizes are also available since the needle diameter should match the diameter of the hair shaft to be treated. Smaller needles generally get hotter than larger needles. Client pain can be reduced by selecting the largest needle possible.

Stainless steel is the standard material from which needles are made; however, one company markets a gold plated needle which is termed "hypoallergenic." Sometimes the electrologist may use multiple needles at a time to speed the treatment. A computerized electrolysis machine is used to sequentially administer energy to the needles in the proper order and for the specified length of time.

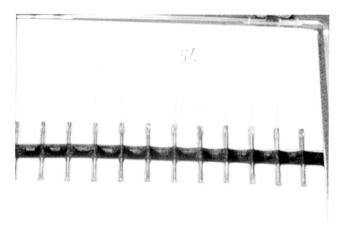

Figure 32.7 Single-use electrolysis needles are recommended to prevent the inadvertent transmission of contagious diseases.

NEEDLE INSERTION TECHNIQUES

The needle must be properly inserted into the follicular ostia to insure destruction of the hair follicle without cutaneous scarring. The most popular technique for needle insertion is known as the forehand technique. The needle holder is held much like a pencil between the thumb and forefinger. The removal forceps are then placed between the needle holder and thumb of the same hand. This allows the free hand to be used for stretching the skin. Skin stretching is important to open the follicular ostia for needle insertion.

The needle is always inserted parallel to the hair shaft opposite to the direction of hair growth. Hairs may exit the skin at angles varying between 10° and 90°. The needle must be inserted at the same angle as hair growth. If the hair is long and lays on the skin surface, it should be clipped to gain a better appreciation of its exit angle. The needle should also always be inserted below the hair shaft. These steps are necessary to destroy the follicle without scarring the surrounding skin.

It is important that needle insertion occurs to the proper depth. A general rule is that coarse hairs have deeper follicles than fine hairs. A slight dimpling of the overlying skin and resistance means that the bottom of the follicle has been reached and the needle should be withdrawn slightly until the dimpling disappears. A proper needle insertion should be painless and bloodless for the client. Shallow needle insertions may result in pain and scarring for the client.

ELECTROLYSIS HAIR REMOVAL TECHNIQUES

Once the hair has been treated, the needle should be withdrawn at exactly the same angle as it was inserted. The forceps held between the thumb and needle holder are now positioned 90° to the hair shaft for epilation. The hair should be grasped firmly and gently slide out of the follicle, if the treatment has been properly performed. Resistance in removing the hair means that the hair has been epilated and not treated with electrolysis, thus regrowth may occur.

ELECTROLYSIS ADVERSE REACTIONS

Electrolysis must be properly performed to minimize client scarring. Table 32.3 summarizes the pointers that must be followed for successful electrolysis (26). Care must also be taken to perform the procedure under sanitary conditions to prevent the spread of bacterial and viral infection (27).

Table 32.3 Method for Electrolysis Scar Prevention

1. The treated hair should be pulled effortlessly from the follicular ostia.
2. The needle size should be the same as the hair diameter.
3. The skin should be dry.
4. The skin should not be blanched following treatment.
5. The current should only flow when the needle has been completely inserted in the follicular ostia to the level of the follicle.
6. The needle should only be removed when the current has stopped.
7. The same follicular ostia should not be re-entered or treated twice.

The real concern regarding electrolysis is the lack of regulation, as 23 states do not require licensing for electrologists. This lack of licensing means that training and health standards are apt to vary tremendously between salons. Improper techniques can result in permanent scarring while failure to adequately sterilize equipment can result in the transmission of bacterial and viral infections. If a good operator with superior health standards can be found, electrolysis may be useful in a female with a few unwanted facial hairs on the upper lip or chin. This technique is not suitable for removal of large hairy areas, such as the male beard, as only 25 to 100 hairs can be removed per sitting.

BLEACHING

Bleaching is not a method of hair removal, but is included in this section because it can make unwanted hair less apparent. Commercial products are available for bleaching hair; however a home-made bleach can be made by mixing 40 ml of hydrogen peroxide with 7 ml of 20% ammonia. The bleach is left in contact with the hair until the color is removed, about five to ten minutes. This product is irritating to the skin and should not be used around the eyes or mucous membranes.

Hair bleaching is most appropriate in the female patient who notes excess pigmented hair on the arms, upper lip, or jawline. The hair may be pigmented due to a Hispanic, Mediterranean, or Middle Eastern genetic background. Bleaching may be the most acceptable alternative when shaving produces an unacceptable regrowth appearance and the area is too large for waxing.

> Hair bleaching is most appropriate in the female patient who notes excess pigmented hair on the arms, upper lip, or jawline.

LASER

Lasers have revolutionized professional hair removal and are presently poised to enter the consumer market, as well. Home lasers may become commonplace as the safety and reduced cost of these devices make them more appealing. Laser hair removal is clearly more permanent and more effective than any other method. Many different types of lasers and light sources can be used to destroy hair growth, including normal-mode ruby, neodymium:yttrium-aluminum-garnet (Nd:YAG), diode, and intense pulsed light (IPL).

Even though laser hair removal is considered permanent, the FDA definition of permanent is a stable decrease in the number of terminal hairs for a period longer than one complete hair cycle at a given site. This does not mean that the hair is all gone! This is why it takes several treatments to completely remove the hair and some hair may regrow, but it is finer and less pigmented. How much hair reduction occurs depends on the treatment type, the hair location, and the color of the hair. Persons with deeply pigmented hair do the best, but persons with red, blonde, gray, or white hair may not get as much reduction requiring treatments every three months.

> Laser hair removal works best in deeply pigmented hair meaning patients with red, blonde, gray, or white hair achieve as much hair growth reduction.

In order for the hair to be permanently removed, complete destruction only occurs when both the germinative cells in the hair bulb and the stem cells in the hair bulge area are destroyed. This topic is discussed in the hair chapter in more detail. The melanin in the hair serves as the target for the laser energy. This means that selective thermolysis is used to damage the hair growth. The hair melanin functions to absorb energy in the range of 600 to 1100 nm and is known as the chromophore. The energy is then released by melanin as heat. This allows the light energy to penetrate to the bottom of the hair follicle and rapidly heat the water thus cooking and destroying the hair. Hairs in the telogen resting cycle cannot be treated with laser hair removal, accounting for the multiple treatments needed to achieve a satisfactory result. A variety of laser and light devices can be used for permanent hair removal as long as they follow the concept of selective thermolysis.

SUMMARY

The hair removal techniques discussed here should be used in combination with wet shaving, discussed in chapter 31, to assist the patient concerned about hirsutism. Every hair removal technique has pluses and minuses that should be evaluated in light of the needs of the patient and the risk versus benefit ratio. In the case of laser hair removal, the cost and the suitability of the hair for selective photolysis should also be considered. These hair removal techniques should be combined with medical treatment, where appropriate, in the hirsute patient.

REFERENCES

1. Bhaktaviziam C, Mescon H, Matolsky AG. Shaving. Arch Dermatol 1963; 88: 242–7.
2. Lynfield YL, MacWilliams P. Shaving and hair growth. J Invest Dermatol 1970; 55: 170–2.
3. Brooks GJ, Burmeister F. Preshave and aftershave products. Cosmet Toilet 1990; 105: 67–9.
4. Hollander J, Casselman EJ. Factors involved in satisfactory shaving. JAMA 1937; 109: 95.
5. Elden HR. Advances in understanding mechanisms of shaving. Cosmet Toilet 1985; 100: 51–62.
6. Strauss J, Kligman AM. Pseudofolliculitis of the beard. Arch Dermatol 1956; 74: 533–42.
7. Spencer TS. Pseudofolliculitis barbae or razor bumps and shaving. Cosmet Toilet 1985; 100: 47–9.

8. Richards RN, Uy M, Meharg G. Temporary hair removal in patients with hirsuitism: a clinical study. Cutis 1990; 45: 199–202.
9. Blackwell G. Ingrown hairs, shaving, and electrolysis. Cutis 1977; 19: 172–3.
10. Scott JJ, Scott MJ, Scott AM. Epilation. Cutis 1990; 46: 216–17.
11. Wright RC. Traumatic folliculitis of the legs: a persistent case associated with use of a home epilating device. J Am Acad Dermatol 1992; 27: 771–2.
12. Dilaimy M. Pseudofolliculitis of the legs. Arch Dermatol 1976; 112: 507–8.
13. Wagner RF. Physical methods for the management of hirsutism. Cutis 1990; 45: 319–26.
14. Breuer H. Depilatories. Cosmet Toilet 1990; 105: 61–4.
15. de la Guardia M. Facial depilatories on black skin. Cosmet Toilet 1976; 91: 37–8.
16. Halder RM. Pseudofolliculitis barbae and related disorders. Dermatol Clin 1988; 6: 407–12.
17. Goldberg HC, Hanfling SL. Hirsutism and electrolysis. J Med Soc NJ 1965; 62: 9–14.
18. Richards RN, Meharg GE. Cosmetic and medical electrolysis and temporary hair removal. Ontario: Medric Ltd., 1991: 17–18.
19. Richards RN, Meharg GE. Cosmetic and medical electrolysis and temporary hair removal. Ontario: Medric Ltd., 1991: 24–5.
20. Hinkel AR, Lind RW. Electrolysis, thermolysis and the blend. California: Arroway Publishers, 1968: 181–7.
21. Fino G. Modern electrology. New York: Milady Publishing Corp., 1987: 35–69.
22. Cipollaro AD. Electrolysis: discussion of equipment, method of operation, indications, contraindications, and warnings concerning its use. JAMA 1938; 110: 2488–91.
23. Wagner RF, Tomich JM, Grande DJ. Electrolysis and thermolysis for permanent hair removal. J Am Acad Dermatol 1985; 12: 441–9.
24. Hinkel AR, Lind RW. Electrolysis, thermolysis and the blend. California: Arroway Publishers, 1968: 199–223.
25. Gior F. Modern electrology. New York: Milady Publishing Corporation, 1987: 32–3.
26. Richards RN, Meharg GE. Cosmetic and medical electrolysis and temporary hair removal. Ontario: Medric Ltd., 1991: 85–6.
27. Petrozzi JW. Verrucae planae spread by electrolysis. Cutis 1980; 26: 85.

SUGGESTED READING

Alster TS, Tanzi EL. Effect of a novel low-energy pulsed-light device for home-use hair removal. Dermatol Surg 2009; 35: 483–9.

Casey AS, Goldberg D. Guidelines for laser hair removal. J Cosmet Laser Ther 2008; 10: 24–33.

Dierickx CC. Photoepilation (Chapter 21). In: Blume-Peytave U, Tosti A, Whiting DA, Trueb RM, eds. Hair growth and disorders. Springer, 2008: 427–45.

Fodor L, Menachem M, Ramon Y, et al. Hair removal using intense pulsed light (EpiLight): patient satisfaction, our experience, and literature review. Ann Plast Surg 2005; 54: 8–14.

Gault D. Treatment of unwanted hair in auricular reconstruction. Facial Plast Surg 2009; 25: 175–80.

Gold MH, Bell WE, Teresa DF. Long-term epilation using the epilight broad band, intense pulsed light hair removal system. Dermatol Surg 2008; 23: 909–13.

Görgü M, Aslan G, Aköz T, Erdogan B, ASVAK Laser Center. Comparison of alexandrite laser and electrolysis for hair removal. Dermatol Surg 2000; 26: 37–41.

Liew SH. Laser hair removal: guidelines for management. Am J Clin Dermatol 2002; 3: 107–15.

Littler CM. Hair removal using an Nd: YAG laser system. Dermatol Clin 1999; 17: 401–30.

Ort RJ, Dierickx C. Laser hair removal. Semin Cutan Med Surg 2002; 21: 129–44.

Pickens JE, Zakhireh M. Permanent removal of unwanted hair. Aesthetic Surg J 2004; 24: 442–5.

Ramos-el-Silva M, de Castro MCR, Carneiro LV. Hair removal. Clin Dermatol 2001; 19: 437–44.

Spencer JM. Clinical evaluation of a handheld self-treatment device for hair removal. J Drugs Dermatol 2007; 6: 788–92.

Tatlidede S, egemen O, Saltat A, et al. Hair removal with the long-pulse alexandrite laser. Aesthetic Surg J 2005; 25: 138–43.

Traversa E, Machado-Santelli GM, Velasco MVR. Histological evaluation of hair follicle due to papain's depilatory effect. Int J Pharm 2007; 335: 163–6.

Zoumaras J, Kwei JSS, Vandervord J. A case review of patients presenting to royal north shore hospital, with hair removal wax burns between January and November 2006. Burns 2008; 34: 254–56.

33 Hair and photoprotection

Photoprotection as it pertains to hair is not a common topic addressed by the dermatologist. After all, hair is nonliving and as such requires no protection from UV radiation, because carcinogenesis of the hair shaft itself is not possible. If hair proteins are altered by sun exposure, damaged hair can be removed and replaced by new growth. Thus, at first glance, the whole issue of photoprotection for the hair might seem irrelevant; however, patients frequently consult the dermatologist for advice on hair growth and appearance problems. Hair photoprotection is an important part of maintaining the cosmetic value of the hair shaft. This chapter will focus on the chemical effects of UV radiation on the hair shaft, hair photoaging, intrinsic hair UV photoprotective mechanisms, and the use of hair sunscreens. The whole science of hair and photoprotection is currently in its infancy and an area of focused research within the hair care product and salon industries.

HAIR AND UV RADIATION

Much of the understanding regarding hair and how it interacts with UV radiation has come from the textile industry. Natural fibers, such as wool, cotton, silk, and rayon, discolor when exposed to sunlight. White fabrics tend to take on a light brown/yellow color, a process known as photoyellowing (1,2). The same chemical process of photoyellowing can also occur in natural unprocessed human hair. Human hair contains two pigments, eumelanin and pheomelanin, accounting for the brown and red hues seen in hair, respectively. A third melanin pigment, known as oxymelanin, is found in unprocessed human hair that has been exposed to sunlight. Oxymelanin is an oxidative photodegradation product. While the presence of this photodegraded melanin decreases the cosmetic value of the hair, it also chemically affects hair dye and permanent wave solution interaction with the hair shaft. Most importantly, the amount of oxymelanin present equates with the degree of hair shaft photoaging.

> Oxymelanin is a photodegradation pigment that accounts for photoyellowing in hair.

UV radiation also damages the hair lipids. It is for this reason that photodamaged hair is dull and dry. Intact hair lipids are required to coat the hair shaft imparting shine and manageability. Manageability is the ease with which the hair shaft can be styled. Hair that is devoid of intact lipids is subject to static electricity, fractures easily with combing friction, and appears frizzy.

HAIR PHOTOAGING AND ENDOGENOUS PROTECTION

In order to understand hair photoaging, it is necessary to understand how UV radiation interacts with the proteins of the hair shaft. Hair is a complex nonliving structure with an outer cuticle that provides a hard protective barrier for the inner cortex. The cortex is composed of fibrillar proteins, which are responsible for the mechanical strength of the hair shaft. Melanin pigments are contained in the cortex embedded in an amorphous protein matrix. Sometimes the hair shaft may contain a medulla, but the function of this inner structure is largely unknown and is found less frequently in mature hair shafts. Sunlight damages the strength of the hair shaft by increasing the scission of the cystine disulfide bonds. The hair disulfide bonds prevent the hair shaft from fracturing with minimal trauma. Thus, the primary photoaging effect of sunlight on hair is physical weakening of the shaft.

> The protein structure of the hair is damaged by UV radiation.

The second major effect of sunlight on the hair shaft is oxymelanin production, as previously mentioned. While oxymelanin leads to pigment dilution and lightening of hair color, it is the pigments within the hair shaft that provide the only source of endogenous photoprotection. The natural pigments actually prevent disulfide bond disruption, preserving the strength of the hair shaft, even though a hair color change occurs. In other words, chemical alterations in the hair pigment function to protect the protein structural backbone of the hair. Hair contains the original pigment sunscreen, which is an area of rapid technical development in the commercial skin sunscreen industry.

The third major effect of sunlight on hair is bleaching, or lightening, of the hair color (3). Brunette hair tends to develop reddish hues due to photo-oxidation of melanin pigments while blonde hair develops photoyellowing. The yellow discoloration is due to photodegradation of cystine, tyrosine, and tryptophan residues within the blonde hair shaft (4). Furthermore, hair treated with permanent or semipermanent hair dyes may also shift color when exposed to UV radiation (5).

TOPICAL HAIR PHOTOPROTECTION

Until recently, the main approach to topical exogenous hair photoprotection was no different from skin photoprotection. UVB and UVA sunscreens were added to formulations designed for hair use, such as instant conditioners, styling gels, and hair sprays. The main problem with this topical approach to hair photoprotection was the failure to create an even film protecting the entire surface area of every hair on the head. This is virtually impossible since the collective surface area of the hair on a human head is huge. Another challenge is creating a sunscreen formulation that will adhere to the hair cuticle. Furthermore, coating each and every hair shaft with an equal thickness of sunscreen without making the hair appear limp or greasy is a cosmetic challenge no hair care product has yet overcome.

A photoprotection rating system has been proposed for hair care products known as an HPF or hair protection factor (6). This is similar to the concept of SPF, or skin protection factor, except that tensile strength assessments of the hair shaft are used for grading instead of sunburn assessment. HPF ratings follow a logarithmic scale from 2 to 15. At present, this system has not caught on because skin care products labeled with an SPF are considered over-the-counter (OTC) drugs. Hair care products are true cosmetics and do not wish to be included in the sunscreen monograph or subject to the regulations governing OTC drugs. This dilemma led cosmetic researchers to question whether photoprotection could be imparted to the hair shaft through another means, perhaps through the internal structure of the hair shaft.

INTRINSIC HAIR PHOTOPROTECTION

An analysis of the internal structure of the hair shaft led to some interesting insight into possible mechanisms of photoprotection. The natural color of the hair shaft results from a combination of visible light absorption and light scattering abilities of the pigment granules distributed within the cortex. Exposure of the hair to sunlight leads to lightening of the hair color, known as bleaching, and ultimately damage to the fiber itself, as previously discussed. The pigment lightening is obvious when looking at a woman with long brown hair. The distal hair tips have a reddish hue while the proximal hair shafts have a brown hue. This loss of pigment and the resultant amino acid changes appear to predispose the hair shaft to more accelerated photoaging. This led the cosmetics industry to question whether alterations in hair color could be used to enhance intrinsic hair photoprotection.

Industry hair researchers have demonstrated that unpigmented hair is much more susceptible to UV-induced damage than pigmented hair, meaning that the color granules are providing some protection from oxidative damage. Hair protein degradation is induced by light wavelengths from 254 to 400 nm (7). Chemically, these changes are thought to be due to ultraviolet light–induced oxidation of the sulfur molecules within in the hair shaft (8). Oxidation of the amide carbon of polypeptide chains also occurs producing carbonyl groups in the hair shaft (9). This is explained by the fact that the rate of cystine disulfide bond breakage due to environmental exposure is greater for unpigmented than pigmented hair. Thus, white hair and advanced gray hair are more susceptible to the damaging effects of UV radiation than youthful pigmented hair. Even though it has been traditionally held that hair dyes are damaging to the hair shaft, the photoprotective effects of replacing hair shaft pigments may offset some of this damage.

Pigmented hair is much less susceptible to UV photodamage than pigmented hair.

METHODS OF ENHANCING INTRINSIC PHOTOPROTECTION

If natural pigments within the hair shaft provide photoprotection, it may be possible to preserve the hair cosmetic value with synthetic pigments deposited on the cuticle and within the cortex via hair dyes. There are two types of hair dyes that

can artificially increase the hair shaft pigments: semipermanent and permanent hair dyes.

Semipermanent hair dyes are composed of a combination of dyes, such as nitrophenylenediamines, nitroaminophenols, and aminoanthraquinones. These dyes are left on the hair for 25 minutes and used in combination to arrive at the final desired color. As might be imagined, there is damage that occurs to the hair fibers upon dyeing. However, as the hair is exposed to longer periods of UV radiation, the initial damaging effect of the dyeing procedure is outweighed by antioxidant effect of the color deposited on and in the hair shaft. Thus, white hair that is undyed exhibits more mechanical strength damage from UV radiation than semipermanently dyed hair after four days of exposure. This means the darker the hair dye color, the more photoprotection provided. The semipermanent hair colors are a mixture of dyes designed to create the desired final color. Usually, a mixture of reds and blues are used to create brown. It is interesting to note that the red pigments produce better photoprotection than the blue pigments. This is probably due to the red dyes absorbing the more energetic part of the UV spectrum than the blue dyes.

This same effect was also observed with permanent hair dyes. Permanent hair dyes penetrate more deeply into the hair shaft creating color because of an oxidation/reduction reaction. They too act as photoprotectants; however, the permanent hair dyes are more damaging due to the hydrogen peroxide and ammonia used to allow the chemicals to penetrate the hair shaft. It is somewhat paradoxical that the more alkaline dyes, which produce more cuticular and structural hair shaft damage, provide better photoprotection. This is due to the ability of permanent hair dyes to act as passive photofilters by reducing hair fiber protein damage through incident light attenuation. The dye molecule absorbs light energy, which promotes it to a more excited state, followed by a return to ground state via radiative and nonradiative pathways. This is the mechanism by which hair dyes can function as antioxidants to prevent hair weakening through disulfide bond dissolution (Fig. 33.1).

Brown permanent hair dyes provide excellent photoprotection.

SUNSCREEN CONTAINING HAIR CARE PRODUCTS

There are a variety of hair care products, in addition to hair dyes, which can provide some hair photoprotection. These include shampoos, instant conditioners, deep conditioners, and hair styling products. Some of the higher priced prestige shampoos are incorporating sunscreens into their formulations designed for dyed hair. As mentioned previously, since UVA radiation alters the color of dyed hair, these shampoos are marketed as products that extend the life of the hair dye. They may prevent dyed blonde hair and dyed brunette hair from developing red hues or brassy overtones. Certainly, the delivery of photoprotection from a shampoo is challenging, since the surfactant must be completely rinsed from the hair prior to styling. It is my opinion that these products do indeed contain added chemical sunscreens, such as oxybenzone or

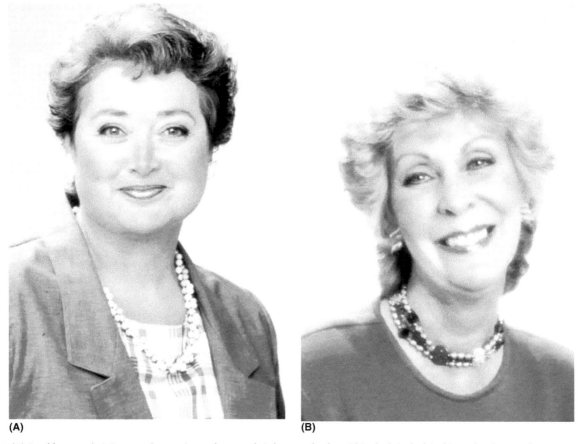

(A)   **(B)**

Figure 33.1 (**A**) Dyed brunette hair is more photo resistant than gray hair because the dye within the hair shaft is able to absorb UV radiation preventing hair protein damage. (**B**) Dyed blonde hair is more susceptible to photodamage than dyed brunette hair.

octyl methoxycinnamate, but their ability to coat and protect the hair is limited.

A better approach to hair photoprotection is through the use of conditioners. Some of the newer conditioners based on silicones, such as dimethicone, can indeed deposit a thin film of both conditioner and sunscreen on the hair shaft. While it is likely that the film will not evenly coat each hair shaft, sunscreens have better substantivity when applied in this manner. Instant conditioners that are applied immediately following shampooing and rinsed prior to towel drying are not as effective as deep conditioners that remain on the hair for 15 to 30 minutes. The longer the conditioner remains on the hair shaft, the more likely the added sunscreen ingredient will adhere to the hair. Thus, the contact time of the conditioner with the hair will determine the degree of photoprotection obtained, to some extent.

Styling products that are applied following drying of the hair are probably the most effective in terms of delivering photoprotection. These include blow drying conditioners, styling gels, and hair sprays. Blow drying conditioners are massaged through the hair when wet, just prior to drying to act as a protectant against heat damage. If they are massaged thoroughly through the hair, they may provide excellent photoprotection. Styling gels that may be applied to only certain areas of the hair, such as the hair shaft roots or tips, may not provide much protection due to limited contact. This is also the case with hair sprays that are applied as a thin film to a finished hair style.

Sunscreen containing hair sprays and conditioning sprays can reduce hair UV damage.

The degree of photoprotection offered by a hair care products is minimal at best. A more thorough, thicker application will result in better photoprotection, but this is difficult given the massive surface area of a head of hair. Many currently available sunscreen actives are not substantive to hair, meaning that they do not stick or adhere to the hair well preventing sunscreen deposition and facilitating removal. A better approach to hair photoprotection may be the use of clothing, such as a hat, scarf, or umbrella. Much research and development remains in the realm of hair photoprotection.

SUMMARY

New insights into semipermanent and permanent dyes as a means of hair photoprotection are intriguing. Many of the female patients who present to the dermatologist for suggestions regarding hair growth are mature with gray hair. The temptation is to bleach the hair, thus removing any remaining pigment granules to produce hair color lightening. Hair that is gray or bleached possesses fewer pigment granules than brown hair and is thus more susceptible to photoaging. Darker hair colors are more resistant to photodegradation. Thus, it may be beneficial to mature women who enjoy the outdoors to dye their hair a darker color to prevent hair shaft weakening from

UVA exposure. At the present time, hair dye is the best sunscreen available. Sunscreen containing shampoos and conditioners offer limited photoprotection at best.

REFERENCES

1. Launer HF. Effect of light upon wool. IV. Bleaching and yellowing by sunlight. Textile Res J 1965; 35: 395–400.
2. Inglis AS, Lennox FG. Wool yellowing. IV. Changes in amino acid composition due to irradiation. Textile Res J 1963; 33: 431–5.
3. Tolgyesi E. Weathering of the hair. Cosmet Toilet 1983; 98: 29–33.
4. Milligan B, Tucker DJ. Studies on wool yellowing. Part III sunlight yellowing. Text Res J 1962; 32: 634.
5. Berth P, Reese G. Alteration of hair keratin by cosmetic processing and natural environmental influences. J Soc Cosmet Chem 1964; 15: 659–66.
6. Nacht S. Sunscreens and hair. Cosmet Toilet 1990; 105: 55–9.
7. Arnoud R, Perbet G, Deflandre A, Lang G. ESR study of hair and melanin-keratin mixtures: the effects of temperature and light. Int J Cosmet Sci 1984; 6: 71–83.
8. Jachowicz J. Hair damage and attempts to its repair. J Soc Cosmet Chem 1987; 38: 263–86.
9. Holt LA, Milligan B. The formation of carbonyl groups during irradiation of wool and its releance to photoyellowing. Textile Res J 1977; 47: 620–4.

SUGGESTED READING

Draelos ZD. Sunscreens and hair photoprotection. Dermatol Clin 2006; 24: 81–4.
Hoting E, Zimmerman M. Sunlight-induced modifications in bleached, permed, or dyed human hair. J Soc Cosmet Chem 1997; 48: 79–91.
Hoting E, Zimmerman M, Hilterhaus-Bong S. Photochemical alterations in human hair: I. Artificial irradiation and investigation of hair proteins. J Soc Cosmet Chem 1995; 46: 85–99.
Jachowicz J. Hair damage and attempts at its repair. J Soc Cosmet Chem 1987; 38: 263–86.
Pande CM, Albrecht L. Hair photoprotection by dyes. J Soc Cosmet Chem 2001; 52: 377–89.
Tolgyesi E. Weathering of hair. Cosmet Toilet 1983; 98: 29–33.

34 Alopecia and cosmetic considerations

The practicing dermatologist frequently encounters patients who express concerns regarding hair loss. Generally, patients state that their usually thick, shiny, and manageable hair has become thin and difficult to style. If this is the dermatologist's first consultation with the patient, verifying the degree of hair loss is difficult. It is estimated that an individual must lose approximately 50% of their hair before an unacquainted observer can examine the scalp and note a reduction in the hair shaft number. In the hair cosmetic industry, the number of hairs required for hair fullness is listed in Table 34.1. Notice that the lighter the hair color, the greater the number of hairs that are required for visually thick hair.

Red hair requires fewer shafts than blond hair to appear full since red hair shafts have the thickest diameter while blond hair shafts are the thinnest. This is of interest, since more blond and brown haired patients seem to present for hair loss issues than black or red hair, in my practice. Nevertheless, hair loss is a complex dermatologic problem mediated by internal and external factors. It may be difficult for the dermatologist to know where to begin when assisting the distressed patient who is complaining of hair loss. An algorithm must be in mind when the patient requests help in order to efficiently and logically address the problem. This chapter describes my approach to the patient with diffuse, nonscarring hair loss, which can be addressed medically and cosmetically. Scarring causes of hair loss are beyond the scope of this book and unfortunately must be addressed by the use of hair prostheses, discussed in a prior chapter (1).

EVALUATION OF EXTERNAL VS. INTERNAL HAIR LOSS CAUSATION

It is of utmost importance to begin an evaluation of the hair loss patient by differentiating internal versus external factors. Generally, internal causes of hair loss result in shedding of the complete hair shaft, including the bulb. If the bulb is elongated, the hair has been shed during the anagen phase, indicating anagen effluvium. On the other hand, if the bulb is club shaped, the hair has been shed during the telogen phase, indicating telogen effluvium.

> Patient hair loss must be evaluated for external and internal causes.

External causes of hair loss resulting from grooming practices or cosmetic chemical hair treatments weaken the hair shaft so that breakage occurs. These broken hair shafts do not contain the bulb. However, abnormally formed hair shafts, found sporadically or in association with genodermatoses (trichoschisis, trichorrhexis invaginata, pili torti, monilethrix, and trichorrhexis nodosa) can also result in decreased hair shaft strength and subsequent breakage. Examination of several plucked hairs under the microscope is necessary to ensure normal hair structure.

Hair loss can be easily distinguished from hair breakage by performing 10 hair pulls over various areas of the scalp. The hair pull is performed by grasping the hair shaft close to the scalp with the fingers and firmly pulling over the length of the shaft. Removed hairs are examined for the presence and formation of the bulb. If more than six hairs are removed per pull, excessive hair loss is present. This procedure also provides an opportunity to ascertain that no localized areas of total hair loss are present, allowing elimination of tinea capitis, alopecia areata, and so on as the cause.

EVALUATING THE MAGNITUDE OF HAIR LOSS

Hair pulls in the office can be misleading, especially if the patient has shampooed prior to being examined and has removed the loose or broken hairs. It may prove difficult to get an accurate estimate of the magnitude of the hair loss from the patient, since most are not aware that a normal individual may lose approximately 100 to 125 hairs per day. If grooming of the hair is infrequent, shampooing may cause a loss of up to 200 hairs.

> Normal hair loss is around 100 to 125 hairs per day.

Information on the magnitude of the loss can best be obtained by having the patient collect all hair lost for four consecutive days and place each day's loss in separate envelopes, noting days on which shampooing was performed. The hair should be brushed or combed over the sink and the hair collected from the sink and also from the brush or comb. Hairs should also be removed from the drain following shampooing. The dermatologist can examine each day's loss noting both the amount and presence or absence of the hair bulb.

INTERNAL CAUSES OF HAIR LOSS

Once it has been determined that the hair loss is indeed in excess of 100 hairs per day and that normally formed hairs are being shed diffusely from a nonscarred scalp with an intact bulb, anagen effluvium and telogen effluvium must be considered. Anagen effluvium is generally due to internally administered medications, such as chemotherapy agents, which act as cell poisons and disrupt the growing hair follicle. Telogen effluvium, on the other hand, is due to an increased number of hair follicles prematurely exiting the anagen phase or hair cycle synchronization (2). Premature anagen exit can be due to medications, such as coumarin or heparin, while hair cycle synchronization occurs during pregnancy and with oral contraceptive use.

The causes of diffuse, nonscarring telogen hair loss to be considered are summarized in Table 34.2. Most of these

Table 34.1 Number of Hairs by Hair Color for Hair Fullness

Blond: 140,000 hairs
Brown: 110,000 hairs
Black: 108,000 hairs
Red: 90,000 hairs

Table 34.2 Internal Causes of Diffuse, Nonscarring Alopecia

1. Hormonal causes: postpartum, oral contraceptives, menopause, hormone supplementation
2. Physical stress: surgery, illness, anemia, rapid weight change
3. Emotional stress: psychiatric illness, death of family member
4. Endocrinopathy: hypothyroidism, hyperthyroidism, hypoparathyroidism, hyperparathyroidism
5. Oral medications:
   a. blood thinning agents: heparin, coumarin
   b. retinoids: high-dose vitamin A, isotretinoin, etretinate
   c. antihypertensive agents: propranolol, captopril
   d. miscellaneous: quinacrine, allopurinol, lithium carbonate, thiouracil compounds

considerations can be eliminated by a review of systems and some basic laboratory work. Anemia, thyroid abnormalities, and many illnesses can be evaluated by obtaining a complete blood count with differential, thyroid panel, and chemistry panel to include liver function studies. If deemed clinically necessary, an antinuclear antibody can also be obtained to rule out any collagen vascular diseases. A complete history can determine the nature of any severe physical or emotional stress and document the ingestion of prescription or over-the-counter medications or vitamin supplements.

Physical or Emotional Stress

Surgeries, febrile illnesses, and severe emotional stresses must be evaluated by the dermatologist for the past six months. In many cases, a three-month delay is present between the actual event and the patient's onset of hair loss. Furthermore, there may be another three-month delay prior to the return of noticeable hair regrowth. Thus, the total hair loss and regrowth cycle can last six months or possibly longer. Patients should be educated as to when a reasonable regrowth can be expected.

Diet Considerations

Hair loss due to rapid weight loss is not uncommon. Many times patients embark on franchised diet programs administered under the direction of a physician with prescribed meals and dietary supplements. Sometimes patients are told that vitamin supplements purchased as part of the weight loss program are necessary to prevent hair loss associated with dieting. From a dermatologist's standpoint, however, the vitamins cannot prevent hair loss associated with a rapid, significant weight loss.

Hormonal Considerations

Hormonal causes of hair loss deserve special attention in the female patient. Many women do not realize that hair loss can present postpartum or following discontinuation of oral contraceptives. It is important to remind the female patient that hair loss may be delayed by three months following a hormonal status change and another three to six months may be required for regrowth to be fully appreciated.

Menopausal women with decreased ovarian estrogen production may also experience diffuse hair thinning, generally more prominent over the top of the head with bitemporal recession. A thin strip of hair at the anterior hairline is usually spared. A follicle-stimulating hormone (FSH) level can be obtained to document the onset of menopause, although menopausal hair thinning may be present even though FSH levels are not low. Institution of estrogen replacement can prevent further loss, but has not been shown to promote regrowth. Other treatments such as topical minoxidil may be indicated.

Lastly, it is important to rule out any hormonal abnormalities in the female patient. Inquiring as to the regularity of menses and the presence of infertility problems can uncover ovarian hormonal failure or the presence of excess endogenous androgens. Questions should also be directed as to whether the patient is ingesting oral steroids with androgenic effects. If necessary, hormone levels such as free testosterone and dehydroepiandrosterone sulfate (DHEA-S) can be drawn and an endocrinologic evaluation initiated (3). A more detailed discussion of hormonally induced hair loss is beyond the scope of this book (4,5).

EXTERNAL CAUSES OF HAIR LOSS

Shed hairs without a hair bulb are considered broken hairs. Hair breakage is generally due to external factors; however, abnormalities in hair shaft formation must be eliminated. Table 34.3 contains the technical terms used to describe hair shaft abnormalities and a definition of the term (6). Trichoschisis, trichorrhexis invaginata, pili torti, and monilethrix are all abnormalities intrinsic to the hair shaft (7). Trichoptilosis and trichonodosis may be due to cosmetic manipulation of the hair. Trichorrhexis nodosa may be due to intrinsic abnormalities or cosmetic manipulation. All of these conditions predispose the hair to breakage, which can become magnified by extensive grooming, chemical waving procedures, or permanent dyeing.

> The hair shaft should be examined under the microscope in the alopecia patient to evaluate intrinsic malformations in the hair shaft and abnormalities due to cosmetic procedures.

Gross Hair Shaft Evaluation

Once it has been determined that the primary cause of hair loss is breakage, the patient's scalp hair should be grossly examined to assess the state of the hair shafts. An overall impression should be formed:

1. Does the hair have shine?
2. Does the hair feel soft?
3. Does the hair lay in an orderly fashion?
4. Is there an evidence of hair styling aid being used?
5. Does the hair color appear natural and match the patient's eyebrows, eyelashes, and body hair?
6. Is the hair curly or straight?
7. How long is the hair and when was it last cut?

Table 34.3 Structural Hair Shaft Abnormalities

Intrinsic abnormalities
1. Trichoschisis: a clean, transverse fracture across the hair shaft through both cuticle and cortex. Congenital forms seen in trichothiodystrophy characterized by hair with an abnormally low sulfur content
2. Trichorrhexis invaginata: a nodular expansion of the hair shaft in which a ball in socket joint is formed, also known as bamboo hair. Congenital forms seen in Netherton's syndrome
3. Pili torti: a flattened hair shaft that is twisted through 180° on its own axis
4. Monilethrix: elliptical nodal swellings along the hair shaft with intervening, tapering constrictions that are nonmedullated

Extrinsic abnormalities
1. Trichoptilosis: a longitudinal splitting or fraying of the distal end of the hair shaft, also known as split ends
2. Trichonodosis: knotting of the hair shaft

Intrinsic or extrinsic abnormalities
1. Trichorrhexis nodosa: small, beaded swellings associated with a loss of the cuticle. Congenital forms seen in argininosuccinic aciduria and Menkes disease, but may also be due to cosmetic hair shaft manipulation

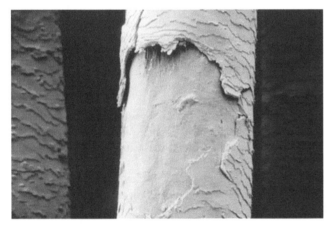

Figure 34.1 Weathered hair is characterized by cuticle loss.

Hair Shine

Hair possessing an intact cuticle with closely overlapping cuticular scales is shiny, healthy hair. It is the smoothness of the overlapping scales that promotes light reflection, interpreted by the eye as shine. Normal grooming processes such as combing and brushing result in loss of cuticular scales, which is more pronounced at the distal hair shaft (8). This process is known as "weathering" and is accelerated by overly aggressive grooming and chemical processing (9,10) (Fig. 34.1).

Hair Softness

Hair softness, also due to an intact cuticle, creates a smooth hair shaft surface. Permanently waved or dyed hair must have a disrupted cuticle in order to allow penetration of the waving lotion or dye. Thus, chemically processed hair never feels as soft as virgin hair, even though hair conditioners attempt to temporarily smooth the disrupted cuticle. Harsh feeling hair is an evidence of cuticular damage.

Hair Frizziness

Hair that has been chemically processed is also prone to static electricity. This allows the hair to appear frizzy and unruly, especially at the distal hair shafts. Generally, chemicals applied to the hair penetrate better at the distal hair shaft due to less cuticular scale. A well-educated cosmetologist is aware of this fact, especially when processing long hair, and will apply the chemicals to the scalp first and then dilute the product prior to applying the solutions to the distal hair shafts. Overprocessed hair appears frizzy and is severely weakened.

Use of Styling Aids

It is important not to be misled when evaluating hair shine, softness, and frizziness by the use of hair styling aids such as hair spray, mousse, and styling gels. These products usually contain a polymer which forms a thin film over the hair shafts imparting shine and stiffness. Combing the hair will remove the polymer film which will appear as tiny white flakes throughout the hair, but the true state of the hair shafts can be better appreciated.

Use of Hair Coloring

Unfortunately, some patients who dye their hair will not openly admit that they use hair coloring. Furthermore, many patients do not know what kind of dye has been applied to the hair and whether any bleaching has occurred. This means that the dermatologist must rely on his or her powers of observation.

Hair color should be compared with eyelashes, eyebrows, or other body hair. (It is possible to dye the eyelashes and eyebrows.) If the scalp hair color is lighter than hair of other body parts, bleaching has occurred. If regrowth is present at the scalp, a permanent hair color has been used. If the color appears to gradually vary from the proximal hair shaft to the distal hair shaft with the presence of some grayish hairs, a semipermanent hair color has been used. If the hair has a yellowish cast, a metallic hair color has been used. These guidelines can be used to initiate conversation when obtaining a patient history.

Degree of Curl

The degree of curl the hair possesses should also be evaluated since tightly curled hair is more prone to breakage. It should also be determined whether the curl is natural or due to permanent waving. Hair that has been chemically waved appears straight at the scalp and curlier at the ends. Hair that is naturally curly will have an even curl throughout the length of the hair shaft. If the hair has been chemically waved, the type of permanent wave and length of processing should be obtained either from the patient or from the salon. These factors cannot be determined by visual examination.

Hair Length

Lastly, it is important to note the length of the hair and ask the patient when it was last cut. Longer hair is subject to more weathering, and so an increased breakage is expected. Patients also evaluate hair loss by the amount of hair in the brush or sink; longer hair shafts will create a larger lump than shorter hair shafts even though the same number of hairs has been lost. Thus, patients with longer hair tend to overestimate their actual loss. Hair which has been cut frequently shows less evidence of damage than infrequently cut hair. If the damaged hair shaft ends have been removed prior to visiting the dermatologist, the full extent of hair damage may not be appreciated; however, chemical processing damages the whole hair shaft and the evidence of damage will reappear shortly.

Microscopic Examination of a Hair Shaft

The gross findings should be confirmed by a microscopic examination of a shed hair shaft. The cuticular scales should be examined to note if weathering is present. The decrease or absence of scales can confirm the gross observation that the hair is dull, harsh, and frizzy. If the cuticular scales are greatly decreased at the distal hair shaft, trichoptilosis results from exposure of the soft medulla. If trichonodosis is observed, hair twisting or teasing may be the cause of the knots predisposing the hair to breakage. If trichorrhexis nodosa is present, and not part of a genodermatosis, this suggests an extensive cuticular loss.

COSMETIC TECHNIQUES FOR MINIMIZING THE HAIR LOSS

Hair grooming includes cleansing, drying, combing, brushing, and styling of the hair. While any manipulation of the hair shaft can cause breakage, loss can be minimized by recommending proper grooming practices to the patient.

Proper grooming practices can minimize hair loss.

Hair Cleansing

Cleansing the hair should be done only when hair has dirt or excess sebum. If sebum production is minimal and the patient has a sedentary lifestyle, daily washing is not necessary for good hygiene. Patients should select a shampoo appropriate for their hair type: normal, oily, dry, fine, damaged, or chemically treated. These labels usually appear on the outside of the shampoo bottle. If the patient with normal to minimal sebum production insists on daily shampooing, a dry hair shampoo with less detergent action should be recommended. Aggressive removal of sebum results in hair that tangles readily, appears dull, and attracts static electricity.

Hair Conditioning

An instant conditioner or a cream rinse can be valuable in minimizing hair loss by detangling the hair, especially long hair (11). Patients who have excess sebum production may prefer a cream rinse over a conditioner. All formulations of instant conditioners are good at detangling hair by smoothing the cuticle and reducing friction. However, if the hair has been severely damaged and the cuticular scales are sparse with the presence of trichoptilosis, only a protein-containing conditioner can penetrate the hair shaft and temporarily mend split ends. This is due to the substantivity of protein conditioners for hair keratin.

Hair Drying

It is best if the hair is allowed to dry without externally applied heat; however, many patients wish to speed up the drying process or style their hair while drying. Heat-damaged hair from

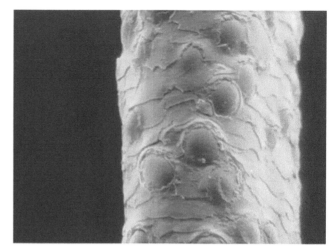

Figure 34.2 Bubble hair forms when the hair is rapidly heated and the water within the hair shaft turns to highly energetic steam and exits the hair shaft creating a bubble.

improper dryer use appears frizzy and curly at the ends. It may also develop an abnormality known as "bubble hair" (12) (Fig. 34.2). Any tension applied to the burned hair shaft will cause the hair to break in tiny fragments, some of which can be crushed between the fingers. Heat damage can be avoided by using the lowest heat setting and holding the nozzle at least 6 inches from the scalp. A specially designed vented blow-drying brush should be used to prevent high temperatures along the brush.

Hair Combing and Brushing

Hair shafts are subject to fracture most when they are wet, due to increased elasticity. It is much easier to stretch a wet hair shaft to the breaking point than a dry one. Therefore, hair should be initially detangled with the fingers and slightly dried prior to detangling with a wide toothed comb. Brushes should not be used for detangling. Combing and brushing should be kept to a minimum. The idea that 100 brush strokes a day is beneficial to the hair is mistaken. Combs should be selected for their smooth, widely spaced teeth so that they glide freely through the hair. Brushes should have widely spaced bristles with rounded tips for the same reasons. Whether the bristles are synthetic or natural is less important than the spacing of the bristles.

Hair shafts are most subject to fracture when wet due to increased elasticity and stretching of the hair beyond the breaking point.

Hair Styling

Hair styles should be loose to minimize breakage and not require excessive hair pins or combs. All hair pins should be rubber coated with smooth edges so that the hair is not broken as the clasp is closed. Unfortunately, the clasp must hold the hair tightly or it will not remain in place. Rubber bands should not be used in the hair as they are difficult to remove.

There are several common presentations of patients who are experiencing hair breakage due to hair styling. The first is the patient who wears her or his hair in a pony tail or braid, and claims decreased hair growth. Examination of the hair shows hair shafts fractured at the same distance from the scalp. This is due to repeated breakage where the hair clasp is placed. A second presentation is the patient who wears braids on the scalp, also known as cornrows, and notes thinning at the front hairline. In this instance, the hair is broken due to maximum tension at the front hairline; traction alopecia may also be present. The third presentation is the patient who has had hair extensions glued or woven into their natural hair. The weight of the extensions can cause hair breakage and traction alopecia. It may be necessary to question the patients on hair styling practices as they may wear their hair differently on the day they visit the dermatologist.

Hair Appliances
Burning of the hair and subsequent breakage can also be caused by heated hair appliances: curling irons, crimping irons, straightening irons, and heated curlers. Most patients prefer to use these appliances at their hottest setting as this produces the tightest, longest lasting curl, but also induces hair damage to the greatest extent. This burning is minimized if a lower heat setting is chosen. Hair that is burned with a heated appliance appears frizzy at the ends.

Permanent Hair Coloring
Darkening the natural hair color is less damaging than lightening the natural hair color as the original eumelanins and pheomelanins are not removed. Any lightening of the hair color requires the use of bleaching to remove the existing pigments. In general, the more the bleaching required to achieve the final hair color, the weaker the hair shaft at the end of the chemical process. Many patients erroneously think that if the bleached blonde hair is redyed to its darker original color, it will be healthier. This is not true. Any further dyeing only contributes to additional weakening of the hair shaft.

Permanent Waving of Hair
Permanent waving of the hair is more damaging than dyeing since the protein structure of the hair shaft is actually degraded and reconstructed in a new form. Damage can be minimized, however, by wrapping the hair loosely around larger curlers. This results in a looser, shorter lasting curl, but breakage is minimized (Fig. 34.3).

The processing time can also be shortened which decreases the degree of bond breaking. The processing time is checked by performing a "test curl." The test curl is a rod, usually selected at the nape of neck, where the hair is periodically unwound to determine if the desired amount of curl has been achieved. Not all cosmetologists use a test curl, but it is highly recommended. It is also recommended that the test curl not be placed at the nape of the neck, but rather at the front hairline. Traditionally, the nape of the neck is chosen because hair here is more difficult to permanently wave than in any other area of the scalp. If the appropriate amount of curl is present at the nape, then the rest of the scalp will also be curled. However, hair at the front hairline curls more readily and may be overprocessed by the time the nape has curled. This accounts for patients noting more breakage at the anterior hairline.

Many patients both permanently dye and wave their hair. While the damage produced by these procedures is additive,

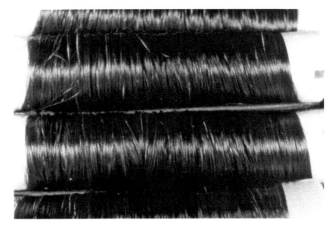

Figure 34.3 A proper technique for wrapping hair around mandrels for permanent waving procedure.

it can be minimized by allowing 10 days between procedures and permanently waving the hair first followed by dyeing the hair.

CAMOUFLAGE TECHNIQUES FOR FEMALE PATTERN HAIR LOSS
Female pattern hair loss affects susceptible women beginning at puberty with noticeable thinning present by age 40. These women present with hair loss over the entire scalp, but the thinning is most prominent over the frontoparietal areas with sparing of a thin fringe along the anterior hair line. This pattern was first illustrated by Ludwig (13). Camouflaging hair loss over the top of the scalp presents a greater challenge than that over the sides of the scalp. Cosmetic methods of camouflaging female androgenetic alopecia should be combined with appropriate medical treatments (14). Only cosmetic approaches for androgenetic alopecia are discussed: hair styling, hair styling products, hair permanent waving, hair coloring agents, hairpieces, and hair additions.

Hair Styling
Careful hair style selection can minimize the appearance of female pattern hair loss. Since the hair is thinned predominantly on the top of the head, styling techniques should be aimed at adding volume and fullness in this area. The perception of thick hair is based on the distance that the hair stands away from the scalp, but hair styling and styling products can create the illusion of fullness.

Two styling techniques are valuable for creating the illusion of hair volume: curling and back combing. Curled hair does not lay as close to the scalp as straight hair and therefore appears fuller. Temporary curls can be created by heat styling with a blow dryer and a round brush, setting wet hair on rollers, wrapping hair around heated rollers or a curling rod, and forming pin curls close to the scalp. Tighter curls will yield more hair fullness.

Back combing involves combing the hair in the opposite direction from which it would normally lay on the scalp. In most women, the hair pattern is such that the hair on the top of the scalp lays forward. Combing the hair backward from the front of the head to the crown lifts the hair creating the illusion of volume. The hair will not stay in this unnatural position for long; therefore, styling aids are necessary for the hair to hold this shape.

Teasing is another technique, popular in the 1960s "beehive" hair styles, the change of which used to create volume. Teasing involves combing the hair from the distal to proximal hair shaft using a fine-toothed comb or teasing brush to create tangles between the hair shafts. These tangles, or "rats" as they are known, allow the hair to stand away from the scalp. Teasing, however, can result in the disruption of the hair shaft cuticle and accelerate hair breakage. It is important to avoid hair breakage in areas where the hair is already thinned.

Hair Styling Products

Hair styling products can aid in creating the illusion of fullness by allowing the hair to stand away from the scalp. Available styling products include styling gels, sculpturing gels, mousses, and hair sprays. Styling gels, sculpturing gels, and mousses are generally applied to towel-dried hair while hair sprays are used to improve the hold of a finished hair style. Sculpturing gels provide a stiffer hold than styling gels, which provide a better hold than mousses.

A small amount of gel or mousse is massaged into the base of the hair shafts and then the hair is dried with a blow dryer while combing the hair away from the scalp. This will increase the ability of the hair to stand away from the scalp creating the illusion of volume. The styling products lose their hold once the hair is combed or gets wet, so reapplication is necessary each time the hair is styled.

Hair spray can be used to keep the final hair style in place. For example, after back combing the hair, it can be liberally sprayed to allow the hair to fall backward instead of forward on the forehead.

Permanent Waving

Permanent waving of the hair increases the apparent hair volume allowing less amount of hair to cover more area of scalp due to increased curl. Thus, a permanent wave in the frontoparietal area can nicely camouflage the female pattern hair loss. However, chemical curling damages the hair shaft by decreasing its strength, degrading its structure, and causing protein loss. This damage can be minimized if the permanent wave is performed with care.

Hair shaft damage can be decreased by wrapping the hair loosely around larger curling rods resulting in a looser curl that is shorter lasting, but also less likely to fracture the hair shaft. Another method of decreasing hair shaft damage is to shorten the processing time, which decreases the degree of bond breaking. It is also advisable to allow as much time as possible between permanent waving procedures.

Dyeing

Hair color lightening can be an effective camouflage technique for female pattern hair loss because it blends very well with a fair scalp. Of all the hair coloring types available, only permanent hair dyes can achieve color lightening, but permanent hair dyes also can cause damages to the hair shaft most.

Hairpieces

A valuable hairpiece in the female with androgenetic alopecia is a hair thickener, which sits on top of the head, to provide additional hair in the frontoparietal region. The hair is wefted to a mesh through which the patient can pull her own hair to both anchor the hairpiece and provide a natural appearance. This type of hairpiece costs between $30 and $100, depending on whether it is constructed of synthetic or natural human hair.

Hair Additions

Hair additions can nicely camouflage frontoparietal thinning, but must be used cautiously as the weight of the hair addition can result in traction alopecia, only augmenting hair loss. Hair additions can be expensive, depending on the time required to complete the hair style, and are not appropriate for all patients.

CAMOUFLAGE TECHNIQUES FOR MALE PATTERN HAIR LOSS

The same basic camouflage techniques described previously for female pattern hair loss also apply to male pattern hair loss. However, male pattern hair loss does not spare a thin strip of hair at the anterior hairline (15). This makes recreation of a natural appearing anterior hair line more challenging.

COSMETIC TECHNIQUES FOR DAMAGED HAIR

Unfortunately, cosmetically damaged hair cannot be repaired by the body. However, cosmetic remedies may allow the hair to assume an acceptable appearance until new growth occurs. Table 34.4 lists cosmetic suggestions for the common hair problems.

The initial step in advising a patient on cosmetic remedies for hair problems is to ensure that he or she is using the appropriate shampoo. Patients with light-colored hair may note a greenish discoloration following swimming in a pool with copper-contaminated water from copper-containing algicides or copper pipes (16). Low water pH, chlorinated water, and copper contamination all must be present for the hair discoloration to occur. This problem is most pronounced in individuals with bleached hair as the copper is readily absorbed due to the increased content of cysteic acid and other anionic sulfonate groups (17). The use of special shampoos (Clairol, Metalux) or 2% penicillamine shampoos have been reported to be effective in removing the abnormal color (18). Green hair may also be seen after using copper- contaminated tap water (19), and some tar-based shampoos. Special shampoos can aid in removing the undesirable hue.

Shampoo selection is also important for chemically treated hair, which is dry and more subject to static electricity and tangling than healthy hair. Patients can achieve an improved feel and manageability if a conditioning shampoo is selected. Patients with fine, chemically treated hair, however, may find that a conditioning shampoo works well for about one to two weeks and then leaves the hair limp and without ability to hold a curl. This is due to excess conditioner on the hair shaft, which is inadequately removed by the mild shampoo. Shampooing with a deep cleaning detergent shampoo once weekly will prevent conditioner buildup. Patients should be encouraged to allow their hair to begin drying prior to combing, since wet hair is more elastic and more subject to fracture.

It is recommended that patients with chemically treated hair use an instant conditioner following shampooing. The optimal instant conditioner should contain hydrolyzed animal protein. For severely damaged hair, a deep conditioner is recommended every two weeks, although too frequent application will render the hair limp. Patients who have a permanent

Table 34.4 Cosmetic Suggestions for the Common Hair Problems

Problem	Possible cosmetic cause	Possible cosmetic solution
Hair texture		
Fine, limp hair	Overconditioning	Use instant oily hair conditioner
Coarse, unmanageable hair	Underconditioning	Use deep conditioner
Fine, frizzy hair	Underconditioning	Use instant conditioner for dry hair
Hair contour		
Too curly	Underconditioning	Use instant conditioner for dry hair
Too straight	Overconditioning	Use instant conditioner for oily hair
Hair color		
Early graying, less than 15%	Normal process	Vegetable or synthetic semipermanent dye or stain
Yellow-gray hair tones	Gradual loss of eumelanin pigments	Temporary rinse applied following shampooing
Hair grow out	New undyed hair growth	Touch up dye to roots, not entire hair shaft
Undesirable permanent dye hair color	Dyeing of previously chemically treated hair	Use semipermanent dye to tone undesirable shade until grown out
Green hair	Copper in swimming pool water	Wear swim cap, treat pool water, use special shampoo
Hair thinning		
Total scalp	Numerous medical problems	Wig
Top of scalp	Male or female pattern baldness	Partial hair piece, spot permanent wave; use of styling gels, sculpturing gels, or mousse
Decreased length	Slower growth rate, hair breakage	Remove damaged hair to halt inevitable breakage
Hair breakage		
Trichoptilosis	Loss of cuticle on distal hair shaft	Cut damaged hair or use an instant conditioner containing hydrolyzed animal protein for temporary repair
Trichoclasis	Styling trauma	Avoid tight hair clasps and use ball-tipped styling combs and brushes
General shaft fragility	Overprocessed hair	Use semipermanent instead of permanent hair dyes, use short permanent wave processing time
Hair appearance		
Dull	Cuticle irregularities	Use styling glaze or leave-in conditioner
Lack of body	Fine hair texture	Hair permanent wave, styling gel, or sculpturing gel to increase hold
Hair texture		
Dry, rough	Overshampooing, permanent wave process time to long	Deep conditioner, shorten permanent wave processing time, do not repeat permanent wave for 3 months
Greasy, slick	Overconditioning or inadequate shampooing	Avoid conditioning shampoos and deep or oily hair conditioners

wave will note that heavy conditioners tend to relax the curl, which may or may not be desirable.

Damaged chemically treated hair should be subjected to as little physical stress as possible. Permanent waving alone decreases hair strength by 15%. Styling, including combing and brushing, should be kept to a minimum. Tight hair clasps and hair styles that pull on the hair shaft should be avoided. Patients should be encouraged not to sleep with brush-type plastic rollers in their hair. Curling irons that clamp the hair to the heated rod should be avoided. In other words, anything that might result in hair breakage should be minimized since chemically treated hair is more likely to demonstrate trichoptilosis and trichoclasis. Recommended styling procedures include the use of a round, ball-tipped brush to curl the hair while blow drying and heat-set rollers.

Permanent waving decreases hair strength by at least 15%.

Shine, or gloss, can be restored to chemically damaged hair with a hair glaze or leave-in conditioner. Additional shine and hold can be achieved with a styling gel for minimal hold or a sculpturing gel for maximal hold. These products work best when applied sparingly to damp hair and massaged throughout the hair prior to styling.

Many patients undergo another chemical process to improve the appearance of damaged hair. For example, a patient who notes that her permanently dyed hair does not hold a curl may undergo a "conditioning" permanent wave. The end result is more hair damage and further problems. Patients are better advised to opt for an attractive wig, which may cost no more than a permanent wave, until new hair growth occurs.

COSMETIC TECHNIQUES FOR MEDICAL HAIR CONDITIONS

Numerous inherited medical hair conditions (trichorrhexis nodosa, trichorrhexis invaginata, pili annulati, etc.) exhibit a variety of hair shaft defects. The end result of all these conditions is a fragile hair shaft lacking shine or grow slowly. Defective hair shafts should not undergo permanent dyeing or waving procedures. The end result will be cosmetically poor and the hair shaft will fracture more readily. However, temporary or semipermanent hair dyes may be used; these coat or minimally penetrate the hair shaft without causing severe internal shaft damage.

Hair manipulation, including shampooing, combing, brushing, and curling, should be minimized. Patients generally do best with a short, straight hair style. Infrequent shampooing with a conditioning shampoo, followed by an instant conditioner, decreases breakage and increases manageability.

If the quality of the scalp hair is poor, patients may wish to investigate the possibility of wearing a hair piece.

SUMMARY

Alopecia is a physically and emotionally disabling condition for many patients. The dermatologist may find it challenging to assist patients with hair loss because of the relatively little knowledge that is available in medical textbooks on the subject and the lack of exposure to hair care issues during residency. This chapter has distilled the medical and cosmetic treatment of alopecia down to each basic step. Familiarity and personal customization of these guidelines can make assisting patients with hair issues rewarding and productive.

REFERENCES

1. Bergfeld WF. Scarring alopecia. In: Roenigk RR, Roenigk HR, eds. Dermatolgic Surgery, Principles and Practice. New York, NY: Marcel Dekker, 1989: 759–79.
2. Headington JT. Telogen effluvium. Arch Dermatol 1993; 129: 356–63.
3. Redmond GP, Bergfeld WF. Diagnostic approach to androgen disorders in women. Cleve Clin J Med 1990; 57: 423–32.
4. Sperling LC, Heimer WL. Androgen biology as a basis for the diagnosis and treatment of androgenic disorders in women. I. J Am Acad Dermatol 1993; 28: 669–83.
5. Sperling LC, Heimer WL. Androgen biology as a basis for the diagnosis and treatment of androgenic disorders in women. II. J Am Acad Dermatol 1993; 28: 901–16.
6. Whiting DA. Structural abnormalities of the hair shaft. J Am Acad Dermatol 1987; 16: 1–25.
7. Camacho-Martinez F, Ferrando J. Hair shaft dysplasias. Int J Dermatol 1988; 27: 71–80.
8. Wolfram L, Lindemann MO. Some observations on the hair cuticle. J Soc Cosmet Chem 1971; 2: 839.
9. Rook A. The clinical importance of "weathering" in human hair. Br J Dermatol 1976; 95: 111.
10. Robbins C. Weathering in human hair. Text Res J 1967; 37: 337.
11. Menkart J. Damaged hair. Cutis 1979; 23: 276–8.
12. Detwiler SP, Carson JL, Woosley JT, et al. Bubble hair. J Am Acad Dermatol 1994; 30: 54–60.
13. Ludwig E. Classification of the types of androgenetic alopecia (common baldness) occurring in the female sex. Br J Dermatol 1977; 97: 247–54.
14. Bergfeld WF. Etiology and diagnosis of androgenetic alopecia. In: DeVillez RL, ed. Clinics in dermatology. Vol. 6. Philadelphia: JB Lippincott, 1988: 102–7.
15. Hamilton JB. Patterned long hair in man: types and incidence. Ann NY Acad Sci 1951; 53: 708.
16. Roomans GM, Forslind B. Copper in green hair: a quantitative investigation by electron probe x-ray microanalysis. Ultrastruct Pathol 1980; 1: 301–7.
17. Zultak M, Rochefor A, Faivre B, Claudet MH, Drobacheff C. Green hair: clinical, chemical, and epidemiologic study. Ann Dermatol Venereol 1988; 115: 807–912.
18. Person JR. Green hair: treatment with a penicillamine shampoo. Arch Dermatol 1985; 121: 717–18.
19. Nordlund JJ, Hartley C, Fister J. On the cause of green hair. Arch Dermatol 1977; 113: 1700.

SUGGESTED READING

Chartier MB, Hoss DM, Grant-Kels JM. Approach to the adult female patient with diffuse nonscarring alopecia. J Am Acad Dermatol 2002; 47: 809–18.
De Lacharriere O, Deloche C, Misciali C, et al. Hair diameter diversity. Arch Dermatol 2001; 137: 641–6.
Feughelman M. Morphology and properties of hair (Chapter1). In: Johnson DH, ed. Hair and hair care. Marcel Dekker, Inc., 1997: 1–12.
Feughelman M. Physical properties of hair (Chapter2). In: Johnson DH, ed. Hair and hair care. Marcel Dekker, Inc., 1997: 13–32.
Feughelman M, Willis BK. Mechanical extension of human hair and the movement of the cuticle. J Cosmet Sci 2001; 52: 185–93.
Fiedler VC, Alaiti S. Treatment of alopecia areata. Dermatol Clin 1996; 14: 733–7.
Gamez-Garcia M. Cuticle decementation and cuticle buckling produced by Poisson contraction on the cuticular envelope of human hair. J Cosmet Sci 1998; 49: 213–22.
Gamez-Garcia M. Plastic yielding and fracture of human hair cuticles by cyclical torsion stresses. J Cosmet Sci 1999; 50: 69–77.
Gamez-Garcia M. The cracking of human hair cuticles by cyclical thermal stresses. J Cosmet Sci 1998; 49: 141–53.
Gummer CL. Cosmetics and hair loss. Clin Exp Dermatol 2002; 27: 418–21.
Harrison S, Sinclair R. Optimal management of hair loss (alopecia) in children. Am J Clin Dermatol 2003; 4: 757–70.
Hermann S. Hair 101. GCI. 2001: 14.
Price VH. Treatment of hair loss. Drug Ther 1999; 341: 964–73.
Ross EK, Shapiro J. Management of hair loss. Dermatol Clin 2005; 23: 227–43.
Rushton DH, Morris MJ, Dover R, Busuttil N. Causes of hair loss and the developments in hair rejuvenation. Int J Cosmet Sci 2002; 24: 17–23.
Shapiro J, Wiseman M, Lui H. Practical management of hair loss. Can Fam Physician 2000; 46: 1469–77.
Sinclair RD. Healthy hair: what is it? J Investig Dermatol Symp Proc 2007; 12: 2–5.
Swift JA. Human hair cuticle: biologically conspired to the owner's advantage. J Cosmet Sci 1999; 50: 23–47.
Swift JA. Letter to the editor(The cuticle controls bending stiffness of hair). J Cosmet Sci 2000; 51: 37–8.
Wolfram LJ. Human hair: a unique physicochemical composite. J Am Acad Dermatol 2003; 48(6 Suppl): S106–14.

35 Seborrheic dermatitis

Seborrheic dermatitis, which is considered a severe case of symptomatic dandruff, is one of the most challenging conditions for the dermatologist to treat because it is a chronic relapsing disease. While the exact etiology is known to be the overgrowth of fungal organisms such as *Malassezia globosa* and *M. restricta*, the reason for some exhibiting the inflammatory condition and others not is unknown. Proper treatment requires both prescription agents and proper shampoo selection to prevent recurrence. The biggest challenge is recurrence since these organisms are normal flora on the scalp, but can reproduce rapidly in the absence of an intact immune system using sebum as food for growth. The sebum is broken down into free fatty acids that cause scalp irritation and signs and symptoms of seborrheic dermatitis. Seborrheic dermatitis is frequently seen in immunosuppressed persons and elderly individuals, especially after myocardial infarction, stroke, and the onset of Parkinson's disease. It is interesting to note that the signs and symptoms of seborrheic dermatitis can be elicited by applying oleic acid, a free fatty acid, to the scalp of susceptible individuals in the absence of fungal organisms. This means that scalp hygiene is key to the prevention of seborrheic dermatitis.

> The signs and symptoms of seborrheic dermatitis can be reproduced by placing oleic acid on the scalps of susceptible individuals.

SHAMPOO SELECTION FOR SEBORRHEIC DERMATITIS

The treatment for seborrheic dermatitis may include a variety of prescription antifungals, such as ketoconazole, either orally for five days accompanied by sweating to allow the ketoconazole to reach the skin surface via eccrine secretions or topically. Many other topical antifungals, such as clotrimazole, terbinafine, and ciclopirox, may also be used. Usually topical corticosteroids are added to reduce the inflammation induced by the *Malassezia* produced free fatty acids. It is interesting to note that topical corticosteroid alone will alleviate the symptoms of seborrheic dermatitis without an antifungal. However, the symptoms will rapidly return without the use of something to decrease the *Malassezia* population. This is where shampoos become important in aiding treatment and preventing recurrence.

> Shampoos are important in aiding the treatment and prevention of seborrheic dermatitis.

Seborrheic dermatitis cannot be adequately controlled without proper shampoo selection. Effective shampoo ingredients include sulfur, tar, selenium sulfide, zinc pyrithione,

and salicylic acid. Sulfur shampoos have fallen out of favor because they can stain light colored hair yellow, but sulfur pomades are still used in persons with kinky hair both on the hair and scalp to control fungal growth since shampoo frequency is weekly or biweekly. Sulfur is a potent antifungal and will maintain scalp hygiene without the need to shampoo, but scalp scale will accumulate because the physical removal of the dander with scrubbing is absent. For this reason, the accumulation of scalp scale in African American individuals cannot be used as a definitive marker for seborrheic dermatitis, although the two observations are many times related.

Tar shampoos are some of the most effective cleansers in seborrheic dermatitis. This is because tar is a naturally occurring anti-inflammatory agent. By definition, anti-inflammatory agents decrease the white blood cell population in a given skin area. Inflammation in the skin always occurs for a reason, but the dermatologist may not be able to determine the cause. Many skin conditions are treated with anti-inflammatory agents nonspecifically without understanding the etiology. Psoriasis and seborrheic dermatitis are excellent examples. Anti-inflammatories can only control symptoms and not produce a cure. While chasing the white blood cells out of the skin with tar in seborrheic dermatitis produces remission of the scaling and itching associated with the condition, it is also a carcinogen for the same reason. The carcinogenicity of tar has been a source of controversy discussed on some consumer websites. Tar is a carcinogen, but purified tar with the creosote removed is less of a carcinogen. The newer dandruff shampoos use purified tar because it does not stain fabric washcloths, it has a more pleasant odor, and it is less of a carcinogen. Interestingly, it is also less effective in treating seborrheic dermatitis.

> Small particle zinc pyrithione dandruff shampoos can decrease fungal colonization on the scalp.

Selenium sulfide and zinc pyrithione are two ingredients with similar effects on the scalp. They also function as antifungal and anti-inflammatory agents. Zinc pyrithione is felt to be a better anti-inflammatory than selenium sulfide due to the known benefits of zinc on the skin. An antifungal can only be effective, however, if it is present on the scalp. The newer dandruff shampoo formulations use smaller particle size zinc pyrithione allowing more particles to be present in the bottle with the same percentage of the active ingredient. It is only the particle edge that touches the scalp which is effective in preventing fungal growth so the smaller particle formulations are more effective. Also, the formulations that leave behind the small zinc pyrithione particles in the follicular ostia are more effective. Since this is the most sebum-rich area of the scalp, the follicular ostia contain more *Malassezia* organisms representing the target site for zinc pyrithione deposition.

Finally, salicylic acid is useful in seborrheic dermatitis to remove scalp scale and function as an anti-inflammatory, since it is of the salicylate family. Salicylic acid shampoos are most efficacious in patients who have seborrhiasis, an overlap condition of seborrheic dermatitis and psoriasis. Another discussion of shampoos for this purpose is found in the chapter on psoriasis.

Even though most dermatologists focus on the active agent in the shampoo, the workhorse of the shampoo is really the detergent. The detergents are what remove the sebum nutrient source for the *Malassezia* and physically break apart the skin. The detergents are applied with vigorously rubbing and massaging, which further removes the skin scale. Shampooing is both a chemical and a physical process that prevents the recurrence of seborrheic dermatitis and this cannot be overlooked. Most dandruff shampoos contain excellent foaming agents and strong surfactants. The foaming allows the detergent to be effectively spread over the hair and scalp for more thorough sebum removal, up to a point. While consumers associate abundant foam with good cleansing, foaming agents can be added in any quantity desired by the formulator. Clean hair foams better than dirty hair, so patients should not use this as a criterion for efficacious shampoo selection.

> Many seborrheic dermatitis patients apply shampoo to the hair only and do not clean the scalp adequately.

Seborrheic dermatitis is a condition of the scalp and not the hair. Many patients with this disease are focused on hair beautification, apply shampoo only to the hair, and do not clean the scalp adequately. Remind patients that shampoo is primarily to clean the scalp and not the hair. Proper shampoo technique should be to apply a half dollar dab of shampoo to the palm and rub into the scalp thoroughly. Leave the shampoo on the scalp while washing the rest of the body. This increases contact time between the active ingredient in the shampoo, such as tar or zinc pyrithione, and the scalp thereby increasing efficacy. The shampoo can then be worked through the hair and rinsed immediately. Gently scrubbing with a scalp brush or the fingernails is necessary to remove the skin scalp and clean every portion of the scalp. The frequency of shampooing is determined by the scalp sebum production. Oily scalp may require daily shampooing while dry scalp may only require twice weekly shampooing. One of the biggest contributing factors to seborrheic dermatitis is poor scalp hygiene.

CONDITIONERS FOR SEBORRHEIC DERMATITIS
Conditioning the hair is very important in the seborrheic dermatitis patient. Most dandruff shampoos do not do a good job of beautifying the hair. They attempt to remove sebum thoroughly from the scalp, but overdry the hair. This leaves the hair dry, brittle, rough, frizzy, hard to style, dull, and susceptible to humidity and static electricity. All of these problems can be overcome by proper conditioning.

Treatment conditioners containing zinc pyrithione are available for dandruff. The conditioner leaves behind zinc pyrithione in the follicular ostia in greater concentration than the zinc pyrithione–containing dandruff shampoo. This may be helpful in preventing the growth of *Malassezia*, but many women do like the feel of their hair after using this type of conditioner. These products are well accepted by men with shorter hair, however. Women using dandruff shampoos should definitely be encouraged to use a conditioner. Conditioners do not worsen seborrheic dermatitis as they do not increase *Malassezia* growth and do not interfere with prescription medications.

> Conditioners do not worsen seborrheic dermatitis.

Instant conditioners are the best way to overcome the reduced aesthetics of dandruff shampoos. Dandruff shampoos tend to overcleanse the hair and the conditioner can restore hair shine. Instant conditioners are applied immediately following shampooing and rinsed before leaving the shower and towel drying the hair. The instant conditioner should be rubbed generously onto every hair shaft by pulling the fingers through the hair multiple times from proximal to distal end. If possible, the conditioner should be left in contact with the hair for three to five minutes, perhaps while shaving in the shower. It should be rinsed with cool water, which leaves more conditioner residue behind to beautify the hair.

> Rinsing an instant conditioner with cool water can increase the amount of dimethicone left on the hair to improve appearance in patients using dandruff shampoos.

The two best conditioning agents for persons with seborrheic dermatitis are dimethicone and the polyquaternium compounds. Both coat the hair shaft and smooth the cuticle, which increases hair shine. They also provide a protective coating over the hair to minimize the effects of humidity and static electricity. The conditioner can protect the hair from heat damage due to the use of hair dryers, curling irons, hot curlers, crimping irons, or heated hair straightening devices. Conditioners can reduce combing friction decreasing hair breakage and improve the softness of the hair. Instant conditioners can be combined with leave-in conditioners applied after towel drying the hair to increase hair beautification. There are not special leave-in conditioners for seborrheic dermatitis patients and a thorough discussion of this topic can be found in the chapter on hair conditioners.

GROOMING PRACTICES
Grooming practices are important to increase the success of treatment in seborrheic dermatitis patients. Combing and brushing gently can help to dislodge skin scale, but aggressive scalp manipulation should be avoided. The most important activity to avoid in seborrheic dermatitis patients is scalp scratching. Unfortunately, pruritus is the most bothersome symptom of seborrheic dermatitis and may be the main reason for which the patient seeks treatment. Scalp scratching must be stopped immediately to prevent hair damage. It is impossible to scratch only the scalp; the hair is scratched at the same time. In only 45 minutes, the entire cuticle can be removed from a hair shaft. Once the cuticle is removed, it cannot be restored and the hair devoid of the cuticle will readily fracture and break. This is why many seborrheic dermatitis

patients complain of poor hair growth. The hair is growing fine since seborrheic dermatitis does not generally affect the hair shaft; but the hair is damaged cosmetically by scalp scratching giving the impression of poor hair growth.

Topical prescription corticosteroids to alleviate itching are probably the best solution to poor hair quality in seborrheic dermatitis patients. This will work better than any high priced hair procedure or concoction to beautify the hair. It may seem too simple, but the key to great looking hair in the seborrheic dermatitis patient is itch control.

> The key to great looking hair in the seborrheic dermatitis patient is alleviating pruritus.

OTC TREATMENTS

A variety of over-the-counter (OTC) scalp treatments, based on salicylic acid and hydrocortisone, are available for seborrheic dermatitis. These treatments may not be sufficient for alleviating pruritus, but may be used in the maintenance phase of disease. Salicylic acid can remove some of the skin scale, but is probably more effective in patients with a psoriasis/seborrheic dermatitis overlap condition where the skin scale does not slough from the scalp properly. Once it has been well treated, 1% hydrocortisone solutions can aid in the control of itching.

> OTC seborrheic dermatitis treatments contain salicylic acid and hydrocortisone.

Seborrheic dermatitis is a challenging condition to treat, but the judicious selection of shampoos and conditioners can prolong remission and increase hair beauty. Both are important to the patient, as well as the dermatologist who will understand the hair care market and offer patients better advice.

36 Psoriasis and hair

Dermatologists are preoccupied most with improving scalp psoriasis to alleviate itching and reduce scaling. While these are important goals, patients with scalp psoriasis are also concerned with the health and appearance of their hair. Most patients will not have beautiful hair until the psoriasis has been treated, but providing advice on hair beautification during the early phase of treatment can be helpful in building a strong physician–patient relationship and encouraging compliance. This chapter discusses the psoriasis patient and hair care practices.

SHAMPOOS

A variety of shampoos are available to meet the needs of the scalp psoriasis patient. These shampoos are considered over-the-counter (OTC) drugs and list an active agent on the label, which is the distinct packaging attribute of all OTC drugs. The limitations of OTC drugs are that they can only contain one active agent and this agent must be selected from a list of approved active agents on a monograph that is set forth by the government. There is no psoriasis scalp monograph; so all of the active agents for psoriasis shampoos are taken from the dandruff shampoo monograph. This monograph has limited ingredients for selection, which is why most shampoos for psoriasis are basically dandruff shampoos, even though the etiology of psoriasis is much different from that of seborrheic dermatitis.

> Psoriasis shampoos are basically dandruff shampoos, even though psoriasis and seborrheic dermatitis have different etiologies.

Psoriasis treatment shampoos usually contain a very strong detergent to deliver the active agent to the scalp and to remove as much sebum as possible. While this is important to improving scalp psoriasis, this type of shampoo does not beautify the hair. Thus, psoriasis shampoo selection is a balance between optimizing scalp treatment while not damaging the hair. Sodium laureth sulfate or sodium lauryl sulfate are the two main cleansers in the shampoos. A new trend is to eliminate the sulfates from shampoos, since they are considered "unnatural" ingredients. Sulfates are the most important synthetic detergents in all body and hair cleansers today and eliminating them for replacement by another detergent is really immaterial, since cleansers remain in contact with the skin for a brief period of time before removal and are not ingested.

In additional to the detergent, psoriasis shampoos may contain sulfur, tar, botanicals, salicylic acid, zinc pyrithione, and selenium sulfide. Sulfur is an antifungal and antibacterial. Some dermatologists believe that bacterial-induced inflammation may worsen psoriasis, which may point to the value of sulfur shampoos. Furthermore, many patients have psoriasis that overlaps with seborrheic dermatitis and may find the antifungal properties important, but for the most part sulfur is not a good ingredient in shampoos. It stains light colored hair and is damaging to the hair shaft. Tar can similarly stain light colored hair, if it has not been purified to remove the creosote. However, creosote is one of the most potent anti-inflammatory agents in the complex naturally occurring mixture known as tar. Creosote is also carcinogenic. Botanical anti-inflammatory concoctions blending green tea, lavender, chamomile, tea tree oil, and oatmeal extract are also on the market. It is unlikely that these ingredients have much effect separate from their detergent vehicle in improving scalp psoriasis.

> Salicylic acid is the most useful shampoo ingredient for scalp psoriasis.

Salicylic acid is in my opinion the most helpful ingredient in scalp psoriasis. It is an oil-soluble substance that can mix with scalp sebum to cause the thick collected scalp corneocytes to exfoliate. Unless the scalp scale is removed, prescription topical treatments do not physically touch the scalp and cannot provide improvement. It is the chemical effect of the detergents on the scalp scale and the physical effect of scrubbing that provide most of the improvement, which are augmented by the exfoliating effect of the salicylic acid. Salicylic acid can also function as a mild anti-inflammatory, but the brief contact of the salicylic acid with the scalp may minimize this effect. Unfortunately, salicylic acid is not a hair-friendly substance. It can remove scalp skin scale and also hair cuticular scale. This means that a conditioner must be used following shampooing to smooth the cuticle and restore the softness and luster of the hair.

Zinc pyrithione and selenium sulfide are the last two ingredients that can be used in scalp psoriasis. Selenium sulfide is not used as much because it is an orange ingredient that is fairly expensive and difficult to formulate. Its efficacy is similar to zinc pyrithione, but zinc pyrithione is a better anti-inflammatory agent. New grinding technology has allowed very small size zinc pyrithione particles to be produced that can deposit in the follicular ostia. This technology may be worthwhile in psoriasis, since this delivery may provide longer lasting anti-inflammatory effects. The zinc pyrithione is also antifungal, providing benefit in patients with seborrhiasis, an overlap between seborrheic dermatitis and psoriasis.

> Rotating shampoos in the psoriasis patient is very important as use of one shampoo may create cosmetic scalp and hair issues.

Rotating shampoos in the psoriasis patient is very important as use of one shampoo may create cosmetic scalp issues. Many

Table 36.1 Sample Shampoo Regimens for Patients
with Scalp Psoriasis

(A) Sample Scalp Psoriasis Daily Shampoo Regimen

Monday	Salicylic acid shampoo
Tuesday	Conditioning shampoo
Wednesday	Zinc pyrithione shampoo
Thursday	Conditioning shampoo
Friday	Salicylic acid shampoo
Saturday	Conditioning shampoo
Sunday	Conditioning shampoo

(B) Sample Scalp Psoriasis Thrice Weekly Shampoo Regimen

Monday	Salicylic acid shampoo
Tuesday	No shampoo
Wednesday	Conditioning shampoo
Thursday	No shampoo
Friday	Zinc pyrithione shampoo
Saturday	No shampoo
Sunday	No shampoo

(C) Sample Scalp Psoriasis Twice Weekly Shampoo Regimen

Monday	Salicylic acid shampoo
Tuesday	No shampoo
Wednesday	No shampoo
Thursday	Conditioning shampoo
Friday	No shampoo
Saturday	No shampoo
Sunday	No shampoo

psoriasis patients wish to shampoo daily to optimize scale removal, which can create dry hair issues. A possible shampoo regimen to maximize scalp and hair appearance might be as listed in Table 36.1. Patients with drier hair and less scalp scale may wish to shampoo twice or thrice weekly and possible regimens are also presented in Table 36.1. Using a hair conditioner is very important in all regimens to maintain the cosmetic beauty of hair, the next topic of discussion.

CONDITIONERS

Conditioners are very important in the psoriasis patient to beautify the hair while minimizing the presence of disease. Some of the newer zinc pyrithione dandruff hair conditioners are worthwhile in the psoriasis patient as these instant conditioners applied after shampooing can leave behind additional zinc pyrithione in the follicular ostia to decrease inflammation and the colonization of the scalp by malassezia species. This type of conditioner should be used once or twice weekly. A standard instant conditioner that is applied immediately following shampooing should be used the rest of the time. Instant conditioners can leave behind dimethicone during the rinse phase to minimize the damaging effect of the psoriasis shampoo surfactant. The instant conditioner will provide more hair benefits if left on the hair for a longer period of time in the bath. A possible recommendation might be to have the patient shampoo first in the shower and rinse, then apply the instant conditioner. The conditioner should be left on while bathing the rest of the body or shaving and then rinsed just before leaving the shower. This allows more time for the conditioner to coat the hair shaft and smooth the cuticle. Instant conditioner

Leave-in conditioners can function as a scalp moisturizer to lubricate skin scale and reduce scalp itching.

can also be rubbed into the scalp to soften the psoriatic scale and rinsed.

Once the instant hair conditioner is rinsed, the hair is towel dried and a leave-in conditioner that is not removed is applied. These are creams providing additional dimethicone to further smooth the cuticle. The cream should be massaged through the hair and lightly rubbed into the scalp. The leave-in conditioner can function as a scalp moisturizer to lubricate scalp scales and reduce the scalp itching. Once the hair has dried, further conditioning can be provided with a dimethicone-containing hair serum. These are clear liquids, also known as products to control hair frizz; they further smooth the cuticle. The hair serum should be applied daily to keep the hair moisturized, but can also be applied to the scalp as a moisturizer. Skin moisturizers are frequently used by psoriasis patients to make the skin feel smoother and softer and can also be used to lubricate the scalp in the form of hair serums.

GROOMING PRACTICES

Patients with scalp psoriasis are very self-conscious of their hair and sometimes have elaborate grooming practices that can be detrimental to disease treatment. Aggressive combing and brushing are sometimes used on a daily basis to decrease the amount of scalp scale. Psoriasis patients sometimes mistakenly think that they can brush out all of the scalp disease. Since psoriasis exhibits the Koebner phenomenon, where trauma to the scalp increases the inflammation and resultant scaling, combing and brushing of the scalp are not recommended. The hair should be gently groomed and the scalp manipulated as little as possible. Psoriasis patients may also wish to permanently dye, wave, or straighten their hair with chemicals that can also be damaging to the scalp. One way to minimize inflammation is to pretreat the scalp with a clobetasol solution or gel on the night prior to and after the chemical hair procedure. This can aid in reducing the inflammation preventing a flare of psoriasis. In general, advise psoriasis patients to minimize manipulation of the scalp.

Aggressive combing and brushing should be avoided to decrease scalp trauma, which may worsen scalp psoriasis.

OTC TREATMENTS

OTC treatments for scalp psoriasis are available in plenty to alleviate scaling and itching. Again, since only one active agent can be present, most psoriasis scalp solutions have either hydrocortisone or salicylic acid. The prescription formulations at higher concentrations utilizing fluorinated corticosteroids are more effective, but understanding the OTC market is important to the dermatologist. OTC salicylic acid solutions can formulate with up to 2% salicylic acid, which should be applied directly to the scalp and not to the hair. OTC topical corticosteroid solutions can contain up to 1% hydrocortisone, which is only effective in the thinnest of plaques. The best efficacy is achieved by using the 2% salicylic acid in the morning and 1% hydrocortisone in the evening for patients with limited funds or those who are in the maintenance phase of treatment.

SUMMARY
This chapter has evaluated the use of OTC drugs and hair care products in patients with psoriasis. It is important for the dermatologist to skillfully transition the patient from prescription products to OTC treatments as the disease improves. Treatment can be supplemented by the careful selection of shampoos and hair conditioners to optimize scalp psoriasis treatment.

37 Aging hair issues

Hair ages differently than other body structures because it is one of the few nonliving tissues that is constantly renewed, the only other similar structure being the nails. Hair care becomes important as aging progresses because damage to the hair is irreversible and the average hairs on a mature head are three years old. This means that the effect of any cosmetic procedure gone awry will be present for a long time. Changes that occur as the follicle matures include a decrease in rapidity of hair growth, a reduction in the diameter of the hair shaft, and a failure to pigment the hair shaft. All of these observations are consistent with a loss of follicle vigor. Since hair growth requires high-energy output, this decreased vigor is consistent with the slowing of other body activities with age, but the senescence of the hair shaft is particularly visible. Gray hair is the first sign of maturity noticed by both men and women.

This chapter addresses methods of maintaining the hair in a state of health. Much of the information regarding hair behavior is obtained from the textile literature, especially the processing and dyeing of wool fabrics. Human hair experiences most of the same phenomenon exhibited by wool and extrapolations can be made with accuracy. Healthy hair is full, shiny, soft, and manageable. It resists static electricity, maintains the desired hairstyle, and bounces with movement. Since hair is nonliving, hair care becomes very important, especially with maturity. This chapter presents nine concepts important when considering the unique needs of aging hair.

HEALTHY HAIR IS NATURAL HAIR

Many mature women are dissatisfied with the appearance of their hair and seek cosmetic alterations, such as hair dyeing or permanent waving. These procedures work well on hair that grows quickly because the hair damaged by the chemical process is removed and not reprocessed repeatedly. This is not the case with aging hair that has a slower growth rate. Hair manipulations of all types should be kept to a minimum and as much time as possible be allowed between chemical processing. The hair should be protected when outdoors at all times by wearing a hat or scarf. Sun, wind, and humidity are the enemies of aging hair. It may be hard to convince the mature woman that the less she does to her hair the better! It is just too simple to believe.

> Sun, wind, and humidity are the enemies of aging hair.

TRIM HAIR FREQUENTLY

Many mature patients are hesitant to cut their hair, since the hair growth rate slows down decreasing the maximal achievable length. If the hair shafts have been damaged by too much manipulation and chemical processing, no special shampoo or pricey conditioner can restore hair beauty. For these patients, the overall hair appearance can be improved by removing 1 to 2 inches from the distal hair shafts every other month depending on the rate of hair growth. This trims away split ends, formed when the missing cuticle exposes the softer internal cortex, and creates fresh hair ends that are less frizzy, more likely to maintain a curl, and less subject to static electricity. Trimming also eliminates the irregularity of broken hairs that creates the illusion of fuller, healthier hair. Frequent haircuts are recommended to improve hair appearance.

TREAT UNDERLYING SCALP CONDITIONS

The health of the hair is directly related to the health of the scalp. Many mature patients have postmenopausal itchy scalp, seborrheic dermatitis, or scalp folliculitis. When assessing the hair of a mature patient, do not forget to assess the scalp. Any pruritic scalp disease will cause hair problems. It is possible to remove all of cuticular scale from a hair shaft with only 45 minutes of continuous scratching with the fingernails. Most patients will not scratch their scalp continuously for 45 minutes, but the hair shaft effects of scratching are additive. 45 minutes can easily be added up if the patient scratches 5 minutes a day for 9 days. For this reason, it is important to treat scalp itching and any other scalp conditions noted on physical examination.

AGING HAIR AND HEAT EXPOSURE

It is common for mature individuals to applying external heat to speed hair drying and prevent chilling of the body. While the blow dryer is an excellent way to rewarm a wet head, the heat can permanently damage the protein structure of the hair. Once the water has evaporated from the outside of the hair shaft, overdrying of the hair can occur where the water within the shaft turns to steam and exits the hair shaft creating a loss of cuticular scale, known as "bubble hair" (Fig. 34.2 in a previous chapter is a scanning electron micrograph demonstrating the bubbles created by the energetic steam.). Unfortunately, the condition is permanent and bubble hair results in a weakening of the mature hair shaft and eventual breakage. For this reason, aging hair should be dried until very slightly damp, but not completely dry to avoid bubble hair. The dermatologist can easily detect the presence of hair shaft damage, such as bubble hair, by grasping the hair 1 inch from the end with one hand and pulling on the hair ends with the other. If the hairs break, hair damage from bubble hair or other causes may be present.

AGING HAIR AND CHEMICAL PROCESSING

Chemical processing becomes an important part of grooming in aging hair. Gray hair is dyed to bring back a more youthful color and also permanently waved to make the hair appear thicker and fuller. Both procedures damage aging hair, but most mature women are resistant to giving up chemical processing. For many, the hairdresser is a weekly social outing that is an enjoyable part of retirement. Chemical processing can be continued with maturity as long as the hairdresser realizes that the aging hair will process more quickly than youthful hair.

This is because aging is smaller in diameter allowing easier penetration of the chemicals and the slower growth rate means that the same hair is reprocessed repeatedly. Already chemically processed hair processes more rapidly with each subsequent chemical exposure due to the already damaged cuticle.

Overprocessing of aging hair by leaving the permanent wave solution on too long or the hair bleach on too long is the most common problem I see in my office. It is easy to avoid if the beautician is aware of the issues. When the processing time is completed, the beautician must attend to the patient immediately rather than allowing another 10 to 15 minutes to pass while she attends to other customers. Unfortunately, there is no way to undo the damage caused by overprocessing. This means that the mature patient must pick a beautician who is careful in her technique and experienced in treating aging hair.

> Overprocessing of aging hair leads to hair breakage and poor manageability.

SHAMPOOS FOR AGING HAIR
Many mature patients who present to the dermatologist have already severely damaged their hair and permanent restoration is not possible. Yet, it is important to counsel the patient on how to optimize hair appearance until new growth occurs. One method of minimizing hair damage is to select a shampoo designed to remove sebum and simultaneously beautify the hair, known as a conditioning shampoo. Conditioning shampoos, also known as 2-in-1 shampoos, perform two separate functions based on the difference in shampoo to water ratio during the washing and rinsing phases. During the washing phase, the shampoo is applied to damp hair and massaged into the scalp. In this phase, the shampoo quantity is high and the water quantity is low resulting in detergent cleansing primarily of the scalp, but also the hair. Following completion of the cleansing phase, the shampoo is rinsed from the hair progressively lowering the amount of shampoo and increasing the amount of water. During this rinse phase, a thin layer of conditioner is left behind to coat each hair shaft thus minimizing damage.

CONDITIONERS FOR AGING HAIR
Conditioners are very important in aging hair to preserve the architecture of the cuticle and make the hair soft and shiny. As the rapidity of hair growth slows down with age, the hair is cut less frequently. This means that mature patients must take better care of their hair and the damage resulting from any unsuccessful cosmetic manipulation will be longer lasting. Conditioners place a coating over the hair shaft that can be protective against the heat damage from blow dryers and heated hair styling appliances. Conditioners also decrease hair grooming friction thereby minimizing hair breakage. Mature patients should first condition with an instant conditioner that is applied in the shower immediately following shampooing. The conditioner is then rinsed with cool water and the hair is towel dried. When the hair is mildly damp, a quarter-sized amount of leave-in cream conditioner containing dimethicone should be dispensed into the hand and stroked through the hair in an attempt to cover every hair shaft. More should be applied to the distal hair shaft and less to the proximal hair shaft. The hair should then be allowed to air dry to minimize heat damage. When the hair is almost dry,

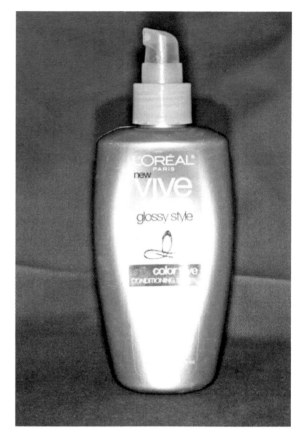

Figure 37.1 An example of a hair conditioning spray for dyed hair containing photoprotection.

a hair serum should be applied with two to four squirts into the palm and again rubbed gently through the hair. The stepwise application of these conditioners will protect the hair and enhance its ability to shine. The conditioner will also improve the ability of the hair to hold a style.

STYLING PRODUCTS FOR AGING HAIR
Once the hair has been shampooed, conditioned, and dried, it is ready for styling. Hair styling is best done when the hair is almost dry. Whatever the hair configuration be, the instant the hair shaft goes from wet to dry, it will determine the final shape of the hair. For this reason, it is best to style almost dry hair. The hair should be handled gently, since wet hair is more prone to breakage than dry hair. Another layer of hair serum containing dimethicone should be applied at this point. A hair conditioning spray containing sunscreen, most commonly benzophenone, can also be applied to minimize UV damage to the hair (Fig. 37.1). The hair can then be finger styled or styled with a curling iron or hot rollers set on low to avoid heat damage. Finally, once styled, the hair can be sprayed with a flexible-hold pump hair spray.

> Aging hair should be manipulated as little as possible to prevent hair breakage from hair styling.

HAIR STYLES FOR AGING HAIR
The hair style selected for aging hair should be simple and require little hair manipulation. Combing and brushing frequently fracture the fine hair shafts characteristic of aging hair (Fig. 37.2). Combs should be wide toothed and brushing

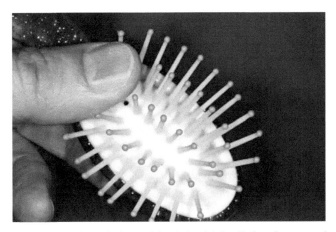

Figure 37.2 A wide toothed smooth bristle brush is less likely to fracture weak aging hair shafts.

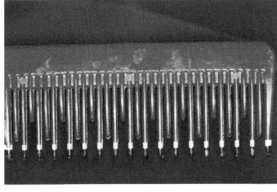

Figure 37.3 Combs with broadly spaced teeth will style hair while minimizing hair shaft cuticle damage.

should be avoided, if possible (Fig. 37.3). The hair should only be styled when dry and handled minimally when wet, since wet hair is more susceptible to hair breakage. Elaborate hair styles requiring teasing, pulling, clasps, barrettes, rubber bands and the like are not recommended because hair breakage will be increased. Hair styles that can only be achieved with permanent waving or frequent hair setting are also not advised. Simple is again the most important consideration when selecting a hair style to optimize the appearance of aging hair.

SUMMARY

It is important for the dermatologist to understand the needs of aging hair. Mature men and women want to look their best at any age and hair is an important part of appearance. While aging hair is not as forgiving as youthful hair, it can be carefully groomed and styled to optimize appearance. It is most important not to undergo risky procedures that might end up in a disastrous cosmetic result because scalp hair growth slows with age and it is not as easy to cut away the unattractive hair in anticipation of regrowth.

38 Damaged hair issues

One of the most common problems the dermatologist faces is the patient who is experiencing hair loss, which can result from either medical or cosmetic causes. No matter what the cause of the hair loss, premature hair breakage is an important contributing factor. Hair is protein and anything that weakens the protein structure will cause the hair to fracture with minimal trauma. Patients are usually seeking medical help to determine how to strengthen their hair and sometimes resort to body building permanent waves or hair-strengthening hair dyes or expensive hair conditioners with caviar. The truth is that once the nonliving hair is damaged it cannot be permanently repaired. Furthermore, any additional cosmetic manipulations will result in more problems. The best and simplest answer for the patient who wishes to restore hair beauty is to cut the hair off and allow new hair to grow, avoiding the cosmetic mistakes of the past. This is excellent advice, but usually not well received by the patient.

This chapter discusses 10 easy tips to be shared with patients, in search of elusive great looking hair. Providing these ideas will help the patient minimize problems and perhaps allow them to feel that their problems were seriously addressed by the physician. These tips are summarized in Table 38.1 and can be easily placed in a handout for patient distribution.

HAIR MANIPULATION

Manipulate the hair as little as possible (Fig. 38.1).

There is a misnomer among hair stylists that the more you do to the hair, the healthier it becomes. This is not true. There is no such thing as a "body restoring permanent wave" or a "strengthening hair dye." The more you dye or perm the hair, the weaker it becomes. The more you comb, brush, curl, twist, clip, tease, braid, etc. the hair, the more damage it incurs. This damage is permanent, since the hair is nonliving. Basically, any manipulation of the hair shaft results in the possibility of cuticular damage, which is known in the hair care industry as "weathering." Weathering is visible even on the healthiest head of hair as a tightly overlapped intact cuticle on the newly grown proximal hair shaft, with a disrupted, sometimes absent cuticle on the older distal hair shaft. Weathering is basically the sum of chemical and physical environmental insults on the hair shaft, which can be minimized through reduced manipulation.

HAIR COMB SELECTION

Select a wide-toothed comb with Teflon coated tips (Fig. 38.2).

One of the most common insults the hair receives on a daily basis is grooming. This grooming is usually done with a comb. Thus, it is important to select a comb that decreases hair breakage by minimizing the friction between the hair and the teeth of the comb. For this reason, a comb should have broadly spaced smooth teeth, preferably Teflon coated, to reduce combing friction. A comb that tends to grab the hair shafts as they pass through the tangled hair increases hair shaft fracture,

usually at the point where cuticular scale is most disrupted or completely absent.

Combing friction is also maximal when the hair shafts are tangled. Unfortunately, the most common reason for combing the hair is to remove tangles. This means that the hair should be protected from situations that might cause hair tangles, such as wind, unconscious hair twisting, or teasing. The most effective way to reduce hair combing friction, besides proper comb selection, is application of a conditioner.

HAIR STYLING

Select a vented ball-tipped styling brush (Fig. 38.3).

The second most commonly used grooming implement is a brush and it too requires careful selection. The main goal again is to reduce friction between the brush and the hair shafts. Natural bristle brushes or brushes with a dense arrangement of bristles have recently become popular since they fit quite nicely with the current "back to nature" trend and the use of botanicals in the hair care industry; however, these brushes maximize hair breakage. A better option is to select a brush design, known as a blow-drying brush, for general grooming needs. These brushes possess vents or openings on the brush head to prevent heat from building up between the hair and the brush head. The widely spaced bristles are also plastic and ball tipped to minimize friction. If drawing the brush across the palm of the hand causes discomfort, the brush is not recommended for use on the hair.

HAIR GROOMING

Do not comb hair when wet (Fig. 38.4).

Hair is much more likely to fracture when wet than dry. For this reason, it is advisable to gently detangle hair following shampooing from the distal ends to the proximal ends with the fingers, not attempting combing or brushing until the hair is almost dry. Many persons feel that the hair must be styled wet in order to attain the desired style. This is only partially true. Hair will set in the position in which it is placed the instant that the last water molecule evaporates from the hair shaft. This means that the hair is optimally styled just before it is completely dry. Thus, it is best to finger-detangle the hair wet and then allow it to almost dry prior to styling to prevent hair breakage.

HAIR DRYING

Allow hair to air dry avoiding heated drying appliances (Fig. 38.5).

Many people prefer to speed the drying process by applying heat to the hair shaft to speed up the evaporation of water. This can be done with a hand-held blow dryer or a hooded professional salon dryer. Heat is also used to style the hair shafts in the form of heated rollers or a curling iron. Unfortunately, any type of heat that is applied to the hair shafts can permanently damage the protein structure of the hair.

Table 38.1 Care Instructions for Damaged Hair

1. Manipulate the hair as little as possible
2. Select a wide-toothed comb with Teflon coated tips
3. Select a vented ball-tipped styling brush
4. Do not comb hair when it is wet
5. Allow hair to air dry avoiding heated drying appliances
6. Avoid scratching the hair and scalp
7. Select a conditioning shampoo
8. Apply an instant conditioner after each shampooing
9. Consider use of a deep conditioner once weekly
10. Cut away damaged hair shafts

It is important to distinguish between the water that resides on the outside of the hair shaft when the hair is wet and the water that resides inside the hair shaft to act as a plasticizer. Hair dryers attempt to speed evaporation of the water on the outside of the hair shaft and heating styling appliances attempt to rearrange the water deformable bonds within the hair shaft. Remember that water is the plasticizer of all of the keratin-based structures of the body including the skin, hair, and nails. When the hair is rapidly exposed to high temperatures, the water within the shaft turns to steam and exits the hair shaft creating a loss of cuticular scale and a condition known as

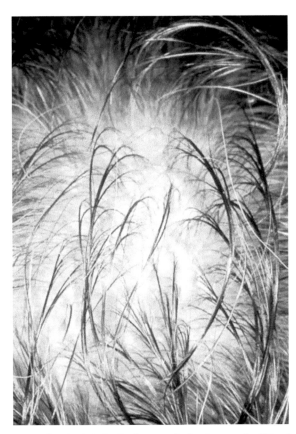

Figure 38.1 Thinning hair that has been manipulated too much will break and appear even thinner.

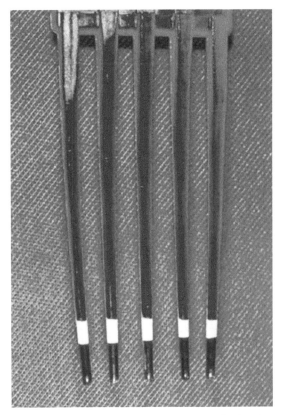

Figure 38.2 A wide-toothed comb should be used especially when detangling the hair after shampooing to minimize hair shaft breakage.

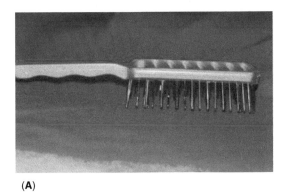

(A)

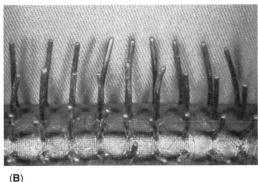

(B)

Figure 38.3 (**A**) A vented ball-tipped blow-drying brush is demonstrated that minimized hair breakage from grooming. (**B**) A brush without ball tips is demonstrated representing a poor-grooming brush choice.

"bubble hair." Under scanning electron microscopy it is actually possible to see the bubbles created by the energetic steam. Unfortunately, the condition is permanent and bubble hair results in a weakening of the hair shaft that contributes to breakage.

The dermatologist should be aware that many patients who present with hair loss may be experiencing hair breakage due to bubble hair. While it is not possible to see bubble hair under a light microscope, it is possible to have the patient collect four days worth of hair loss, by placing each day's loss in a separate bag. The dermatologist can examine these bags to determine the ratio of broken hairs without the hair bulb to shed telogen hairs containing the hair bulb. If the number of broken hairs exceeds 20%, the patient is experiencing hair

breakage. At this point, the dermatologist should inquire as to the use of heated hair drying and styling appliances and make some recommendations; however, most patients will not discontinue the use of heat.

Even though all forms of heat are damaging to the hair shaft, it is possible to minimize damage by altering the abrupt manner in which the hair contacts heat. Bubble hair is more likely to occur if the hair shaft at room temperature is suddenly exposed to high heat. If the hair exposure to the heat is gradual, the damaging effect is not as great. Thus, a gradual temperature increase is recommended. This means that hair dryers can be safely used if the nozzle blowing out hot air is held at least 12 inches from the hair, allowing the air to cool prior to touching the hair shaft. Hair dryers also should be started on low heat to initially warm the hair prior to drying at higher temperatures.

Heat hair rollers and curling irons can be used safely if allowed to cool prior to application to the hair. These thermostatically controlled devices tend to slightly overheat, which can induce bubble hair immediately on hair contact. Heated styling devices should be unplugged for 1 to 2 minutes prior to placing them in contact with the hair. If possible, the styling devices should be operated on a low, rather than high, temperature setting. If the device does not have multiple temperature settings, the temperature of the metal or plastic that contacts the hair can be lowered by placing it in a damp towel. Many patients prefer to use styling heated devices at a high temperature setting, since the high temperature results in the rearrangement of more water deformable bonds and a tighter, longer-lasting curl. Hair that has been heat damaged appears wavy and friable to the human eye.

SCALP SCRATCHING

Avoid scratching the hair and scalp (Fig. 38.6).

It is not usual for patients with seborrheic dermatitis to present with the complaint of hair loss. Medically, it is difficult to reconcile how a fungal infection of the skin of the scalp could alter hair growth from the hair follicles located deep within the dermis and in the superficial subcutaneous tissue. The answer to hair loss in the seborrheic dermatitis patient lies in having

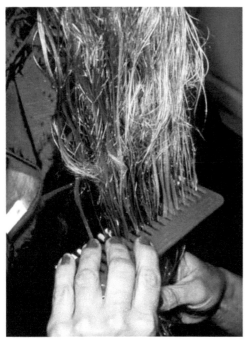

Figure 38.4 Freshly shampooed hair is tangled and fragile creating a situation conducive to hair shaft fracture.

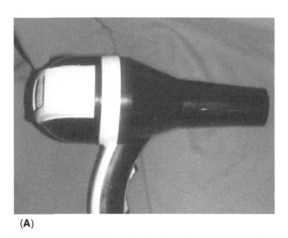

(A)

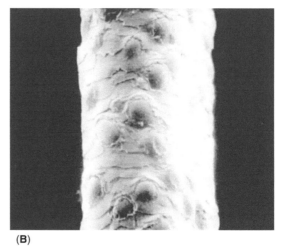

(B)

Figure 38.5 (**A**) Blow drying the hair can lead to heat damage and a condition known as bubble hair. (**B**) An electron micrograph of bubble hair illustrating the bubbles or lumps in the hair shaft created by escaping steam.

the patient collect all hairs lost while shampooing or grooming over a 24-hour period in a bag. Examination of these hairs will reveal absence of the cuticle and hair shaft fracture. Remarkably, it is possible to remove the entire cuticle from the hair shaft with 1 hour of vigorous scratching. Most patients will not

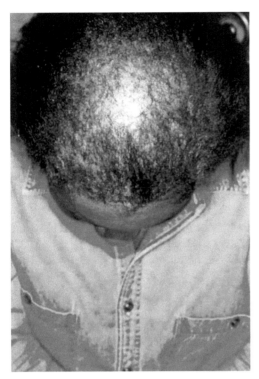

Figure 38.6 Scratching of the scalp can lead to increased hair breakage only magnifying the hair loss characteristic of a scarring alopecia.

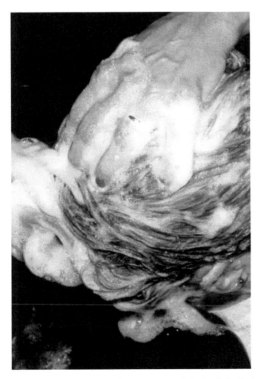

Figure 38.7 Use of a conditioning shampoo can minimize hair shaft damage due to shampoo detergents.

scratch their scalp continuously for 1 hour, but the effects of scratching are additive to the hair shaft. One hour can easily be achieved if the patient scratches 10 minutes a day for 6 days. Usually patients are intending to scratch only the itching present on the scalp, but it is impossible to scratch the scalp without scratching the hair shafts, as well.

Thus, the solution to hair loss in the seborrheic dermatitis patient is to treat the underlying disease. Many times I have treated my patients complaining of hair loss aggressively for scalp pruritus in addition to my standard hair loss workup. Fingernail damage to the hair shaft will result in dull, unmanageable, broken hair that performs poorly. Stopping hair shaft damage from scalp itching is key to solving the cause of hair loss in some patients.

SHAMPOO SELECTION

Select a conditioning shampoo (Fig. 38.7).

Unfortunately, many patients who present to the dermatologist have already severely damaged their hair and therefore, a permanent restoration is not possible. Yet, it is important to counsel the patient on how to optimize the appearance of their damaged hair until new growth occurs and the damaging cosmetic procedure has been discontinued. One such method of minimizing hair damage is to select a conditioning shampoo. There is no doubt that sebum is the optimal hair conditioner and all synthetic conditioners are a poor substitute, however, patients do not like the greasy, flat appearance sebum imparts to the hair shaft. This led to the introduction of shampoos designed to remove sebum from the hair. Remember that the original intention of shampoo was to remove sebum, skin scale, environmental dirt, and apocrine and eccrine secretions from the scalp. Patients forget that shampoo is to cleanse the scalp and not the hair when they are in the shower.

The need to improve the hair while cleansing the scalp has led to the development of conditioning shampoos. The main ingredient in this technology is silicone, a light-weight, clear oil that can coat the hair shaft and smooth the disrupted cuticular scale. This technology was pioneered as part of the Pantene line of shampoos (Procter & Gamble, Cincinnati, Ohio), still manufactured today. These shampoos were originally known as 2-in-1 shampoos, since they both cleansed the scalp and conditioned the hair. They are available for all types of hair including dry, normal, oily, and chemically treated. Silicone is instrumental in these formulas since it can coat the hair shaft without leaving the greasy appearance of sebum. The silicone also significantly reduces the friction of combing and brushing, minimizing hair breakage. Thus, patients with hair loss or chemically damaged hair may benefit from the use of a silicone-containing conditioning shampoo.

CONDITIONER SELECTION

Apply an instant conditioner after each shampooing (Fig. 38.8).

Silicone technology has also been applied to instant conditioners. Instant conditioners are products applied immediately following shampooing in the bath or shower. They are left on the scalp for a short period of time and then thoroughly rinsed from the hair, hence the name "instant" conditioner. Since these products do not contain a surfactant designed to remove

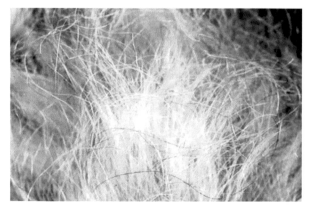

Figure 38.8 An instant conditioner is important to prevent tangles from developing among the hair shafts predisposing to hair shaft breakage.

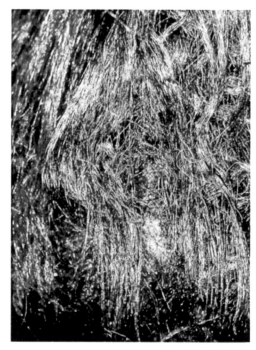

Figure 38.9 Deep conditioners are especially important in chemically straightening African-American hair to prevent hair shaft breakage.

oils from the scalp, they can focus on augmenting the effect of a previously applied conditioning shampoo. Instant hair conditioners usually incorporate cyclomethicone, dimethicone, or amodimethicone as their active agent, in addition to quaternary ammonium compounds. Amodimethicone is a cyclic silicone that appears to have more substantivity for hair keratin. This means that it sticks to the cuticle better and resists water rinsing, thus providing longer-lasting conditioning. Quaternary ammonium compounds, also known as quats, are excellent at decreasing static electricity, which produces unmanageable frizzy hair.

While these important ingredients function to smooth the loosened cuticular scale and increase hair shine, they also reduce friction. By doing so, it is easier to detangle freshly washed hair, thus reducing hair breakage during the hair drying process. Hair conditioners also decrease the grooming friction between the comb and brush and the hair fibers. Hair conditioners also provide a protective coating over the hair shaft that can protect from heat damage and the effects of UV radiation.

In short, one of the best recommendations the dermatologist can provide to the patient who experiences hair loss is to use an instant conditioner following shampooing. Use of this product will prolong hair longevity, no matter what the underlying cause of hair loss may be. No fabrics are sold without a fabric finish, which improves with wear and imparts shine to the fabric. It is actually the removal of the fabric finish that changes a soft cotton t-shirt into a stiff faded rag with repeated visits to the wash machine. These same changes occur with hair. Restoring the softness of fabric by using a fabric softener in the wash machine or dryer is analogous to applying an instant conditioner to the hair.

DEEP CONDITIONERS

Consider use of a deep conditioner once weekly (Fig. 38.9).

Occasionally it is necessary to impart more conditioning benefits to the hair fiber than an instant conditioner can deliver. This is especially the case in hair that has underdone chemical processing, such as permanent dyeing, bleaching, permanent waving, or chemical straightening. These procedures all intentionally disrupt the cuticular scale in order to reach the cortex and medulla of the hair shaft to induce a change in color or configuration. Once the cuticle has been disrupted with chemical processing, it can never be fully restored. Thus, there is a trade off for the patient between the cosmetic value of chemically treating the hair shaft and its reduced ability to function optimally. Some of the damage can be minimized by using what is known as a deep conditioner.

Deep conditioners are applied to hair for 20 to 30 minutes outside the bath or shower. They can be used both at home and in a salon. There are basically two types of deep conditioners: oil treatments and protein packs. Oil treatments are usually used for kinky hair that has been straightened. The process of lye straightening hair results in decreased hair water content, which reduces the hair shaft elasticity and predisposes to hair breakage. Apply a heavy oil to the hair shaft is much like moisturizing the skin in that it attempts to both smooth the cuticle and prevent further water loss from the hair shaft. In general, oil treatments are not used for straight hair, since the heavy oil leaves the hair limp and difficult to style.

Protein packs represent a second type of deep conditioner and can be used for all hair types. These conditioners are formulated as creams or lotions and are a variation on the instant conditioner, except that they remain on the hair longer prior to rinsing. Protein packs may contain silicones and quaternary ammonium compounds, as previously discussed, but they also contain some form of hydrolyzed protein. Usually, collagen from animal sources is used, but any hydrolyzed protein will do. The protein can diffuse into the hair shaft through the cuticular defects created by the chemical treatment. The protein can impart some strength to the hair shaft and also smooth the cuticular scale more thoroughly than an instant conditioner.

For patients who have chemically processed hair, I recommend a deep conditioner once every one to two weeks in addition to an instant conditioner after shampooing.

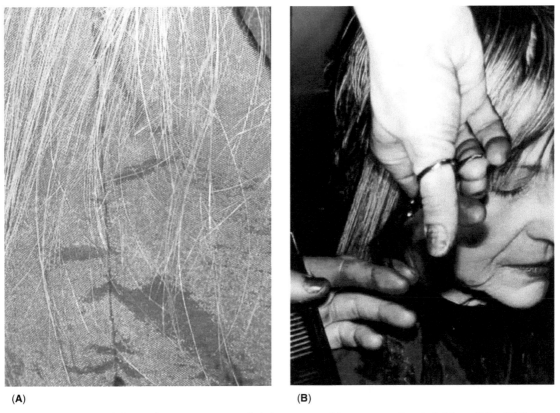

(A)   **(B)**

Figure 38.10 (**A**) Broken irregular hair shafts must be cut away to restore the hair to a presentable appearance, since the hair is nonliving. (**B**) Patients with thinning hair may be tempted to decrease the frequency of hair trimming. Hair trimming should be performed on an approximately six-week basis to keep the hair looking full and healthy.

HAIR TRIMMING

> Cut away damaged hair shafts (Fig. 38.10).

Many patients who are losing their hair are reluctant to cut their hair. I believe that they feel they should hang onto all their hair in case no more grows. Unfortunately, hair that has been damaged by too much chemical processing and too little conditioner application cannot be restored. For these patients, the overall appearance of the hair can be improved simply by removing 1 to 2 inches from the distal hair shafts. This trims away the split ends and creates new hair ends that are less frizzy, more likely to maintain a curl, less subject to static electricity. Trimming also eliminates the irregularity of broken hairs that creates a thin appearance. In short, removal of the damaged hair can create the illusion of fuller, healthier hair. Of course, the newly exposed ends must receive proper care or they too will develop an unattractive cosmetic appearance with time.

SUMMARY

Even though hair is a nonliving substance, proper care can allow it to resist breakage that contributes to hair loss. Much of the product development regarding hair care has been the adaptation of textile processing techniques to the human hair fiber. When hair is thought of as a fabric, it is easy to understand how proper handling of the hair fiber and limited exposure to damaging chemicals and environmental variables can influence its cosmetic performance. This section has presented some ideas for the dermatologist to use when assisting patients concerned about medical or cosmetic hair loss.

SUGGESTED READING

Robbins C. Hair breakage during combing. I. Pathways of breakage. J Cosmet Sci 2006; 57: 233–43.

Robbins C. Hair breakage during combing. II. Impact loading and hair breadage. J Cosmet Sci 2006; 54: 245–57.

Robbins C, Kamath Y. Hair breakage during combing. IV. Brushing and combing hair. J Cosmet Sci 2007; 58: 629–36.

IV Nail: Introduction

The nails are interesting structures. Perhaps they are vestiges of claws used by animals for eating and self-protection. Maybe, they are necessary for protection of the highly innervated tissues of the fingertips. Perhaps nails are there just for nothing more than cosmetic adornment! Certainly, there are a myriad of products to improve the appearance of the nails from something as simple as a nail clipper to something as complex as a polymerized acrylic prosthesis placed on the nail for elongation. It is said that nails can tell a lot about the individual. Grease-stained fingernails indicate work as an auto mechanic while yellowed fingernails may indicate excessive cigarette smoking. Clean well-trimmed fingernails may indicate physical health and excellent hygiene while misshapen fingernails may indicate an underlying dermatologic disease. Nails can be a clue to a lung or renal disease that may be lurking inside the body as of yet undiagnosed except by the skillful eye of the dermatologist! There is no doubt that nails tell an unspoken story about the life of a person.

Given this preoccupation with nails, the cosmetic industry has found a ripe opportunity. There are products designed to bleach discolored nails and moisturize brittle nails. There are nail polishes to coordinate nail color with clothing, moods, or fashion trends. Some nail prostheses are designed to be worn only for one day or for months at a time in short, medium, long, and excessively long lengths. The prostheses have become an art form for many with elaborate painting, jewels, or sculptures stuck to the natural nail plate. And, these manipulations are not only performed on the fingernails, but also on the toenails, creating 20 little canvases for artistic expression.

Besides the cosmetic intrigue, nails also have specific grooming and hygiene needs. It is said that outside of the mouth, the skin beneath the nails is one of the dirtiest areas on the human body. Indeed, many diseases are passed from the hands to the mouth, eyes, or nose with the aid of the fingernails. This means that nail hygiene can assume paramount importance in both sexes and in persons of all ages. There are specific needs for nails in children and also in nail disease, including nail dystrophy and nail psoriasis. This section of the book covers all of these areas to provide a compendium of nail cosmetics in nail health and disease.

39 A problem-oriented approach to fingernail issues

Nail problems are perplexing for the dermatologist and in many ways more challenging than skin problems, since the nails are nonliving (Fig. 39.1). The renewal time for the stratum corneum is a mere two weeks, but it takes three to six months to grow a new fingernail and 6 to 12 months to grow a new toenail. This means the time between treatment and visible results is prolonged creating problems with unrealistic patient expectations. Nevertheless, the nails are an important appearance attribute nonverbally communicating our sex, personal care habits, occupation, hobbies, and habits. While the nails function primarily to protect the tender fingertip and facilitate manipulation of small items, modern society assigns paramount importance to the appearance of nails as a manner of determining social status. Persons who perform manual labor cannot maintain long nails, while individuals who work in managerial positions use longer nail length as one method of indicating occupational success. Women spend both time and money pursuing long brightly colored prosthetic fingernails and toenails as nonverbal body art to display social standing.

Nail adornment is an interesting topic, because it allows expression of subtle personality characteristics. Is red nail polish an indication of an extrovert while a clear nail polish an indication of an introvert? Are damaged nails from biting an indication of a nervous timid personality? This reasoning further extends into the concern over nail disease. Do the yellow/green thickened nails of fungal infection indicate a contagious condition? Are the pitted nails characteristic of psoriasis socially associated with ill health? Certainly, the hands and nails are the second area of visual contact when meeting a new individual after the face. There can be no doubt that nails say a great deal about who we are and what we aspire to be.

This chapter takes a problem-oriented approach to nail cosmetic problems and issues of nail disease. It begins by dividing nail issues into those pertinent to the fingernails, toenails, and unique issues in children. Common patient cosmetic problems are presented with a discussion of the issues and products that may cause and improve the condition. Since most cosmetic problems require that the damaged nail grow until replaced by new normal growth, identifying the problem and suggesting solutions is paramount. Nail disease, on the other hand, can be challenging to treat; yet, cosmetic interventions may provide a temporary solution until new nail appears. This chapter links nail cosmetics and nail cosmetic procedures to the problems they create and camouflage (Table 39.1).

NAIL DISCOLORATION

Nail discoloration is a common cosmetic concern (Table 39.2) (1–4). The normal nail plate is transparent, allowing the nail bed to be visualized as pink through the proximal nail plate with the air interface allowing the nail to appear white at the distal free edge. With advancing age and the onset of nail disease, the nail plate becomes less transparent and more translucent making the nail bed appear paler and giving the impression of reduced blood flow. The aging nail may also be yellowed, either from a poorly formed nail plate or staining from environmental substances, such as nicotine, foodstuffs, cleaning fluids, pigmented cosmetics, etc. (Fig. 39.2). Nail growth also slows down increasing the renewal time for the nail plate and the opportunity for nail staining. The easiest camouflage for nail discoloration is the use of nail polish, which is also the most common nail cosmetic for adornment. Discolored nails can also be treated by bleaching.

Nail Polish

Nail polish, also known as nail enamel, is a pigmented coating applied to the nail plate. It was introduced in the 1920s when lacquer technology was developed in the automobile industry to replace slow-drying oil-based paints. The basis of nail polish is nitrocellulose created by reacting cellulose fiber, from cotton linters or wood pulp, with nitric acid. The boiled nitrocellulose is dissolved in organic solvents, which evaporate leaving a hard, glossy film known as a lacquer (5). In 1930, Charles Revson developed the idea of adding pigments to the clear lacquer to form an opaque, colored nail polish and founded the cosmetic company, Revlon, in 1932.

> Nail polish can be used to camouflage nail discoloration.

Nail polish consists of pigments suspended in a volatile solvent to which film-formers have been added (Fig. 39.3). The ingredients are listed in Table 39.3 (6). Nitrocellulose is the most commonly employed primary film-forming agent in nail lacquer because it produces a shiny, tough film that sticks well to the nail plate. The film is oxygen permeable, which is felt to be important to nail plate health. This is the advantage of using nail polish to camouflage nail discoloration, instead of artificial nail prostheses, which are oxygen impermeable. Thus, nail polish places an inert protective coating on the nail plate that does not produce damage.

> Toluene-sulfonamide-formaldehyde resin found in many nail polishes is a common allergen.

A secondary film-forming resin must be added, however, to make the nail polish film flexible, otherwise it would crack with movement of the nail plate. The main resin used to enhance the nitrocellulose film was toluene-sulfonamide-formaldehyde; however, this resin is allergenic and found on the standard dermatology patch test tray. Nail polishes labeled "hypoallergenic," meaning reduced allergy, should not use this resin. This resin is still widely used, however, some individuals are sensitive to this substance, which is found on the standard dermatology patch test tray. The resin has been eliminated in

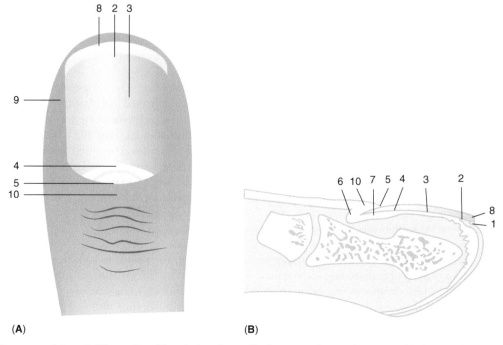

Figure 39.1 Normal anatomy of the nail: (**A**) top view; (**B**) sagittal section. 1, distal groove; 2, hyponychium; 3, nail bed; 4, distal border of lunula; 5, cuticle; 6, proximal matrix; 7, distal matrix; 8, free edge; 9, lateral nail fold; 10, proximal nail fold. *Source*: Reproduced from Richert B, Di Chiachio N, Haneke E. Nail Surgery. Informa Healthcare, 2010.

Table 39.1 Nail Cosmetics

Nail cosmetic	Main ingredients	Function	Adverse reactions
Nail polish	Nitrocellulose, toluene-sulfonamide resin, plasticizers, solvents, and colorants	Add color and shine to nail plates	Allergic contact dermatitis to toluene-sulfonamide resin, nail plate staining
Nail hardener	Formaldehyde, acetates, acrylics, or other resins	To increase nail strength and prevent breakage	Allergic contact dermatitis to formaldehyde
Nail enamel remover	Acetone, alcohol, ethyl acetate, or butyl acetate	Remove nail polish	Irritant contact dermatitis
Cuticle remover	Sodium or potassium hydroxide	Destroy keratin that forms excess cuticular tissue on nail plate	Irritant contact dermatitis
Nail bleach	Hydrogen peroxide	Remove nail plate stains	Irritant contact dermatitis
Nail polish drier	Vegetable oils, alcohols, or silicone derivatives	Speed drying time of nail polish	Practically none
Nail buffing cream	Pumice, talc, or kaolin	Smooth ridges in nails	Practically none
Nail moisturizer	Occlusives, humectants, and lactic acid	Increase water content of nails	Practically none

some hypoallergenic nail enamels and replaced with a polyester resin or cellulose acetate butyrate, but sensitivity is still possible and the enamel is less resistant to wear, meaning it is readily removed from the nail plate with friction (7).

Nail lacquers also contain other ingredients, such as plasticizers like dibutyl phthalate and dioctyl phthalate, which function to keep the product soft and pliable in the bottle. It should be mentioned that the phthalates have recently come under criticism for their possible estrogenic side effects. Some states are considering legislation to remove this family of ingredients, which is also used for preservative purposes, from the market. However, there is little evidence that phthalates have caused health issues in humans.

All of the ingredients discussed are then dissolved in a solvent, such as N-butyl acetate and ethyl acetate, leaving a colored film on the nail plate. Toluene and isopropyl alcohol may be added to act as diluents to keep the lacquer thin and lower its cost. To this vehicle, a variety of coloring agents and specialty fillers can be added to determine the final cosmetic appearance of the nail polish. Coloring agents, such as organic colors, can be selected from a Food and Drug Administration (FDA) approved list of certified colors. Inorganic colors and pigments may also be used, but must conform to low heavy metal content standards (8). These colors can be suspended within the lacquer with suspending agents, such as stearalkonium hectorite, to produce colors ranging from white to pink to purple to brown to orange to blue to green.

Table 39.2 Nail Discoloration Causes

1. Aging nail plate with poor keratin production
2. Nicotine staining from cigarette smoking
3. Handling fruits (peaches, oranges, tomatoes, strawberries) and vegetables (yellow squash, beets, pumpkin) with carotenoids that are colored yellow, orange, or red
4. Nail polish staining from red and orange nail polish
5. Solvent contact, such as turpentine, glutaraldehyde, formaldehyde, etc.
6. Poor internal health (respiratory disease, cancer chemotherapy, heart disease)
7. Contact with pigmented products, such as hair dye, self-tanning preparations, facial foundations, etc.
8. Yellow nail syndrome
9. Onychomycosis

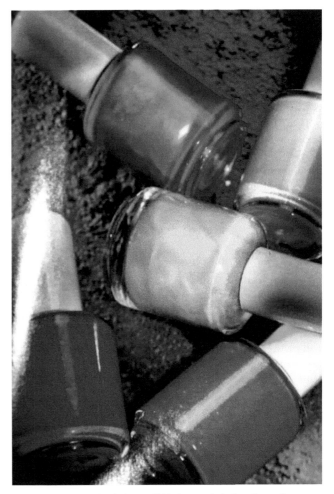

Figure 39.3 Nail polish is available in a myriad of modern colors.

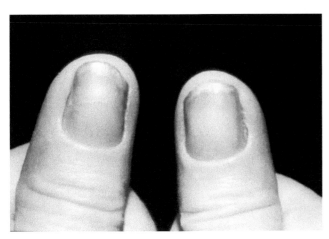

Figure 39.2 Discolored nail plate.

Specialty fillers, such as guanine fish scale, bismuth oxychloride, or titanium dioxide-coated mica, can be added to give a frosted appearance, due to enhanced light reflection. Chopped aluminum, silver, and gold can be added for a metallic shine. For optimal nail discoloration camouflaging, the nail polish should be opaque and properly applied. The technique for nail polish application is discussed next.

Nail Polish Camouflaging Technique

> Nail polish does not damage the nail plate, but nail polish remover dehydrates the nail plate.

Nail polish must be properly applied to camouflage the underlying discolored nail plate. Proper application ensures longevity of the camouflage. This is important because it is not the nail polish that damages the nail plate, but rather the nail polish remover. Proper application requires three layers of nail polish: a base coat, pigmented nail enamel, and a top coat (Table 39.4). The base coat ensures good adhesion to the nail plate and prevents polish chipping. It contains no pigment, less primary film-former, more secondary film-forming resin and is of a lower viscosity since a thinner film is desirable. The second layer is the actual pigmented nail enamel. The top coat, or third layer, provides gloss and resistance to chipping.

Table 39.3 Nail Polish Ingredients

1. Primary film-former (nitrocellulose, methacrylate polymers, vinyl polymers)
2. Secondary film-forming resin (formaldehyde, p-toluene sulfonamide, polyamide, acrylate, alkyd and vinyl resins)
3. Plasticizers (dibutyl phthalate, dioctyl phthalate, tricresyl phosphate, camphor)
4. Solvents and diluents (acetates, ketones, toluene, xylene, alcohols)
5. Colorants (organic D&C pigments, inorganic pigments)
6. Specialty fillers (guanine fish scale or titanium dioxide-coated mica flakes or bismuth oxychloride for iridescence)
7. Suspending agents

Table 39.4 Nail Polish Application Technique

1. Base coat: clear polish designed to seal nail plate with a thin coat of film-former
2. Nail enamel: pigmented polish producing an opaque film to camouflage underlying discolored nail plate
3. Top coat: thin clear polish containing sunscreen to prevent polish color fading, add high shine, and prevent removal of nail enamel
4. Nail polish drier: liquid that speeds up the drying of the nail polish by encouraging evaporation of the solvent

It contains increased amounts of primary film former, more plasticizer and less secondary film-forming resins. Some top coats may contain sunscreen, to prevent the nail lacquer but do not contain pigment. Finally, a nail polish drier, consisting of vegetable oils, alcohols, and silicone derivatives may be brushed or sprayed over the completed nails to induce rapid hardening of the enamel by drawing off the nail polish solvent.

These three consecutive coats increase the ability of the nail polish to stay on the nail plate, a characteristic known as nail lacquer "wear." The wear of the nail polish is determined by the film hardness, water resistance, adhesion to the nail, and ability to resist abrasion. Since it is the nail polish remover that damages the nail plate, it is desirable for the nail polish to remain on the nail plate as long as possible.

Nail Polish Staining

Nail polish containing D&C Reds No. 6, 7, 34, or 5 Lake can temporarily stain the nail plate yellow.

It is important to remember that nail polish can also stain the nail plate (Fig. 39.4). The nail staining occurs when the polish pigment is dissolved rather than suspended. It is most common with deep red nail polishes containing D&C Reds No. 6, 7, 34, or 5 Lake (9). The nail plate will be stained yellow after 7 days of continuous wear, but the stain will fade without treatment in approximately 14 days, once the enamel has been removed. Scrapping of the nail plate with a scalpel blade can be used to confirm that only the nail surface has been stained, an important distinction in nail pigmentation abnormalities (10).

French Manicure Camouflage

A camouflage technique known as the French manicure, which artistically utilizes a variety of colors of nail polish to simulate the normal nail plate, can be remedy for nail discoloration (Fig. 39.5). First, the nail is painted with a white opaque base coat to cover the discoloration. A light pink enamel is added to the entire nail plate to simulate the nail bed. Finally, a white enamel is applied to the distal nail tip, simulating the nail free edge. A clear top coat is applied last to prevent color fading and minimize enamel chipping (Fig. 39.6). French manicures can

be performed professionally by a manicurist or at home with prepackaged kits available at mass merchandisers.

Nail Bleach

It is possible to bleach superficial stains out of the nail plate. For example, food and nicotine stains can be removed with the high volume peroxide found in nail bleach; however, irritant contact dermatitis can occur (11). A safer alternative to nail

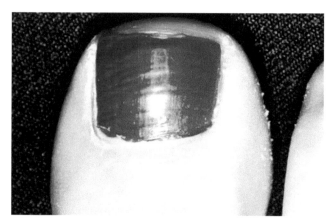

Figure 39.4 Nail plate staining can occur with deep red nail polish.

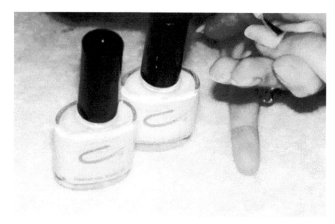

Figure 39.5 White and pink nail polishes are used to simulate a healthy natural nail plate.

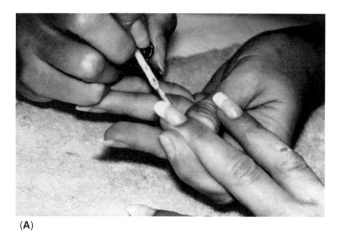

(A)

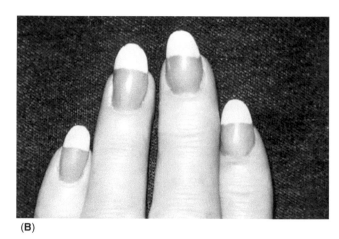

(B)

Figure 39.6 A French manicure is an effective way to camouflage discolored, unattractive nails. (**A**) Colored enamels are artistically applied to the nail plate. (**B**) The finished appearance of the decorated nails.

bleach is nail filling. This technique is discussed next and can also be used to treat ridged nails.

NAIL RIDGING

> Nail ridging can be minimized with nail files or nail buffing creams.

Another common nail problem, seen primarily in persons 40 years and older, is nail ridging. Longitudinal nail ridging is common as the nail bed ages and can be likened to gray hairs on the head. The ridge represents a group of nail matrix cells that are no longer producing a quality smooth nail plate, much like a gray hair produced by an aging follicle that no longer manufactures pigment. Typically, the ridge is permanent, as more ridges appear with advancing age (12). Fortunately, the ridge is only on top of the nail plate and can be removed by sanding or buffing the nail plate along with any nail plate discoloration that may be present.

The nail plate is best sanded with a series of three nail files (Table 39.5). The first nail file is coarse and should sand the nail ridge until smooth. This is best determined by rubbing the treated nail with the finger pad of the same nail from the opposite hand. Once the nail is smooth, it is then filed with a finer file to increase smoothness and finally filed to achieve a high shine. Usually, the three files are sold together for under $5 in mass merchandisers and labeled as cleaning, conditioning, and shining files. Each time the nails are cut, the filing sequence must be repeated, as new nail growth will contain the longitudinal ridge (Fig. 39.7).

If the patient does not wish to perform the filing at home, this sequential filing routine can be included as part a regular manicure. The technique can be used by both men and women to minimize longitudinal ridges, remove nail plate discoloration, and restore a more youthful appearance to the nail plate.

Table 39.5 Nail Filing Technique for Nail Ridging

1. Cleaning file: coarse file to grind the nail plate leaving a rough surface
2. Conditioning file: finer file to remove nail dust
3. Shining file: smooth file to add high shine to nail plate

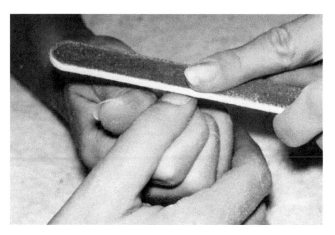

Figure 39.7 Demonstration of the filing technique to smooth out nail ridges.

An alternative to nail filing is the use of a nail buffing cream to smooth nail plate ridges. Nail buffing creams contain finely ground pumice, talc, kaolin, or precipitated chalk as abrasives. Waxes are also added to increase the nail shine (13).

A variant of nail ridging is the habit tic deformity. In this condition, the nail is characterized by horizontal ridges, instead of longitudinal ridges, down the nail center. It results from a repeated picking trauma to the nail and is most common when the thumbnail is manipulated by the first fingernail of the same hand. In most patients, it is a subconscious behavior in individuals who like to keep their hands moving. It is a hard habit to break. Some success can be achieved by offering another object for manipulation, such as a smooth stone, a strand of beads, a piece of cloth, or a compressible ball. The patient can select a comforting object to manipulate in their pocket, instead of nail picking. The ridges can be smoothed once the nail picking stops with the same sequential filing technique described for the longitudinal ridges.

NAIL SPLITTING

> Nails split due to loss of nail plasticity from lack of water.

In addition to nail ridging, the nails may also split for many reasons, but primarily due to loss of nail plasticity. Water is the plasticizer of the nail plate allowing it to bend and rebound with trauma. Since the hands grasp, type, write, dig, scratch, squeeze, etc., the nails are subject to more trauma than any other nonliving portion of the body. It is no wonder then that the nails split. The best method to prevent nail splitting, also known as onychorrhexis, is to preserve the water content of the nail plate. No one exactly knows how much water should be in the nail plate, since underhydration results in the cracking of the keratin and overhydration results in the softening of the nail keratin, both of which result in a nail plate less resistant to trauma. The best sources available state that the normal nail contains about 16% water, becoming soft with saturation at 30%. The water content of nail keratin is proportional to relative humidity being 7% at 20% relative humidity and 30% at 100% relative humidity (14).

There are several different techniques of addressing nail splitting issues, sometimes also termed brittle nails, in patients (15–17). The obvious explanation is that the nails should be protected from trauma of all types, but this is not a practical advice. Table 39.6 lists some of the cosmetic methods for helping patients minimize nail plate splitting and fracture (18).

Due to the nonliving nature of the nail plate, once the water is lost, it can never be fully replaced. Thus, patients with nail splitting should be advised to prevent nail dehydration at all costs (19,20). Hand washing is the obvious cause of nail plate dehydration, lending credence to the concept that the nails should not be washed unless dirty focusing the cleansing on the hands only. Another cause of nail plate dehydration is the use of waterless hand sanitizers. These products contain triclosan, an antibacterial agent, in a rapidly evaporating vehicle. The vehicle efficiently removes water from the nail plate to a greater degree than traditional soap and water. For this reason, hand sanitizers should be avoided to prevent nail splitting.

Table 39.6 Methods to Minimize Nail Plate Splitting and Fracture

1. Minimize water loss from nail plate
   a. Wash hands, not nails, if not soiled
   b. Avoid waterless hand sanitizers
   c. Eliminate antibacterial soaps and cleansers with triclosan
   d. Wear gloves when using cleaning solvents, hair dyes, and hair permanent wave solutions
2. Apply nail moisturizers to trap and bind water within the nail plate
   a. Use nail moisturizer with petrolatum to trap water and glycerin to attract water to the nail plate
   b. Increase the water-binding sites on nail keratin with urea or lactic acid
3. Increase oral biotin intake
4. Apply a fibered nail polish
5. Apply a nail hardener, but use with caution

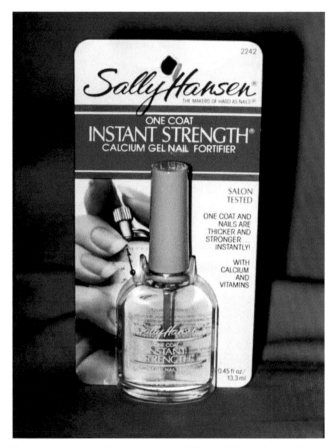

Figure 39.8 An example of a commercially available nail-strengthening product.

Nails are also dehydrated by the use of cleaning fluids that contain ammonia, bleach, and strong detergents (21). Contact with these substances may be necessary, but gloves should be worn to protect the nails from dehydration. It is worthwhile reminding the patient that only one contact with strong surfactants is necessary for dehydration to occur. Thus, consistency in hand protection is important.

> Nail moisturizers temporarily increase nail plate hydration by increasing water binding sites on nail keratin.

Nail moisturizers may temporarily increase nail plate hydration to prevent splitting. The products are usually creams or lotions containing occlusives, such as petrolatum, mineral oil, lanolin, etc (15). Humectants, such as glycerin, propylene glycol, and proteins, may also be added. Alpha-hydroxy acids, lactic acid, and urea are active ingredients used to increase the water-binding capacity of the nail plate. A well-formulated nail moisturizer should contain substances from all of the aforementioned groups to maximally treat the dehydrated nail plate.

A possible solution to nail splitting is oral supplementation with biotin (22). A variety of commercial products are available in tablet form. Biotin was originally used to prevent hoof splitting in racehorses by veterinarians and then adapted to humans. It is possible biotin deficiency may occur in the elderly where biotin transport across the gastrointestinal mucosa may be decreased. Furthermore, the highest concentration of biotin is found in egg whites, and elderly individuals typically limit their egg consumption due to elevated cholesterol issues. For this reason, it may be worthwhile for the physician to consider a biotin supplement (250 mg per day) in persons with brittle, splitting nails (22). There is no evidence that topical biotin added to nail moisturizers has a similar beneficial effect. There is also no evidence that topical gelatin, calcium, iron, botanical extracts, biological extracts, etc. are effective in treating brittle nails (23).

Nail cosmetics can also be used to prevent nail splitting. Nail polishes, as previously discussed, can increase the thickness of the nail plate thereby improving the ability of the nail to resist trauma. Since nail polish forms a flexible film, it can bend as the nail is deformed increasing resistance to fracture. The nail polish can add further strength to the nail by containing 1% nylon or rayon fibers. These polishes, termed fibered nail polishes, add further flexibility to the nail plate. They can be used as an alternative top coat in persons with extremely brittle nails. Nail polish may actually prevent nail plate dehydration by preventing detergent contact with the nail plate acting as a protectant and decreasing nail water vapor loss from 1.6 to 0.4 mg/cm²/hour (24).

> The main active ingredient in nail hardeners is the allergen formaldehyde.

Finally, products known as nail hardeners are available (Fig. 39.8). The main active ingredient in nail hardeners is formaldehyde, originally used in concentrations greater than 10% resulting in onycholysis, subungual hyperkeratosis, reversible subungual hemorrhage, and bluish discoloration of the nail plate (25–27). Formaldehyde is also a cause of allergic contact dermatitis (28,29). Recognition of this problem led to regulation prohibiting formaldehyde in concentrations greater than 5% in nail hardener preparations manufactured for interstate sale, as mandated by the U.S. FDA. Free formaldehyde in concentrations of 1–2% is still used, but acetates, toluene, nitrocellulose, acrylic and polyamide resins, substances found in the nail polishes previously discussed, are now used to structurally reinforce the nail plate.

Once the nail plate has split, there is little that can be done except to address the issues listed in Table 39.6 and wait for a new nail plate to grow. Sometimes the nail will split into the nail bed causing pain and bleeding. This can be aided with a nail repair technique called the tea bag repair.

Repairing Split Nails

A split nail can be repaired with a tea bag until new growth occurs.

A technique that can be safely recommended to patients to repair a painful split nail is the tea bag repair. This method can be used to repair a broken nail where the break occurs proximal to the nail free edge resulting in the removal of the nail from the nail bed. This type of broken nail is painful and a site of injury for infection. While the medical solution to this problem is new nail growth, a cosmetic repair can be helpful in alleviating pain and preventing infection. This technique utilizes a tea bag and clear nail polish and can be performed at home by the patient. The tea bag is cut and the tea leaves emptied to obtain the surrounding fiber paper. A small piece of fiber paper is cut to fit over the nail break and an additional 2 mm around the break. The broken nail is pushed back into place and covered with a layer of clear nail polish. The fibered paper is placed on the break and embedded in the clear nail polish followed by two to three extra coats. This technique reinforces the break with fibered paper held in place by nail polish as a semipermanent band aid until healing can occur.

This repair can be repeated, as the nail grows as often as necessary. It uses commonly found materials costing little. Most patients who experience this type of painful broken nail wear their nails too long. The easiest suggestion to remedy recurrent broken nails is to cut the nail such that the free edge cannot be visualized over the fingertip as viewed from the palm of the hand. While the patient may not take kindly to the suggestion that she wear shorter nails, this is the only clinically reproducible method for reducing broken nails of this type.

NAIL PEELING

Cutting the nail plate with a sharp scissors perpendicularly to the nail plate can prevent nail peeling.

Nail peeling, also known as onychoschizia, is lamellar splitting of the nail. The keratin peels from the nail tip in layers weakening the nail and catching on clothing. This condition is most commonly due to poor nail manicuring techniques. If the nail is not cut sharply perpendicular to the nail plate, nail peeling can occur. The steps in performing a nail manicure to prevent nail peeling are reviewed.

The main goal of a manicure is proper trimming of the nails to maintain a strong, healthy nail plate. The nail should be rounded at the tip for aesthetics, but the corners should be left square to maximize strength. Too sharp an arc extending from the lateral to medial nail margin will weaken the nail structurally resulting in nail plate fracture. Ideally, the nail plate should not be cut, but filed frequently with an orange stick to avoid cracking the nail plate through shearing forces generated by scissors or clippers. However, most patients groom their nails

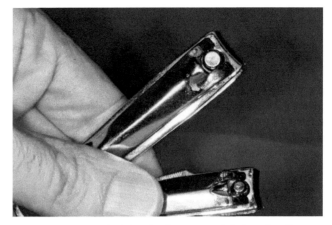

Figure 39.9 Properly designed nail cutters to minimize nail peeling.

infrequently necessitating cutting. Cutting should be done with a pair of curved nail clippers, since scissors may not cut the nail plate squarely (Fig. 39.9). An angle on the distal nail plate predisposes to nail peeling. Any remaining sharp edges should be filed with a diamond dust file (30). Under no circumstances should the cuticle be removed or traumatized as this may precipitate the formation of paronychia, onychomycosis, or onychodystrophy.

Nail peeling can also be minimized with nail polish. Once the nail is properly cut, a thin coat of clear nail polish is placed at the distal free edge and underneath the free edge. This placement protects the nail tip from the trauma that results in nail splitting. However, it should be mentioned that the removal of nail polish may also contribute to onychoschizia (31). Nail polish removers are liquids designed to strip nail polish from the nail plate. They may contain solvents such as acetone, alcohol, ethyl acetate, or butyl acetate. These solvents break down the nail polish film, but also dehydrate the nail plate contributing to brittle nails and nail peeling. Conditioning nail enamel removers are available, containing fatty materials such as cetyl alcohol, cetyl palmitate, lanolin, castor oil, or other synthetic oils. It is thought that these oily substances act as occlusive nail moisturizers retarding water evaporation, but they cannot totally prevent nail plate dehydration, if used frequently. Thus, nail polish should be properly applied, as discussed under the title, nail splitting.

ONYCHOLYSIS

The most common cosmetic cause of onycholysis is nail prostheses.

Onycholysis is removal of the nail plate from the nail bed, usually due to trauma. Onycholysis can also be seen in nail fungal infection, a condition known as onychomycosis. However this discussion will focus on onycholysis related to the use of cosmetic nail products.

The most common cause of onycholysis is the use of artificial nails, also known as nail prostheses. Onycholysis occurs because the bond between the artificial nail and the natural nail plate is stronger than the adhesion between the natural nail and nail bed (Fig. 39.10). Thus, minor trauma rips the nail

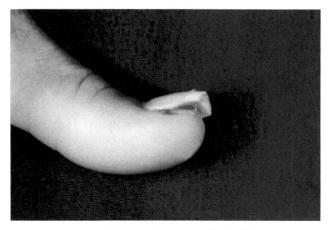

Figure 39.10 Onycholysis between the natural nail bed and the nail prosthesis.

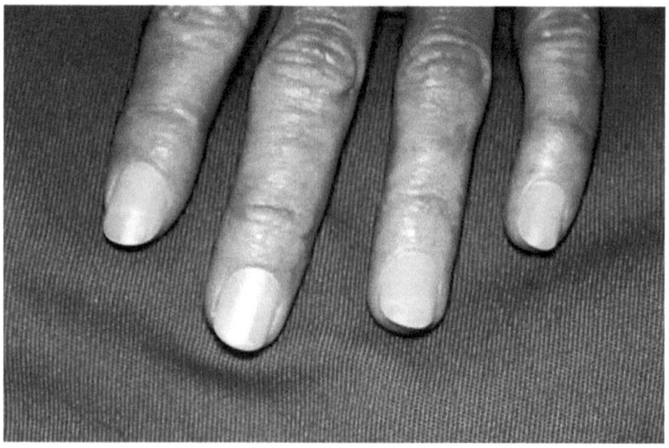

Figure 39.11 Press-on nails are the simplest at home application of nail prostheses.

from the nail bed, an injury that cannot be repaired until new nail growth occurs. Onycholysis can also occur due to sensitivity to the methacrylate polymer (32,33).

In addition to onycholysis, many patients are appalled at the broken, thinned, yellowed appearance of their nails following sculpture removal. This is due to interference with the nail's normal vapor exchange, nail plate trauma during the removal process, and damage to the underlying nail bed (34). While nail prostheses are extremely popular among women of all ages, they present an opportunity for the onset of nail disease. This section examines nail prostheses and their relevant dermatologic issues.

Preformed Nail Prostheses

The original artificial nail was a preformed piece of plastic that was glued over the natural nail plate with a methacrylate-based adhesive (35) (Fig. 39.11). These nails are still popular today and available in a variety of styles: precolored, uncolored, precut, and uncut. Preformed nails come in press-on, preglued forms and in forms requiring glue application, but the nails usually pop off before onycholysis can occur with trauma. The nails also come in a variety of sizes and shapes to match the patient's natural nail plate (36). Even with the variety available, most patients do not find a suitable preformed nail accounting for the increasing popularity of custom-made nail prostheses discussed next.

Custom Nail Prostheses

Sculptured nails are custom-made nail prostheses created on a template attached to the natural nail plate.

Custom-made nail prostheses are known as sculptured nails, an increasingly popular method of obtaining long, hard nails. The word "sculptured" is used since the custom-made artificial nail is sculpted on a template attached to the natural nail plate. The sculpted nail fits perfectly and, if well done, can be hard to differentiate from a natural nail. These sculptured nails are the most common cosmetic cause of onycholysis in women who present to the dermatologist.

The application technique is summarized in Table 39.7 (Fig. 39.12). The entire process takes 2 hours to create a set of

Table 39.7 Sculptured Nail Prosthesis Technique

1. All nail polish and oils are removed from the nail
2. The nail is roughened with a coarse emery board, pumice stone, or grinding drill to create an optimal surface for sculpted nail adhesion
3. An antifungal, antibacterial liquid, such as decolorized iodine, is applied to the entire nail plate to minimize onychomycosis and paronychia
4. The loose edges of the cuticle are either trimmed, removed, or pushed back depending on the operator
5. A flexible template is fit beneath the natural nail plate upon which the elongated sculpted nail will be built
6. The acrylic is mixed and applied with a paint brush to cover the entire natural nail plate and extended onto the template to the desired nail length. A clear acrylic is used over the natural nail plate attached to the nail bed so that the natural pink color shows through. A white acrylic is used from the nail plate's free edge distally
7. The nail prosthesis is sanded to a high shine
8. Nail polish, jewels, decals, decorative metal strips, and air brushed designs may be added, depending on the fashion tastes of the patient

10 fingernails. Originally, methyl methacrylate was the monomer used to fashion the nail, but its use has been discontinued due to its sensitizing potential. Currently, liquid ethyl or isobutyl methacrylate are utilized as the monomer and mixed with powdered polymethyl methacrylate polymer. The product is allowed to polymerize in the presence of a benzoyl peroxide accelerator and a formable acrylic is made which hardens in seven to nine minutes (37). Usually, hydroquinone, monomethyl ether of hydroquinone, or pyrogallol is added to slow down polymerization (38). The acrylic is then shaped to the length and fingernail style desired by the patient. The bond formed between the acrylic and the natural nail plate is extremely strong, since the nail plate is chemically and sometimes physically etched with a drill to increase the surface area over which polymerization can occur. It is for this reason that trauma usually separates the natural nail plate from the nail bed.

Many patients are not aware that the finished nail sculptures require more care than natural fingernails. With

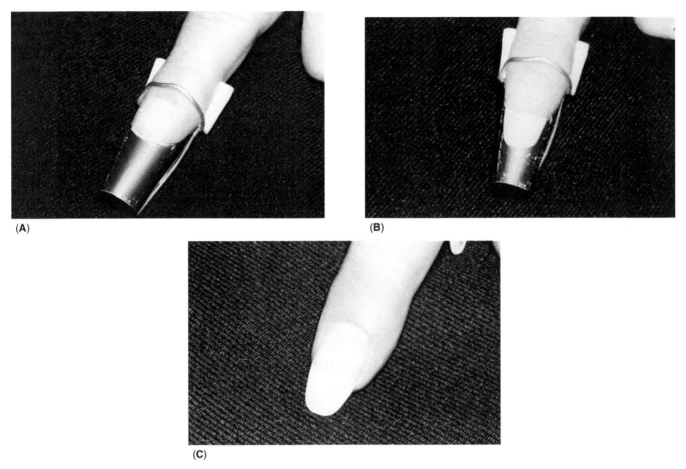

Figure 39.12 (**A**) A form is placed beneath the natural slide over which the nail prostheses will be formed. (**B**) The polymerized acrylate is formed over the natural nail plate and the form to create the illusion of nail length. (**C**) The finished appearance of the nail sculpture.

continued wear of the sculpture, the acrylic loosens from the natural nail, especially around the edges. These loose edges must be clipped and new acrylic should be applied approximately every three weeks, to prevent development of an environment for infection. The sculpture grows out with the natural nail plate, and more polymer material must be added proximally, depending on the nail growth rate. This procedure is known as "filling." Failure to undergo filling every 2 to 3 weeks will result in creation of a lever arm that predisposes to traumatic onycholysis or damage to the natural nail plate. If necessary, the sculptured nails can be removed by soaking in acetone.

Damage to the natural nail plate still occurs with nail sculpture use, even if the patient is conscientious. After two to four months of wear, the natural nail plate becomes yellowed, dry, and thin. Most operators prefer to allow the patient's natural nail to grow and act as a support for the sculpture. However, the nails become thin, bendable, and weak. For this reason, it is not advisable to wear sculptured nails for more than three months consecutively with a month's rest between applications.

Nail Sculptures with Preformed Tips

Preformed tips allow the creation of excessively long nails that can increase the chance for onycholysis.

A less time-consuming and less expensive method to make custom nail prostheses is to combine custom-made nail sculptures with preformed artificial tips (Fig. 39.13). This involves applying the liquid acrylic to the natural nail and embedding a preformed nail tip at the distal end. This method is used for patients who wish to have extremely long nails or nails embedded with numerous jewels. The possibility of developing traumatic onycholysis is enhanced with this variation due to the extreme length of the nails.

Photo-Induced Onycholysis

Photo-induced onycholysis can occur when patients on photosensitizing oral medications use photobonded sculptured nails.

A variation on nail sculptures, known as photobonded nails, can precipitate photo-induced onycholysis. This nail technique utilizes a UV cured acrylic sculpted on the natural nail. The nail is exposed to a magnesium light for one to two minutes. This technique is similar to restorative dental bonding, however a patient on photosensitizing oral medications, such as tetracycline or doxycycline, may experience photo-onycholysis (39) (Fig. 39.14). When the onycholysis does not involve the distal nail plate and nail sculptures are present, the physician should inquire as to the use of photobonded nails. In addition to photo-onycholysis, nails may get allergic contact dermatitis also.

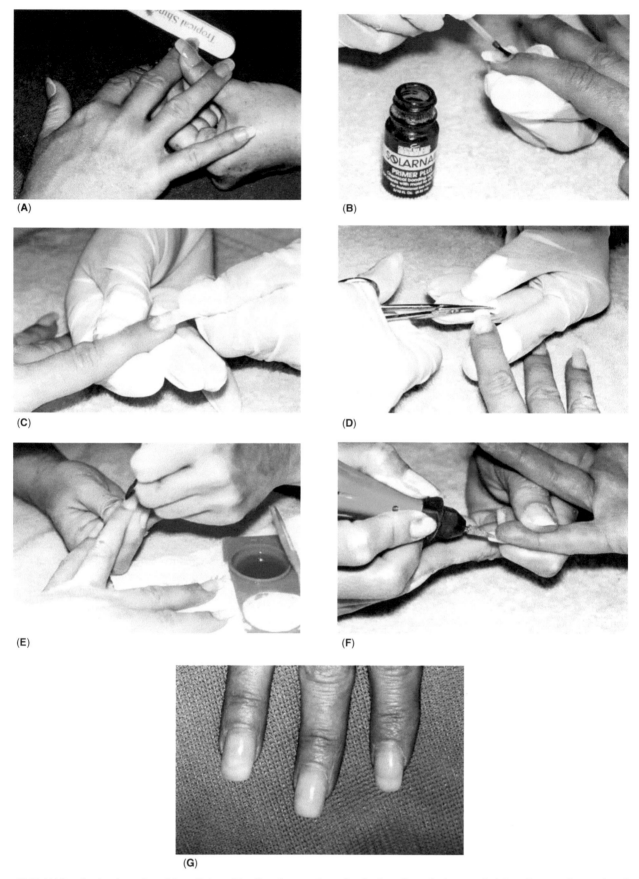

Figure 39.13 (**A**) Roughening the surface of the nail plate with a file to increase the surface for the nail prosthesis to attach. (**B**) Application of an antifungal solution to the natural nail plate to prevent infection. (**C**) Methacrylate-based glue is used to stick in the artificial nail to the natural nail plate. (**D**) Trimming of the artificial nail plate with scissors to the desired length. (**E**) Mixing of the powdered polymethyl methacrylate with the liquid isobutyl methacrylate to create a formable acrylic to fill the distance between the natural nail plate and the proximal nail fold. (**F**) A drill is used to smooth the natural nail plate in the prosthesis. (**G**) The finished appearance of a nail prosthesis.

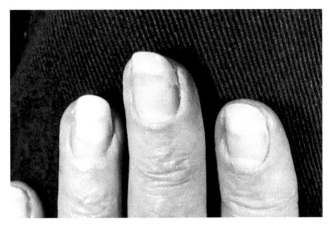

Figure 39.14 Photo-induced onycholysis.

ALLERGIC CONTACT DERMATITIS

Nail polish allergy may be observed not only in the fingers, but also around the eyes.

Patients with proximal nail fold erythema and edema, fingertip tenderness and swelling, and/or eyelid dermatitis should be evaluated for allergic contact dermatitis to nail products (40). The most common cause of allergic contact dermatitis of this type is nail polish allergy. The North American Contact Dermatitis Group determined that 4% of positive patch tests were due to toluene sulfonamide–formaldehyde resin used in nail polish, as discussed previously. Patients who are allergic to the toluene sulfonamide–formaldehyde resin should consider using hypoallergenic nail polish containing the alternative polyester resins, which are less allergenic (41). Even though the allergic reaction is most commonly due to wet nail enamel, Tosti et al. found 11 out of 59 patients who were patch test positive to wet polish, also reacted to the dried enamel (42). Allergic reactions can be severe necessitating time lost from work (43).

Patch testing to verify allergy to toluene sulfonamide/formaldehyde resin can be performed using the standard patch test tray or the patient's bottle of nail polish. Nail polish can be tested "as is," but should be allowed to thoroughly dry as the volatile solvent can cause an irritant reaction if not allowed to evaporate rapidly. The toluene sulfonamide/formaldehyde resin can be also tested alone in 10% petrolatum (44). Patients who are allergic to this resin should select hypoallergenic nail polishes (45).

The second most common cause of nail area allergic contact dermatitis is allergy to the methacrylates, which are used to glue artificial nails and create sculptured nail prostheses. Even though methyl methacrylate is no longer used, isobutyl, ethyl and tetrahydrofurfuryl methacrylate are still strong sensitizers (46,47). It is important to remember the polymerized, cured acrylic is not sensitizing, only the liquid methacrylate monomer (48). Therefore, a careful nail operator, who avoids skin contact with the uncured acrylic, can avoid sensitizing the patient. Patch testing should be performed in suspected sensitized individuals with methyl methacrylate monomer, 10% in olive oil, and methacrylate acid esters, 1% and 5% in olive oil and petrolatum (49).

CUTICLE PROBLEMS

A large proportion of cosmetic nail issues arise from the removal or trimming of the cuticle.

Cuticle problems are varied and can range from paronychial infection to irritant contact dermatitis. Most cuticle problems arise from removal of the tissue, since it is considered cosmetically unattractive. Perhaps the true reason the cuticle is removed, is to aid the nail artist in more easily painting the fingernails or applying nail prostheses. The cuticle can be removed chemically or physically. Chemical cuticle removers are formulated as liquids or creams and contain an alkaline substance to digest the keratin (50). They may contain sodium or potassium hydroxide, a common cause of irritant contact dermatitis, in a 2–5% concentration with propylene glycol or glycerin added as a humectant. Milder preparations can be made with trisodium phosphate or tetrasodium pyrophosphate, but they are also less effective (51).

A variant of cuticle removers are known as cuticle softeners. These are quaternary ammonium compounds in a 3–5% concentration, sometimes combined with urea, designed to soften the cuticular protein and facilitate mechanical removal. Mechanical removal consists of either trimming the softened cuticle or pushing the cuticle back with a plastic or wood stick. Aggressive physical removal of the cuticle can damage the nail matrix cells resulting in nail dystrophy, which can be temporary or permanent based on the severity of the injury.

Both chemical and physical cuticle removal results in breaking the watertight seal the cuticle provides between the proximal nail fold and the nail plate. Removal of the cuticle creates a potential space for water and other liquids to reside. Since it is difficult to dry this area, water accompanied by body warmth creates an environment for the growth of bacteria and yeast. Usually, the yeast colonization occurs first, setting the stage for subsequent bacterial infection and a paronychia. If the cuticle has been removed, isopropyl alcohol (rubbing alcohol) or acetic acid (vinegar) can aid in the evaporation of the water, preventing paronychial formation. Treatment with a medium-potency topical corticosteroid combined with a topical antifungal can aid in the resolution of a paronychia. However, if the lesion is draining pus, an oral antibiotic may be necessary.

The solution has to allow the cuticle to remain in place to prevent a paronychia, since it performs an important anatomic function. The physician may wish to establish a relationship with a nail technician who is willing to groom the nails without removing the cuticle. This is especially important in the patient who experiences recurrent or chronic paronychia.

INGROWN FINGERNAILS

Proper nail grooming can minimize the recurrence of ingrown nails.

Another frequently encountered medical nail problem is an ingrown fingernail. Ingrown fingernails are most commonly due to improper fingernail cutting. Most people with ingrown fingernails either bite their nails or cut their fingernails too short. Most people like to cut their fingernails in a gentle arc with the longest part of the nail in the center of the finger. This grooming method causes trouble at the sides of the fingernail where improper cutting can leave nail fragments that may ingrow.

The best way to cut fingernails is straight across with no curve. This leaves the sides longer making the nail too long to ingrow. If the nail should ingrow, I prefer to wrap a piece of Teflon dental tape beneath the ingrown nail lifting it out to the skin surface. Regular dental floss can also be used, but the Teflon is less likely to break and is smoother at the edges preventing skin trauma. The dental tape is then covered by an adhesive dressing, which can be replaced as necessary.

SUMMARY

An understanding of common nail problems and their treatment through medical and cosmetic techniques is important to the physician. Nail cosmetics can both cause disease and provide valuable camouflaging benefits. It has been said that nails are an indicator of social status, age, sex, and general health. Perhaps nail cosmetics are popular since they can conceal the underlying truth. The physician should never be hesitant to remove nail polish or an artificial nail in the office to adequately diagnose disease. For this reason, it is worthwhile to invest a dollar in a bottle of acetone-containing nail polish remover. The nail polish remover can be placed on a cotton ball and stroked over the nail to remove polish or poured into a crucible to soak off an artificial nail. It is important never to miss a diagnosis because of failure to visualize the natural nail plate.

REFERENCES

1. Mautner G, Scher RK. Yellow nail syndrome. J Geriatric Dermatol 1993; 1: 106–9.
2. Nelson LM. Yellow nail syndrome. Arch Dermatol 1969; 100: 499–500.
3. Venencie PY, Dicken GH. Yellow nail syndrome. J Am Acad Dermatol 1984; 10: 187–92.
4. Samman PD, White WF. The "yellow nail" syndrome. Br J Dermatol 1964; 76: 153–7.
5. Wimmer EP, Scholssman ML. The history of nail polish. Cosmet Toilet 1992; 107: 115–20.
6. Wing HJ. Nail preparations. In: deNavarre MG, ed. The chemistry and manufacture of cosemtics. Wheaton: Allured Publishing Corporation, 1988: 983–1005.
7. Schlossman ML. Nail-enamel resins. Cosmet Technol 1979; 1: 53.
8. Schlossman ML. Nail polish colorants. Cosmet Toilet 1980; 95: 31.
9. Samman PD. Nail disorders caused by external influences. J Soc Cosmet Chem 1977; 28: 351.
10. Daniel DR, Osmet LS. Nail pigmentation abnormalities. Cutis 1980; 25: 595–607.
11. Wilkinson JB, Moore RJ. Harry's cosmeticology. 7th edn. New York: Chemical Publishing, 1982: 371.
12. Lewis BL, Montgomery H. The senile nail. J Invest Dermatol 1955; 24: 11–18.
13. Cohen PR, Scher RK. Nail changes in the elderly. J Geriatic Dermatol 1993; 1: 45–53.
14. Mast R. Nail products. In: Whittam JH, ed. Cosmetic safety a primer for cosmetic scientists. New York: Marcel Dekker, Inc, 1987: 265–313.
15. Scher RK. Brittle nails. Int J Dermatol 1989; 28: 515–16.
16. Kechijian P. Brittle fingernails. Dermatol Clin 1985; 3: 412–29.
17. Silver H, Chiego B. Nail and nail changes. III Brittleness of nails (fragilitas unguium). J Invest Dermatol 1940; 3: 357–73.
18. Samman PD. Nail disorders caused by external influences. J Soc Cosmet Chem 1977; 28: 351.
19. Finlay AY, Frost P, Keith AD, Snipes W. Effects of phospholipids and water on brittleness of nails. In: Frost P, Horwitz SN, eds. Cosmetics for the dermatologist. St. Louis: CV Mosby, 1982: 175–80.
20. Finlay AY, Frost P, Keith AD, Snipes W. An assessment of factors influencing flexibility of human fingernails. Br J Dermatol 1980; 103: 357–65.
21. Cohen PR, Scher RK. Geriatic nail disorders: diagnosis and treatment. J Am Acad Dermatol 1992; 26: 521–31.
22. Hochman LG, Scher RK, Meyerson MS. Brittle nails: response to daily biotin supplementation. Cutis 1993; 51: 303–5.
23. Wing HJ. Nail preparations. In: Navarre MG, ed. The chemistry and manufacture of cosmetics. 2nd edn. Wheaton: Allured Publishing Company, 1988: 994–6.
24. Mast R. Nail products. In: Whittam JH, ed. Cosmetic safety a primer for cosmetic scientists. New York: Marcel Dekker, Inc, 1987: 265–313.
25. Jawny L, Spada FJ. Contact dermatitis to a new nail hardener. Arch Dermatol 1967; 95: 199.
26. Paltzik RL, Enscoe I. Onycholysis secondary to toluene sulfonamide formaldehyde resin used in a nail hardener mimicking onychomycosis. Cutis 1980; 25: 647–8.
27. Donsky HJ. Onycholysis due to nai hardener. Canadian Med Assoc J 1967; 96: 1375–6.
28. Lazar P. Reactions to nail hardeners. Arch Dermatol 1966; 94: 446–8.
29. Huldin DH. Hemorrhages of the lips secondary to nail hardeners. Cutis 1968; 4: 709.
30. Engasser PG, Matsunaga J. Nail cosmetics. In: Scher RK, Daniel CR, eds. Nails: therapy, diagnosis, surgery. Philadelphia: WB Saunders Company, 1990: 214–15.
31. Wallis MS, Bowen WR, Guin JD. Pathogenesis of onychoschizia (lamellar dystrophy). J Am Acad Dermatol 1991; 24: 44–8.
32. Goodwin P. Onycholysis due to acrylic nail applications. J Exp Dermatol 1976; 1: 191–2.
33. Lane CW, Kost LB. Sensitivity to artificial nails. Arch Dermatol 1956; 74: 671–2.
34. Baden H. Cosmetics and the nail. In diseases of the hair and nails. Yearbook Publishers, 1987: 99–102.
35. Baran R. Pathology induced by the application of cosmetics to the nails. In: Frost P, Horwitz SN, eds. Cosmetics for the dermatologist. CV Mosby, 1982: 182.
36. Brauer EW. Selected prostheses primarily of cosmetic interest. Cutis 1970; 6: 521–4.
37. Barnett JM, Scher RK, Taylor SC. Nail cosmetics. Dermatol Clin 1991; 9: 9–17.
38. Viola LJ. Fingernail elongators and accessory nail preparations. In: Balsam MS, Sagarin E, eds. Cosmetics, science and technology. 2nd edn. New York: Wiley-Interscience, 1972: 543–52.
39. Fisher AA. Adverse nail reactions and paresthesia from photobonded acrylate sculptured nails. Cutis 1990; 45: 293–4.
40. Scher RK. Cosmetics and ancillary preparations for the care of the nails. J Am Acad Dermatol 1982; 6: 523–8.
41. Adams RM, Maibach HI. A five-year study of cosmetic reactions. J Am Acad Dermatol 1985; 13: 1062–9.
42. Tosti A, Buerra L, Vincenzi C, et al. Contact sensitization caused by toluene sulfonamide-formaldehyde resin in women who use nail cosmetics. Am J Contact Dermatitis 1993; 4: 150.
43. Liden C, Berg M, Farm G, et al. Nail varnish allergy with far-reaching consequences. Br J Dermatol 1993; 128: 57–62.
44. deGroot AC, Weyland JW, Nater JP. Unwanted effects of cosmetics and drugs used in dermatology. 3rd edn. New York: Elsevier, 1994: 526.
45. Shaw S. A case of contact dermatitis from hypoallergenic nail varnish. Contact Dermatitis 1989; 20: 385.
46. Marks JG, Bishop ME, Willis WF. Allergic contact dermatitis to sculptured nails. Arch Dermatol 1979; 115: 100.
47. Fisher AA. Cross reactions between methyl methacrylate monomer and acrylic monomers presently used in acrylic nail preparations. Contact Dermatitis 1980; 6: 345–7.
48. Fisher AA, Franks A, Glick H. Allergic sensitization of the skin and nails to acrylic plastic nails. J Allergy 1957; 28: 84.
49. Baran R, Dawber RPR. The nail and cosmetics. In: Samman PD, Fenton DA, eds. The nails in disease. 4th edn. Chicago: Yearbook Publishers, 1986: 129.
50. Brauer E. Cosmetics: the care and adornment of the nail. In: Baran R, Dawber RPR, eds. Diseases of the nail and their management. Oxford: Blackwell, 1984: 289–92.
51. Wilkinson JB, Moore RJ. Harry's cosmeticology. 7th edn. New York: Chemical Publishing, 1982: 369–72.

SUGGESTED READING

Baran R. Nail cosmetics: allergies and irritation. Am J Clin Dermatol 2002; 3: 547–55.

Baran R, Schoon D. Nail beauty. J Cosmet Dermatol 2004; 3: 167–70.

Barnett JM, Scher RK, Taylor SC. Nail cosmetics. Dermatol Clin 1991; 9: 9–17.

Chang RM, Hare AQ, Rich P. Treating cosmetically induced nail problems. Dermatol Ther 2007; 20: 54–9.

Draelos ZD. Nail cosmetics issues. Dermatol Clin 2000; 18: 675–83.

de Berker DAR. Nails. Medicine 2004; 32: 32–5.

De Wit FS. An outbreak of contact dermatitis from toleuneseulfonamide formaldehyde resin in a nail hardener. Contact Dermatitis 1988; 18: 280–3.

Egawa M, Ozaki Y, Takahashi M. In vivo measurement of water content of the fingernails and its seasonal change. Skin Res Technol 2005; 12: 126–32.

Haneke E. Onychocosmeceuticals. J Cosmet Dermatol 2006; 5: 95–100.

Heising P, Austad J, Talberg HJ. Onycholysis induced by nail hardener. Contact Dermatitis 2007; 57: 280–1.

Kanerva L, Estlander T. Allergic onycholysis and paronychia caused by cyanoacrylate nail glue, but not by photobonded methacrylate nails. Eur J Dermatol 2000; 10: 223–5.

Lazzarini R, Duarte I, de Farias DC, Santos CA, Tsai AI. Frequency and main sites of allergic contact dermatitis caused by nail varnish. Dermatitis 2008; 19: 319–22.

Militello G. Contact and primary irritant dermatitis of the nail unit diagnosis and treatment. Dermatol Ther 2007; 20: 47–53.

Mowad CM, Ferringer T. Allergic contact dermatitis from acrylates in artificial nails. Dermatitis 2004; 15: 51–3.

Norton LA. Common and uncommon reactions to formaldehyde-containing nail hardeners. Semin Dermatol 1991; 10: 29–33.

Rich P. Nail cosmetics. Dermatol Clin 2006; 24: 393–9.

Rich P. Nail cosmetics and esthetics. Skin Pharmacol Appl Skin Physiol 1999; 12: 144–5.

Scher RK. Cosmetics and ancillary preparations for the care of nails. Composition, chemistry, and adverse reations. J Am Acad Dermatol 1982; 6(4 Pt 1): 523–8.

Schoon D. Nail varnish formulation (Chapter 20). In: Baran R, Maibach HI, eds. Textbook of cosmetic dermatology. 2nd edn. Martin Dunitz, 1988: 213–18.

Schoon D, Baran R. Cosmetics for nails (Chapter 44). In: Paye M, Barel AO, Maibach HI, eds. Handbook of cosmetic science and technology. 2nd edn. Informa Healthcare USA, Inc., 2007: 593–6.

Slodownik D, Williams JD, Tate BJ. Prolonged paresthesia due to sculptured acrylic nails. Contact Dermatitis 2007; 56: 298–9.

Vilaplana J, Romaguera C. Contact dermatitis from tosylamide/formaldehyde resin with photosensitivity. Contact Dermatitis 2000; 42: 311–12.

Wimmer E. Nail polishes (Chapter 27). In: Rieger MM, ed. Harry's cosmetology. 8th edn. Chemical Publishing Co., 2002: 573–88.

Yokota M, Thong HY, Hoffman CA, Maibach HI. Allergic contact dermatitis caused by tosylamide formaldehyde resin in nail varnish: an old allergen that has not disappeared. Contact Dermatitis 2007; 57: 277.

40 Understanding and treating brittle nails

There is one condition that is more challenging to treat than bullous pemphigoid or granuloma annulare, and it is simply known as "brittle nails." Most dermatologists have had this experience: the patient who has been treated for a major skin condition during an office visit asks as a quick end-of-visit aside for advice on her brittle nails. While at first glance brittle nails may appear to be a simple problem, treatment for this common condition is perplexing. It may even be argued that brittle state is a variant of normal change associated with aging and should not even be considered a problem worthy of treatment. Nevertheless, a few ideas on why brittle nails occur and how to effectively minimize the problem are worthwhile.

This chapter examines the physiology behind brittle nails and presents suggestions on how to prevent the condition. Nail problems are particularly challenging to treat, since the non-living nail cannot be healed and can only be replaced by new growth. This new growth occurs slowly, requiring six months or longer for a new fingernail to be produced. Treating nail problems never results in immediate gratification requiring faith on the part of the patient, who eventually heeds to the dermatologic advice for a positive outcome.

NAIL PHYSIOLOGY

Brittle nails are the equivalent of xerotic eczema. Water is the plasticizer of both the nails and the skin. Dehydrated nails become brittle and fractured while dehydrated skin cracks and flakes exposing the underlying nerve endings to the environment, precipitating itching. While topical corticosteroid anti-inflammatories accompanied by moisturizers are the mainstay of eczema treatment, only moisturizers can be used in the treatment of brittle nails. A barrier composed of corneocytes and intercellular lipids maintains the water content of the skin at 30%. Healing of the skin usually occurs within two weeks, which is the turnover time for the stratum corneum. Simply put, the nails do not heal.

At 30% water content, the nails are overhydrated and soft, which is different from skin. The optimal water content for the nails is 16%, but this varies with ambient humidity. Under conditions of 20% relative humidity, the water content of the nails drops to 7%. Proper hydration is key, as water allows the nails to bend without fracturing. Problems arise when the water is lost, because it is not possible to permanently replace the water. Nail soaking results in enhanced water loss, not rehydration.

> The water content of a proper nail is 16%.

PREVENTING BRITTLE NAILS

The best treatment for brittle nails is prevention of damage to the newly growing nail plate. Nails become dehydrated with exposure to surfactants and solvents. When the hands are washed, so are the nails. Once piece of advice for patients is to wash their hands, but avoid placing surfactant on the nails unless they require cleansing. Hand sanitizers, which are replacing hand washing, are very damaging to the nail plate. The combination of the rapidly evaporating vehicle and the triclosan both cause water loss. All soaps and household cleansers cause nail water loss making glove protection of the nails essential.

> Dehydration from nail exposure to surfactants and solvents is the most common cause of brittle nails.

STRENGTHENING BRITTLE NAILS

Many cosmetic techniques are available to strengthen nails, as this is a profitable market. The common products are nail hardeners that contain formaldehyde. Formaldehyde works to harden nails by cross-linking the keratin protein. While this cross-linking makes the keratin harder, it can also paradoxically make the nails more brittle. Thus, nail hardeners are not recommended for strengthening brittle nails.

Perhaps the best way to strengthen brittle nails rests with nail polish. Nail polish places a protective film over the nail plate that thickens the nail. The flexible nail polish polymer, which may be toluene sulfonamide resin or polyester, also increases nail flexibility and acts as a barrier to nail water contact. Problems arise, however, when the nail polish must be removed. Both acetone-containing and acetone-free nail polish removers dehydrate the nail plate. Thus, nail polish can be used in the treatment of brittle nails, but should be removed as infrequently as possible (Fig. 40.1).

Some also advocate the use of nail prostheses in brittle nail treatment. While it is true that artificial nails can protect the underlying nail plate, removal of the prostheses is always traumatic to the nail. With prolonged wearing, oxygen transport is decreased and the nail weakens. While prostheses can be worn for a limited time, continued use for the treatment of brittle nails is not recommended.

> Nail polish may be helpful in placing a polymer coating over brittle nails to increase flexibility.

DIET AND BRITTLE NAILS

Some also believe that brittle nails can be improved through dietary modification. Nails are pure protein, thus adequate protein intake is necessary for healthy nails. Many strict vegetarians find their nails to be one of the first places to show the effects of incomplete protein ingestion. Biotin has also been implicated as necessary for healthy nails. Egg whites are the richest source of biotin and many individuals do not consume eggs. Nutritionists also believe that biotin absorption across the small intestine decreases with advancing age. This is the rationale for providing biotin supplementation as part of nail health in mature individuals.

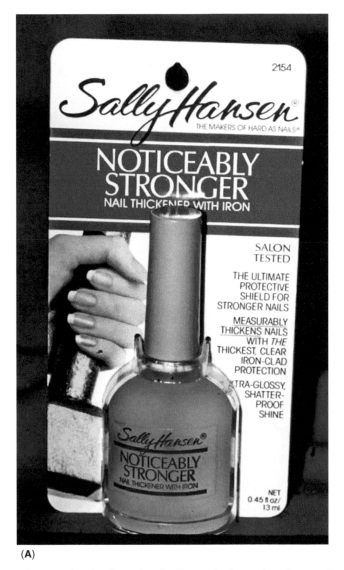

(A)

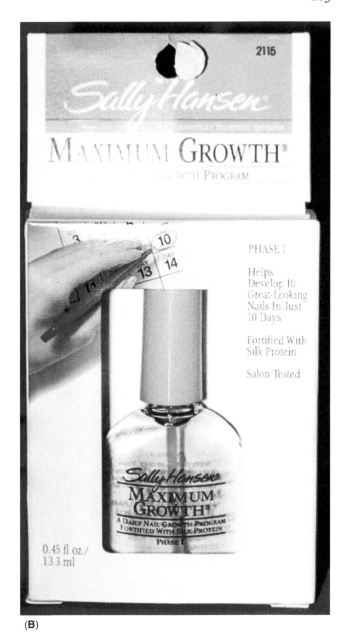

(B)

Figure 40.1 (**A, B**) Nail growth and nail-strengthening products that are primarily nail polishes, but contain other ingredients to support their marketing claim.

The use of biotin in human nails was adapted from the veterinary use of biotin in racehorses. If the hoof of a racehorse splits, it ends the career of the animal. Veterinarians supplement horse diets with biotin believing that it prevents hoof cracking. Whether biotin is useful in humans to prevent nail splitting has not been proven in large double-blind placebo controlled studies.

Adequate protein intake is necessary for good nail plate formation, which may not be present in strict vegetarian diets.

NAIL MOISTURIZATION

Perhaps the best way to treat dehydrated brittle nails is with a moisturizer. Two ingredients have the greatest efficacy: urea

and lactic acid. Both urea and lactic acid are classified as humectants because they increase the water-holding capacity of the nail. This occurs from the digestion of nail keratin that opens up water-binding sites and enhances hydration. The hydration is only temporary, however, requiring continued moisturizer application.

The urea concentration should be between 5 and 20%. And 20–40% urea digests too much of the nail keratin and softens the nails. Remember that 40% urea is used to avulse toenails. The lactic acid concentration should be between 5 and 10%. Twice-daily application of the urea or lactic acid preparation is sufficient, as too frequent application will damage the nail plate. More frequent use of nonmedicated moisturizers rich in glycerin and petrolatum can be used each time the hands are washed.

Urea and lactic acid are humectants that increase nail hydration by opening up water-binding sites on nail keratin.

Table 40.1 Brittle Nails Summary

Nails require hydration for flexibility
Too much or too little nail water causes problems
Nail polish and nail prostheses provide only temporary nail strength improvement
Biotin may be a useful dietary supplement
Any change in nail treatment will take 3–6 mon to see results
Avoid nail exposure to triclosan, solvents, household cleaners
Wear gloves
Apply urea or lactic acid to increase water-binding sites on nail keratin

SUMMARY

Brittle nails are indeed a perplexing problem. The basic concepts surrounding brittle nails are summarized in Table 40.1. Prevention is as important as treatment for brittle nails. This article has presented the nail physiology accounting for brittle nails and ideas for prevention. Prevention is perhaps the best treatment, but other options have also been discussed. It is hoped that this article has demystified brittle nails offering insight for the next patient challenge.

SUGGESTED READING

Baran R, Schoon D. Nail fragility syndrome and its treatment. J Cosmet Dermatol 2004; 3: 131–7.
Kechijian P. Brittle fingernails. Dermatol Clin 1985; 3; 421–9.
Stern DK, Diamantis Smith E, Wei H, et al. Water content and other aspects of brittle versus normal fingernails. J Am Acad Dermatol 2007; 7: 31–6.

41 Cosmetics in nail disease

Cosmetics can be of use in nail disease to provide camouflaging or to restore a damaged nail plate to functionality. Anyone who has had a nail torn or ripped can identify with the pain associated with nail damage. Many persons with nail disease experience this same type of discomfort until the nail can be repaired. Since nails are nonliving, nail repair can take three to six months depending on the rate of growth; however, in the case of nail disease no improvement may be expected for longer. The cosmetic solutions for nail problems are summarized in Table 41.1.

PSORIATIC NAILS

One of the most common nail diseases seen by the dermatologist is nail psoriasis characterized by minor as nail pitting to dramatic nail plate disintegration. The severity of nail disease in nail psoriasis is quire variable. Minor nail pitting results in the irregularity of the nail plate. This can be easily corrected by applying a thin layer of nail sculpture polymer over the nail plate in a procedure known as "shellacking." The term comes from the shellac shiny finish placed over wood to seal the porous material and provide a waterproof protective covering. Shellacking provides the same benefits to psoriatic nails. Just like in the nail prostheses, previously discussed in chapter 39, liquid ethyl or isobutyl methacrylate are utilized as the monomer and mixed with powdered polymethyl methacrylate polymer. The shellac is allowed to polymerize in the presence of a benzoyl peroxide accelerator and a formable acrylic is made which hardens in seven to nine minutes (1). The acrylic is then painted over the fingernail in a thin coating and not used to elongate the fingernail. The acrylic can be pigmented with any color desired to camouflage the underlying nail to create a smooth shiny fashionable nail appearance for persons with mild nail psoriasis. The coating also strengthens the nail and prevents further pits from occurring due to reduced nail trauma.

For persons with more severe nail psoriasis involving breakdown of the entire nail plate, cloth wraps can be used to strengthen and create a nail plate for adornment. A simple nail acrylic will not be able to create a smooth surface and the nail will not be strong enough to resist flaking and cracking. Cloth wraps provide reinforcement across the entire nail plate, but are most appropriate for female patients (Fig. 41.1). A cloth wrap is created by placing a layer of acrylic over the nail plate, as described previously. Before acrylic dries, a piece of silk or linen material is placed in the acrylic sized to fit the nail. Once this dries in place, another layer of acrylic is placed on top to imbed the cloth between two acrylic layers (Fig. 41.2). The nail can then be painted to camouflage the cloth. This technique is very effective in severely dystrophic female psoriatic nails.

Shellac or cloth wraps can be used to camouflage the nail pitting characteristic of psoriasis.

MYCOTIC NAILS

Mycotic nails combine nail thickening, subungual debri, and nail discoloration. The nail thickening and subungual debri can be minimized by proper pedicuring. The nails should be soaked for at least 30 minutes in a pan of warm water with a few drops of liquid dishwashing detergent. The soaking will soften the dystrophic nail plate and subungual debris. The nail can be trimmed with a double action nail cutter and the subungual debri can be removed with a nail spatula. Certainly, an oral antifungal therapy should be considered, but a nail prosthesis can be used temporarily. One of the easiest ways to camouflage the abnormal mycotic nail bed is to employ a French manicure, which is appropriate for both male and female patients. A French manicure utilizes a number of colored nail enamels to simulate the natural appearance of unpainted nail. Initially, the nail is painted with an unpigmented opaque base coat to cover the discoloration. A light pink enamel is then added to the entire nail plate followed by white enamel to the tip, simulating the nail free edge. Lastly, a clear top coat is applied to prevent enamel chipping. French manicures can be performed professionally by a manicurist or with kits available for home use. This type of artistic recreation of a normal nail plate is effective following a pedicure in patients with mycotic nails (Fig. 41.3).

A French manicure can restore a discolored mycotic nail to a more normal appearance in male and female patients.

NAIL DYSTROPHY

Nail dystrophy is an inherited or acquired nail condition involving all 20 nails or selective fingernails and toenails. The cause of the condition is poorly understood, but nail dystrophy can be a presenting finding of several dermatologic conditions that are beyond the scope of this text. One method that can be used to camouflage dystrophic nails is known as "photobonding." Photobonded nails are a variation on cured acrylic sculptured nails, which has been discussed in chapter 39. Photobonding refers to light curing of the acrylic instead of chemical curing. More recently, photobonded nails are referred to as "gel nails" because the acrylic is a clear gel squeezed out of a tube and allowed to dry under a magnesium light for one to two minutes. This same type of photobonding is used in dentistry to seal children's teeth protecting them from decay. However, photo-onycholysis and paresthesias have been reported as a result of this procedure (2). In summary, photobonding is an excellent solution to male or female nail dystrophy resulting in a smooth nail plate with a restored nail shape.

Photobonding can smooth the surface and restore shape to dystrophic nails.

Table 41.1 Cosmetic Techniques for Damaged Nails

Damage	Possible cosmetic cause	Possible cosmetic solution
Nail color		
Yellowish stain	Nail polish containing D & C Reds No. 6, 7, 34, 5 Lake	Discontinue nail polish
Poor nail color	Numerous medical conditions	French manicure technique
Nail Structure		
Onychoschizia lamellina	Nail plate dehydration	Application of lactic acid- or urea-containing cream
Mild median canal dystrophy	Trauma	Sculptured nail with linen wrap
Uneven nail surface contour	Trauma to nail matrix	Artificial or sculpture nails
Nail fragility	Numerous medical conditions, idiopathic	Fiber nail polish
Nail thinning	Nail sculptures worn too long	Remove nail sculptures
Nail dystrophy	Numerous medical conditions, idiopathic	Sculptured nails
Broken nail	Trauma	"Tea bag repair" technique

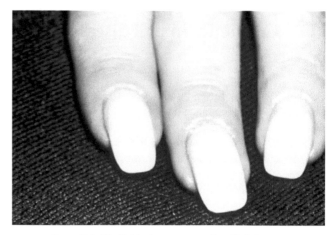

Figure 41.2 The finished appearance of a nail cloth wrap.

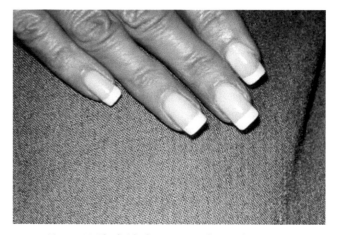

Figure 41.3 The finished appearance of a French manicure.

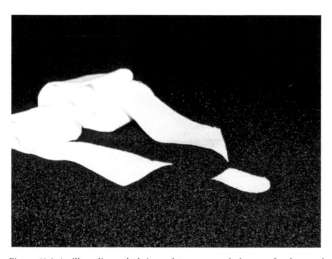

Figure 41.1 A silk or linen cloth is used to create a cloth wrap for damaged nails.

MEDIAN CANAL DYSTROPHY AND HABIT TIC DEFORMITY

Median canal dystrophy and habit tic deformity may result in nail plate damage (3,4). External trauma including nail biting, occupational damage, and exposure to harsh chemicals or solvents may also be problematic (5). Nail biting and habit tic picking are difficult to treat in the unmotivated patient; however, nail enamel can act as a deterrent to manipulation, since picking damages the enamel, which is time consuming to apply.

Nail deformity can also be repaired so that the nail does not catch on clothing or interfere with the use of the hands. A temporary, effective, inexpensive solution known as the "tea bag repair," requires a tea bag and fiber clear nail polish; this is discussed in chapter 39. The broken edges of the nail are reapproximated and the entire nail painted with fiber clear nail polish. A piece of tea bag paper, or other fiber paper, is then cut and shaped to fit over the nail surface and embedded in the wet polish. Several more nail polish coats are subsequently applied. This repair covers the rough broken nail edge and provides strength. The repair can be removed with fingernail polish remover and reapplied as the repair wears. If a more professional solution is desired, the cloth wraps discussed under nail psoriasis can also be used.

A tea bag can temporarily assist patients with median canal dystrophy where the nail edges are not easily approximated.

SUMMARY

Nail surface contour abnormalities result from a variety of medical conditions and may be temporary or permanent. Temporary abnormalities may be seen after the treatment of a paronychia or hand dermatitis, involving the proximal nail fold, or longer lasting, as in psoriasis. For patients who are bothered by poor nail appearance, only sculptured nails can offer a solution. The use of sculptured nails in these patients requires a skilled operator and a motivated patient. Poorly applied or poorly maintained nail sculptures could result in worsening of the nail abnormality. The physician should personally visit a number of nail sculpturing salons and select an operator for patient referral who upholds the highest standards of hygiene. It is also important that the artist work with the physician and accept suggestions for nail grooming. In these patients, the cuticle should never be removed and meticulous care must be taken to avoid contact of liquid acrylic with skin. If a suitable salon cannot be found in the community, patients should not undergo cosmetic nail reconstruction. Patient safety and the cosmetic results are only as good as the skill and intellect of the nail artist.

REFERENCES

1. Barnett JM, Scher RK, Taylor SC. Nail cosmetics. Dermatol Clin 1991; 9: 9–17.
2. Fisher AA. Adverse nail reactions and paresthesia from photobonded acrylate sculptured nails. Cutis 1990; 45: 293–4.
3. Baden HP. The physical properties of nail. J Invest Dermatol 1970; 55: 115–22.
4. Scott DA, Scher RK. Exogenous factors affecting the nails. Dermatol Clin 1985; 3: 409–13.
5. Samman PD. Nail disorders caused by external influences. J Soc Cosmet Chem 1977; 28: 351.

SUGGESTED READING

Baran R. Nail beauty therapy: an attractive enhancement or a potential hazard? J Cosmet Dermatol 2002; 1: 24–9.
Baran R. Nail cosmetics: allergies and irritations. Am J Clin Dermatol 2002; 3: 547–55.
Baran R, Andre J. Side effects of nail cosmetics. J Cosmet Dermatol 2005; 4: 204–9.
Baran R, Schoon D. Cosmetics for abnormal and pathological nails (Chapter 22). In: Baran R, Maibach HI, eds. Textbook of cosmetic dermatology. 2nd edn. Martin Dunitz Ltd, 1998: 233–44.
Dahdah MJ, Scher RK. Nail diseases related to nail cosmetics. Dermatol Clin 2006; 24: 233–9.
Iorizzo M, Piraccini BM, Tosti A. Nail cosmetics in nail disorders. J Cosmet Dermatol 2007; 6: 53–8.
Rich P. Nail cosmetics and camouflaging techniques. Dermatol Ther 2001; 14: 228–36.

42 Children and nail cosmetic issues

SOFT NAILS

The nail plate of children is not as thick or as well keratinized as an adult nail plate. Because the nails are soft, they are easily torn. Traditional nail clippers do not work well on children's nails for this reason. The nail plate cannot be easily broken because it tends to bend. It is better to cut the nails of children with scissors; however, this may be impractical in children who refuse to sit still. Sometimes it is best to simply tear the soft nail plate with the fingers.

Many parents are concerned that the nails of their child become floppy when they grow long. This is normal. I would not advise painting the fingernails with nail polish to make them stronger. Most young children put their fingernails in their mouth and may ingest the nail polish, which is not recommended.

> Soft nails are normal in a child and do not require treatment.

NAILS AND FINGER SUCKING

Continuous wetting of the nail plate from finger sucking can cause unusual nail deformities that may be concerning to parents. The overhydrated nail plate may be very soft and dissolve, but will regrow because the nail matrix remains intact. Further, the overhydrated nail plate may appear an opaque white color. This results from nail keratin hydration, but is reversible once the nail plate returns to its normal state of hydration.

Many parents are concerned about thumb or finger sucking because of dentition and speech problems. Sometimes the child will discard the behavior with maturity, but other children hang onto the habit. The most effective way I have found to break the habit is by painting a thin nail lacquer containing capsaicin on the nail of the digit favored for sucking. The capsaicin is released from the lacquer into the mouth with moisture and creates an unpleasant taste without damaging the mouth. This type of aversion therapy seems to be effective in most children, since thumb and/or finger sucking is a subconscious habit.

> Thumb or finger sucking may be a subconscious habit that can be broken with a taste aversive nail lacquer.

NAIL TRIMMING

Nail trimming can be a big challenge for parents of an active toddler. Several ideas for nail trimming have been presented earlier such as simply tearing the soft nail plate. If this is not possible, the parent can carefully bite the nail away without hurting the child in a playful game followed by filing the nail plate with a soft orange stick (Fig. 42.1). Scissors could scare the child and make nail cutting difficult while awake. The parent could consider cutting the nails carefully with scissors while the child is sleeping, or purchasing a nail clipper specifically designed for children. The arc of an adult nail clipper is too large to trim small nails. Remember, however, that soft nails cannot be broken with a nail clipper.

> The nails of a young child could be trimmed while sleeping.

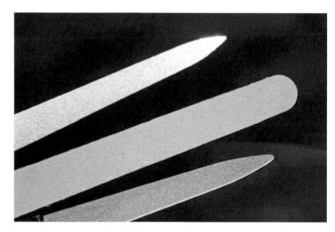

Figure 42.1 Examples of nail files that can be used to groom nails. The recommended orange stick nail file is shown in the middle.

SUMMARY

Nail cosmetics should be largely avoided in children. Children grow fingernails very rapidly so most problems resolve without the need for treatment. The best advice you can give to worried parents is that the nails will normalize as the child matures.

43 Toenails and cosmetic issues

Toenails are most important for protection of the tender tissues at the tip of the toes, yet most women prize them for their cosmetic value rather than their physiologic purpose. Toenails grow slower than fingernails with progressive slowing in growth with advancing age. Regrowth of a new great toenail can take six months to one year requiring patience on the part of the dermatologist and patient while addressing toenail problems. This chapter examines cosmetic issues associated with the toenail and presents cosmetic remedies for consideration.

TOENAIL DYSTROPHY

Toenail dystrophy can take the form of nail thickening, nail ridging, or onycholysis. Many times all of the findings are observed simultaneously. The most common cause of nail thickening is trauma, followed by fungal infection, which is discussed in the next section. Trauma to the toenail that is transmitted to the nail matrix results in the thickening of the nail plate and sometimes horizontal ridging, if the trauma is severe. This trauma occurs usually due to the tip of the toenail receiving a vertical head-on impact from the toe box of the shoe. This trauma can be due to wearing shoes that are too short or the foot moving forward in the shoe during walking, running, or other athletic activity. Patients with a narrow heal and wide-toe spread encounter more problems because the heel of the shoe is too large when a shoe is purchased to accommodate the width of the foot across the base of the toes. The toenail thickening can be remedied by placing a piece of adhesive foam in the shape of figure 8 in the heel of the shoe. This takes up the extra space and holds the foot in place. These shoe inserts can be purchased at most of the shoe stores. Alternatively, tie shoes tend to hold the foot in place better than slip-on shoes, thus shoe selection may also help.

Certain athletic activities also predispose to toenail thickening. These include tennis, where the toe is dragged across the ground during serving, and sports that involve kicking a ball, such as football and soccer. Basketball players also experience toenail thickening when the toe is banged against the toe box with rapid pivoting during blocking and shooting. A solution to toenail thickening in these sports is taken from ballet pointe shoes. Lamb's wool is placed in the tip of the toe shoe to prevent the toenail from digging into the shoe and to prevent toenail injury. Similarly, lamb's wool can be placed in the athletic shoe to prevent toenail thickening. Lamb's wool is preferred over cotton or other textiles because it is stiff, yet soft, and does not pack down in the shoe with wearing.

If the toenail injury is severe, horizontal grooves may also appear in the toenail. It is very hard to camouflage these grooves with nail polish. The best solution to improving appearance in thickened, grooved nails is to file the nail with a sequential file. A sequential file has sand paper of different textures. The coarse file is used first to smooth out the grooves and thin the nail. The remaining finishing files use finer and finer grades of sand paper to progressively shine the nail by smoothing the surface. Filing can improve nail smoothness, but also increase nail transparency by removing the opaque poor quality nail keratin. Once the nail has been filed smooth, nail polish can be applied to achieve a better cosmetic result.

While toenail trauma of the type previously discussed is usually seen in the great toenails, it can also be seen in other toenails for different reasons. For example, in persons with an athlete's toe, where the second toe is longer than the great toe, thickening and ridging will be preferentially seen in this digit. In addition, in persons with a wide foot or a little toe that rolls laterally with walking, the little toenail will also thicken. The little toenail is the second most common toenail to thicken. Usually the thickening is due to the little toe being squeezed out in shoes, especially in shoes with a pointed toe and a high heel. The foot moves forward in the heel and the little toenail is tightly pressed against the toe box. The remedy for this situation is to recommend avoidance of heels and a square toe box with ample room for the little toe. Many patients select their footwear based on fashion. This may not be the best approach. The shoes should be purchased that fit the foot. The foot should not be deformed to fit the shoe! This is how toenail problems arise. The dermatologists have no true effective treatment for shoe-induced toenail trauma except to recommend that the patient select better-fitting shoes.

Severe injury to the toenail can result in onycholysis, which is the lifting of the nail plate from the nail bed. This is especially painful on the toenails because the nail plate continues to be traumatized with walking and other activities. Once the nail plate has been lifted, it cannot reattach, much to the patient's dismay. The nail bed immediately keratinizes when the toenail is lifted so there is no tissue available for reattachment. The best solution is to cut the torn toenail away, but this is not always possible as the toenail may be irregularly attached. The best solution, in a patient who is not methacrylate allergic, is to drip some methacrylate-based super glue beneath the nail plate, pressing and holding the nail plate against the nail bed until the glue has polymerized. This will prevent the nail from ripping further and also reduce pain. It will not help with appearance, since the nail will have an air interface and appear white. Nail polish can be used to camouflage the onycholysis, if the patient desires.

> The most common cause of toenail dystrophy is ill-fitting shoes.

FUNGAL INFECTION

Nail fungus is the most common medical cause of nail dystrophy. The best treatment is oral medication to incorporate an antifungal barrier into the nail plate and prevent further infection spreading from the distal free edge of the nail plate to the proximal nail plate. Terbinafine is most commonly used for this purpose, but the mycotic nail plate must grow out for a normal nail plate to be present. This can take about three to six months or longer, depending on the percentage of the nail plate involved. Some patients may request a cosmetic solution to nail improvement while waiting for the oral antifungal to take effect. Sequential nail filing, as described above for nail dystrophy, may be used to thin the nail plate, which can then be painted with nail polish to camouflage the infection. More deeply pigmented nail polishes, such as burgundy, brown, or black, provide the best camouflage. Alternatively, nail prostheses can be applied to the mycotic nail, a topic discussed later in this chapter under cosmetic issues.

Patients may also be bothered by the smell and appearance of the subungual debris beneath the mycotic nail. This debris can be more easily removed after soaking the foot and nail in water with a triclosan-containing surfactant. Triclosan is found in all deodorant liquid soaps, such as Dial hand soap, or in surgical scrubs, such as Septisol. Advise the patient to add a generous amount of the triclosan-containing surfactant to some warm water until it foams. Soak the foot every evening in the basin for 30 minutes using a nail file to gently remove any loosened nail debris. The odor is in part due to bacterial colonization of the potential space between the nail plate and the nail bed. The triclosan will kill the bacteria thereby reducing odor. This is the same effect triclosan has in deodorant soaps to reduce axillary odor. Manual debridement is also important to remove the keratin food source for organisms growing beneath the nail plate. Finally, clear vinegar can be dropped beneath the nail plate to remove any remaining water and lower the pH beneath the nail to inhibit organism growth. The judicious use of this at-home self-administered pedicure can aid in the treatment of onychomycosis.

A 30-minute soak of mycotic toenails in the triclosan-containing surfactant can reduce nail odor.

INGROWN TOENAILS

Ingrown toenails are another complex dermatologic problem with poor treatment options. One of the most important considerations is to analyze why the ingrown toenail occurred and then take steps to prevent recurrence. Typically, the great toenail ingrowth occurs due to trauma, ill-fitting shoes, improper nail grooming, or cutting the toenails too short. It is important to identify the cause of the ingrown nail to allowing healing to occur and prevent recurrence. I find that educating the patient on proper nail cutting is very helpful. Most people like to cut their toenails in a gentle arc with the longest part of the nail in the center of the toe, similar to the technique used for fingernail cutting. This grooming method causes trouble on the toenails, but not on the fingernails, because the feet are forced into rigid shoes compressing the toenail against the skin.

The best way to cut the toenails when they frequently grow inward and cause pain, sometimes accompanied by infection, is to cut the sides of the nail longer than the center. This arc is opposite to the arc created by the toe pad. When the nail is shorter in the center, and pressure is applied to the nail, the corners of the nail move out, instead of moving in toward the skin. This alternation in nail mechanics prevents the nail from growing inward. It is also more difficult for the sides of the nail to grow inward when they are longer.

Once the nail has ingrown, the best way to encourage the nail to grow properly is to place a small ball of cotton under the nail that is entering the skin. The cotton will elevate the nail and allow it to grow beyond the surrounding edematous tissue. It is easiest for the dermatologist to insert the cotton in small amounts with a toothless Adson–Brown forcep, pushing as far under the nail as possible with minimal pain. If the cotton becomes dislodged, it can be replaced by the patient, who can participate in the process in the office.

Once the nail begins to grow out, the cotton ball can be replaced with Teflon dental tape. The dental tape is placed beneath the nail to continue to lift the nail above the surrounding tissue to prevent a recurrence of the ingrown nail.

Ingrown toenails can be prevented by properly cutting the toenails longer at the edges than at the center.

COSMETIC ISSUES

The use of nail polish in camouflaging toenail issues has already been covered in the preceding discussion, but the use of toenail prostheses is increasing at a rapid rate (Fig. 43.1). Since toenails come in sizes and shapes that are more varied than fingernails, custom-made sculptured nails are popular. The sculptured toenail is made in a fashion similar to sculptured fingernails as detailed in Table 43.1 (1). I recommend that my patients take their own toenail grooming instruments to the nail salon to prevent infection. Toenail instruments may be contaminated with fungi because persons with onychomycosis frequently go to nail salons since they cannot cut their toenails by themselves. This increases the chance of contracting onychomycosis.

The toenail sculptures must be groomed every three weeks, depending on the nail growth, or onycholysis may occur. The loosened polymer must be replaced by a new one to cover the proximal new nail. Allergic contact dermatitis may also occur in methacrylate-sensitive patients even though methyl methacrylate is no longer used; isobutyl, ethyl, and tetrahydrofurfuryl methacrylate are still strong sensitizers (2,3). But it should be emphasized that the polymerized, cured acrylic is not sensitizing, only the liquid monomer (4). Therefore, a careful

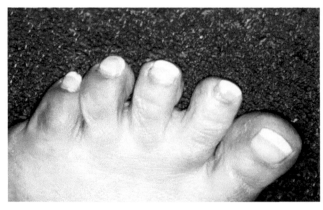

Figure 43.1 An example of toenail prostheses.

Table 43.1 Toenail Nail Sculpture Prostheses

1. The nail is roughened with a coarse emery board, pumice stone, or grinding drill to create an optimal surface for sculpted nail adhesion

2. An antifungal, antibacterial liquid, such as decolorized iodine, is applied to the entire nail plate to minimize onychomycosis and paronychia

3. The loose edges of the cuticle are typically trimmed, removed, or pushed back depending on the operator. The patient with toenail disease should request that this step is not performed

4. A flexible template is fit beneath the natural toenail plate upon which the elongated sculpted nail will be built

5. The liquid methacrylate monomer is mixed with the powdered polymethyl methacrylate polymer in the presence of benzoyl peroxide as an accelerator to yield a formable polymer that is placed using a paintbrush to cover the entire natural nail plate. A clear acrylic is used over the natural nail plate attached to the nail bed so that the natural pink color shows through. A white acrylic is used from the nail plate's free edge distally

6. The final sculpture is sanded to a high shine

7. An air brushed design or stencil may be placed over the toenail, depending on the client wishes

operator who avoids skin contact with the uncured acrylic can avoid sensitizing the patient. Patch testing should be performed in suspected sensitized individuals with methyl methacrylate monomer, 10% in olive oil, and methacrylate acid esters, 1% and 5% in olive oil and petrolatum (5).

Toenail prostheses may be used to camouflage unattractive toenails until new growth occurs.

SUMMARY

Toenails are both functionally and cosmetically important. Thickening, ridging, nail odor, and onycholysis are conditions that cannot be treated by traditional prescription medications. Cosmetic solutions are all that can be recommended until a new toenail grows to replace the damaged nail plate. Since patients want to be empowered to care for their own bodies, the dermatologist must recommend something or the patient will feel that the medical visit was incomplete. This chapter has presented some practical ideas for the treatment of common toenail maladies.

REFERENCES

1. Barnett JM, Scher RK, Taylor SC. Nail cosmetics. Dermatol Clin 1991; 9: 9–17.
2. Marks JG, Bishop ME, Willis WF. Allergic contact dermatitis to sculptured nails. Arch Dermatol 1979; 115: 100.
3. Fisher AA. Cross reactions between methyl methacrylate monomer and acrylic monomers presently used in acrylic nail preparations. Contact Dermatitis 1980; 6: 345–7.
4. Fisher AA, Franks A, Glick H. Allergic sensitization of the skin and nails to acrylic plastic nails. J Allergy 1957; 28: 84.
5. Baran R, Dawber RPR. The nail and cosmetics. In: Samman PD, Fenton DA, eds. The nails in disease. 4th edn. Chicago: Yearbook Publishers, 1986: 129.

Summary

Cosmetics and skin care products can be used as adjuvants to traditional dermatologic care. Healthy skin is characterized by an intact skin barrier, which must be maintained after disease resolution. Moisturizers and cleansers can improve therapeutic outcomes in a wide range of dermatoses from eczema to atopic dermatitis to psoriasis to seborrheic dermatitis to acne. Further, the skin is impacted by the use of ancillary cosmetic treatments of the nails and hair. It is impossible to treat the entire dermatologic patient without understanding the basic care issues created by the use of over-the-counter (OTC) products. This book has provided the basic information needed to create a dermatologic armamentarium that expands traditional therapeutic considerations.

Skin, hair, and nail care information can only be incorporated into a patient's office visit by creating an organized format for their inclusion. The final topic I would like to address in this closing summary is an outline of how I approach my patients requiring assistance in this realm.

It is always important to be objective when making product recommendations. Do not only consider products that are sold in the office. There are excellent formulations sold through dermatologists, mass merchandisers, spa facilities, and boutique outlets. All must be considered and familiarity can only be obtained through personal experience. The wider the knowledge base of the dermatologist, the more valuable becomes the recommendation.

UNDERSTAND THE PURCHASING HABITS OF YOUR PATIENT

The first step in making skin care recommendations is to determine the patient preferred purchase point, which directly determines the cost. Skin care manufacturers intentionally produce products to reach consumers through a variety of markets. Some skin care products are sold exclusively in mass merchandisers, such as grocery stores, drug stores, and discount stores. Skin care products sold through these vendors generally range in price from $2 to $15, although recently some companies are pushing the envelope marketing high price point products in the $30 range. Other skin care products are sold exclusively through cosmetic counters in department stores. Even within the department store market there are products designed for lower-price point department stores and for higher-price point department stores. Lower-price point department stores market cosmetics sell for $10 to $50 as compared to higher price point department store cosmetics that sell for $40 to $200. The most expensive skin care products are sold through boutiques, spas, and medical offices. These products range from $50 to $400 and possibly higher. The envelope on expensive cosmetics is expanding upward and newer pricier technologies are reaching the marketplace. Interestingly enough, some of these exclusive products are manufactured by the same companies that produce items under a different label for sale in mass merchandisers. Generally, boutique products have more attractive, elaborate packaging accompanied by a greater color selection, more expensive fragrances, and innovative specialty additives. Remember that excellent products can be purchased inexpensively!

Another popular route for product purchase is at household parties and individuals who sell door-to-door in their neighborhood. Some of these products are sold through distributors who do not maintain product stock personally, but rather turn their orders into a central distribution center that fulfills and mails the orders. Another model for personal sales requires the salesperson to maintain their own stock and deliver orders personally. This difference is important because the independent salespersons may not take care to maintain fresh stock and may not store the products under optimal conditions. These products generally are in the $4 to $100 range.

Lastly, private label skin care products can be manufactured on a contract basis, generally through small manufacturers. Products can be customized to the needs of the business or simply a standard formulation with a customized label. The price variation in this market is tremendous. It is worthwhile noting that skin care products that are both sold and manufactured in the same state do not need to follow any Food and Drug Administration (FDA) monographs that may apply. All products manufactured and sold between states fall under the FDA jurisdiction, keeping in mind that cosmetics and skin care products are unregulated. Products under FDA regulation are the OTC drugs including sunscreens, antiperspirants, sunscreen-containing moisturizers, acne treatments, and any product that lists an active ingredient. It is important to carefully evaluate these products because smaller cosmetic manufacturers do not have the capital or facilities to undertake product testing.

IDENTIFY THE PATIENT'S UNIQUE SKIN NEEDS

The second step is to understand the specific skin needs of the patient. Begin by determining the patient's skin type: very oily, oily, combination, normal, dry, very dry, etc. Skin care products must be carefully chosen with the skin type in mind. Interestingly, many patients do not know their skin type or have been erroneously assigned a skin type by a salesperson at a cosmetic counter or after reading a book. It is quite straightforward to determine the skin type of a patient based on sebum production. The skin type can be most easily assigned by asking the patient about the amount of sebum production on her and his nose at various time points throughout the day following morning washing.

Sebum production can be assessed by having the patient run her and his finger down the nose several hours following washing. If the patient has flaking skin on the nose all day and no sebum from morning until 5 PM, they have very dry skin.

If the patient has no flaking and no sebum on their nose at 5 PM, they have dry skin. If the patient has minimal sebum on the nose at 5 PM, they have normal skin. If the patient has sebum on the nose at noon, they have oily skin. Finally, if the patient has sebum on the nose one hour following morning washing, they have very oily skin.

The most common skin type found in mature men and women is combination skin. This is understandable given the large sebaceous glands on the central forehead, nose, medial cheeks, and central chin. Combination skin can be assessed by comparing the amount of sebum present on the nose at 5 PM with the amount present on the cheeks. If there is more sebum present on the nose than on the cheeks, the patient has combination skin. Combination skin can be more challenging, since there are differing needs for different facial areas. It may be necessary to use a different cleanser and moisturizer on the central face and another formulation on the lateral face. Thus, the skin could be classified as dry on the lateral face, if no sebum is present at 5 PM, and oily on the nose, if sebum product is present at noon. Any combination of the skin types identified above can be present.

This is a simplistic, but accurate and effective approach to identifying skin type, but there are many other labels on skin care products besides the designation dry, normal, and oily. In fact, there is a current move away from classifying products by skin type and moving toward a problem-oriented approach. For example, products for oily skin may be labeled as appropriate for "acne-prone" skin. Further, products for dry skin may be labeled as developed for "sensitive" skin. This can create confusion in the mind of the patient as to which products to choose. Thus, dermatologist education is important to provide accurate patient recommendations.

TAKE A PRODUCT USE HISTORY
Once the patient purchasing habits and skin needs have been identified, it is necessary to take a product use history. This means asking what products the patient is currently using including facial cleansers, facial moisturizers, body cleansers, and body moisturizers. In addition, cosmeceuticals and skin treatment products (exfoliants, astringents, antiaging serums, home use devices, shaving products, etc.) should also be discussed. Many times the patient has concocted a skin care regimen based on visits to three dermatologists, six cosmetic counters, and four day spas. This leads to skin care product overload. The problems that the patient is experiencing may be due to skin barrier damage from an overzealous approach to skin care. The dermatologist's first goal is to examine the products and arrive at a logical, beneficial skin care regimen.

In any skin care regimen, there are certain common factors such as cleanser, moisturizer, and sunscreen. These products do not need to be duplicated. Examine the patient's regimen eliminating duplications in product use. Look at the ingredients in each product and select the one that you believe will provide the most benefit with the least problems. For example, a glycolic acid cleanser can cause barrier damage when used in combination with an exfoliant, while the benefits of brief skin contact with the glycolic acid cleanser are minimal. The glycolic acid cleanser should be eliminated in favor of a bland moisturizer that will prevent the development of self-induced sensitive skin. Similarly, the sunscreen can also be evaluated.

Select the sunscreen that offers the highest sun protection factor (SPF). While SPF is an indicator of UVB photoprotection, the sunscreens with an SPF of 30+ cannot achieve this SPF rating without some UVA photoprotection. Until the new sunscreen monograph is released with a UVA rating system, SPF can be used indirectly to assess UVA photoprotection. Since UVA radiation is most important in protection against skin cancer and premature photoaging, this is a valuable patient service.

Do not forget to ask patients about their use of devices to include hand-held microdermabraders, rotary or sonicating skin brushes, red light devices, blue light acne treatment devices, home lasers, and hand-held hair removal devices. You may discover some interesting combinations that could be creating skin disease or creating problems with your medical therapy. Exfoliation is the quickest way to make the skin smoother and induce a small amount of edema, minimizing fine lines on the face. Problems arise when patients adopt an aggressive attitude and damage the skin barrier. Several years ago we did a study where computer chips were placed in a face brush to measure the amount of time research subjects used the device for cleansing. Detailed instructions and a demonstration were provided indicating the brush was to be used for 5 minutes twice daily for 2 weeks. As might be expected, some brushes were returned with only 10 minutes total use while others recorded 8 hours of use. Be sure to ask the subject how long they are using the device and for how much time.

Perhaps the hardest area to evaluate is moisturizer use. If one really used all of the "beneficial" ingredients in the cosmeceutical marketplace, it would take 8 hours to complete the applications. I think it is very hard to counsel patients as to which moisturizer is the best. Of course, a sunscreen-containing moisturizer should be used in the morning and a moisturizer without sunscreen should be applied in the evening. Other than that, there are very few absolute recommendations. Nevertheless, patients are looking for instructions that are more detailed. This is difficult given the rapid change in the cosmeceutical marketplace.

I believe that best approach is to look for ingredients in the moisturizer that maintain skin barrier hydration by creating an optimal environment for barrier repair. These ingredients include petrolatum, dimethicone, and glycerin. They represent the workhorse moisturizing ingredients in any formulation. Petrolatum is the premier ingredient for reducing transepidermal water loss, which becomes more aesthetically pleasing when mixed with dimethicone to reduce stickiness. Glycerin, as a humectant, helps the water-holding capacity of the skin. However, these are not new or uncommon ingredients. There is nothing much novel that can be said about this type of a moisturizer from a marketing standpoint. This explains the need to find unusual substances to add to a basic formulation to provide a distinguishing characteristic in a crowded marketplace. It is hoped that this book has clarified some of these issues.

EVALUATE SKIN CARE NEEDS IN LIGHT OF THE PRESENCE OF DERMATOLOGIC DISEASE
Most patients who seek dermatologic care have skin disease of one sort or another accompanied by the inevitable photoaging. Skin care products can be used to supplement the

prescription treatment of most skin disorders. If proper skin care products are not used, disease recurrence and a short remission time are certain. The dermatologist who strives for excellence in patient care not only tries to treat the disease, but goes beyond to consider the prevention aspects of treatment. If a patient has seborrheic dermatitis, a shampoo that reduces scalp sebum and possesses antifungal properties, such as those formulations containing zinc pyrithione in a strong surfactant base, should be advised once the dermatitis component has resolved. If the patient has psoriasis, an excellent moisturizer should be recommended to prevent barrier damage and initiate new psoriatic plaques due to the Koebner phenomenon. It is this type of thinking that combines the prescription realm with the OTC realm to yield superior therapeutic results.

DEVELOP AN ALGORITHMIC APPROACH TO SKIN CARE FOR THE PATIENT

In order to easily combine prescription and OTC products into one treatment plan, it is necessary to develop an algorithmic approach. An algorithmic approach means that a mental checklist has already been imprinted on the brain that can easily be recalled when a patient presents. Each of the chapters in this book has been aimed at providing the material for developing these personal algorithms. Formulations and their effects on the skin, hair, and nails have been discussed. Review of these previously read chapters with this idea in mind may help you personalize your algorithms.

UPDATE PERSONAL AND PATIENT DATABASE, AS NEEDED

Now that you have obtained an understanding of the patient's product use and formulated your recommendation, make a record in the chart. Just like the necessity of documenting the past medical history and the review of systems findings, you must also document your skin care profile. Update this information with each patient encounter. This will allow the most thorough integration of skin, hair, and nail care products into your dermatologic armamentarium.

This text has attempted to take a serious look at the integration of skin care products, cosmetics, hair adornments, and nail cosmetics in the practice of dermatology, thus expanding the realm of disease treatment beyond the diagnosis and treatment into the maintenance phase of healthy skin, hair, and nails. The impact of OTC products on the structures of the external body cannot be ignored. Major developments are taking place at an accelerating pace in this area requiring vigilance on the part of the dermatologist to remain up-to-date. It is my hope that you have enjoyed reading this book and will use it as a foundation for future learning. Perhaps you can sense my enthusiasm and will no longer look at this area with bewilderment, but will accept the challenge!

Index

T - #0567 - 071024 - C292 - 279/216/14 - PB - 9780367382452 - Gloss Lamination